Supra-Gingival Minimally Invasive Dentistry

A Healthier Approach to Esthetic Restorations

Supra-Gingival Minimally Invasive Dentistry

A Healthier Approach to Esthetic Restorations

Jose-Luis Ruiz
Los Angeles Institute of Clinical Dentistry
Los Angeles, CA, USA

WILEY Blackwell

Registered Offices
John Wiley & Sons, Inc., 111 River Street, Hoboken, NJ 07030, USA
John Wiley & Sons Ltd, The Atrium, Southern Gate, Chichester, West Sussex, PO19 8SQ, UK

Editorial Office
111 River Street, Hoboken, NJ 07030, USA

For details of our global editorial offices, customer services, and more information about Wiley products visit us at www.wiley.com.

Wiley also publishes its books in a variety of electronic formats and by print-on-demand. Some content that appears in standard print versions of this book may not be available in other formats.

Library of Congress Cataloging-in-Publication Data

Names: Ruiz, Jose-Luis (Dentist), author.
Title: Supra-gingival minimally invasive dentistry : a healthier approach to esthetic restorations / Jose-Luis Ruiz.
Description: Hoboken, NJ : John Wiley & Sons, Inc., 2017. | Includes bibliographical references and index.
Identifiers: LCCN 2017008998 (print) | LCCN 2017010815 (ebook) | ISBN 9781118976418 (cloth) | ISBN 9781118976425 (Adobe PDF) | ISBN 9781118976432 (ePub)
Subjects: | MESH: Dental Restoration, Permanent–methods | Dental Restoration, Permanent–adverse effects | Minimally Invasive Surgical Procedures–methods | Oral Surgical Procedures, Preprosthetic–methods | Dental Marginal Adaptation | Postoperative Complications–prevention & control
Classification: LCC RK54 (print) | LCC RK54 (ebook) | NLM WU 300 | DDC 617.6/9--dc23
LC record available at https://lccn.loc.gov/2017008998

Cover images: courtesy of Jose-Luis Ruiz

Set in 10/12pt Warnock Pro by Aptara Inc., New Delhi, India

10 9 8 7 6 5 4 3 2 1

Contents

Foreword

I am pleased to have the opportunity to review Dr. Jose-Luis Ruiz's book on conservative dental restorations. I have known Jose-Luis for many years and have been to his office and observed his dentistry, his competent staff, and his overall professionalism. I am impressed with his work ethic, his quality dentistry, and his enthusiasm for the profession.

For years, he has supported and taught the concept of reducing the percentage of crowns placed in the profession, a motive that I share. Many dentists are hesitant to place onlays and veneers, thinking that they are more difficult to place than crowns, and potentially weaker. As with any other clinical procedure, becoming competent with conservative indirect restorations requires a brief period of time and placement of several restorations.

Our research on onlays at the Clinicians Report Foundation has shown that properly made and cemented onlays can be stronger than natural teeth. Additionally, the teeth retain their natural color for years of successful and esthetically pleasing service. Veneers placed on enamel surfaces with only minimal dentin exposed are well known to be among the most beautiful of restorations and have excellent strength and longevity.

You will enjoy reading Jose-Luis's book, and you and your patients will benefit from its contents.

Gordon J. Christensen DDS, MSD, PhD
CEO, Clinicians Report Foundation
CEO, Practical Clinical Courses

Preface

The past three decades have brought a great number of new materials, techniques and devices to dentistry, some of them revolutionary, like adhesive dentistry. Materials that are stronger, more esthetic, with unique features like the ability to set on command, with great mechanical characteristics. Devices offering amazing diagnostic, clinical and manufacturing possibilities. Many of these new materials and devices have promised to make dentistry faster, better, more predictable, and even healthier for patients. But the reality is that while these materials and technology have been implemented, all of the above promises have not truly materialized. Looking at restorative clinical dentistry today shows a small overall improvement in the patient's or dentist's experience. Most dental procedures take longer than with older materials, an example being a simple class II composite. Teeth continue to be cut aggressively for crowns, root canals continue to be performed at amazingly high rates, restorative margins continue to be placed below the gums and patients continue to have pain during and after dental procedures. Is there an actual net gain from all the technological advances?

Tooth-conserving dentistry and partial coverage restorations are strongly advocated by most. Nevertheless, full crowns are still the most popular indirect restoration by far! Why? One reason is the extremely convoluted and demanding techniques advocated by some. Most educators and schools continue to perceive and teach that partial-coverage metal-free restorations, non-gold, are to be used in limited situations, only when "ideal conditions" exist, and so full-coverage crowns are used most of the time. This is mostly due to fear of failure. Some of the most common reasons for these reported failures are the use of new materials with old techniques, the overall lack of understanding and trust in adhesion, and most importantly, the universal acceptance that placing restorative margins subgingivally is out of our control, or often necessary and "normal," and even the belief that placing subgingival margins has important advantages which outweigh the negatives.

Subgingival margins have endless disadvantages to restorative success and patient health. The damage caused by subgingival margins is an under-recognized secret of restorative dentistry. Unknowingly, dentists place subgingival margins unnecessarily every day! Dentists understand the negative consequences of periodontal disease, not only for the longevity of teeth, but also for the overall health of our patients. Defective subgingival margins act as "permanent tartar" affecting the periodontal health of our patients.

The supragingival minimally invasive dentistry approach is a new and innovative approach. It assumes that most subgingival margins are preventable, and all damaged teeth can be restored with a partial-coverage direct or indirect restoration, with the exception of teeth already cut for previous crowns, thus preserving tooth, the health of the pulp and periodontium. This approach recognizes how the continued use of traditional mechanically retained dental techniques is counterproductive to adhesive dentistry, and comes with the negative effects of unnecessary tooth removal and the catastrophic consequences of subgingival margins placement. The innovative supragingival protocol makes supragingival margins possible in most cases. Supragingival restorative margins make adhesive dentistry simple and predictable. This revolutionary approach respects biology, thus making it the most minimally invasive, biocompatible approach in restorative dentistry. It comes with numerous advantages. Supragingival dentistry, by definition, stays above the gum line and makes restorative dentistry easier and faster for the clinician, healthier for the patient, esthetically pleasing, and provides for long-lasting predictable results.

The techniques presented here are not only for the rich and famous, nor for teeth with "ideal conditions", but for all patients and all restorations. Contrary to other adhesive dentistry books available, which show techniques based on an academic approach, this book shows real-world practical techniques and tricks that are easily reproducible, reliable and successful. Research and experience show that even the most damaged teeth can be successfully restored with supragingival minimally invasive partial coverage bonded restorations. This book discusses the indications and the basic rules: "the five principles or rules of supragingival dentistry." With hundreds of pictures and diagrams, this book shows how even in the most complicated cases, supragingival minimally invasive dentistry is not only possible, but a better, healthier choice.

Jose-Luis Ruiz

From the Contributing Editor

During the past three decades, restorative dentistry has gone through a remarkable transition. Conquering adhesion to all dental surfaces, the last one being dentin, with etched enamel equivalent or better bond strengths, has enabled clinicians to perform tooth conserving dentistry that was previously only a century-old dream. This new adhesive approach can totally replace the tooth destructive mechanical approach.

Unfortunately, even with advances in adhesion, old paradigms survive. One is the routine placement of subgingival margins. In this book, Dr. Jose-Luis Ruiz has shown that subgingival margins are undesirable and mostly avoidable. This approach clearly goes against the mainstream theories.

Dr. Ruiz has a great mind for engineering dental restorations. He has recognized the reasons given for resisting change to supragingival restorations and then has come up with many new techniques and choices of materials to help reverse the resistance. My contribution to the book is mostly providing some technical information for the materials and devices employed.

We need more educators like Dr. Ruiz – pioneers willing to stick their necks out for what they feel truly works and is best for patients. I will keep watching future developments from this skilled clinician and educator.

Raymond L. Bertolotti DDS, PhD

Acknowledgments

As with all human endeavors, this work is a continuation of the work of so many amazing professionals who have contributed to the profession of dentistry with their innovation and skill. One such innovator and pioneer in the field of adhesive dentistry is Dr. Raymond Bertolotti. His immense knowledge peppers this book as contributing editor, and his contribution is invaluable. Many images and valuable information were contributed by some of the most prominent researchers and educators in dentistry. I want to thank Dr. Werner Finger, Dr. Jungi Tagami, Dr. Masatoshi Nakajima, Dr. Ilan Rotstein, Dr. Masafumi Kanehira, Dr. Franklyn Tay, Dr. Bruce Crispin, Dr. Rella Christensen, Dr. Gordon Christensen, Dr. Boris Kesselbrener, Dr. Gregory Mar, Dr. Nuria Fernandez, Dr. Renee Kurt, Dr. Patricia Ryan, and Dr. Shigehisa Inokoshi, and Miss Elise Girion for organizing and collating some of my previous works, and any others whom I may have inadvertently omitted, for their kind and priceless contribution.

This book is dedicated to the practicing dental clinician who knows the toil of balancing running a business, a dental team, overheads and a busy schedule. This book and all enclosed techniques are designed for such clinicians who need real-world, simple, practical, reproducible and reliable results.

I want to end by saying that much of my inspiration and drive comes from my parents, Jose-Luis and Diana Ruiz, both prominent lawyers in Mexico. I am also inspired by my brilliant brother Alex Ruiz and my eternal love for my children Robert, Michaela and Mimi.

Jose-Luis Ruiz

Part I

Rationale

1

The Traditional Mechanically Retained Restoration Paradigm: Subgingival Margins are Normal and a Necessary Byproduct of Restorative Needs

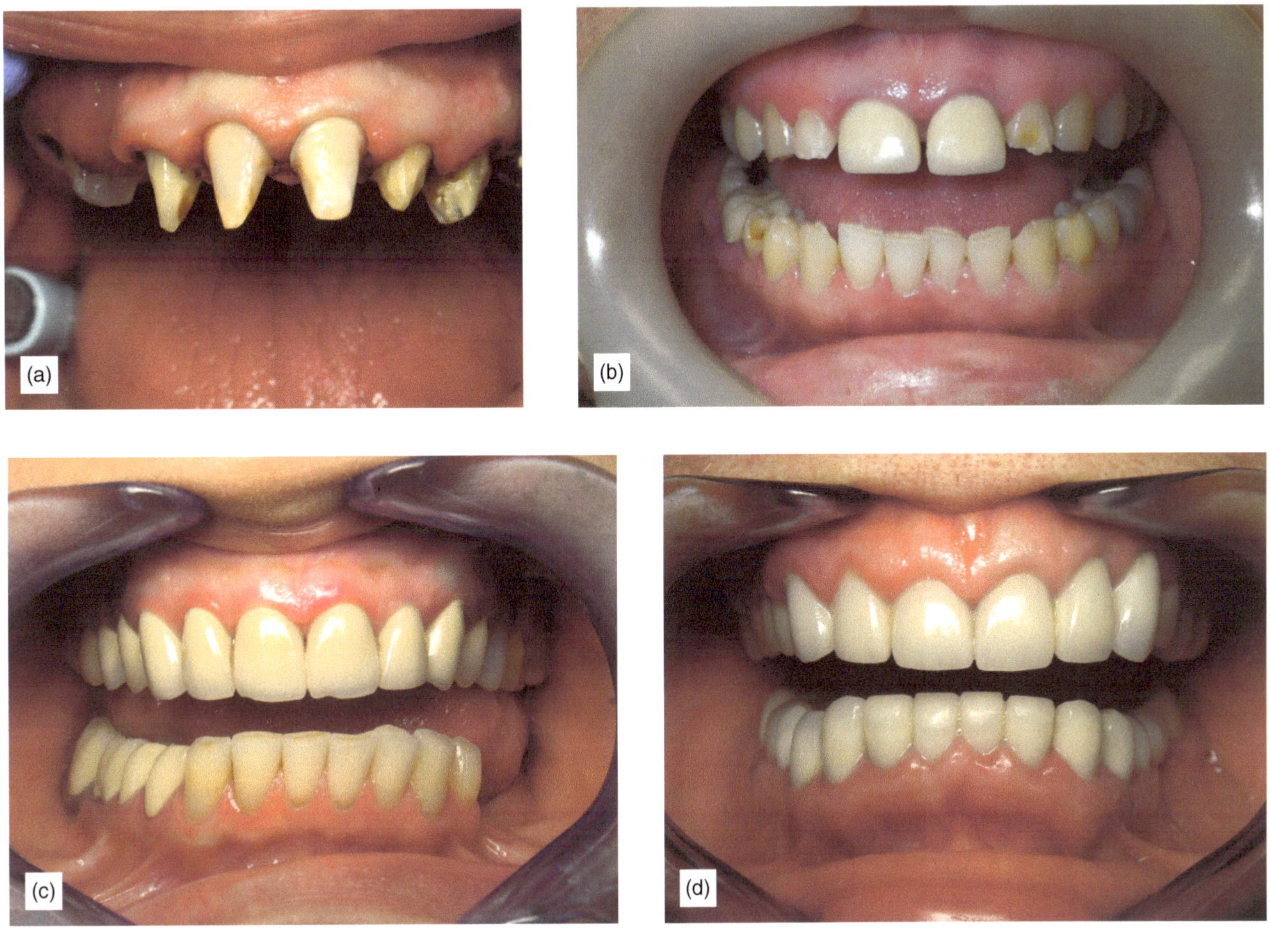

Four images showing periodontal inflammation caused by subgingival margin placement.

Introduction

In traditional mechanically retained dentistry such as full crowns, subgingival margin placement is considered to be normal, necessary, and a byproduct of traditional restorative techniques. The over 37 million crowns placed every year by dentists in the United States [1,2,3] show that it is by far the most popular indirect procedure, regardless of the material used, and is viewed as ideal for most cases, predictable and relatively easy to perform. However, familiarity must not be confused with simplicity [4,5]. Partial coverage supragingival adhesive techniques are often considered to have a more unpredictable outcome, to be more difficult to perform and

Supra-Gingival Minimally Invasive Dentistry: A Healthier Approach to Esthetic Restorations, First Edition. By Jose-Luis Ruiz.

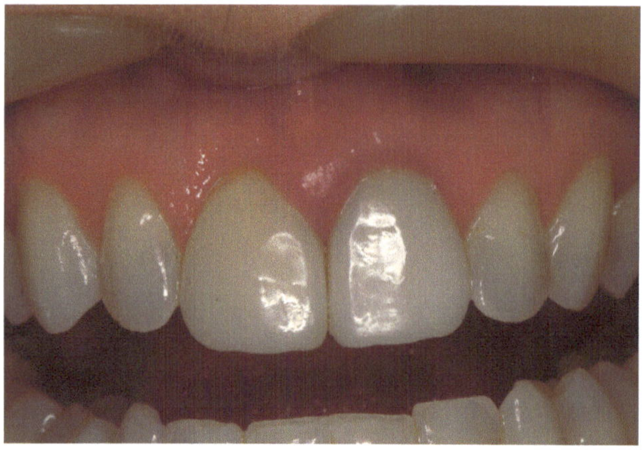

Figure 1.1 Veneer and crown with deep subgingival margins, and poor periodontal health.

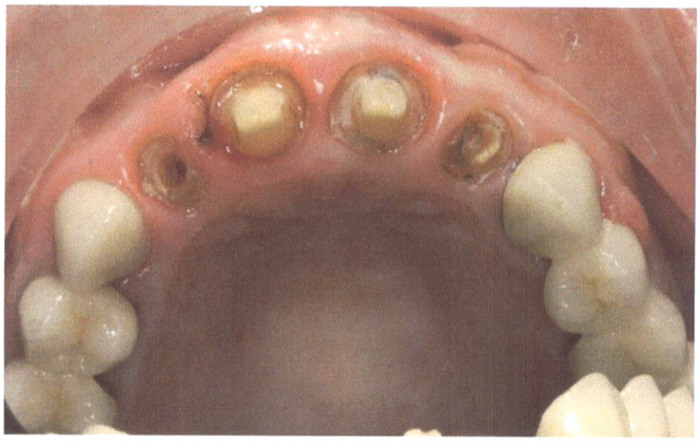

Figure 1.3 Improperly aggressive preparation for a zirconia crown. Both lateral incisors required root canal therapy, owing to damage to the pulp.

less successful in general. It is human nature to think that what we do every day and know well is better than something unfamiliar.

Yes, tooth-colored restorative materials are currently extremely popular, but often these new materials are being used in conjunction with traditional mechanically retained techniques, and some computer-aided designed and manufactured (CAD-CAM) restorations. This often leads to subgingival margin placement. When all ceramic full crowns, inlays, onlays, and veneers are performed using principles and techniques extrapolated from traditional mechanically retained principles such as unnecessary subgingival margin placement, there is a risk of increased failure, postoperative sensitivity, pulp injury, non-esthetic results, and a defective margin. All these outcomes will result in an unhealthy periodontium. This incorrect use of modern restorative and adhesive materials ultimately produces no net benefit to the patient or the dentist (Figures 1.1–1.4).

The negative consequences of periodontal disease are well understood, as they affect not only the longevity of the teeth but also the overall health of our patients. The negative consequences of subgingival deposits of tartar in the ultimate periodontal health of our patients are also understood [6,7]. Overhangs and open margins (in fact, any defective margin, when it is subgingival) have the same effect as permanent tartar on the periodontal health of our patients (Figures 1.5–1.8) [8,9,10,11]. Taking the above statement into account, supragingival restoration margin placement would be ideal, and most clinicians, if asked, would say that this would be their first choice [12]. This prompts the question why are so many crowns, onlays, veneers, and direct class II and many class III restorations being placed with a subgingival margin? The reality is that habit instills the idea that placing margins subgingivally is a "normal" and necessary adverse effect. Subgingival margin placement is so common that it goes undetected and unnoticed. When using traditional mechanically retained restorative principles, it is believed that subgingival margin placement has important advantages, which outweigh

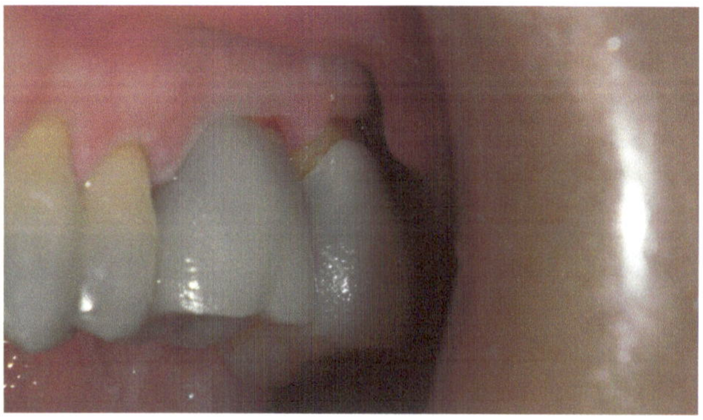

Figure 1.2 Recently completed computer-aided design and fabricated IPS e-max® (Ivoclar) crowns. The patient had severe sensitivity, and the gums were inflamed and bleeding. Some of the margins were deep subgingivally, especially interproximally.

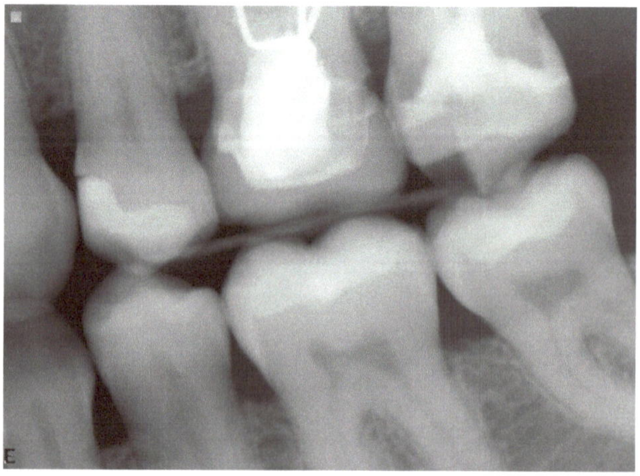

Figure 1.4 Bonded onlays with deep subgingival margins. The extreme difficulty of bonded cementation with bleeding subgingival margins led to catastrophic failure.

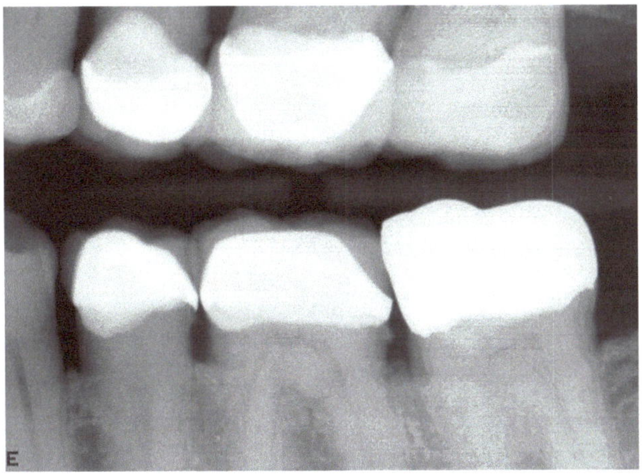

Figure 1.5 Periodontal tartar in proximity to defective crown margins, with similar unhealthy effects.

the negative consequences. Subgingival margin placement should no longer be considered normal or necessary. The continued use of mechanically retained traditional restorative dentistry principles has many disadvantages, and the solution is supragingival minimally invasive adhesive dentistry, which is discussed in subsequent chapters. First, it is important to understand how unnecessary subgingival margin placement happens, and the consequences of such placement.

Subgingival Restorative Margin Placement

Subgingival margin placement is a byproduct of traditional restorative techniques. The majority of these types of restoration include subgingival margin placement, and it often goes unnoticed. There are four primary reasons why the margin is placed subgingivally, and a fifth which is based on misinformation:

1) Mechanical retention and lack of trust in adhesion
2) Traditional restorative techniques, boxes, and cervical clearance

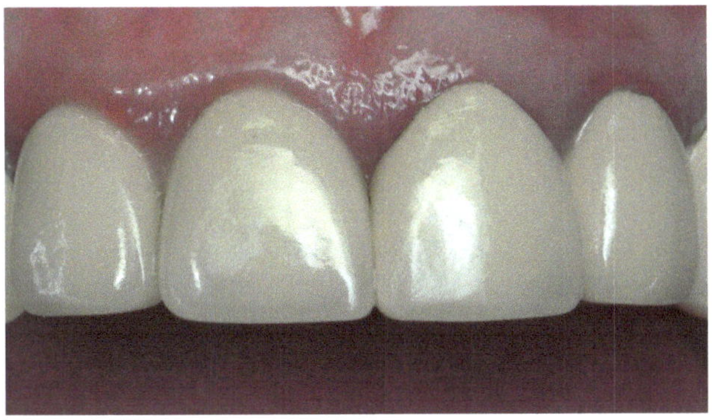

Figure 1.6 This patient was happy and unaware of unhealthy gingiva.

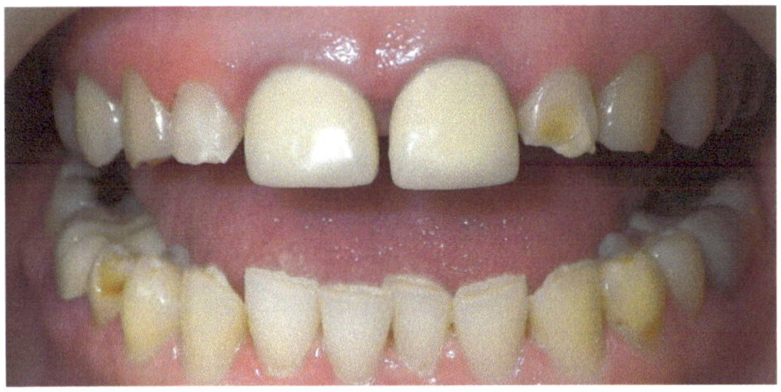

Figure 1.7 Inflamed gums, and poor margin.

3) Subgingival margin placement for esthetic purposes
4) Actual subgingival caries or existing restoration
5) Belief that the tooth will be better off and less likely to have recurrent caries if the margin is placed below the level of the gingiva.

Mechanical Retention and Lack of Trust in Adhesion

Historically, mechanical retention with traditional direct and indirect restorations, amalgams, composites and crowns was necessary [13,14,15,16,17]. For over 100 years, dentistry has relied on mechanical retention to hold restorations in place: axial walls with certain minimum heights, usually 3–4 mm, offsets, boxes, shoulders, and additional mechanical features. Restorations were retained in the tooth primarily by friction before the benefits of adhesion became available. Unfortunately, many dentists still do not fully trust adhesives to support and retain their restorations, and thus they continue to prepare teeth using traditional mechanical features. Even when the caries is supragingival, the need for axial wall and mechanical retention forces a degree of preparation that will invade the gingival sulcus (Figure 1.9). This is most common after the removal of mesial and distal

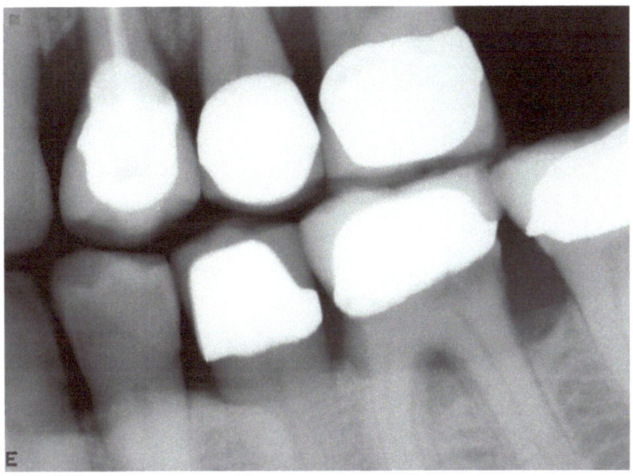

Figure 1.8 X-ray showing severe periodontal damage likely caused by poor fitting subgingival restorations.

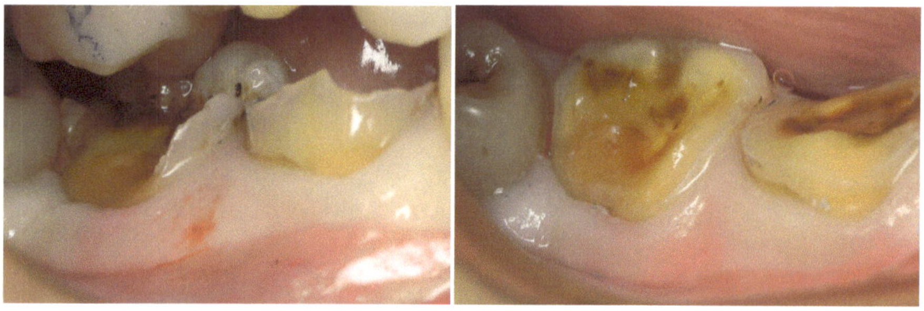

Figure 1.9 Before and after finished adhesively retained onlay preparations. This is most commonly followed by axial reduction for mechanical retention with deep subgingival margins as a byproduct.

caries and old restorations that leave the cavosurface margin already close to or at gum level. A common scenario is when a patient has a short clinical crown, without enough supragingival tooth remaining for a long retentive axial wall. Extension for retention will inevitably lead to a subgingival margin placement (Figure 1.10). An adverse effect of axial reduction is the increase in the amount of tooth reduction. A full crown requires approximately 70% of the clinical crown to be drilled off (Figure 1.11); partial coverage restorations require a fraction of this amount [18,19]. The damage to the pulp by the additional unnecessary drilling (considering that bonded restoration does not require axial reduction) ranges from increased postoperative pain to irreversible pulpitis and pulpal necrosis, correlating with remaining dentin thickness [20,21,22,23,24]. Trust in adhesion and proper supragingival minimally invasive restorative techniques renders mechanical retention unnecessary.

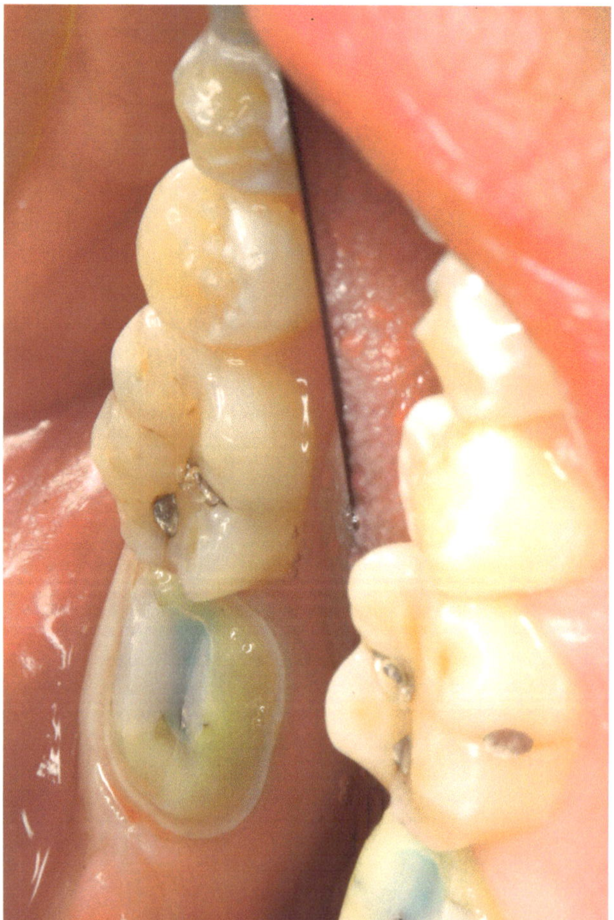

Figure 1.10 Flat tooth showing the inevitable need for subgingival axial walls if resistance and retention are the goal.

Traditional Restorative Techniques, Boxes, and Cervical Clearance

Traditionally, in both direct and indirect restorative dentistry, there has been a need to create clearance with the adjacent tooth facially, lingually, and gingivally, to place a matrix band, take an impression, confirm restoration seal, and so on. Facial and lingual clearance is of concern because of excessive tooth removal, but traditional gingival clearance techniques are the source of subgingival margin placement (Figure 1.12). To gain gingival

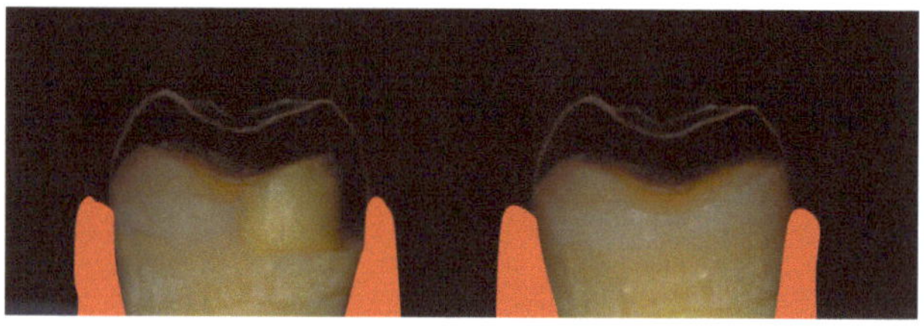

Figure 1.11 The need for mechanical reduction will create subgingival margins; a fully adhesive restoration without axial reduction will stay supragingival.

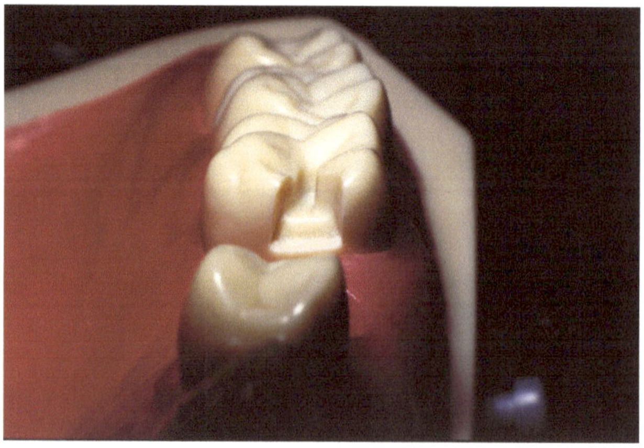

Figure 1.12 A traditional geometric box (courtesy of Dr Boris Keselbrener).

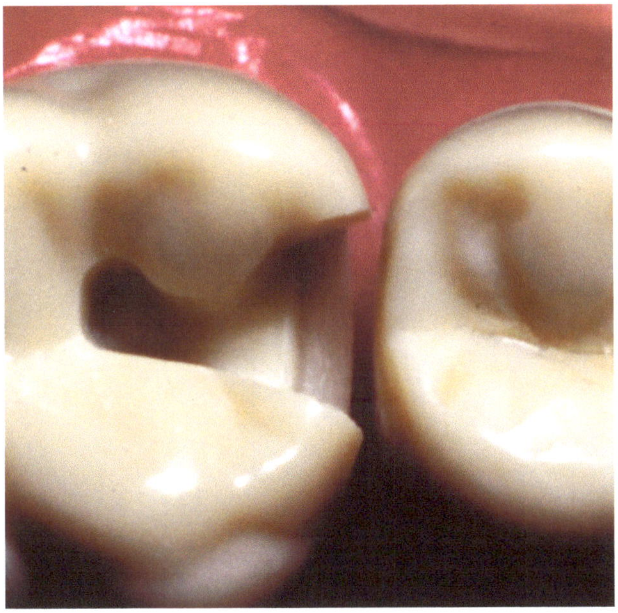

Figure 1.13 Gingival clearance created by dropping box technique (courtesy of Dr Boris Keselbrener).

clearance from the adjacent tooth, dentists have been taught to drop the gingival floor of the box for direct restorations, and the gingival interproximal margin for indirect restorations (Figure 1.13). This technique is extremely counterproductive for any adhesive dentistry procedure, as it leads to subgingival margin placement and causes the loss of the enamel margin, with negative consequences in both cases (Figure 1.14a,b). Techniques such as the "cervical margin separation" can replace the need to drop the margin and go subgingival, as subsequent chapters illustrate.

Subgingival Margin Placement For Esthetic Purposes

The commonly accepted necessity for subgingival margin placement exists purely for esthetic reasons (Figure 1.15a,b). When using porcelain-fused-to-metal (PFM) or any other opacious material, including full or layered zirconia, subgingival margin placement became the norm to hide the esthetically displeasing gingival margin. It is also commonly done when color change is desired, for example in cases of dark teeth, when color change is effected solely with a restoration (Figure 1.16). Although there are currently many highly translucent restorative materials with the ability to blend at the margin area, opacious material continues to be the most popular (Figure 1.17). The placing of subgingival margins for esthetics is mostly habit, even in areas which do not need them (Figure 1.18). The proper use of translucent restorative materials renders subgingival margin placement unnecessary, as the following chapters demonstrate.

Actual Subgingival Caries or Existing Restoration

The only valid reason for a subgingival restorative margin today is when the caries or old restorative materials are already below the gingiva. Nevertheless, subgingival caries and even old restorative materials are usually limited to a small section or sections of the tooth (Figures 1.19–1.21). If only a small area of the tooth is subgingival, managing this area is usually simple and will not usually compromise the ultimate quality or results of the restoration. Unfortunately, the generally accepted concept is that full subgingival margin placement is normal. If one section of the tooth is already subgingival, it may be easy to say "well, it is subgingival

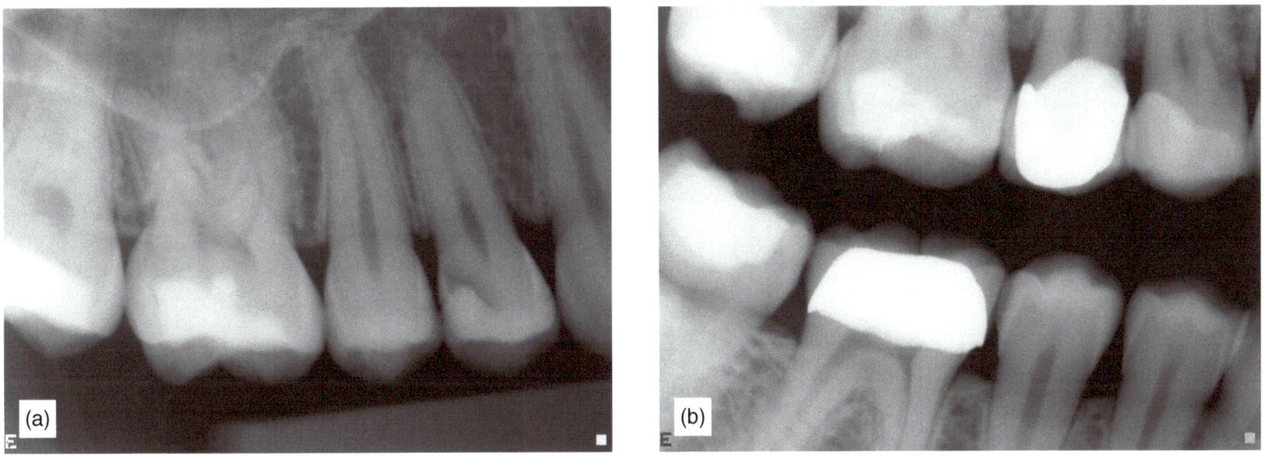

Figure 1.14 (a) Historical progression x-ray showing a small class II cavity on a first premolar, which was diagnosed for direct composite in 2010. (b) In 2015, the patient was seen again with an aggressive subgingival crown on the same first premolar (direct composite on the second premolar was performed by the author 5 years earlier).

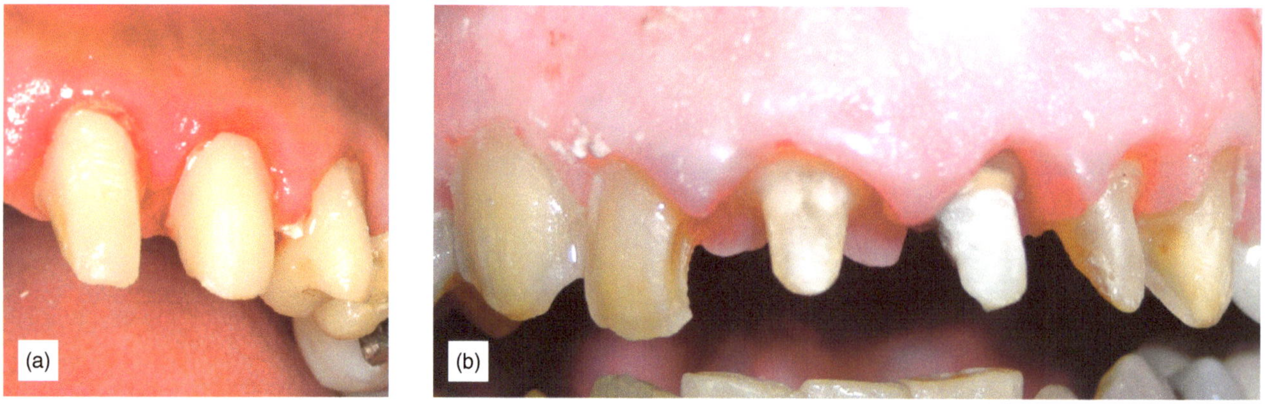

Figure 1.15 (a, b) Crown preparations with traditional subgingival margins.

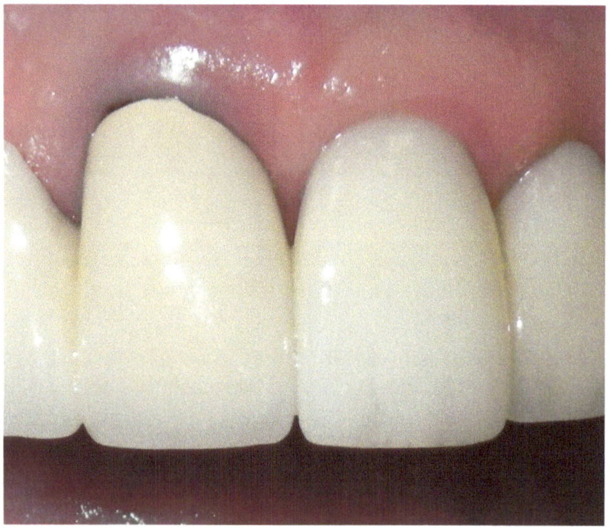

Figure 1.16 It is clear how unsuccessful it is to bury dark margins below the gum. Sooner or later they come out again, revealing uneven gums.

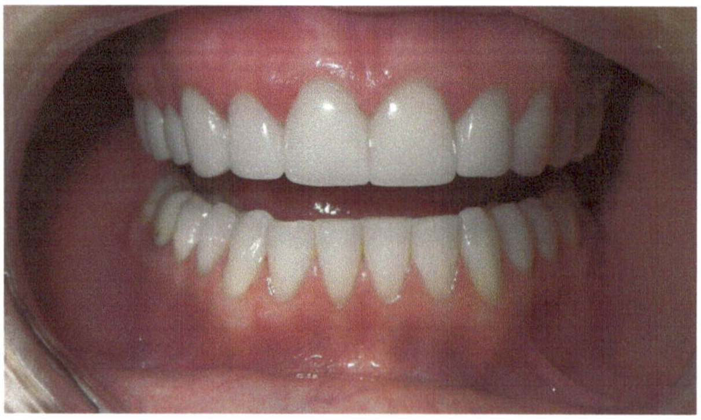

Figure 1.17 A well-known 23-year-old celebrity with recent veneers, showing the effect of unnecessary subgingival margins. Permanent mild periodontitis.

already, let's place the entire margin subgingivally," and although it is not reasonable, this appears to be a common approach. Additionally, sometimes what appears to be a deep subgingival margin can, with high magnification and careful technique, be found to be less subgingival than initially thought (Figure 1.21). Again, the preconception of "it is subgingival already" and subsequent aggressive and careless subgingival preparation can make matters much worse. The first supragingival rule goes a long way towards limiting the use of subgingival margin placement, as is discussed in subsequent chapters.

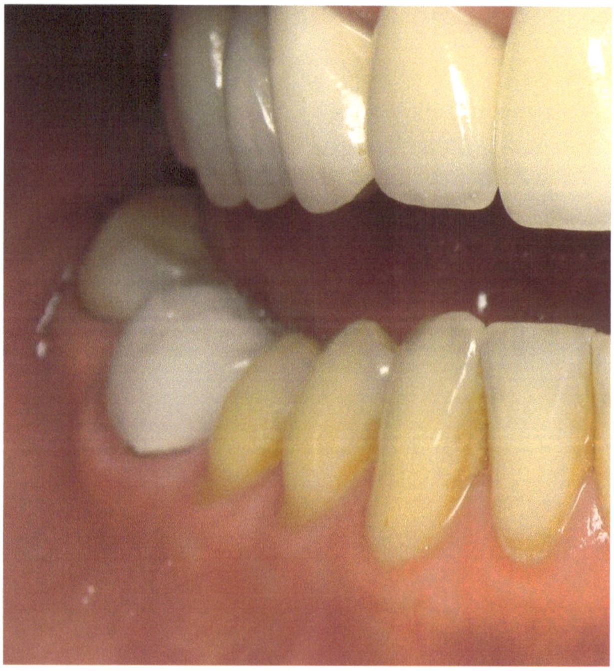

Figure 1.18 Subgingival margins placed unnecessarily on far posterior teeth, showing typical inflammation.

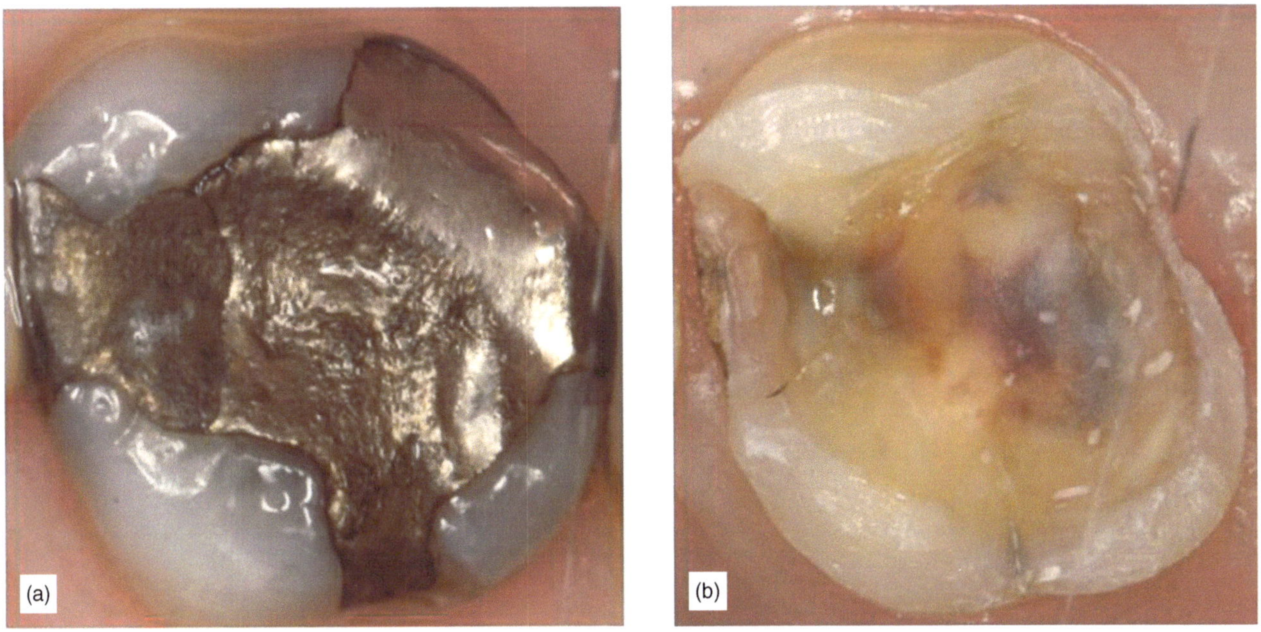

Figure 1.19 (a) Large amalgam filling suggestive of existing subgingival margins. (b) After removal of a large amount of amalgam, showing mostly supragingival margins.

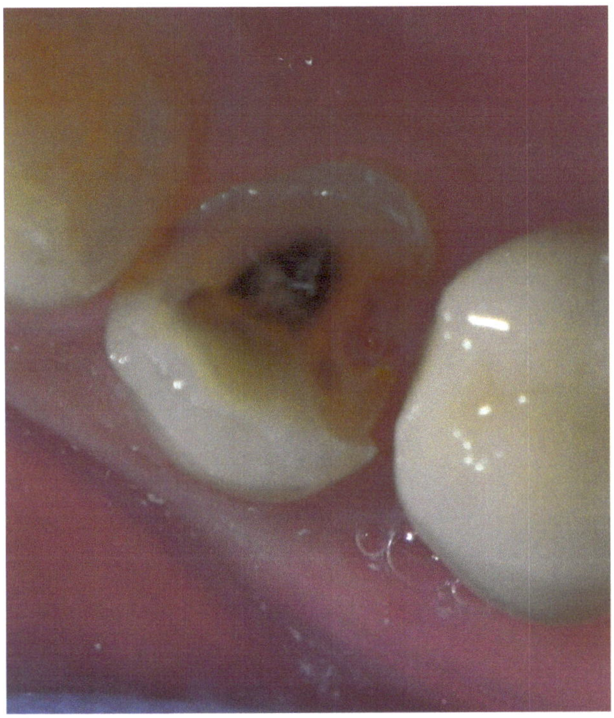

Figure 1.20 A common situation: A tooth with only one area of subgingival decay; the rest of the tooth will be supragingival.

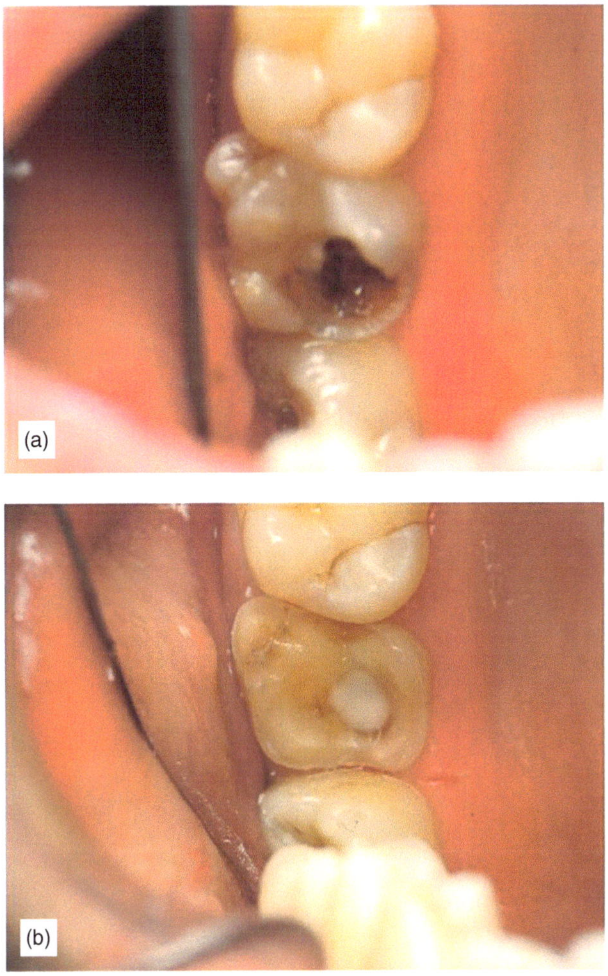

Figure 1.21 (a) A badly decayed tooth, which would suggest extensive subgingival margins. (b) Apparently subgingival margin was supragingival with careful removal of caries.

An Erroneous Belief

The fifth "reason" is the belief that if we place the margin below the gingiva, the tooth will be better off and will be less likely to have recurrent caries. Many patients, and a small percentage of dental professionals, may hold this erroneous belief, but it is important to clarify that it is not based on scientific data. There is no literature available which shows a decrease in recurrent caries, but a great deal of information showing an increase in pathogen levels, inflammation, and plaque accumulation [25].

Familiarity can be confused with simplicity and quality. The following section outlines reasons why traditional mechanically retained dentistry and subgingival margin placement are no longer "normal", necessary, predictable, easier, or more healthy for our patients.

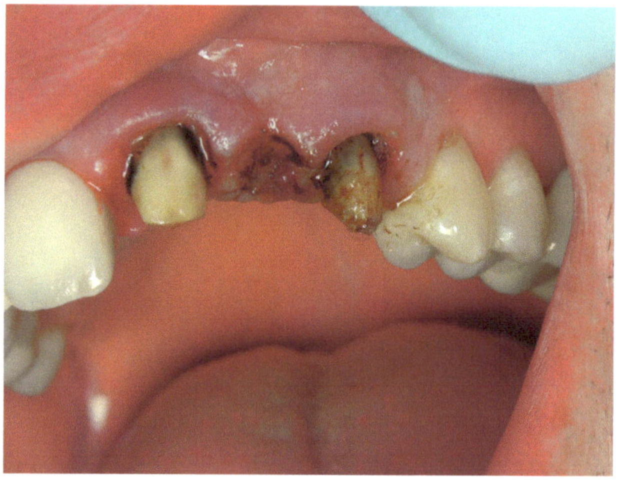

Figure 1.22 After the removal of an old bridge, it is easy to see how difficult the tissue management will be, given the deep subgingival margins.

Mechanically Retained Dentistry with Subgingival Margins is More Difficult

Against common belief, traditional mechanically retained dentistry with subgingival margins is far more complicated than modern supragingival dentistry. For example, a full crown preparation starts with a difficult preparation procedure requiring exact taper and the need to place a preparation margin subgingivally. When performed correctly in an atraumatic way, the first step requires that an initial equigingival margin and then a retraction cord be placed, to expose the subgingival tooth structure. The tooth margin is then prepared (drilled) and placed subgingivally, maintaining a correct taper at all times. After this difficult procedure, the second cord must be placed to take a proper impression of this subgingival margin. This procedure is also very difficult. In fact, it is one of the most difficult and unsuccessful procedures in dentistry, as laboratories around the country can attest from the number of inaccurate impressions they receive (Figures 1.22, 1.23a–c) [26].

The cementation procedure is equally difficult. It is not uncommon to see that the gingiva is inflamed and bleeds easily after the provisional is removed from this subgingival preparation (Figure 1.24). This is usually the consequence of a less than ideal provisional and the patient's poor oral hygiene. With this bleeding gingiva, hemostasis is difficult for cementation. Additionally, it is not uncommon to see the gingiva grow over the preparation, making proper seating of the restoration difficult without aggressive cord packing (Figure 1.25a,b). Cement removal is difficult and unpredictable with subgingival margins, and long-term periodontal trauma can be caused by excess residual cement that is not removed (Figure 1.26).

Subgingival margins are no easier with direct restorations. When using resin composite materials and adhesives, subgingival preparation margins have great disadvantages because, once we work subgingivally,

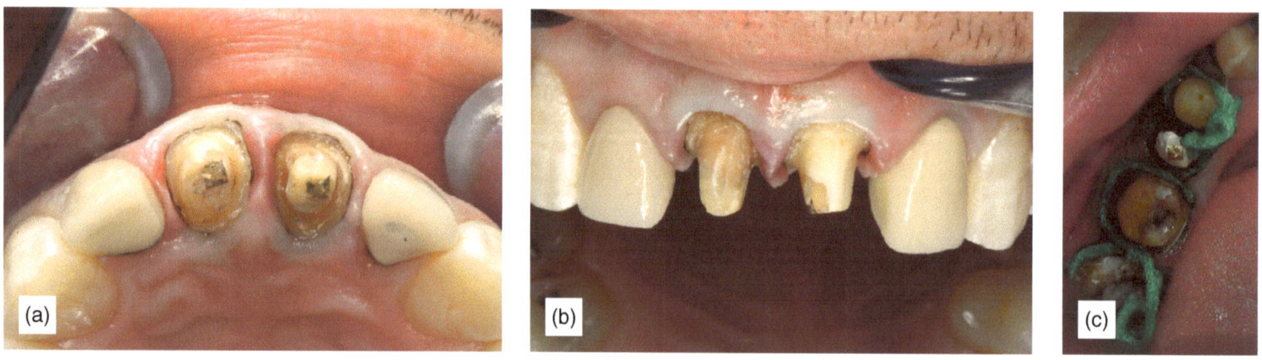

Figure 1.23 (a) Preparations with subgingival margins after cord packing. (b, c) See how blanched and unhealthy the tissue looks, even with careful cord packing procedure.

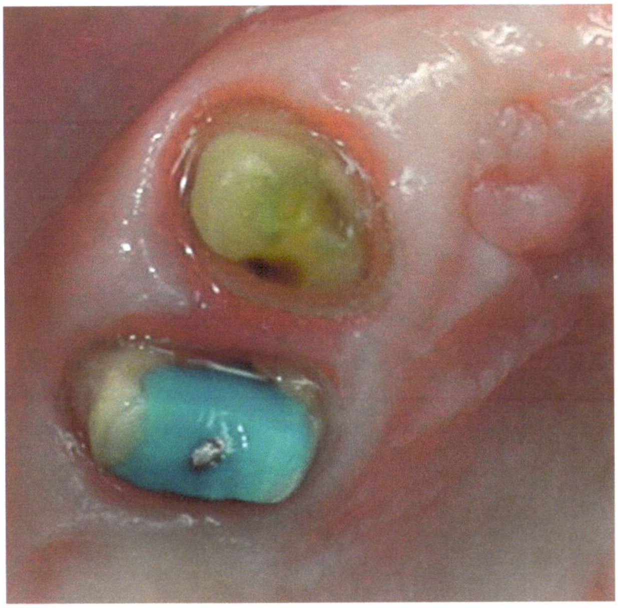

Figure 1.24 Gum after removal of the temporary restoration.

bleeding and moisture control are very difficult. Additionally, it is harder to place matrix bands and wedges with subgingival margins. Finishing and polishing are also considerably more complicated when margins are subgingival (Figures 1.27, 1.28).

Mechanically Retained Dentistry with Subgingival Margins is Less Healthy

As already stated, the negative effects of subgingival margins are not usually considered in dentistry. Traditional mechanically retained dentistry uses multiple techniques and protocols which leave subgingival margins. But what

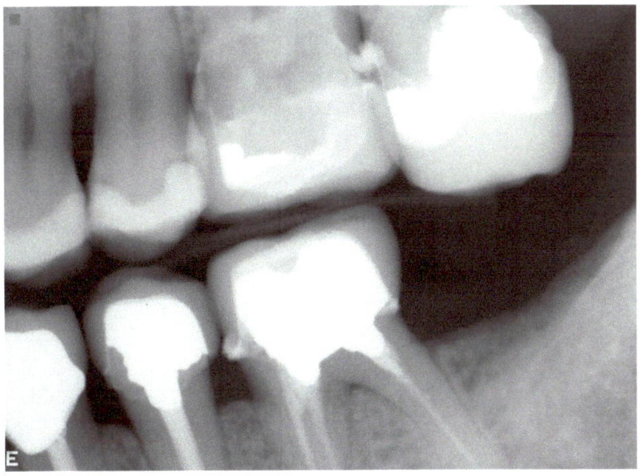

Figure 1.26 Crown showing deep margins with cement.

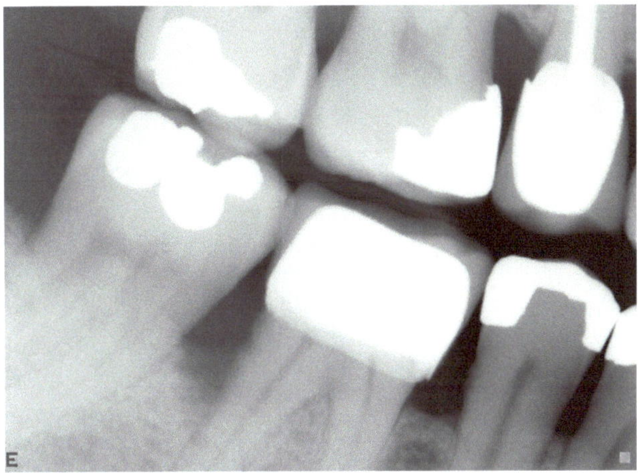

Figure 1.27 Poor margin on deep subgingival class II on first maxillary molar 3, and poor crown margin on lower molar, with bad periodontal consequences.

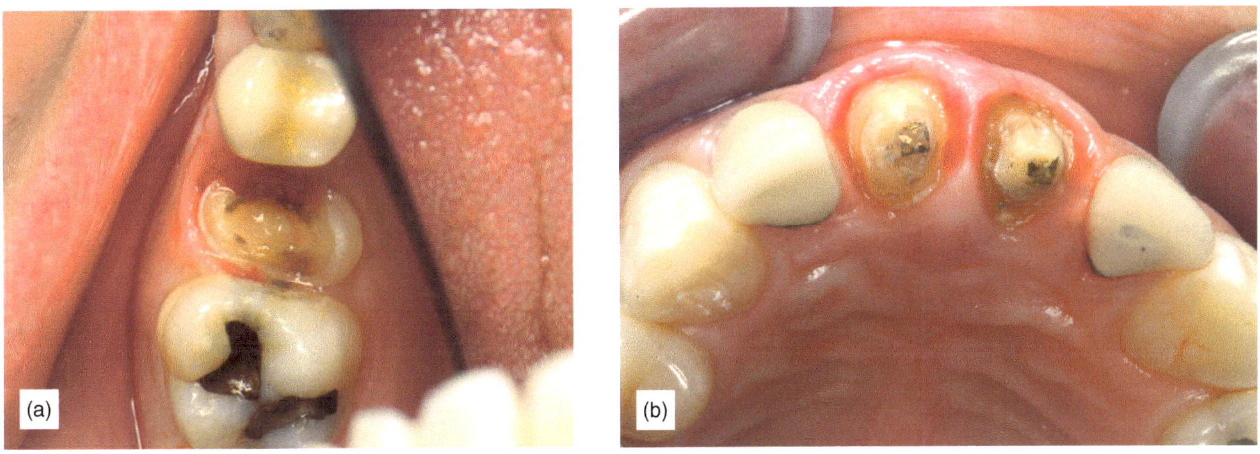

Figure 1.25 (a) Gingiva growing over preparation. (b) After removal of the temporary restoration, inflamed gums can be seen growing over preparation.

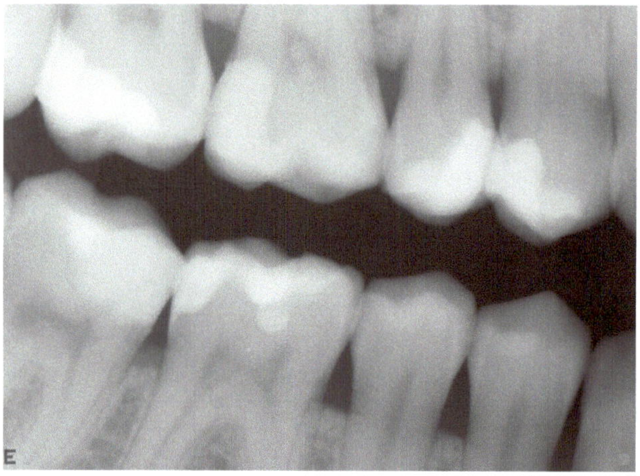

Figure 1.28 Multiple deep margin on a class II composite, showing overhangs, sub-margins, open margins and excess material left behind. Deep subgingival margins are difficult to trim and finish.

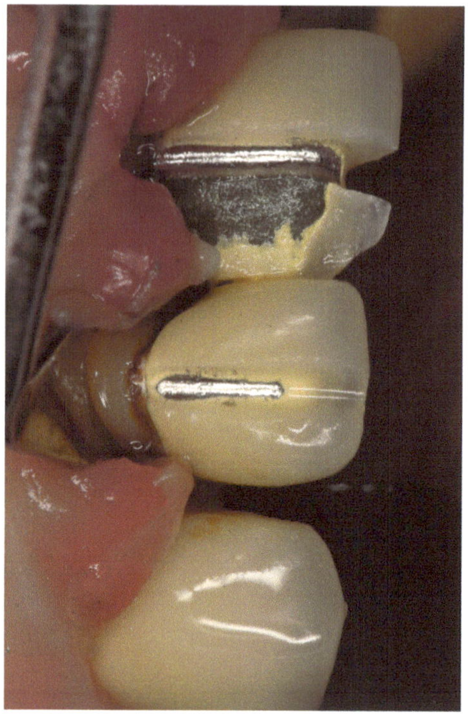

Figure 1.30 Severe gingival inflammation showing the effects of poor margin fit and accumulation of debris and tartar.

are the consequences of these techniques? A subgingival margin will undoubtedly be a factor that will enhance subgingival plaque accumulation. Waerhaug showed, in research with extracted human teeth, that 9 of 10 restorations with subgingival margins were covered with plaque. The conclusion was that "restorations placed below the gingival margin indirectly are strongly involved in the etiology of destructive periodontal disease" (Figure 1.29) [27]. Of course, the worse the margin adaptation, the worse the plaque accumulation. Poor margins lead to what I refer to as "permanent tartar". Permanent tartar is the overhang that traps bacteria and food, becoming destructive to the health of the gingiva (Figure 1.30). It is difficult to see and remove excess cement when it is hidden below the gum line. In another human study, Müller showed that the location of the margin (supragingival, equigingival or subgingival) clearly affects periodontal health [28]. Larato, in a clinical study, found a difference of almost 1 mm in pocket depth between non-restored teeth and teeth with crowns with subgingival margin placement [29]. Beyond research, clinical experience clearly shows the severe damage that subgingival margins cause to the periodontium (Figures 1.31, 1.32). In addition, techniques such as cord packing used

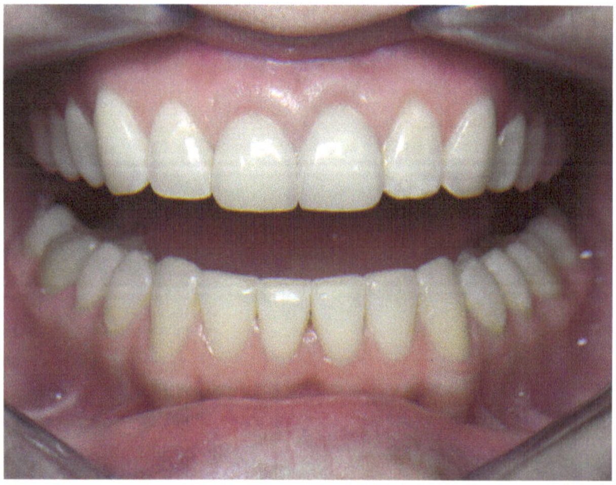

Figure 1.29 A dentist who had some prior subgingival veneers done, clearly showing inflammation on veneers and healthy gums elsewhere.

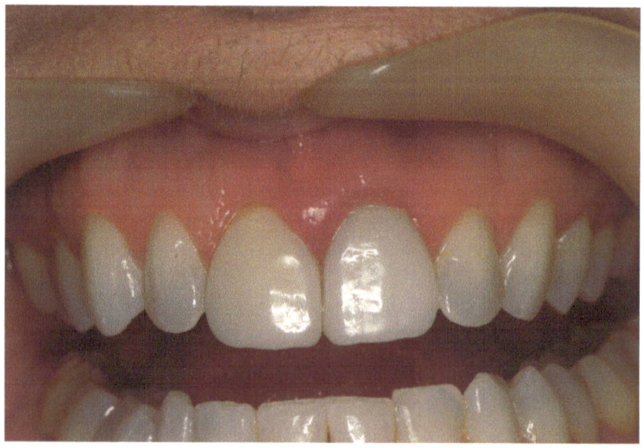

Figure 1.31 Observe the severe inflammation on tooth #9 caused by deep subgingival margin.

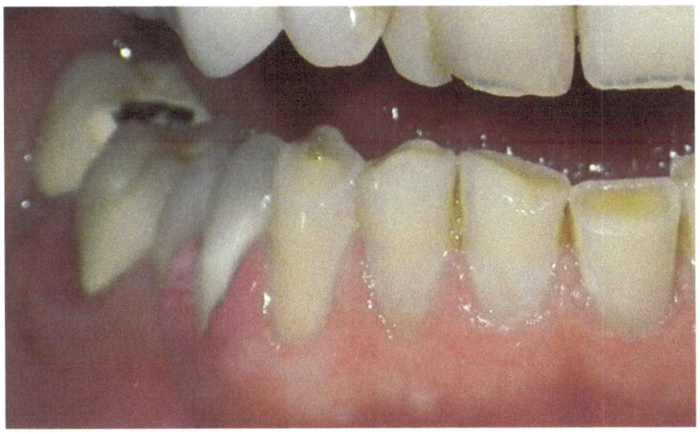

Figure 1.32 Observe the healthy periodontal condition of all non-crowned teeth.

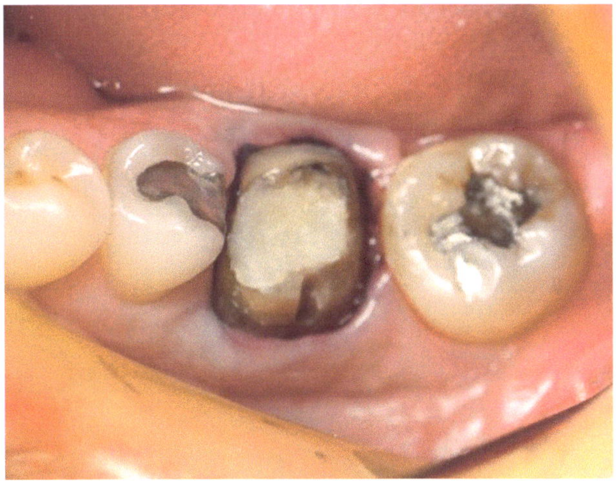

Figure 1.33 Aggressive cord must be placed with deep subgingival margins, causing much irritation.

with traditional subgingival margin placement have the potential to be detrimental to periodontal health [30,31], especially when performed aggressively and incorrectly (Figure 1.33).

Additionally, the more subgingival the restorative margin, the more tooth is reduced. As demonstrated by Shillingburg, "the effect of apical reduction" applies. This means that the more apically the margin is placed, the closer to the pulp the preparation becomes, since a taper in the crown preparation must be maintained (Figure 1.34) [14]. The effects of axial reduction and other mechanical features on the pulpal health are considerable.

Mechanically Retained Dentistry with Subgingival Margins is Less Beautiful

It is interesting that one of the primary reasons given for placing margins subgingivally in dentistry fails so often. Historically, restorative margins have been placed subgingivally because of the desire to hide the unsightly margin of opacious crowns, usually PFM and, more currently, zirconia and IPS e-max® (Ivoclar). Subgingival margins are also placed when the color of the tooth is to be changed by the restorative materials, in cases of dark teeth, or endodontically stained teeth. Unfortunately, this techniques seldom works well (Figure 1.35). First, in the short term, opacious materials are usually unnatural and not attractive; the typical "Chiclet" crown is rarely esthetically pleasing (Figures 1.36a,b, 1.37). Teeth have natural translucency, but when they are covered with an opacious restorative layer unnatural things happen. One effect is that the cervical area of the tooth appears dark because the opacious restoration blocks the light from entering the tooth. The lack of light inside the tooth makes it appear darker or more gray, so the blending of the restoration becomes less predictable. This is the primary reason for the dreaded gray gum around crowns (Figure 1.38). Unhealthy red gingiva is never beautiful.

In the long term, aging and periodontal conditions lead to gingival recession, accelerated by the unhealthy periodontium caused by subgingival margins. When the

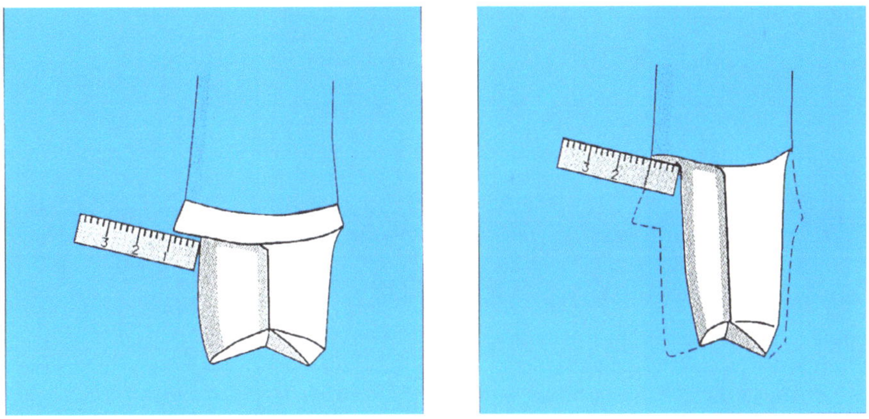

Figure 1.34 The effect of apical reduction.

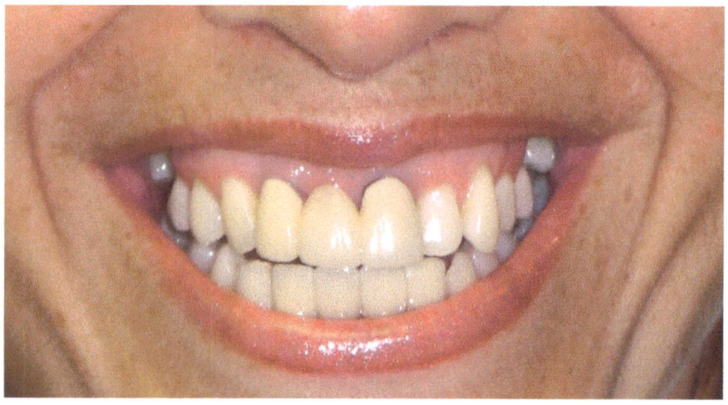

Figure 1.35 Very dark root canal treated tooth with opacious crown, with unesthetic results.

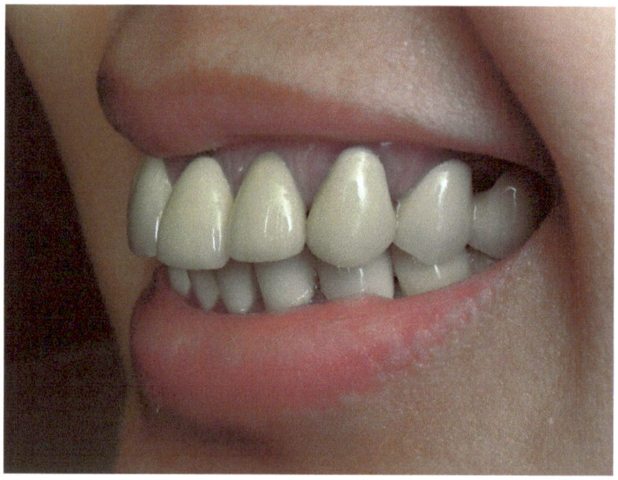

Figure 1.37 This patient was very unhappy with the grayness of the gums on all her crowns.

unsightly margin becomes visible, it often leads to early removal and replacement of the restoration (Figures 1.38, 1.39a,b). Proper use of translucent restorations will render this unnecessary, which is discussed in later chapters.

Mechanically Retained Dentistry with Subgingival Margins is Less Predictable and Less Durable

Because of the long history of crowns and of traditional restorative procedures and rules, it is easy to believe that these procedures are better and more predictable. It is fair to say that almost any procedure, if performed by a master operator, will yield exceptional results. Nevertheless, there are procedures and techniques that are easier to reproduce, and some that are very difficult to reproduce successfully. Traditional crown procedures, such as atraumatic subgingival margin placement, cord packing, subgingival impressions, subgingival cementation cleanup and finishing, are among the most difficult and rarely successful procedures in dentistry. The fact that some of these crowns stay on the tooth for some years past their healthy life, does not mean that they are successful. In the long term, leaky, ill-fitting margins will damage the tooth and the periodontium, and the dentition will have a shorter, less healthy life (Figures 1.40, 1.41a,b) Furthermore, microleakage and recurring caries often go undetected with the more traditional opacious materials (PFM and full

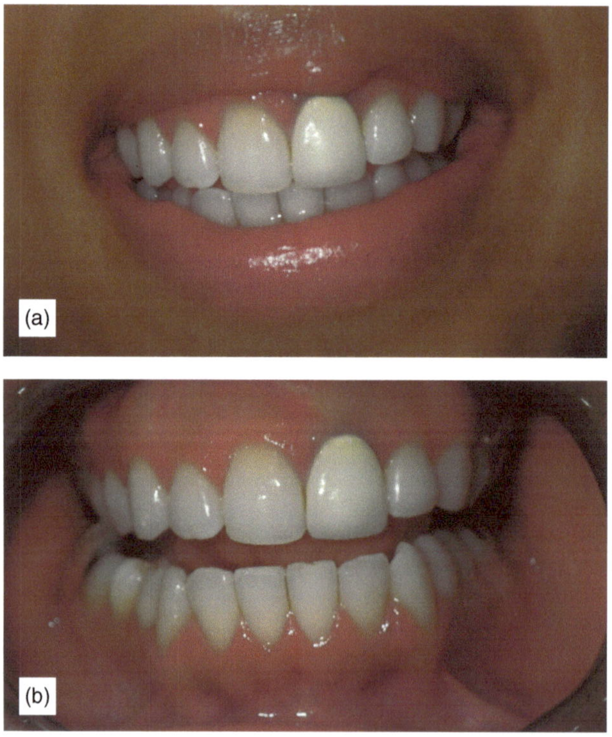

Figure 1.36 (a) Root canal treated tooth restored with opacious crown, leaving a gray margin and "Chiclet"-like tooth. (b) Close-up view of the same tooth; this crown has been replaced three times and each time it ends up showing the margin again.

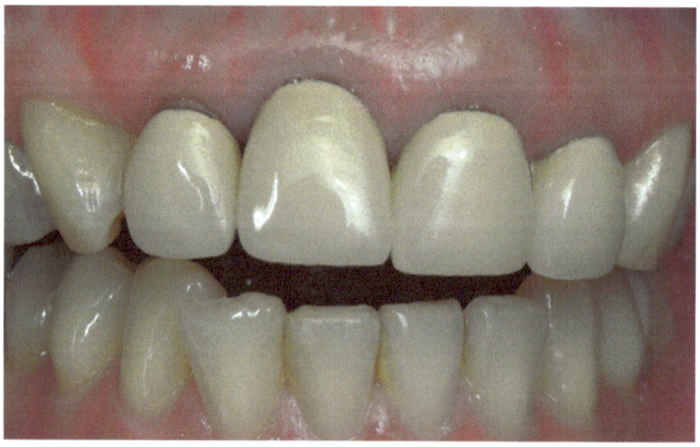

Figure 1.38 This patient complained that the margin used to be acceptable, but the gums have receded and now she does not like the appearance and wants the crowns replaced.

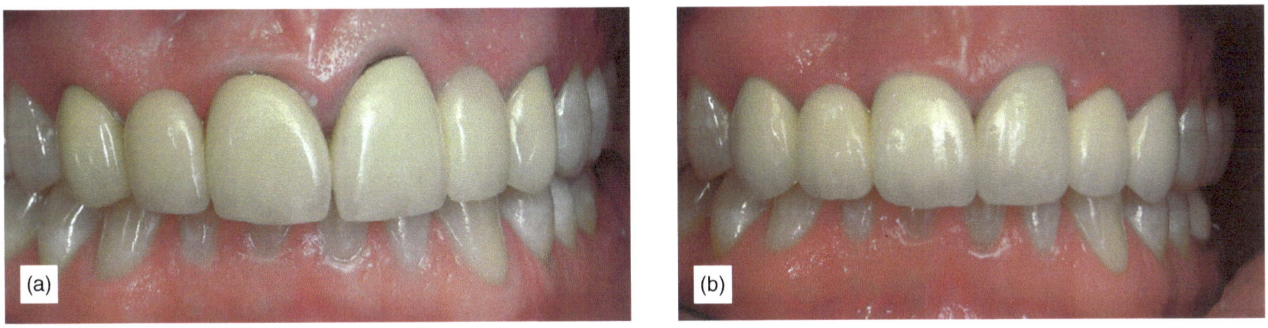

Figure 1.39 (a) These are clinically healthy crowns, but the patient wanted them replaced. (b) After crown replacement – an extremely difficult case, and most likely the gingiva will recede in a few years.

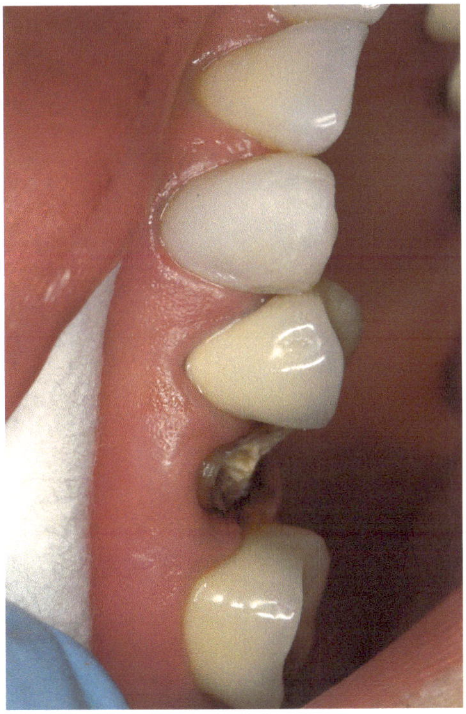

Figure 1.40 After crown removal, what was left of the tooth was not sufficient for a restoration.

zirconia), as opacity make it difficult to discover caries visually, and microleakage and radiopacity make it difficult to assess them radiographically.

Traditional class II and III restorations with boxes, retentive features, and traditional restorative rules which lead to subgingival margins become exponentially more difficult as the margins become more subgingival. Placing matrix (predictably bonding, filling, finishing, and polishing) becomes extremely difficult. Subsequent chapters discuss techniques to minimize and almost eliminate the need for subgingival margins.

Traditional preparation which requires axial wall, boxes, shoulders, and other mechanical retentive features, requires more tooth removal, leads to increasing closeness to the pulp, and increases heat and damage to the pulp. This can increase the need for root canal therapy on teeth treated with crowns, shortening the life of the restoration and the tooth (Figures 1.42, 1.43) [21,22,23,24]. The end result of this is more postoperative pain, unhappy patients, and, ultimately, decreased predictability and longevity. Shorter esthetic life increases the chances of pulpal reaction and necrosis, increases periodontal damage, and limits the ability to repair or replace in a timely fashion. With all of these

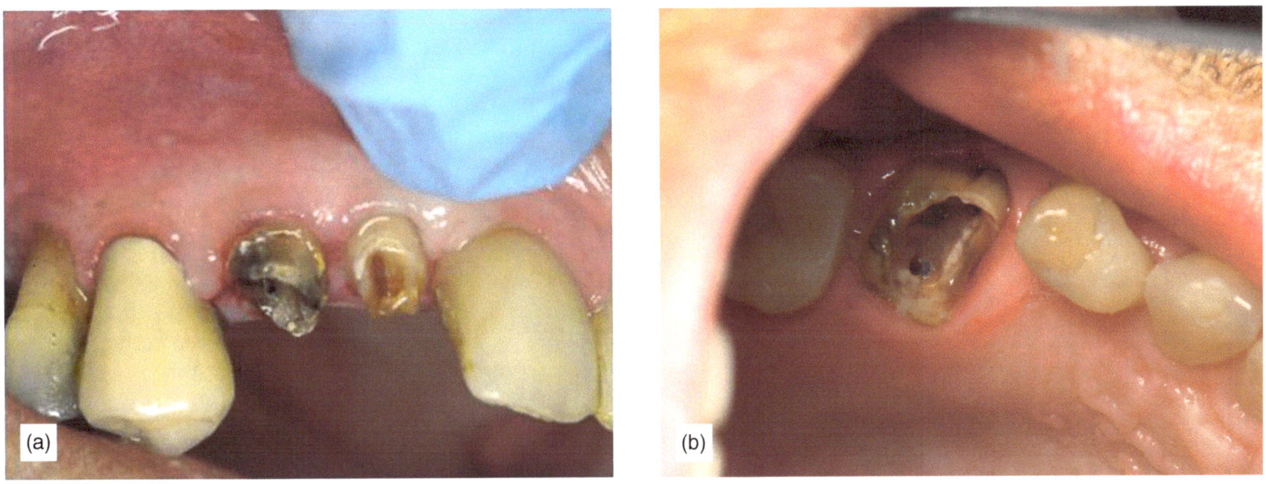

Figure 1.41 (a, b) Crown failure needing root removal.

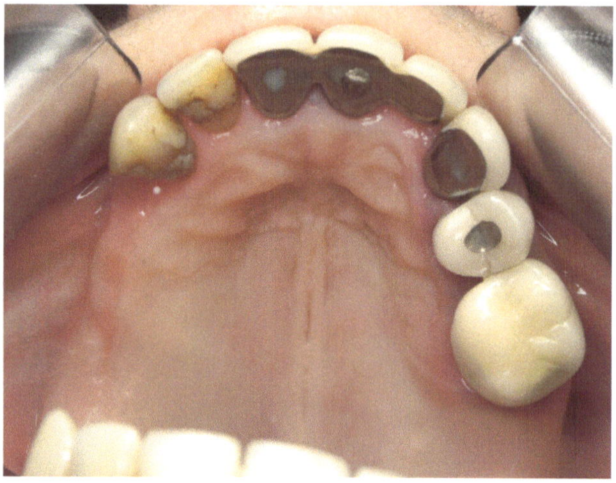

Figure 1.42 There are many little holes on this crown, showing the usual unforeseen common consequence of aggressive preparation.

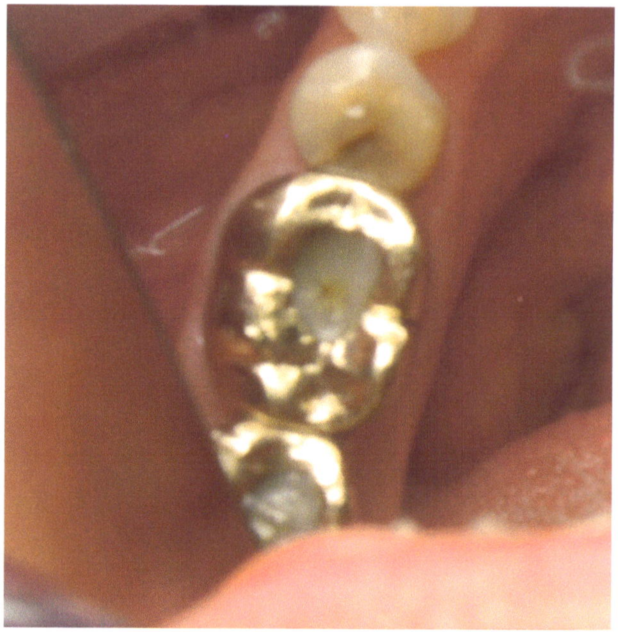

Figure 1.43 Two gold crowns with root canal treatment access holes.

disadvantages, traditional full crowns can hardly be considered successful, predictable or long-lived, even if they can stay in the mouth for many years, well beyond their healthy stage.

Chapter 2 explores the benefits of supragingival minimally invasive adhesive dentistry as a substitute for traditional mechanically retained dentistry with subgingival margins.

References

1 Ruiz JL, Christensen GJ. Myths vs. realities: State of the art indirect posterior restorations. *J Cosmetic Dent*, 2011; 27(3): 63–72.
2 Christensen GJ. Are tooth colored onlays viable alternatives to crowns? *Clinicians Report*, 2012; 5(1): 1, 3.
3 Christensen GJ. The case for onlays versus tooth-colored crowns. *J Am Dental Assoc*, 2012; 143(10): 1141–1144.
4 Ruiz JL, Kurtz R. Are full-coverage crowns overutilized? Supragingival partial-coverage designs as a first option. *Dent Today*, 2014; 33(5): 122, 124–125.
5 Ruiz JL. Anterior and posterior partial-coverage indirect restorations using supragingival dentistry techniques. *J Mass Dent Soc*, 2012; 61(2): 16–19.
6 White DJ. Dental calculus: Recent insights into occurrence, formation, prevention, removal and oral health effects of supragingival and subgingival deposits. *Eur J Oral Sci*, 1997; 105(5 Pt 2): 508–522.
7 Satheesh K, MacNeill SR, Rapley JW, Cobb CM. The CEJ: a biofilm and calculus trap. *Compend Contin Educ Dent*, 2011; 32(2): 30–40.
8 Reitemeier B, Hänsel K, Walter MH, Kastner C, Toutenburg H. Effect of posterior crown margin placement on gingival health. *J Prosthet Dent*, 2002; 87(2): 167–172.
9 Sorensen SE, Larsen IB. Gingival and alveolar bone reaction to marginal fit of subgingival crown margins. *Eur J Oral Sci*, 1986; 94(2): 109–114.
10 Lareto D. Effects of cervical margins on gingiva. *J Calif Dent Assoc*, 1969; 45; 19–22.
11 Feng J, Aboyoussef H, Weiner S, Singh S, Jandinski J. The effect of gingival retraction procedures on periodontal indices and crevicular fluid cytokine levels: a pilot study. *J Prosthodont*, 2006; 15(2): 108–112.
12 Ruiz JL, Christensen GJ. Rationale for the utilization of bonded nonmetal onlays as an alternative to PFM crowns. *Dent Today*, 2006; 25(9): 80–83.
13 Black GV. *The Technical Procedures in Filling Teeth*. Chicago: HO Shepard Co. Printers; 1899, pp. 20–21.
14 Shillingburg HT, Hobo S, Whitsett LD, Jacobi R, Brackett SE (eds). Principles of tooth preparations, in *Fundamentals of Fixed Prosthodontics*, 3rd ed. Quintessence Books; 1997, pp. 119–135.
15 Potts RG, Shillingburg HT Jr, Duncanson MG Jr. Retention and resistance of preparations for cast restorations. *J Prosthet Dent*, 2004; 92(3): 207–212.
16 Shillingburg HT Jr. Conservative preparations for cast restorations. *Dent Clin North Am*, 1976; 20(2): 259–271.
17 Woolsey GD, Matich JA. The effect of axial grooves on the resistance form of cast restorations. *J Am Dent Assoc*, 1978; 97(6): 978–980.

18 AlFouzan, AF, Tashkandi EA. Volumetric measurements of removed tooth structure associated with various preparation designs. *Int J Prosthodont*, 2013; 26(6): 545–548.

19 Edelhoff D, Sorensen JA. Tooth structure removal associated with various preparation designs for posterior teeth. *Int J Periodontics Restorative Dent*, 2002; 22(3): 241–249.

20 Zollner A, Gaengler P. Pulp reactions to different preparation techniques on teeth exhibiting periodontal disease. *J Oral Rehabil*, 2000; 27(2): 93–102.

21 Thomas MS, Kundabala M. Pulp hyperthermia during tooth preparation: The effect of rotatory instruments, laser, ultrasonic devices and airborne particle abrasion. *J Calif Dent Assoc*, 2012; 40(9): 721–731.

22 Davis GR, Tayeb RA, Seymour KG, Cherukara GP. Quantification of residual dentine thickness following crown preparation. *J Dent*, 2012; 40(7): 571–576.

23 Dahl BL. Dentine/pulp reactions to full crown preparation procedures. *J Oral Rehabil*, 1977; 4(3): 247–254.

24 Langeland K, Langeland LK. Pulp reactions to cavity and crown preparation. *Aust Dent J*, 1970; 5(4): 261–276.

25 Padbury A, Eber R, Wang HL. Interactions between the gingiva and the margin of restorations. *J Clin Periodontol*, 2003; 30(5): 379–385.

26 Christensen GJ. The state of fixed prosthodontic impressions: room for improvement. *J Am Dent Assoc*, 2005; 136(3): 343–346.

27 Waerhaug J. Presence or absence of plaque on subgingival restorations. *Scand J Dent Res*, 1975; 83(1): 193–201.

28 Müller HP. The effect of artificial crown margins at the gingival margin on the periodontal conditions in a group of periodontally supervised patients treated with fixed bridges. *J Clin Periodontol*, 1986; 13(2): 97–102.

29 Larato DC. Effects of artificial crown margin extension and tooth brushing frequency on gingival pocket depth. *J Prosthet Dent*, 1975; 34(6): 640–643.

30 Polat NT, Ozdemir AK, Turgut M. Effects of gingival retraction materials on gingival blood flow. *Int J Prosthodont*, 2007; 20(1): 57–62.

31 Fazekas A, Csempesz F, Csabai Z, Vág J. Effects of presoaked retraction cords on the microcirculation of the human gingival margin. *Oper Dent*, 2002; 27(4): 343–348.

2

The Healthier Paradigm: Supragingival Minimally Invasive Adhesive Dentistry – The Benefits

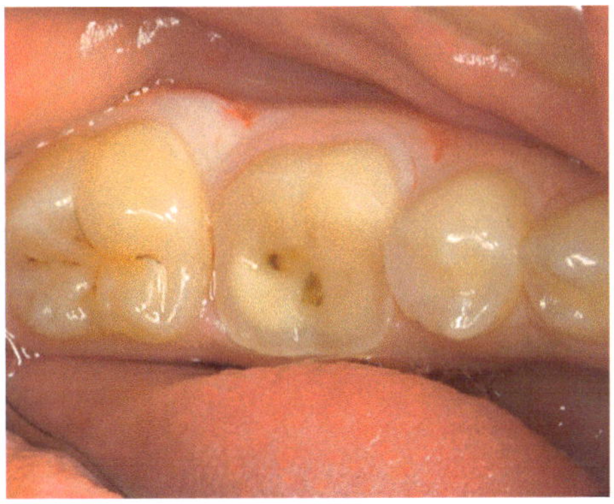

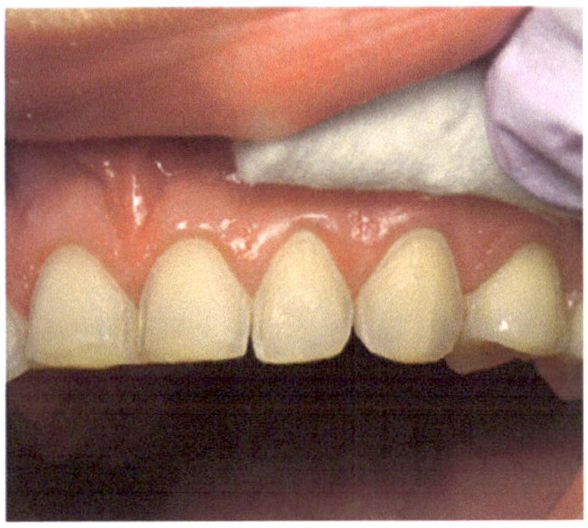

Supragingival margins make preparation, impression, and cementation easier, faster, and more predictable.

Introduction

Subgingival margins are preventable. Nevertheless, most clinicians would say, "I would leave the margins above the gum if I were able!" The previous chapter explained why traditional mechanically retained dentistry considers subgingival margins normal. Supragingival minimally invasive adhesive dentistry is a mode of restorative dentistry which uses a number of modern techniques, and the benefits of adhesive dentistry, to intentionally avoid crowns or any restorative procedure which may cause unnecessary subgingival margin. It strives to retain restorative margins supragingivally and to preserve as much tooth as possible, making it a healthier form of restorative dentistry. With these techniques, it is also possible to limit and repair the damage when subgingival caries or margins are already present.

Supragingival minimally invasive adhesive dentistry comes with numerous advantages. While the desire to stay supragingival in dentistry is universal, the difference is the systematic approach, and the many specialized techniques and absolute commitment to supragingival minimally invasive restorations. Supragingival margins in fact make restorative dentistry easier for the clinician, healthier for the patient, more esthetically pleasing, and provide for long lasting predictable results (Figures 2.1a–g, 2.2a,b).

Esthetic demands from patients led to an increased use of new tooth-colored materials. Adhesives have changed the rules and allow the dentist to provide minimally invasive esthetic dentistry, never considered possible before [1,2,3,4,5]. When initially introduced, bonded restorations posed challenges for dental professionals. Bonded restorations seemed less predictable and filled with complications, such as postoperative sensitivity and restoration fractures, leading to their limited use. Lack of knowledge and trust in adhesion led to less than optimal use of these new tooth-colored materials. Instead of using tooth-conserving adhesion techniques, traditional mechanically retained techniques were employed, which it is often counterproductive.

Over time, newer materials, improved restorative and adhesion techniques, and the realization of previously hidden benefits, especially supragingival margins [6,7,8,9], have allowed these restorations to live up to their full potential [10,11,12]. Adhesion allows for the

Supra-Gingival Minimally Invasive Dentistry: A Healthier Approach to Esthetic Restorations, First Edition. By Jose-Luis Ruiz.

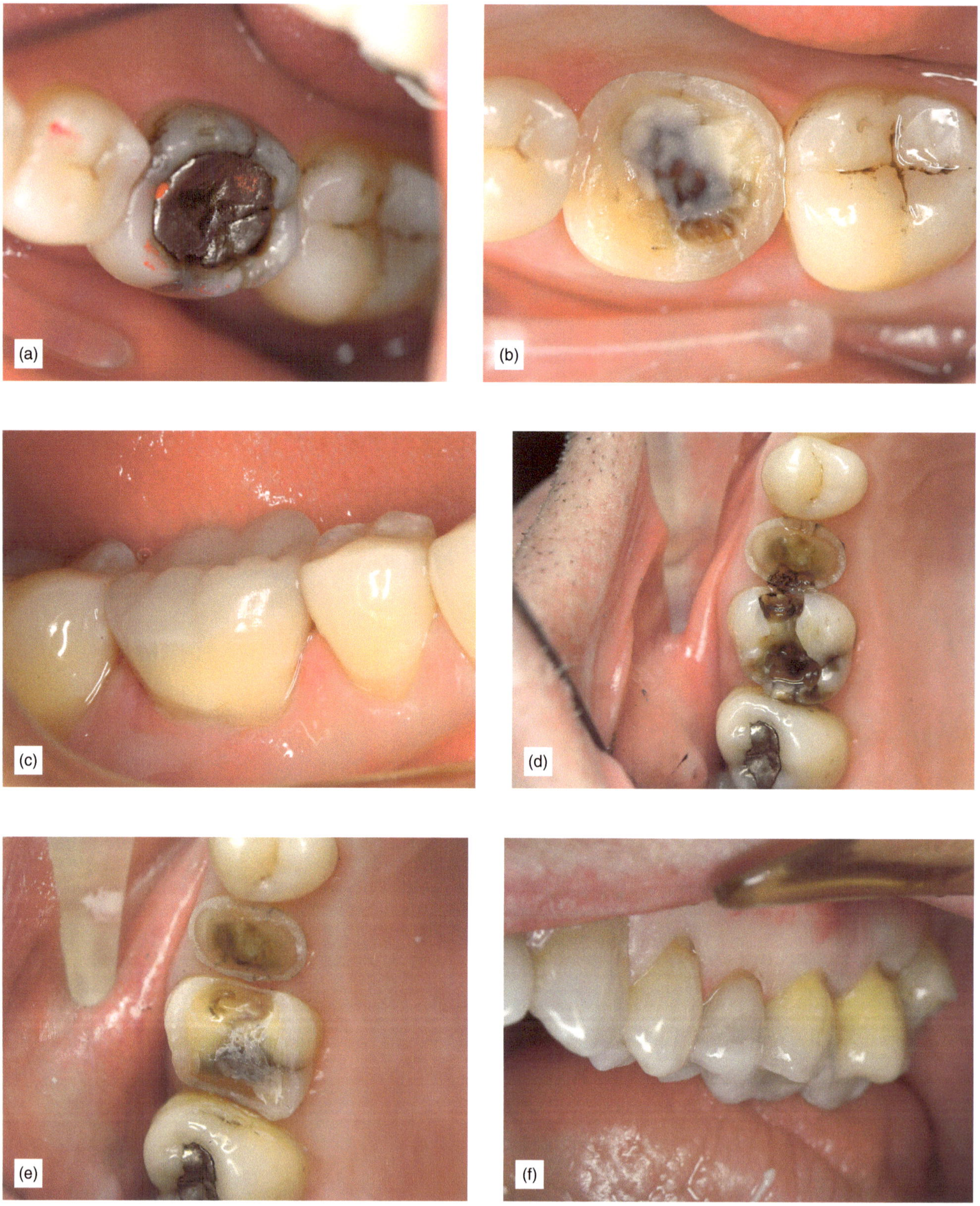

Figure 2.1 (a) Damaged tooth needing an indirect restoration. (b) Undisturbed gingiva during preparation for onlay, showing very little tooth removal. (c) Healthy gingival around finished onlay. (d) Badly damaged teeth. (e) After preparation, with absolutely minimum tooth reduction. (f) Cemented restoration. (*Continued*)

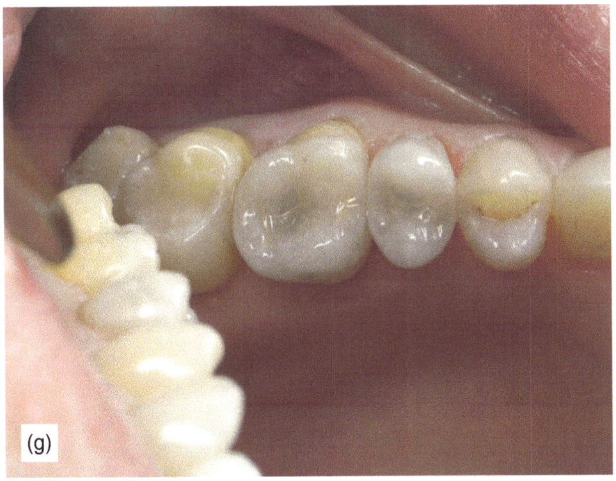

Figure 2.1 (*Continued*)
(g) Occlusal view.

preservation of healthy tooth structure and since remaining dentin thickness correlates with continued tooth vitality [13], bonded restorations preserve the vitality of the tooth (Figure 2.3a–c).

It must be emphasized that although partial coverage bonded restorations such as onlays and veneers are used in dentistry, they are extremely under-used. The overwhelming majority in the profession consider partial coverage bonded restorations as a limited alternative to full crowns, indicated only when a number of requirements are fulfilled (Figures 2.4a,b, 2.5a–d) [14,15,16,17,18]. Keeping restorative margins supragingival has been left to chance, as a suggested option only where possible. In the cases where is not easily achievable, full coverage becomes the preferred choice. Until now, no specific protocol or set of techniques have been advocated to prevent subgingival margins. The supragingival minimally invasive adhesive dentistry approach is different. Progress in understanding adhesive dentistry, added to the great value placed on the health of the periodontium, make supragingival margins a priority, and minimally invasive partial coverage restoration, direct and indirect, becomes the choice in every case, except in teeth already cut for crowns.

While it might be thought that because traditional mechanically retained restorations have a longer history and are thus more predictable, easier and maybe even healthier, the following section presents the argument that supragingival minimally invasive adhesive dentistry is in fact a better restorative alternative for the patient and the dentist. Principles and techniques for supragingival dentistry and a supragingival protocol for achieving supragingival margins are considered in detail in subsequent chapters.

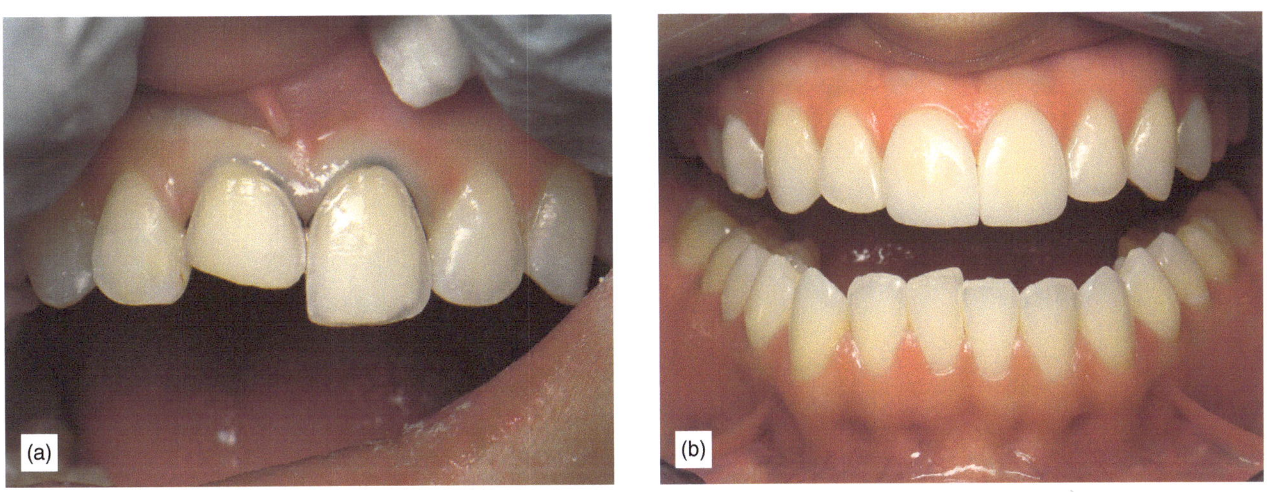

Figure 2.2 (a) Supragingival veneer preparation of a fractured tooth and adjacent central. (b) Healthy undisturbed gingiva around finished veneers.

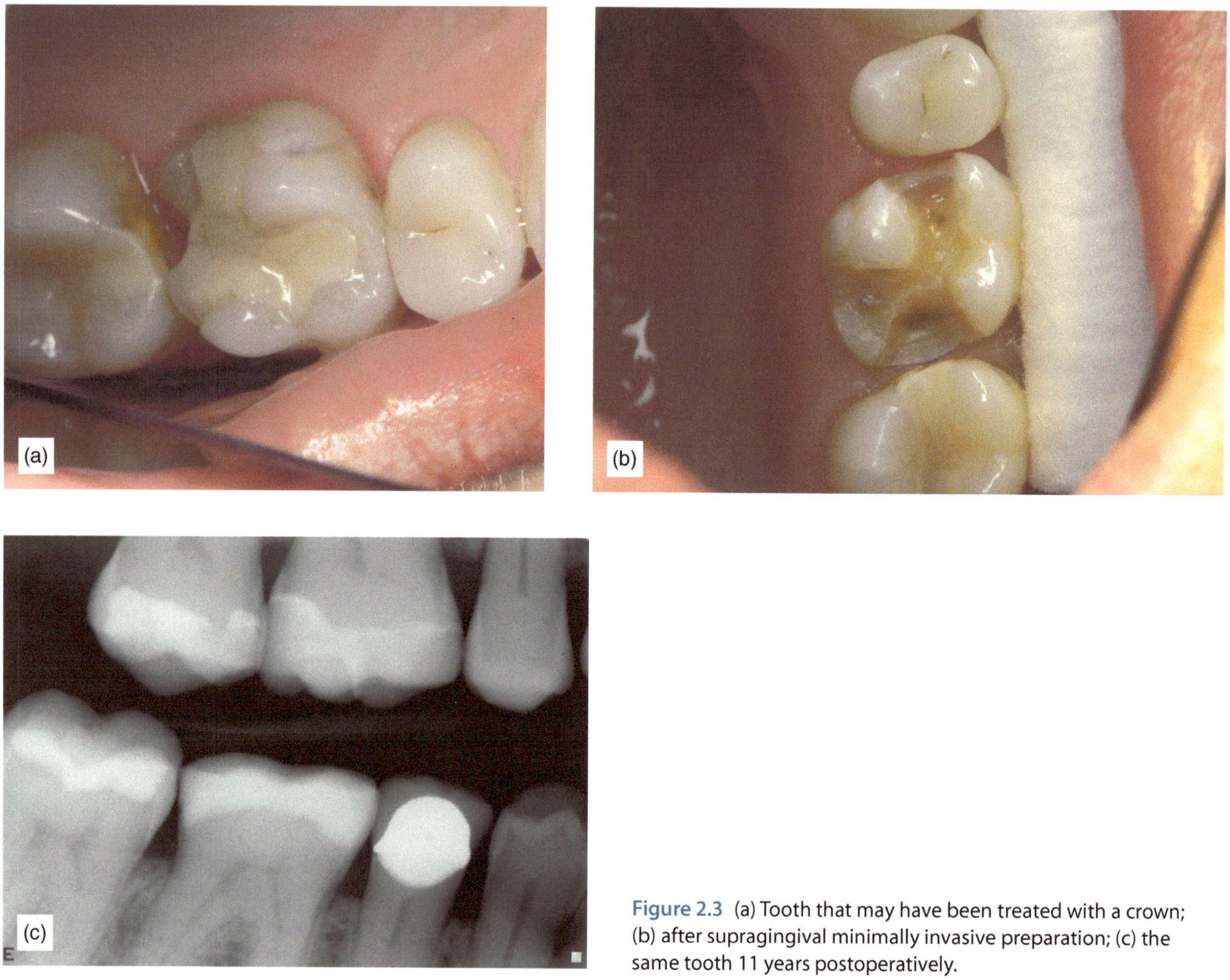

Figure 2.3 (a) Tooth that may have been treated with a crown; (b) after supragingival minimally invasive preparation; (c) the same tooth 11 years postoperatively.

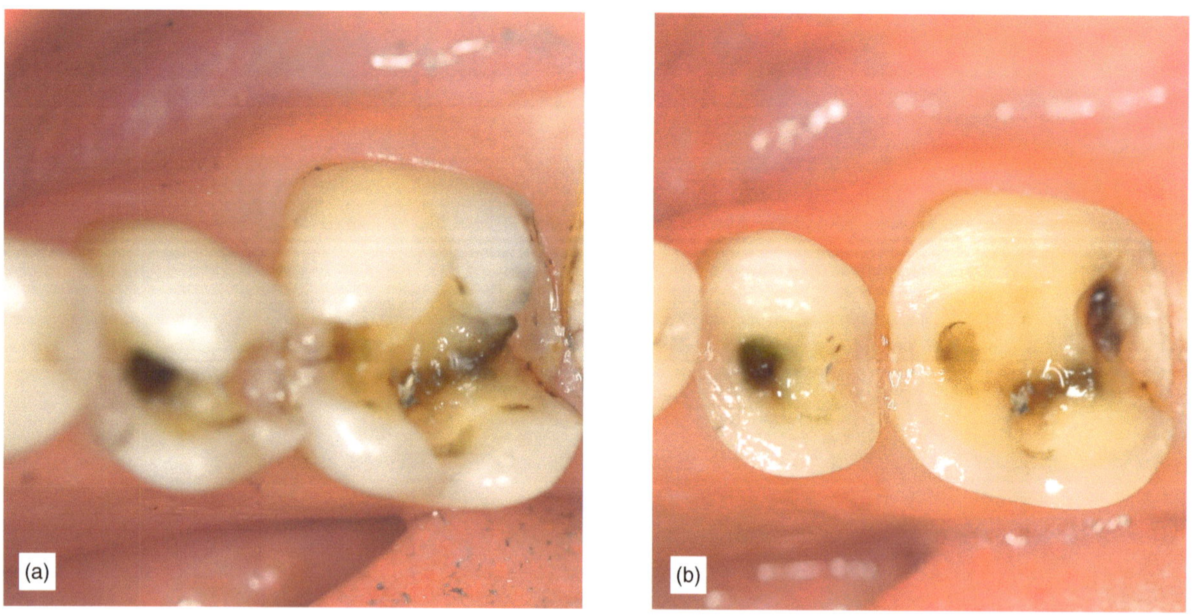

Figure 2.4 (a) Badly damaged teeth usually recommended for full crowns; (b) supragingival onlay preparations.

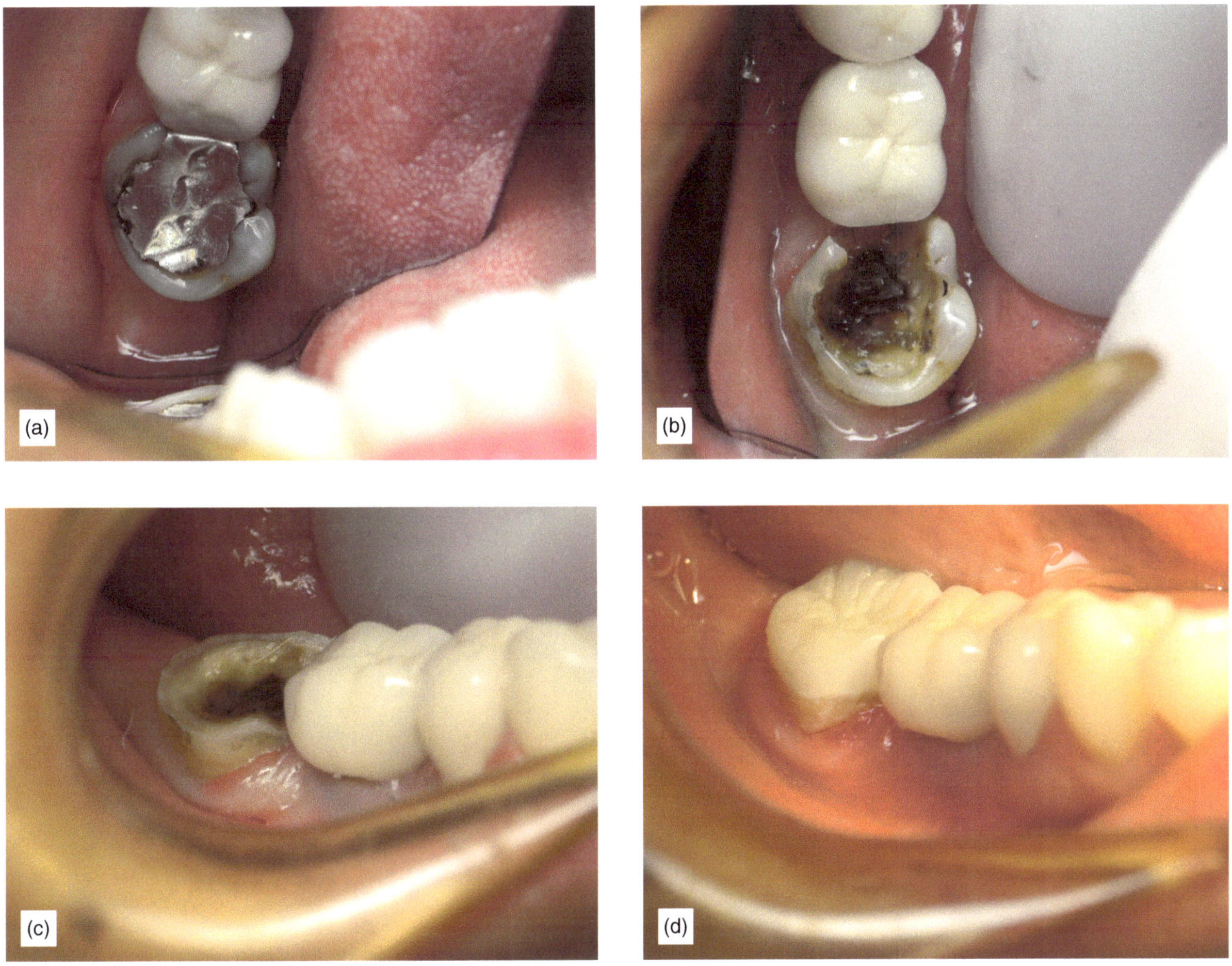

Figure 2.5 Extremely damaged tooth: (a) with amalgam; (b) after amalgam removal, if axial reduction was performed the tooth would end up deeply subgingival; (c) preparation is very supragingival and easy to isolate an event on a second molar; (d) the finished restoration supported by adhesion.

Supragingival Minimally Invasive Adhesive Dentistry is Easier

It may be thought that traditional restorative techniques such as full crowns are easier than partial coverage bonded restorations, but in fact the opposite is true: keeping margins supragingival is key to simple bonded restorations.

The preparation of the tooth for supragingival bonded restoration is considerably more simple. The need for exacting mechanical retention features such as axial reduction with correct taper, and exact boxes, shoulders and offsets during preparations, is eliminated, as adhesive retention is predictable and does not require any retention or resistance forms, thus greatly simplifying the preparation process (Figure 2.6a–c). The very difficult atraumatic subgingival margin placement technique is also eliminated. All of the above make supragingival adhesive dentistry preparation far less complicated and faster to perform correctly, compared with traditional crown preparation (Figure 2.7a,b) [19,20]. Proper preparation leads to easy cementation when the restorative margins are kept supragingival, and the use of a targeted supragingival protocol ensures that the risk of contamination while cementing or bonding is virtually eliminated.

Taking an impression of a subgingival margin is one of the most challenging procedures that dentists perform (Figure 2.8a,b) [21,22,23]. Since subgingival margins are equally difficult to reproduce with digital scanners, digital impressions will also greatly benefit from supragingival margins (Figure 2.9a,b). Supragingival restorative techniques make the task of taking impressions easy, thus making every ensuing step more predictable.

When margins are kept above the gingival level, temporaries are easier to make because the margins are clear

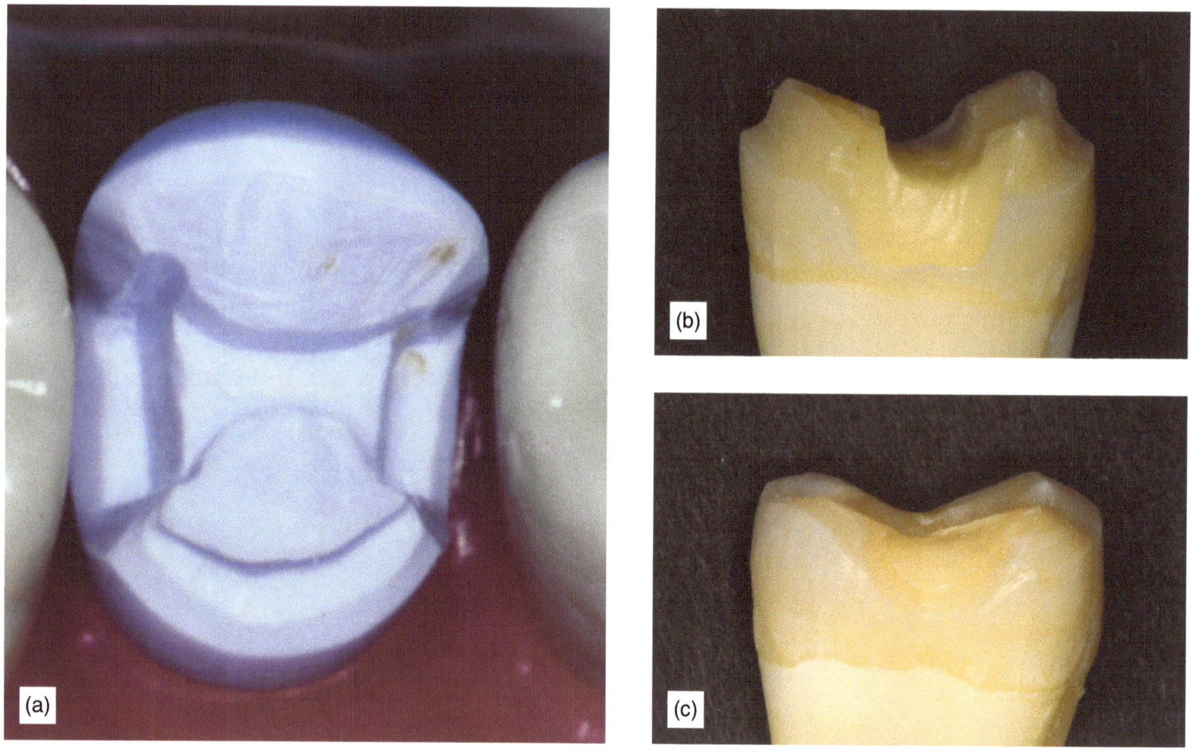

Figure 2.6 (a) Traditional mechanically retained onlay preparation, showing the exacting angles, boxes needed for retention. (b) Compare the increased tooth removal needed for mechanically retained onlay with (c) bonded onlay preparation, showing increased simplicity and tooth preservation.

and visible. Temporary cementation can easily be done on a clean uncontaminated tooth and removal of the temporary cement is easy and predictable, thus allowing for better results, and leaving healthier gingiva at the time of permanent cementation (Figure 2.10a,b).

Final cementation also becomes predictable and stress free. Because there is less room for human error with a more accurate supragingival impression, restorations tend to fit better. There is no need to worry about tissue inflammation, uncontrolled bleeding or placing cord for final cementation, because supragingival temporary restorations allow for healthy tissues (Figures 2.11, 2.12). Margins are away from the gingival tissues, so bonded cementation is cleaner, easier and more successful. Excess cement is more readily visible, making it easier to remove. Since restorative margins are also more accessible, finishing them is easier and leads to better results (Figure 2.13). This is true with direct and indirect restorations.

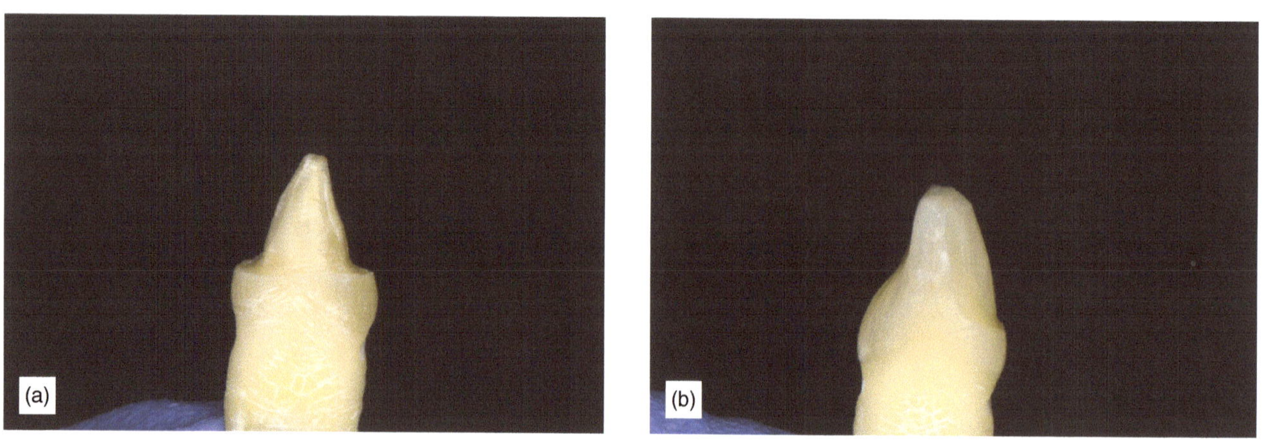

Figure 2.7 Comparison of (a) crown preparation with (b) veneer preparation.

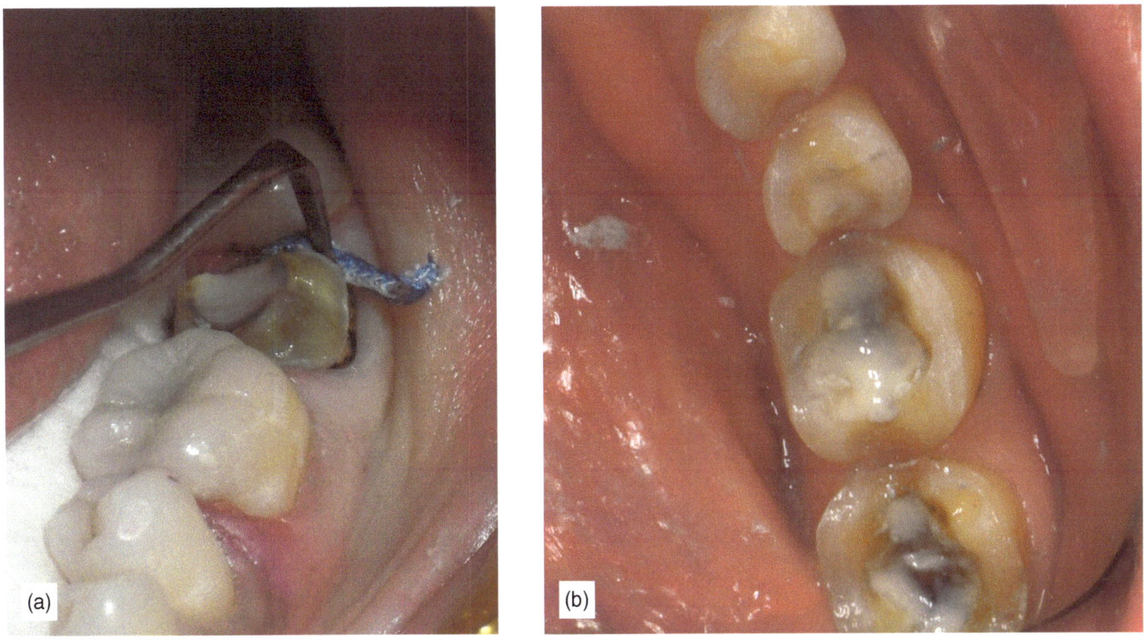

Figure 2.8 (a) Double cord needed for a crown impression. (b) Supragingival margins yield an easy impression, without cord, even in cases involving more than one tooth.

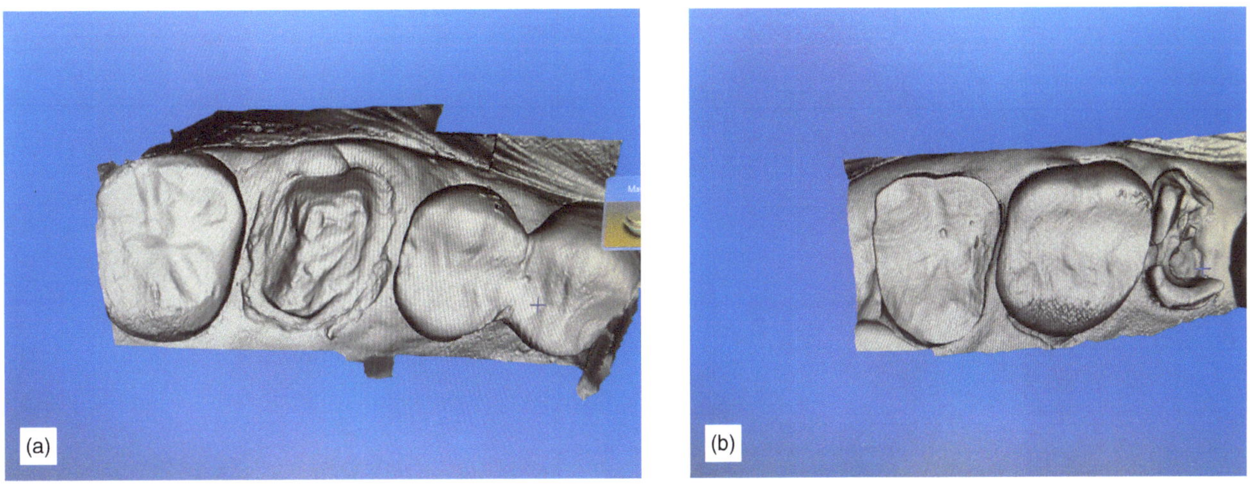

Figure 2.9 (a) It is equally difficult to capture subgingival margin detail with a digital impression, and with polyvinyl siloxane impression material it is sometimes virtually impossible (courtesy of Dr Renee Kurtz). (b) Digital impressions are easy with supragingival margins (courtesy of Dr Renee Kurtz).

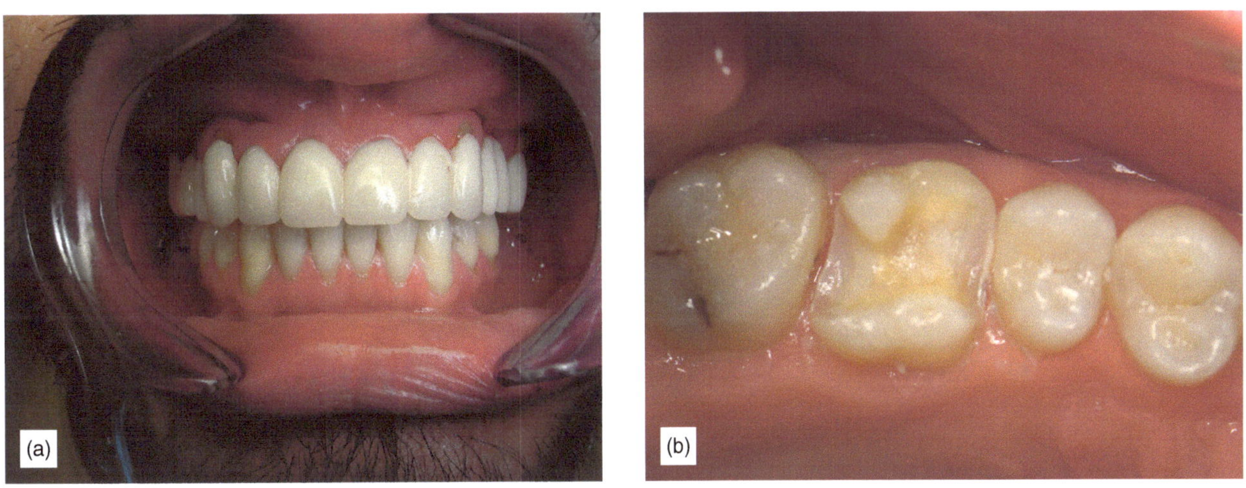

Figure 2.10 (a) Provisional on crown, with unhealthy gums. (b) After the provisional is removed, the gums are healthy.

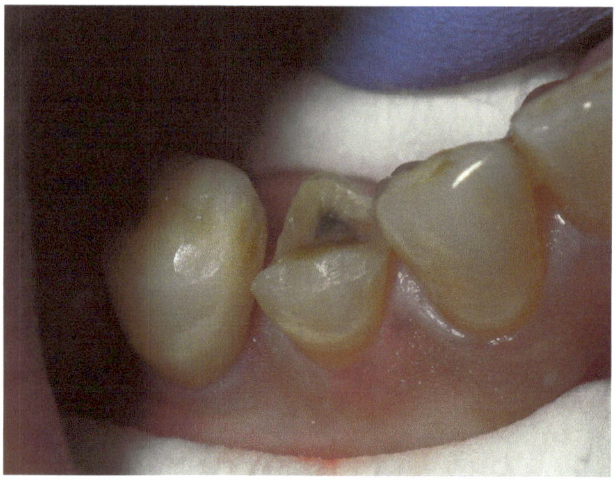

Figure 2.11 Onlay preparation with supragingival margins are easy to isolate and cement.

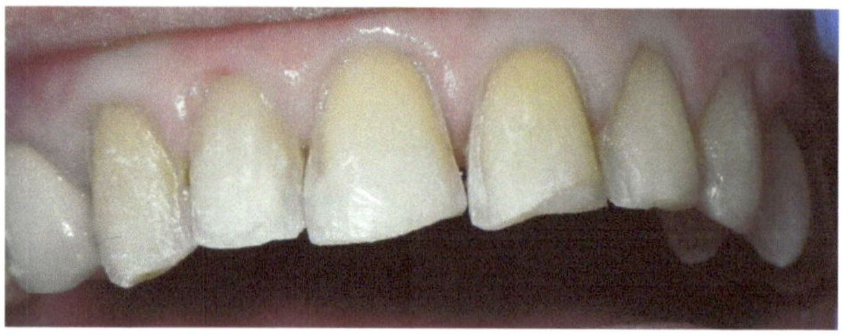

Figure 2.12 Veneer preparation with supragingival margins are easy to isolate and cement.

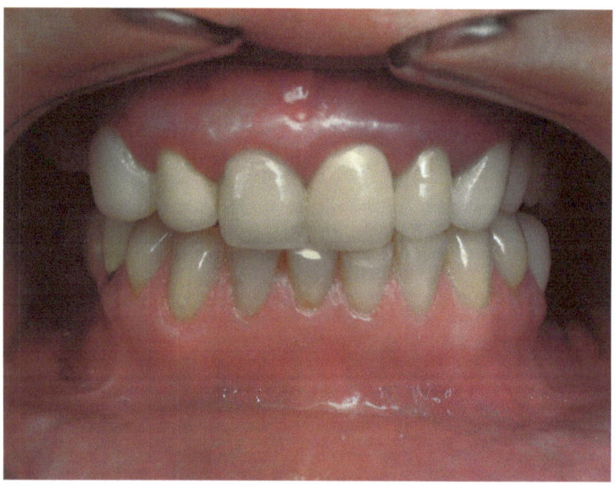

Figure 2.13 Inflamed gingiva on crowns.

Supragingival Minimally Invasive Adhesive Dentistry is Healthier

Not having to compromise or invade the periodontium is one of the chief reasons that supragingival dentistry is healthier for our patients. Poor gingival health is often seen surrounding porcelain-fused-to-metal (PFM) crowns, while supragingival restorations do not affect periodontal health (Figure 2.14). The relationship between subgingival margins and poor periodontal health cannot be overemphasized [24,25,26]. Gingival recession is also less likely to occur when gums are undamaged by subgingival preparation and aggressive cord packing. Supragingival restorative techniques eliminate these problems (Figure 2.15a,b). Even in cases when the clinician may not be able to achieve a perfect marginal fit and smoothness, when the margin is supragingival, the consequences of the imperfect margins are not as devastating to the periodontium. Supragingival defective margins will be more accessible for patients to clean and maintain, and the clinician will be able, at a later date, to realize and perhaps repair the defect because of its better visibility both on x-ray and visually. All of the above provides patients with better quality, healthier dentistry.

Pulpal health is another major benefit of supragingival adhesive dentistry. First, avoiding the need for mechanical retention with the help of adhesion avoids unnecessarily removal of millimeters of healthy tooth and thus overheating and traumatizing the pulp (Figure 2.16a,b). Supragingival bonded dentistry allows the dentist to work away from vital pulp because it does not require axial reduction or any other mechanical retention features. Proximity to the pulp during preparation has been clearly shown to increase both pulp temperature and pulpal changes [27,28,29,30]. Innumerable root canals can be avoided by remaining far away from the nerve during full crown preparation [31].

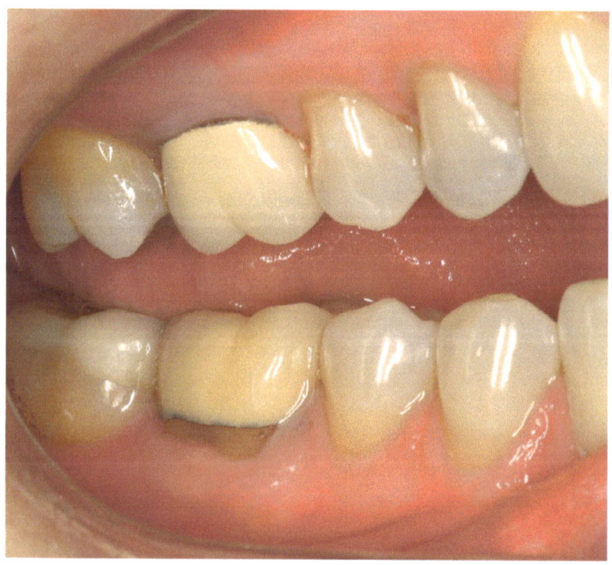

Figure 2.14 Compare periodontal health around the onlay on the lower second molar and the subgingival margin maxillary crown.

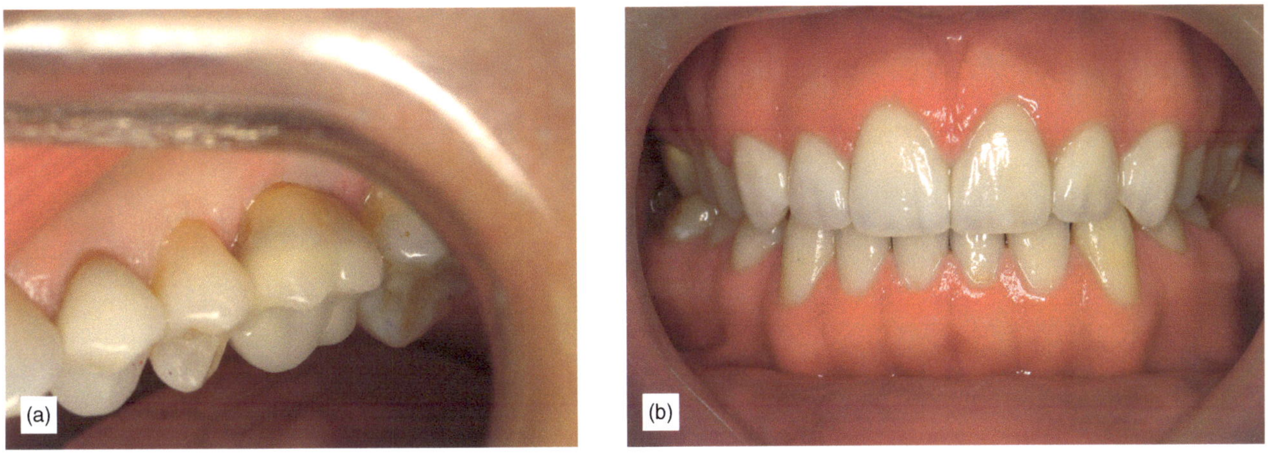

Figure 2.15 (a) Healthy gingiva on onlays with visible supragingival margins. (b) Healthy gingiva on veneers with visible supragingival margins.

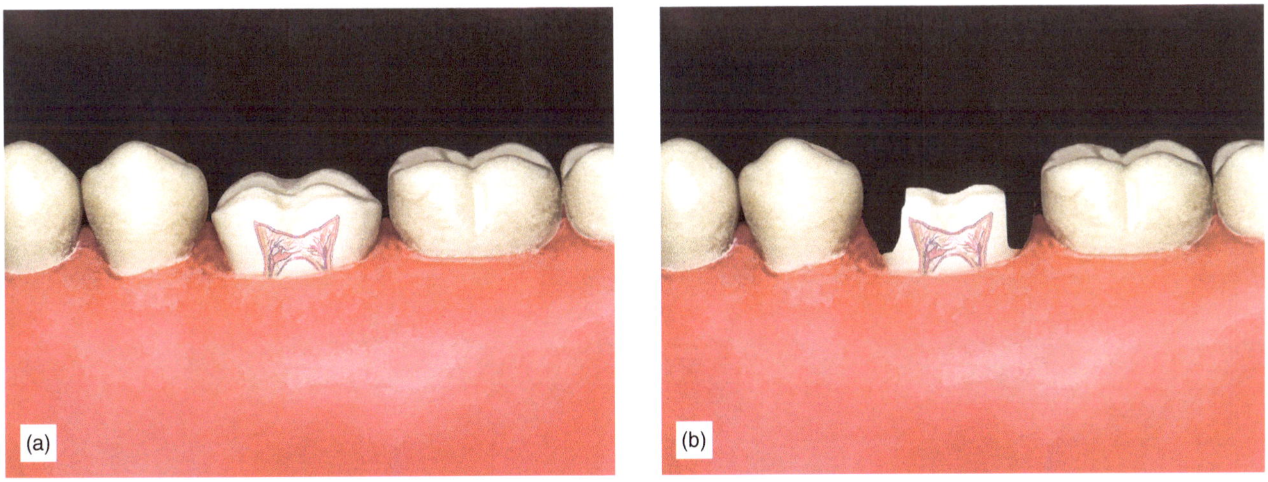

Figure 2.16 Comparison of (a) onlay preparation with only occlusal reduction and (b) crown preparation getting closer to the pulp.

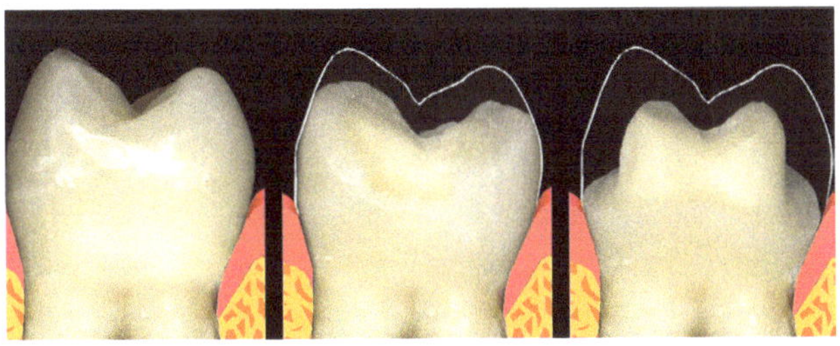

Figure 2.17 My standard tooth reduction comparison: virgin, onlay, crown.

Finally, the value of preserving natural, healthy tooth structure that can be achieved with supragingival minimally invasive adhesive dentistry cannot be stressed enough [7]. The strength of natural, healthy enamel and dentin will always be greater than any other restorative material (Figure 2.17).

Supragingival Minimally Invasive Adhesive Dentistry is More Esthetic

Unlike the traditional approach of hiding the restorative margins subgingivally, supragingival dentistry principles allow for more predictable esthetic results. The correct use of translucent restorative materials to achieve good margin blending is one of the five rules of supragingival restorative dentistry. Translucency is one of the most important aspects of esthetics in dentistry. Teeth have natural translucency, so when translucent material is used correctly, an outcome close to natural can be achieved, resulting in more beautiful natural restorations. Opacious restorations have the opposite effect (Figures 2.18a,b, 2.19a,b). Translucency allows for the ideal blending of tooth and restoration, owing to light passing through the restoration and into the tooth. Enamel and dentin function similar to fiber optic rods.

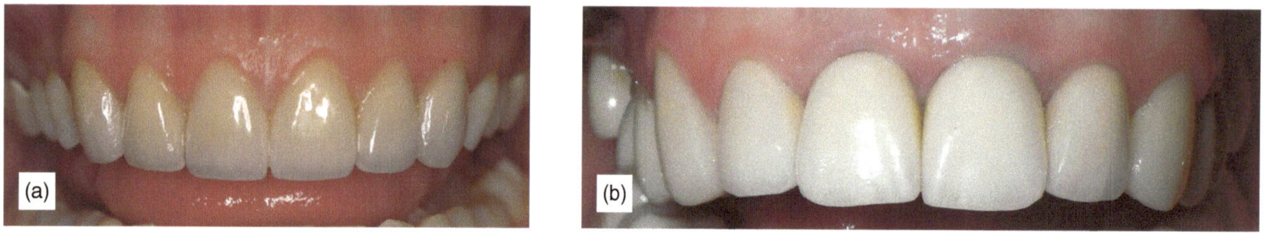

Figure 2.18 (a) Translucent natural-looking veneers. (b) Opacious fake-looking anterior crowns.

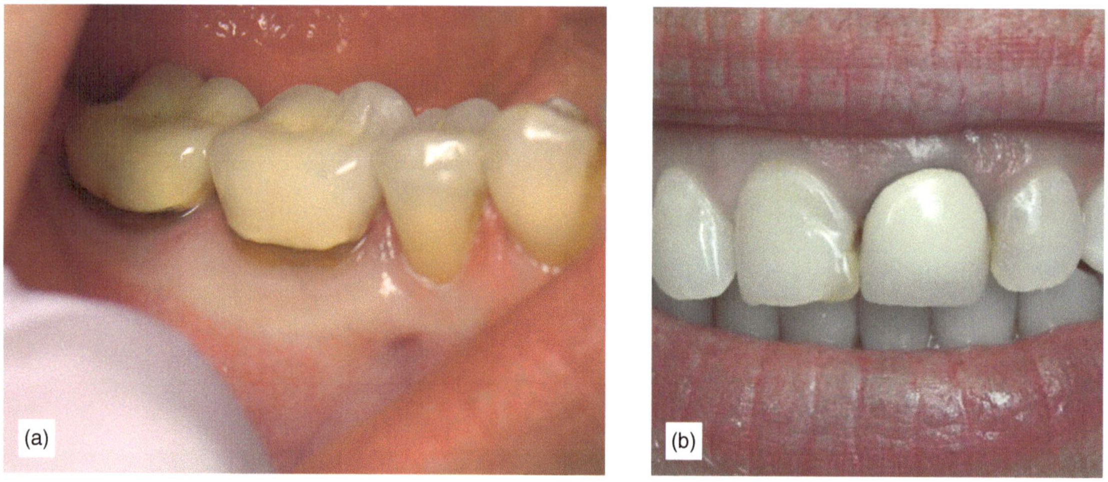

Figure 2.19 (a) Compare the enhanced esthetics of the translucent onlay on the second bicuspid with the opacious molar crowns. (b) Opacious fake-looking anterior crown.

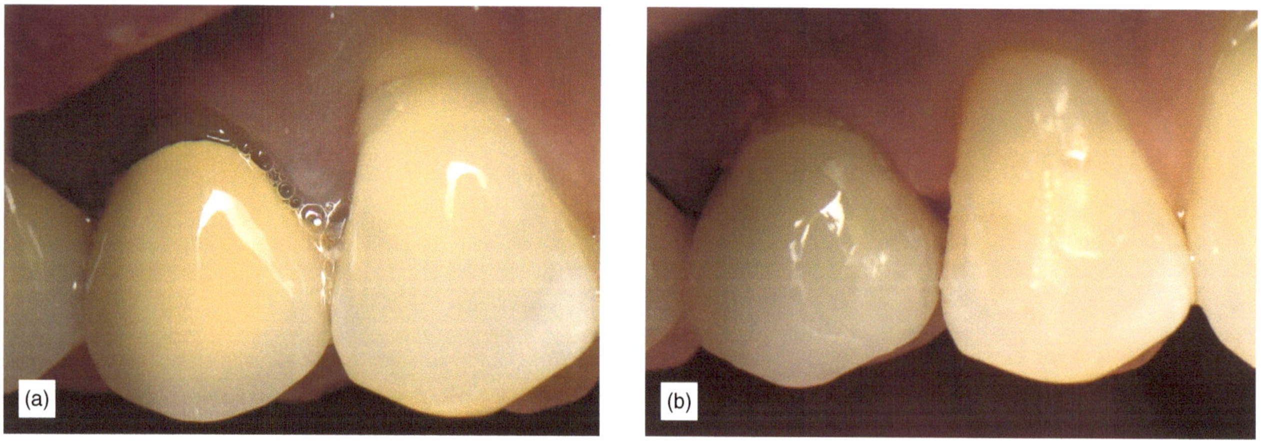

Figure 2.20 (a) Observe how dark the root looks with the opacious crown. (b) Dramatic difference in color after the opacious porcelain-fused-to-metal crown is replaced with translucent ceramic.

When light hits the crown, it travels up through the root [32]. Conversely, when light does not pass though the tooth, the root darkens and appears gray (Figure 2.20).

PFM, full zirconia, layered zirconia, lithium disilicate, composite, feldspathic pressed and layered range from fully opacious to very translucent [33]. Proper use of translucency is key to supragingival dentistry because, when translucent materials are used, the restoration margin will blend with the tooth, creating something of a "contact lens" effect, ensuring that the margin blends neatly. In the esthetic zone, with higher translucency, the margin will virtually disappear (Figure 2.21) [34]. Proper use of translucency while choosing the restorative and luting materials allows for the margin placement to be slightly above the gingiva, even in the esthetic zone, and supragingival in the areas with lesser esthetic requirements. Very beautiful results can be achieved in both posterior and anterior regions when the correct

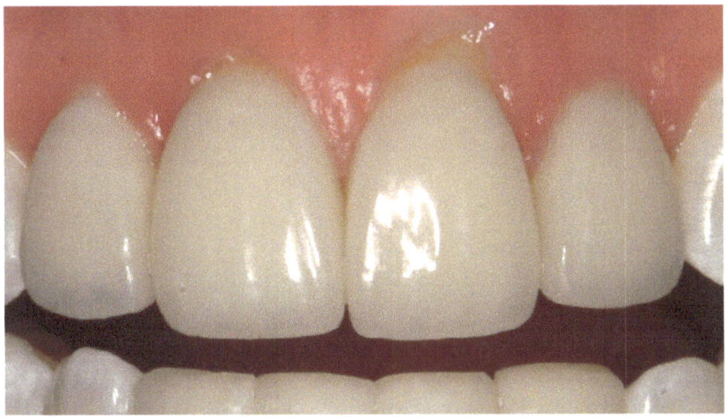

Figure 2.21 Observe that by using translucent porcelain, the restorative margin can blend to an almost undetectable level, similar to the "contact lens" effect.

materials are used appropriately, which is explained in subsequent chapters.

Beautiful gums or gingiva are also part of good esthetics. Supragingival dentistry allows for a more beautiful gingival health. Subgingival margins often lead to slightly or even severely inflamed gingiva, a look which is far from beautiful (Figure 2.22). Supragingival margins allow for perfectly undisturbed, healthy gingiva, which always enhances the final results.

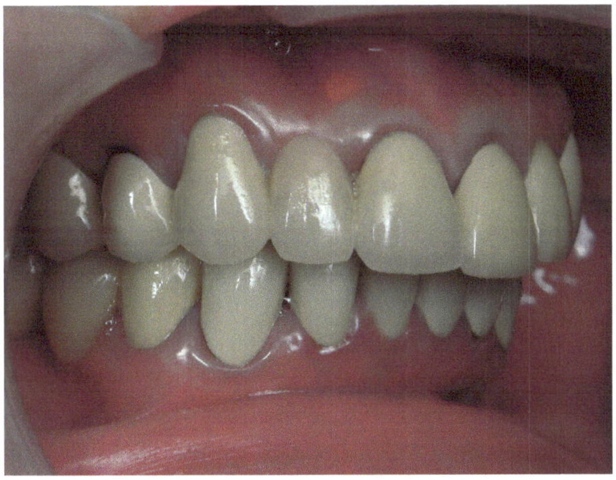

Figure 2.22 Even well-shaped porcelain restorations look bad with ugly gums.

Supragingival Minimally Invasive Adhesive Dentistry is More Predictable and Long Lasting

Many elements must be considered when assessing the real durability of a restoration, the tooth and surrounding tissues. The same supragingival techniques which make this restoration easier, healthier and more esthetic also allow for more predictable, longer-lasting dentistry.

The literature related to the durability of partial coverage bonded onlays and veneers is replete with longevity studies showing excellent results with bonded onlays and veneers, especially when the correct techniques are used. Ruiz and Christensen [35] among other research studies, have shown excellent durability with partial coverage minimally invasive restorations [36,37,38,39,40]. It is my opinion and experience that when using supragingival minimally invasive techniques, the longevity and health of this restoration and surrounding structures can easily outperform any traditional techniques (Figure 2.23a,b). When it comes to longevity, it is important to take occlusion into consideration [41,42], and for that reason this book touches on the subject. Occlusion is also a large factor in preventing sensitivity and adverse pulpal responses.

The short esthetic life of the opacious restorations with subgingival margins is a real problem in dentistry [21] because many restorations in the esthetic zone are replaced, not because of clinical failure but because after the gingiva recedes, the unsightly margin is exposed and the restoration must be replaced. This problem can be avoided altogether by using proper translucency and supragingival techniques. This in fact lengthens the life of restorations in the esthetic zone (Figure 2.24a,b).

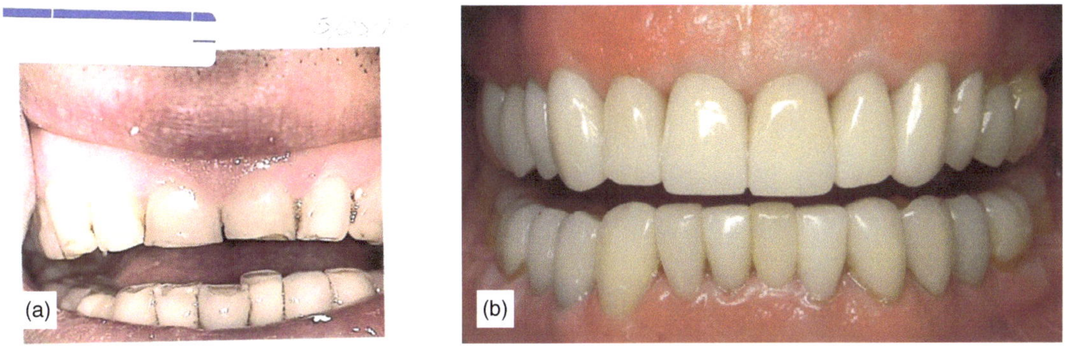

Figure 2.23 (a) Rehabilitation using bonded onlays and veneers in a case with severe wear. (b) The same tooth over 16 years postoperatively.

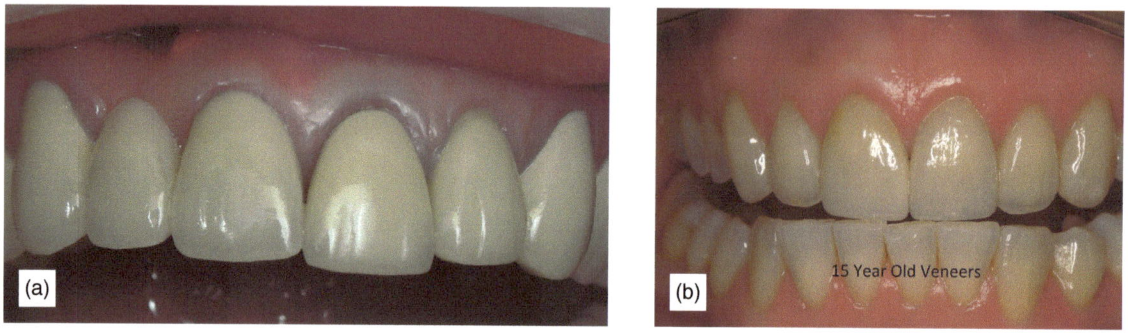

Figure 2.24 (a) This patient was unhappy with gray margins, and requested replacement with clinically acceptable crowns. (b) Veneers at 15 years postoperatively; the margins are visible, but the patient is still happy with the esthetic look.

Patient satisfaction is part of predictable success. Patients do not like to think that their tooth is being drilled down to a nub. When a patient is educated about minimally invasive procedures, they find them to be reassuring and comforting. Equally positive responses from patients are attained when educating them about the benefits of not invading their gingival sulcus and allowing the gingiva to stay healthy using supragingival techniques.

Reparability enhances the longevity of bonded restorations dramatically. Restorative materials such as porcelain and composite can be repaired intraorally with great predictability [43], rather than replacing them (Figure 2.25a–c). In most cases, a repair will add many years of additional service to a restoration.

Traditional restorative techniques with subgingival margin placement and opacious materials hide secondary

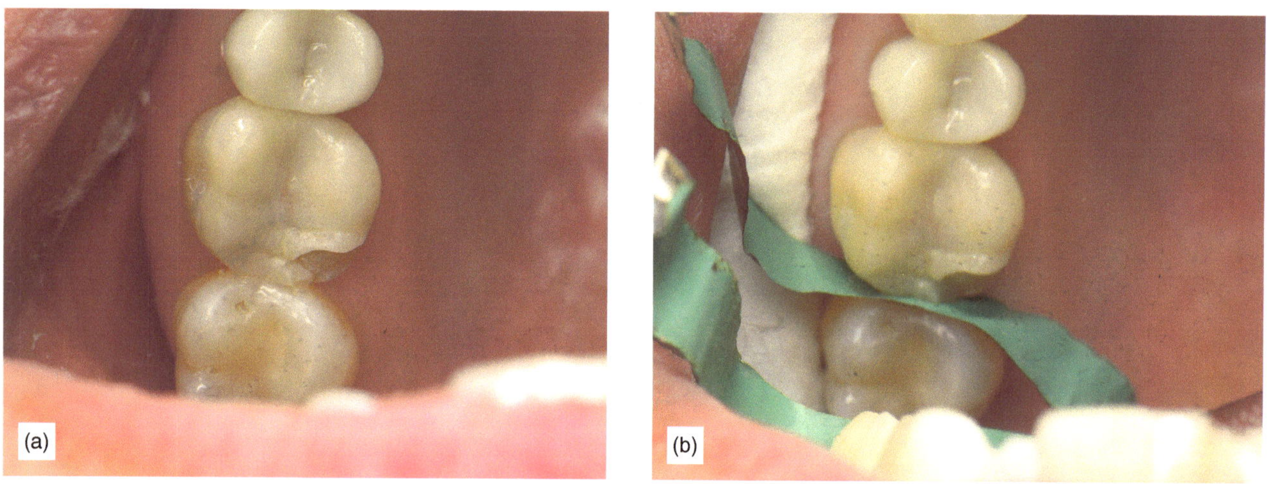

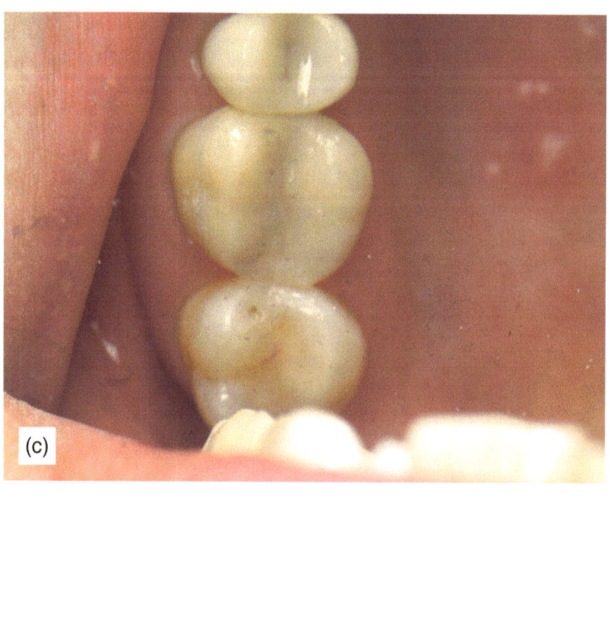

Figure 2.25 (a) A fracture on the distolingual cusp of a ceramic onlay after 10 years. (b) Porcelain repair. (c) The repair will serve the patient a few more years.

caries and marginal leakage, which, in the long term, will allow for irreparable damage to occur. The use of non-metal translucent restorative materials, which blend better at the cavosurface margin area, not only allows for better esthetic results, but also allows the clinician to leave the margin above the gum. When recurring caries or marginal leakage occurs, as it does with all types of restorations, the problem is easier to distinguish in an x-ray of a metal-free restoration. This allows for an earlier intervention. The ability to easily identify caries early and repair or replace the restoration prevents unnecessary root canal work, extensive secondary caries and sometimes the complete loss of a tooth, once again showing supragingival dentistry as the healthier option for the patient.

Regarding durability, it is important to consider not only the durability of the restoration, but also the durability of the surrounding structures. What is more important: the longevity of the restoration, the longevity of the tooth, or both? Of course, patients and dentists would want both to last as long as possible. Undoubtedly, on the larger scale, the longevity of the tooth itself is most important, as that is the ultimate goal. Supragingival minimally invasive bonded restorations are the best choice when considering the health of the restoration and the surrounding tissues.

References

1 Buonocore MG. A simple method of increasing the adhesion of acrylic filling materials to enamel surfaces. *J Dent Res*, 1955; 34(6): 849–853.
2 Fusayama T, Nakamura M, Kurosaki N, Iwaku M. Non-pressure adhesion of a new adhesive restorative resin. *J Dent Res*, 1979; 58(4): 1364–1370.
3 Bertolotti RL. Total etch: The rational dentin bonding protocol. *J Esthet Dent*, 1991; 3(1): 1–6.
4 Calamia JR. The etched porcelain veneer technique. *N Y State Dent J*, 1988; 54(7): 48–50.
5 Bertolotti RL. Adhesion to porcelain and metal. *Dent Clin North Am*, 2007; 51(2): 433–51, ix-x.
6 Ruiz JL. Simplifying the cementation of porcelain onlays. *Dent Today*, 2004; 23(3): 76–79.
7 Ruiz JL. Supragingival dentistry using metal-free restorations. *Dent Today*, 2008; 27: 104–109.
8 Ruiz JL. Anterior and posterior partial-coverage indirect restorations using supragingival dentistry techniques. *J Mass Dent Soc*, 2012; 61(2): 16–19.
9 Ruiz JL, Kurtz R. Are full crowns over utilized? Supragingival partial-coverage designs as a first option. *Dent Today*, 2014; 33(5): 124–125.
10 Magne P, Douglas WH. Rationalization of esthetic restorative dentistry based on biomimetics. *J Esthet Dent*, 1999; 11(1): 5–15.
11 Kramer N, Frankenberger R. Clinical performance of bonded leucite-reinforced glass ceramic inlays and onlays after 8 years. *Dent Mater*, 2005; 21: 267–271.
12 Posselt A, Kerschbaum T. Longevity of 2328 chairside CEREC inlays and onlays. *Int J Comput Dent*, 200; 6(3): 231–248.
13 Zollner A, Gaengler P. Pulp reactions to different preparation techniques on teeth exhibiting periodontal disease. *J Oral Rehabil*, 2000; 27(2): 93–102.
14 Bakeman EM, Kois JC. Posterior, all-porcelain, adhesively retained restorations. *Inside Dentistry*, 2009; 5(5): 20–30.
15 Kois DE, Chaiyabutr Y, Kois JC. Comparison of load fatigue performance of posterior ceramic onlay restorations under different preparation designs. *Compend Contin Educ Dent*, 2012; 33 (Spec No 2): 2–9.
16 Meyer A Jr, Cardoso LC, Araujo E, Baratieri LN. Ceramic inlays and onlays: clinical procedures for predictable results. *J Esthet Restor Dent*, 2003; 15(6): 338–352.
17 Barghi N, Berry TG. Clinical evaluation of etched porcelain onlays: A 4-year report. *Compend Contin Educ Dent*, 2002; 23(7): 657–674.
18 Heymann, HO, Swift EJ, Ritter AV. Indirect tooth color restorations, in *Sturdevant's Art and Science of Operative Dentistry*, 6th ed. Elsevier Mosby, 2013, pp. 280–295.
19 Christensen GJ. Are tooth color onlays viable alternatives to crowns? *Clin Rep*, 2012; 5(1): 1,3.
20 Ruiz JL, Christensen GJ. Myths vs. realities. State of the art indirect posterior restorations. *J Cosmetic Dent*, 2011; 27(3): 63–72.
21 Christensen GJ. Porcelain fused to metal vs nonmetal crowns. *J Am Dent Assoc*, 1999; 130(3): 409–411.
22 Christensen GJ. The state of fixed prosthodontic impressions: room for improvement. *J Am Dent Assoc*, 2005; 136: 343–346.
23 Feng J, Aboyoussef H, Weiner S, Singh S, Jandinski J. The effect of gingival retraction procedures on periodontal indices and crevicular fluid cytokine levels: a pilot study. *J Prosthodont*, 2006; 15(2): 108–112.
24 Larato DC. Effect of cervical margins on gingiva. *J Calif Dent Assoc*, 1969; 45: 19–22.
25 Silness J. Periodontal conditions in patients treated with dental bridges. *J Periodontal Res*, 1970; 5: 6–68.
26 Williams DF, Smith DC. *Biocompatibility of Dental Materials*. Boca Raton, FL: CRC Press; 1982.
27 Thomas MS, Kundabala M. Pulp hyperthermia during tooth preparation: The effect of rotatory instruments, laser, ultrasonic devices and airborne particle abrasion. *J Calif Dent Assoc*, 2012; 40(9): 721–731.
28 Davis GR, Tayeb RA, Seymour KG, Cherukara GP. Quantification of residual dentine thickness following crown preparation. *J Dent*, 2012; 40(7): 571–576.
29 Langeland K, Langeland LK. Pulp reactions to cavity and crown preparation. *Aust Dent J*, 1970; 5(4): 261–276.
30 Dahl BL. Dentine/pulp reactions to full crown preparation procedures. *Oral Rehabil*, 1977; 4(3): 247–254.

31 Valderhaug J, Jokstad A, Ambjørnsen E, Norheim PW. Assessment of the periapical and clinical status of crowned teeth over 25 years. *J Dent*, 1997; 25: 97–105.
32 Hickel R, Brüshaver K, Ilie N. Repair of restorations: criteria for decision making and clinical recommendations. *Dent Mater*, 2013; 29(1): 28–50.
33 Barizon KT, Bergeron C, Vargas MA, Qian F, Cobb DS, Gratton DG, Geraldeli S. Ceramic materials for porcelain veneers: Part II. Effect of material, shade, and thickness on translucency. *J Prosthet Dent*, 2014; 112(4): 864–870.
34 Magne P, Belser U. *Bonded Porcelain Restorations in the Anterior Dentition*. Chicago, IL: Quintessence Publishing; 2002, 168–169.
35 Ruiz JL, Christensen GJ, Sameni A, Vargas L. Clinical performance of bonded ceramic and resin-based composite inlays and onlays using a self-etch bonding system; a 51-month report. *Inside Dentistry*, 2007; 3(5): 62–65.
36 Gresnigt M, Ozcan M. Esthetic rehabilitation of anterior teeth with porcelain laminates and sectional veneers. *J Can Dent Assoc*, 2011; 77: b143.
37 Van Dijken JW, Hasselrot L. A prospective 15-year evaluation of extensive denti-enamel-bonded pressed ceramic coverage. *Dent Mater*, 2010; 26(9): 929–939.
38 Land MF, Hopp CD. Survival rates of all-ceramic systems differ by clinical indication and fabrication method. *J Evid Based Dent Pract*, 2010; 10(1): 37–38.
39 Gurel G. Clinical performance of porcelain laminate veneers: outcomes of the aesthetic pre-evaluative temporary (APT) technique. *Int J Periodont Restorative Dent*, 2012; 32(6): 625–635.
40 Gurel, G. Influence of enamel preservation on failure rates of porcelain laminate veneers. *Int J Restorative Dent*, 2013; 33(1): 31–39.
41 Ruiz JL. Occlusal disease: restorative consequences and patient education. *Dent Today*, 2007; 26(9): 90–95.
42 Ruiz JL. Achieving longevity in esthetics by proper diagnosis and management of occlusal disease. *Contemp Esthet*, 2007; 11(6): 24–27.
43 Christensen GJ. Porcelain fused to metal vs nonmetal crowns. *J Am Dent Assoc*, 1999; 130(3): 409–411.

3

The Supragingival Protocol and Indications: Preventing Subgingival Margins

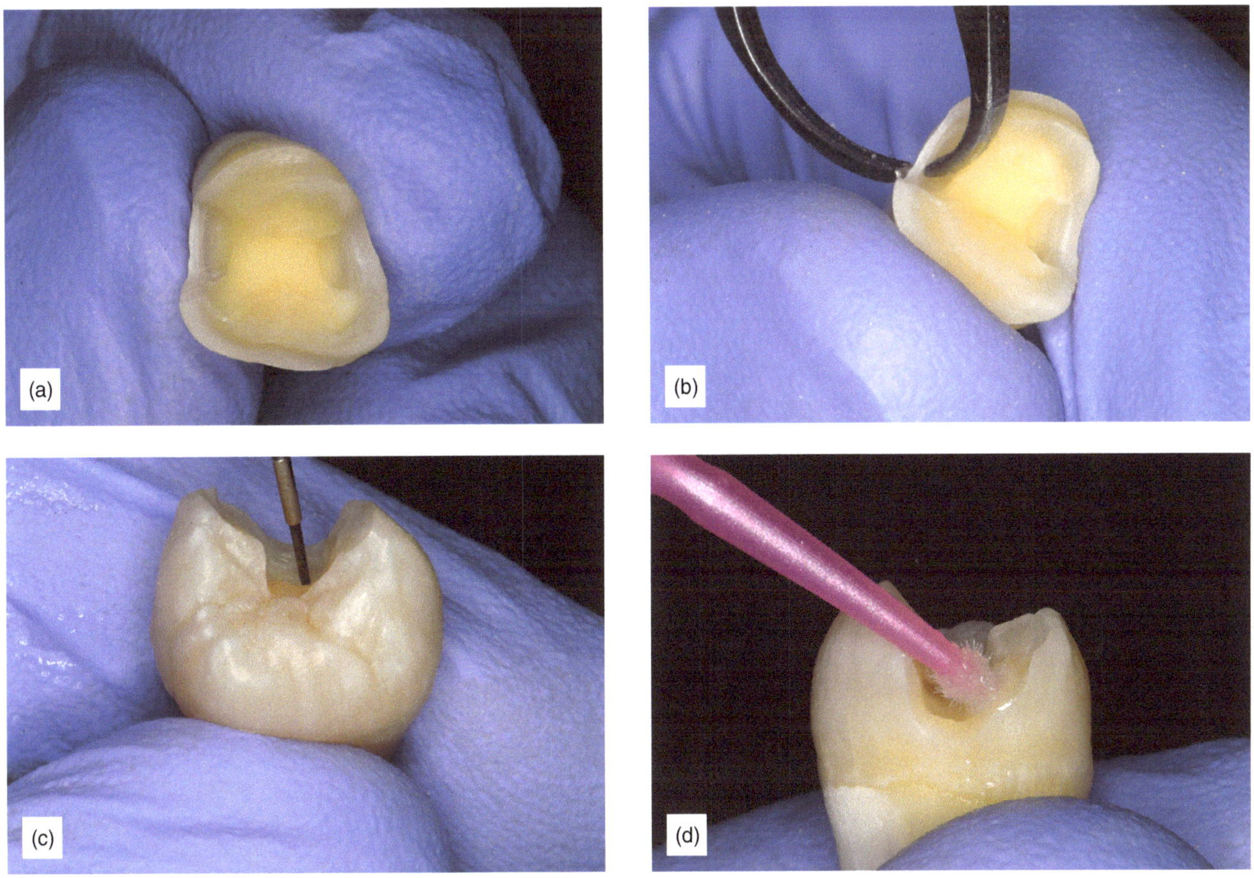

Enamel margin preservation research.

Introduction

Restorative dentists use two approaches to restoring damaged teeth: Direct and indirect. Direct restorations are reserved for teeth where the damage is moderate, the structure of the tooth is not compromised, and it can be safely restored with material with the ability to set or cure immediately in the tooth, such as amalgam or resin-based composite (Figure 3.1). Indirect restorations, on the other hand, are restorations reserved for badly damaged teeth, which may be structurally weak. The full or partial coverage will help to reinforce the tooth and usually requires materials that are fabricated in a laboratory or more recently by computer-aided design and manufacturing. Adhesive dentistry changed the rules rapidly [1,2] and blurred the lines as to when teeth are truly too weak to be restored with a direct technique and when a cusp or cusps are structurally too weak and need

Supra-Gingival Minimally Invasive Dentistry: A Healthier Approach to Esthetic Restorations, First Edition. By Jose-Luis Ruiz.

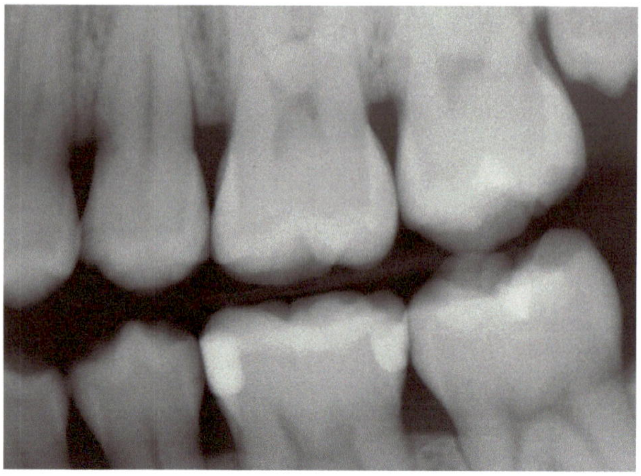

Figure 3.1 X-ray of tooth needing a direct filling.

to be covered (Figure 3.2a,b). Bonded composite has been shown to reinforce tooth structure [3,4]. As shown in Chapter 1, traditionally direct and indirect restorations have been performed using techniques requiring mechanical retention that usually lead to subgingival margins with little regard to the periodontal complications. Direct and indirect restorations can be performed using supragingival minimally invasive techniques.

Full crowns are by far the most popular indirect procedure, as evidenced by the level of usage and the literature [5], and are still considered by most to be the ideal treatment for weak and badly damaged teeth. Adhesively retained partial coverage veneers and onlays have been reserved for limited use only, when several criteria are met [6,7,8,9,10]. The supragingival dentistry approach is a paradigm shift, because it has the unique and intentional goal of using every available technique and clinical trick to intentionally keep restorative margins supragingival and restore the tooth with as little healthy tooth removal as possible [11]. Additionally, unlike traditional dentistry practice, partial coverage supragingival bonded restorations are not limited to easy cases. Research and experience show that even the most damaged teeth can be successfully restored using supragingival minimally invasive partial coverage restorations (Figures 3.3a,b, 3.4a–c).

The Five Principles of Supragingival Dentistry

A supragingival protocol allows the dentist to prevent the unnecessary creation of subgingival margins. When caries or an old restoration are in fact subgingival, then a protocol exists for repairing and isolating the damage, and avoiding further damage to the tooth or the periodontium, employing the great benefits of adhesively retained translucent restoration [12].

The final gingival margin placement has traditionally been a byproduct of restorative mechanical needs, esthetic needs and old restorative rules. The end result of subgingival margins is thus considered normal and necessary. Breaking through this paradigm requires new rules. It is no longer left to chance, but the location of the final gingival margin is intentional and several rules are followed to preserve supragingival margins when possible and to repair subgingival margins when necessary. The implementation of a supragingival protocol to overcome all the traditional reasons why restorative margins end subgingivally and how to minimize or eliminate the need to prepare traditional full crowns are summarized in the five principles of supragingival dentistry. These five principles will help to prevent or greatly minimize subgingival restorative margins with direct and indirect restorations.

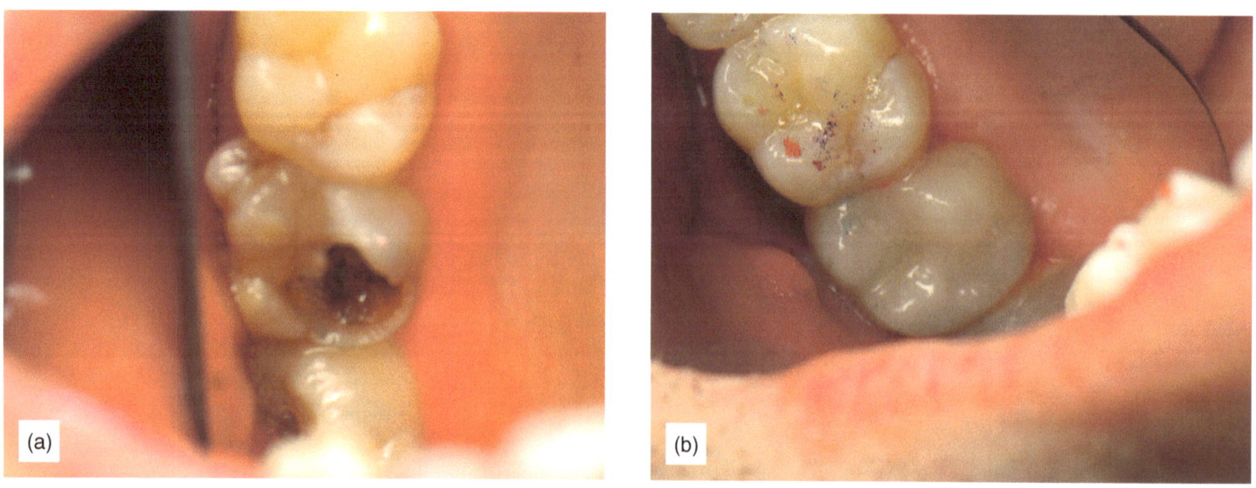

Figure 3.2 (a) Badly damaged tooth needing indirect restoration. (b) Final restoration.

Figure 3.3 (a) Badly damaged tooth. (b) After restoration.

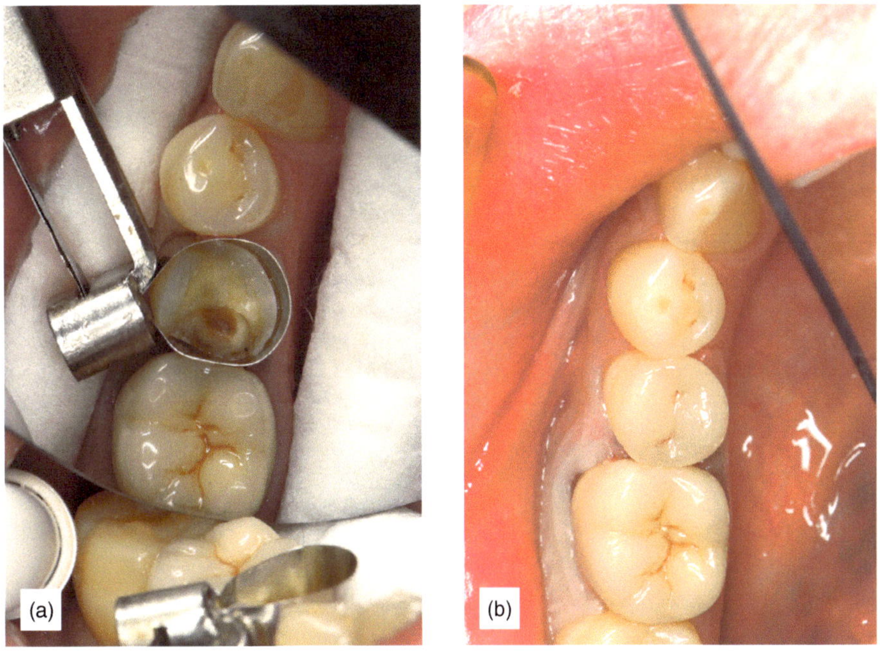

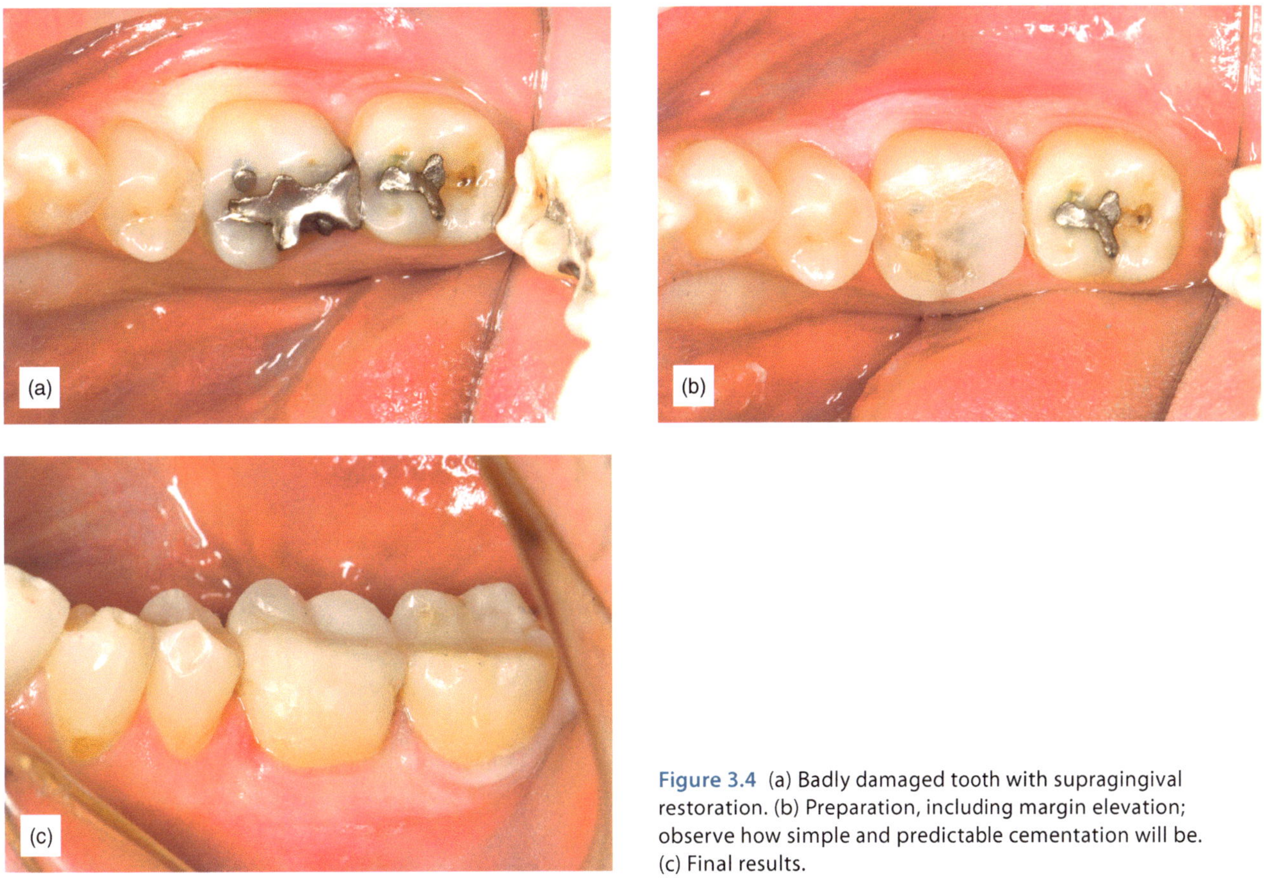

Figure 3.4 (a) Badly damaged tooth with supragingival restoration. (b) Preparation, including margin elevation; observe how simple and predictable cementation will be. (c) Final results.

The First Principle: Careful Removal of Caries and Old Restorative Material Removal Close to the Gingival Margin

Because the gingival margin region of the tooth is so crucial to a successful bonding procedure, it becomes mandatory to take great care while removing caries and restorative material in this region. When the preparation is close to gingival, as much care and respect should be placed as when the bur gets close to the pulp (Figure 3.5a–d). Nevertheless, general acceptance that subgingival margins are inevitable and normal, coupled with the lack of an intentional supragingival protocol can be very influential in the decision about the location of the final preparation margin.

A different attitude exists when working close to the pulp. Restorative dentists take great care, employ special techniques and even different tools, such as spoon excavators and large, round, slow-speed burs, and caries-indicating dyes, to carefully remove caries close to the pulp. The literature and experience show that, with care and the proper technique, pulp exposures can be minimized or avoided [13]. The same extreme care should be applied when the preparation reaches

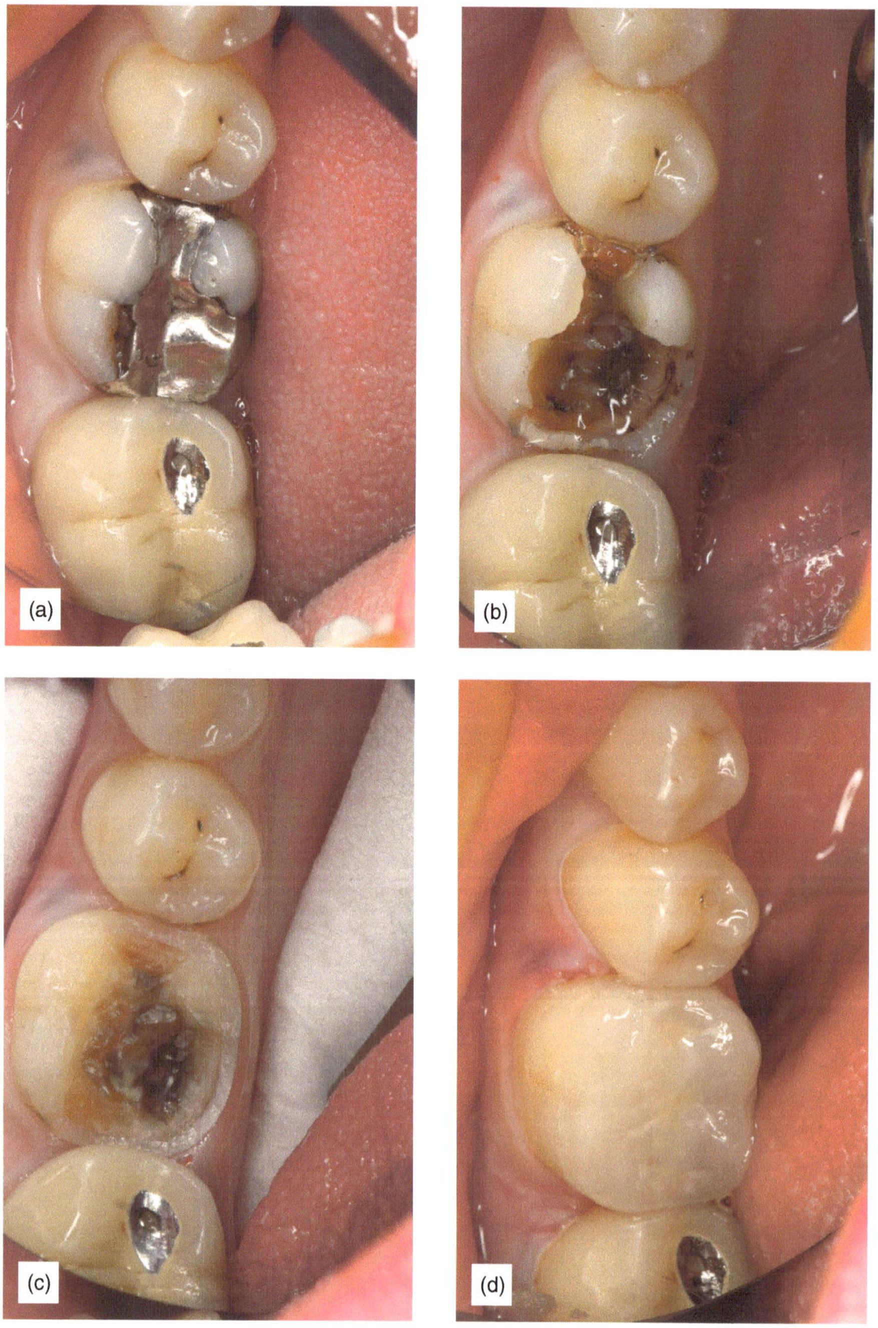

Figure 3.5 (a) A large silver filling with caries. (b) The lingual side of the tooth appears to be deeply subgingival and hopeless for a bonded restoration. (c) With careful technique, the margin was only about 1 mm subgingival and manageable for a bonded restoration. (d) Final supragingival restoration.

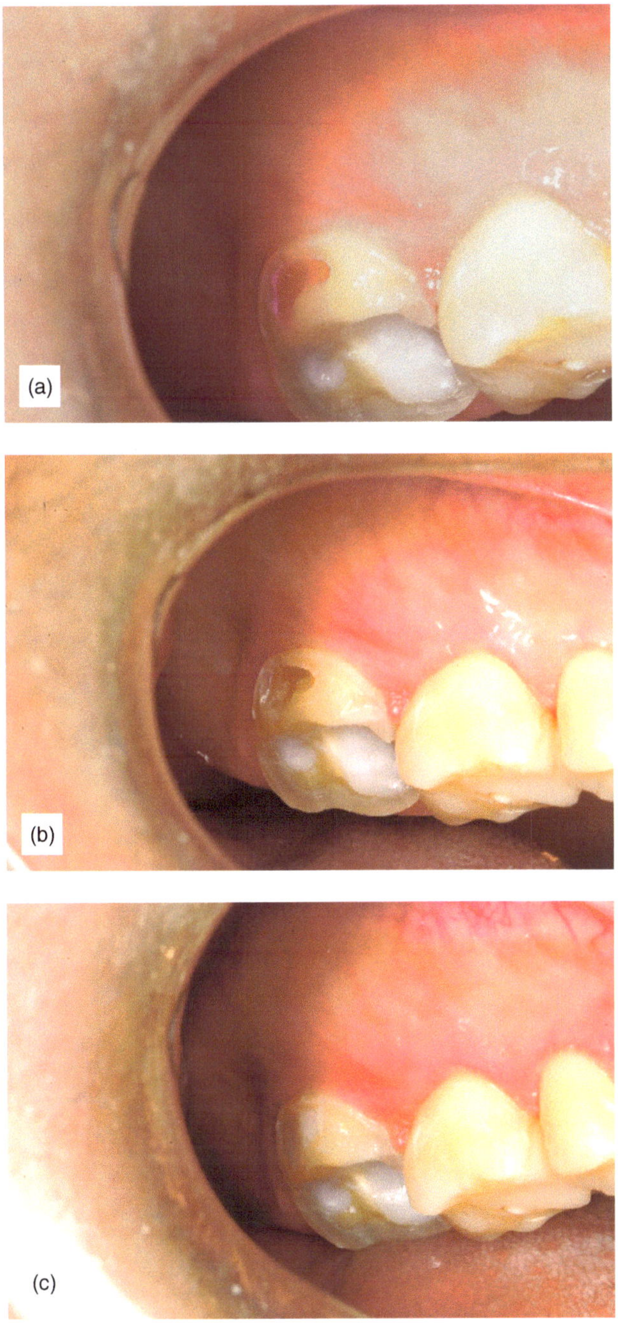

Figure 3.6 (a) A cervical caries close to the gingival margin with a high risk of extending subgingivally. After removal of demineralized enamel, the tooth is stained with caries indicator. (b) After removal of infected dentin, a wall of healthy supragingival enamel is preserved. (c) Careful removal of cervical caries (first principle) combined with enamel preservation (third principle) will allow for subsequent simpler and healthier restorations.

the gingival margin. When such care is taken, this will result in a decrease and even prevention of subgingival margins (Figures 3.6a–c, 3.7a–c). Good illumination and magnification are desirable when working in the marginal area.

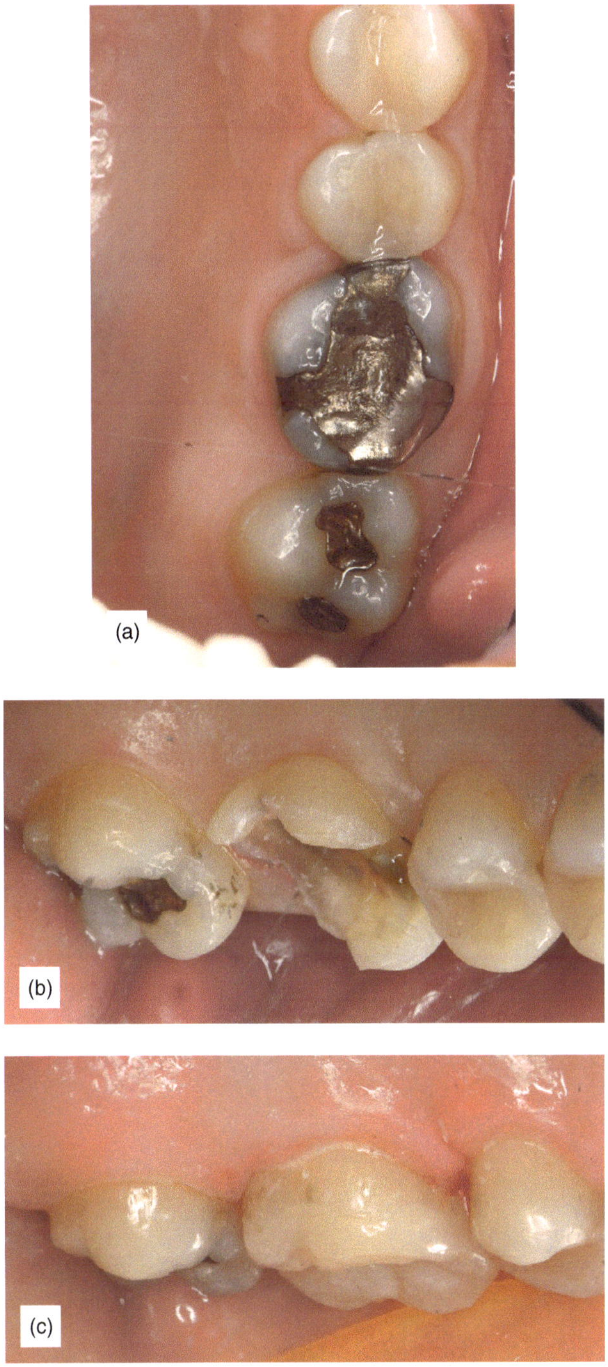

Figure 3.7 (a) Deep gingival margin. (b) Removal of caries completed. (c) Final supragingival restoration.

Even when subgingival caries or restorative material are inevitable, the damage can be limited with careful technique. In this crucial area, 1–2 mm can make all the difference. A slightly subgingival margin of 0.5 mm is manageable, while a subgingival margin of 1.5 mm or more will create many more complications and uncertain results (Figure 3.8a–c).

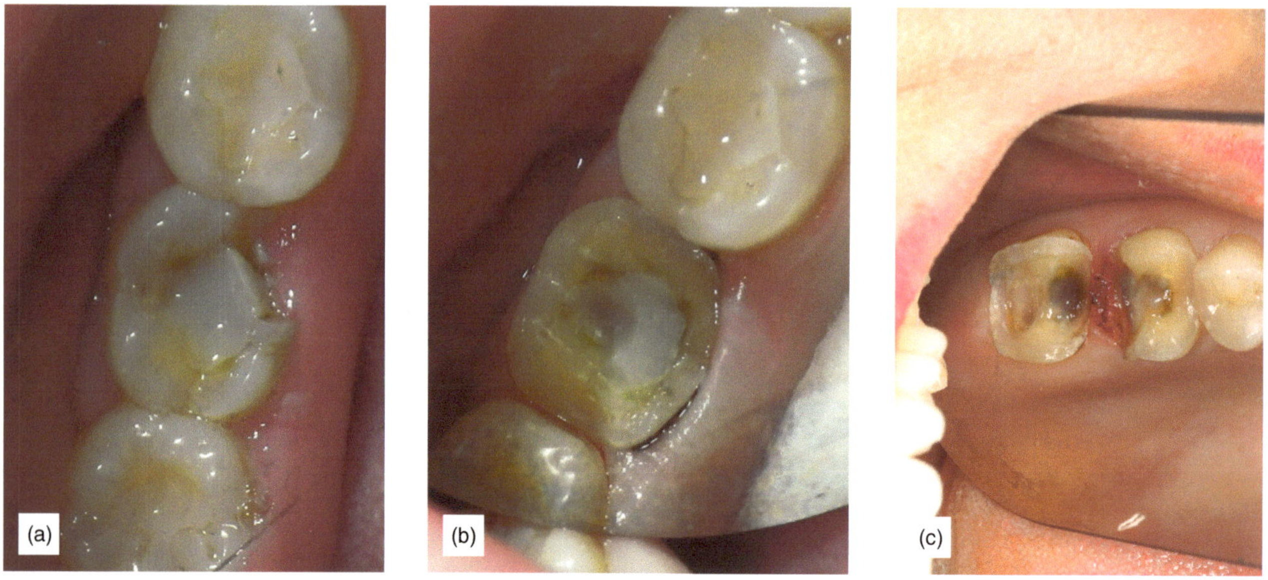

Figure 3.8 (a) An apparently deep subgingival margin. (b) Managed with care, the result will be a slightly (0.5 mm) subgingival margin, easy to manage. (c) A completely different outcome can be expected with subgingival margins deeper than 1.5–2 mm, greatly complicating all subsequent restorative steps, especially bonded cementation.

The following steps are suggested for achieving careful removal of caries and old restorations at or near the gingival margin and to prevent subgingival margins:

1) The use of 3.5–4.5 times magnification when working close to the margin area is most desirable (Figure 3.9).
2) After efficient removal of gross caries, old restorative material and occlusal reduction, the clinician should:
   i) slow down when close to gingival margins
   ii) use a longer diamond for better visibility
   iii) take great care in removing the remaining caries or old restorative materials.
3) Caries indicator stain is indispensable to prevent the removal of non-infected dentin (the detailed technique for the use of caries indicator is given in Chapter 10).
4) Preserve healthy enamel near the gingival margin, including in the absence of dentinal support (enamel margin preservation technique).

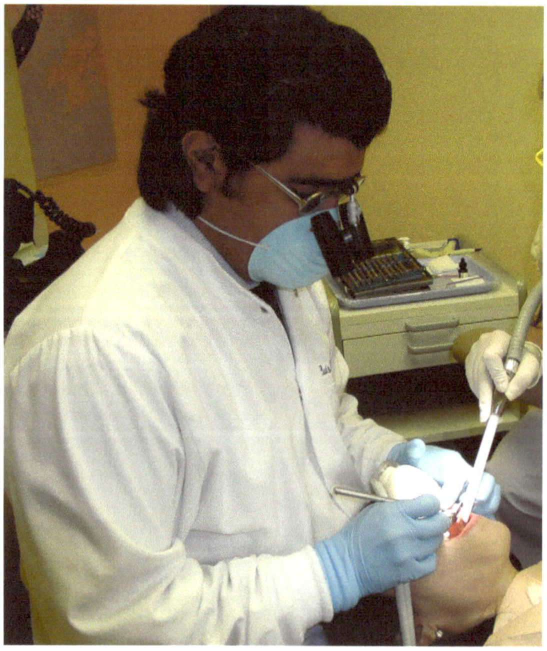

Figure 3.9 Using high magnification (3.5 times and greater) allows for superior visibility and tooth protection.

The Second Principle: Avoid Boxes, Axial Reduction or Counterproductive Mechanical Retention (Trust In Adhesion)

Interproximal boxes and axial reductions are part of the fabric of restorative dentistry [14]. Lack of trust in adhesion make these a part of normal practice. However, trust in adhesion would render mechanical retention obsolete (Figure 3.10a–d). This lack of trust in adhesion, combined with habit and education, makes it normal for the clinician to make a traditional dimension proximal box every time interproximal caries need to be removed, independently of how large the caries may be (Figure 3.11). When a marginal ridge is weak and occlusal coverage of the marginal ridge is needed, a traditional box is the usual way of proceeding. Proximal boxes have also been used as an indispensable part of a mechanically retentive preparation for direct and indirect restorations (Figure 3.12). Nevertheless, proximal

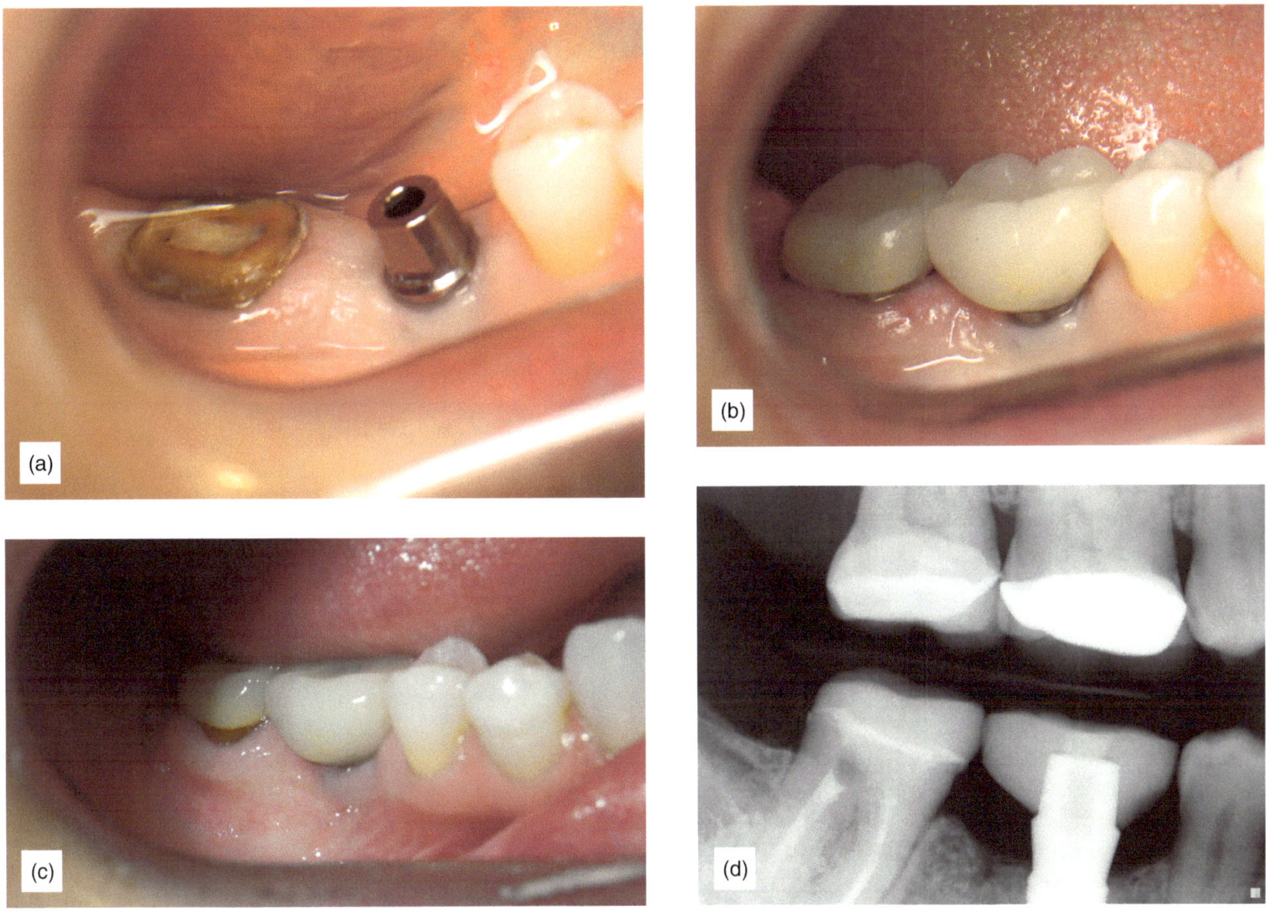

Figure 3.10 (a) Second molar, which had a crown that fractured at gum level. (b) Crown with zero mechanical retention cemented. (c) The same crown 6 years postoperatively. (d) X-ray of the same crown 6 years postoperatively.

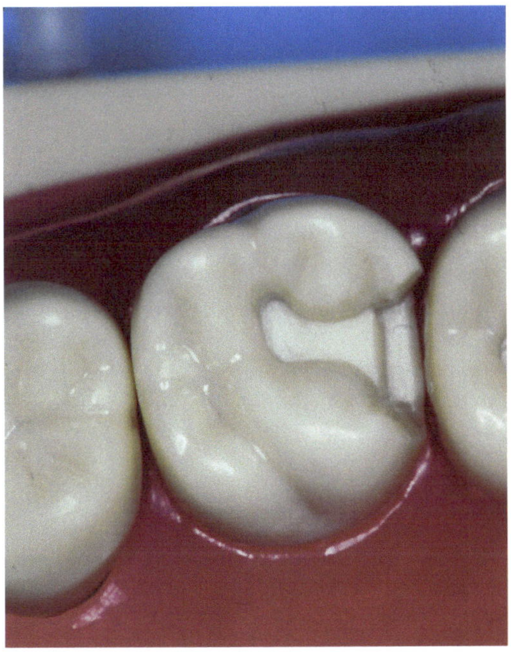

Figure 3.11 Traditional onlay preparation showing aggressive mechanical retention features (courtesy of Dr Boris Keselbrener).

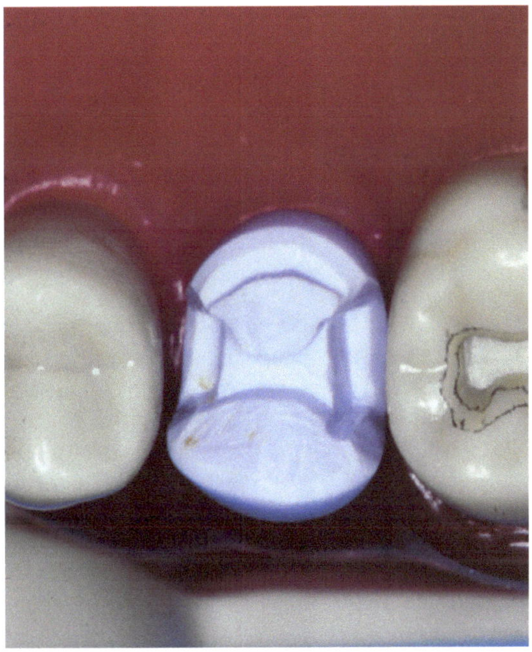

Figure 3.12 Boxes with subgingival margins on x-ray.

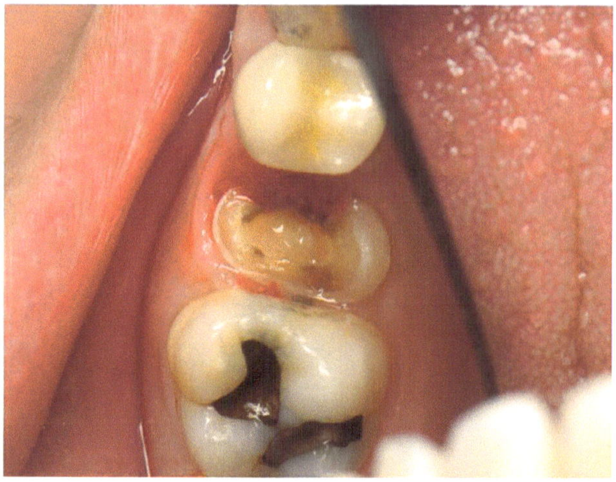

Figure 3.13 Box with bleeding subgingival margin.

boxes have some serious disadvantages. They require a large amount of usually healthy tooth to be removed, and traditional boxes require proximal clearance, including gingival clearance. The universal approach to gaining gingival clearance has been to continue to drop the gingival floor of the box until clearance is achieved. This technique has two negative consequences. First, as the gingival floor is dropped, the margins become subgingival and bleeding will occur (Figure 3.13). Second, the enamel thickness decreases to the point that sometimes it is lost. Both consequences are counterproductive to adhesive procedures. Dropping the box can be substituted with a different technique, the "cervical margins separation technique".

Similarly counterproductive is the preparation of axial walls and ferrules, which often forces margins to go subgingival, for the purpose of retention and resistance forms. Adhesive retention is enough to support any restoration, without the need for mechanical retention. Thus, the proper use and trust in adhesion prevents subgingival margins (Box 3.1; Figures 3.14a–d, 3.15).

During an indirect onlay preparation, proximal boxes can be substituted by a simple U-shaped 2+ mm reduction of the marginal ridge and proximal area, followed by an alternative procedure to create clearance (Box 3.2). Instead of dropping the gingival floor for clearance, a "cervical margin separation technique" can be used to gain the necessary clearance and separation needed for a clean impression (Figure 3.16a–c).

The Third Principle: Enamel Margin Preservation Technique

The idea of preserving the enamel for esthetic or restorative purposes is not new [15,16]. However, a well-entrenched basic rule of cavity preparation is the removal of all unsupported enamel to prevent enamel fracture [17]. It is important to understand that rules like removing enamel without dentinal support applied at a time when dentistry did not have adhesives. Nevertheless, the benefit of preserving some enamel just for the sake of doing so has no great clinical value. On the other hand, the benefits of enamel preservation at the marginal level to allow for a supragingival margin is of

Box 3.1 An alternative technique for substituting a proximal box in direct restoration (slot preparation)

1) If no box has been previously cut, do not cut a traditional box.
2) When caries are present, employ conservative access through the marginal ridge. Avoid the traditional expansion into a box shape (Figure 3.17a).
3) Perform careful caries removal, ignoring undercut formation, and use a caries indicator (Figure 3.17b).
4) Never attempt to create gingival clearance by dropping the gingival floor. It is acceptable to leave cavosurface margins in contact with adjacent tooth.
5) Use a wedge to create enough separation to allow the matrix band to fit, even when the preparation cavosurface margin is in contact with the adjacent tooth (Figure 3.17c).

Cervical margin separation technique

1) In clinical practice, sometimes when the tooth is in contact with the adjacent tooth, passing a thin segmental matrix band can be difficult. If it is not possible to place the matrix, perform a "cervical margin separation technique" rather than dropping the gingival floor.
2) Using a safe-side metal strip, a finishing strip (such as Jiffy® Diamond Strip, Ultradent) or a "mosquito"-shaped bur (such as the Brasseler 8392-016 diamond bur) to create proximal (cervical) separation, using a protection wedge (such as WedgeGuard®, Triodent). It is only necessary to create enough space to allow the matrix band to pass (Figure 3.17d) Attention must be placed to not attempt cervical separation when the tooth is still in heavy contact with adjacent tooth.

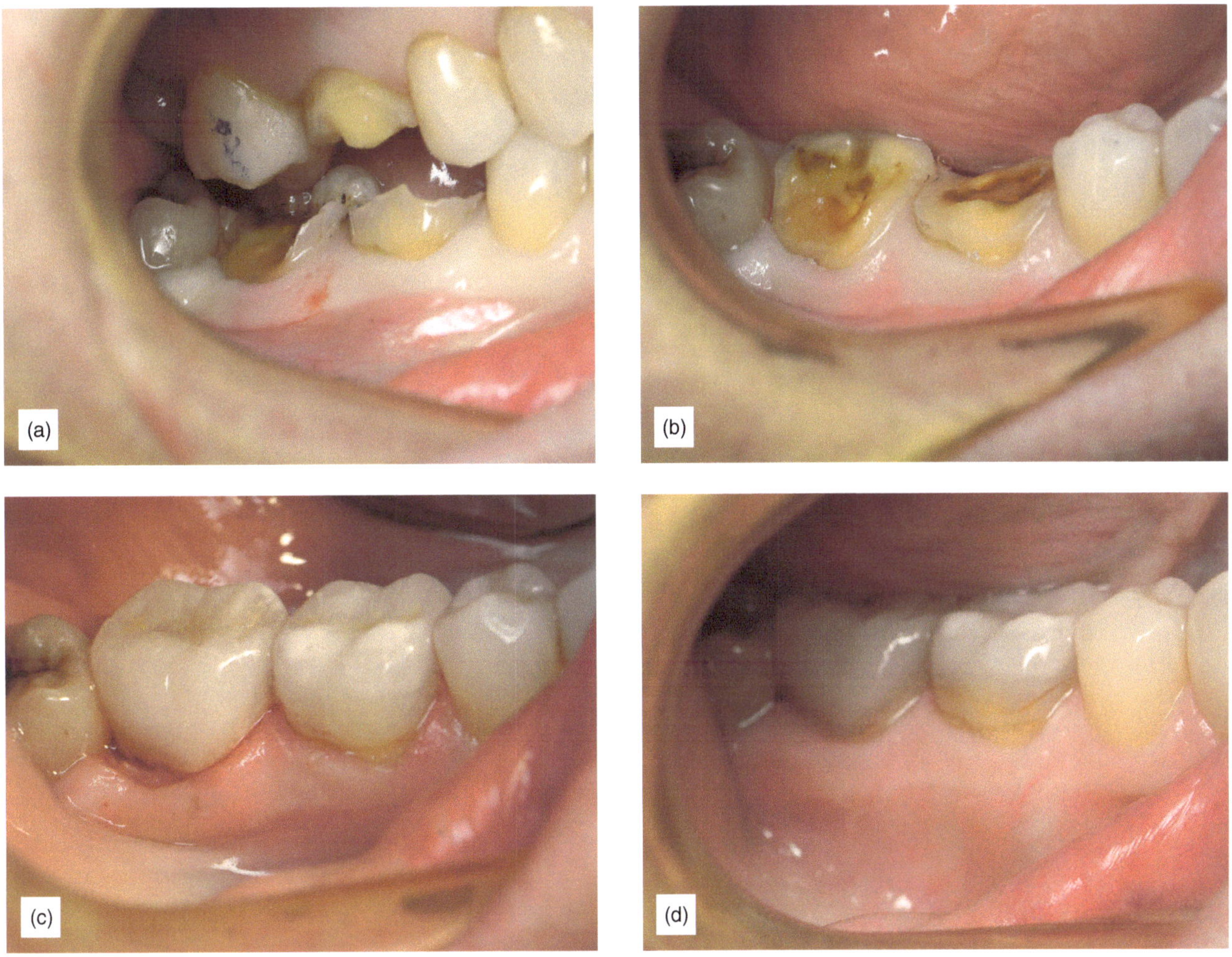

Figure 3.14 (a) Teeth of a very frail patient previously treated for root canal/post/crown plus crown lengthening surgery. (b) After minor preparation, preserving as much tooth as possible and enamel margin. (c) Immediately after cementation. (d) One year postoperatively.

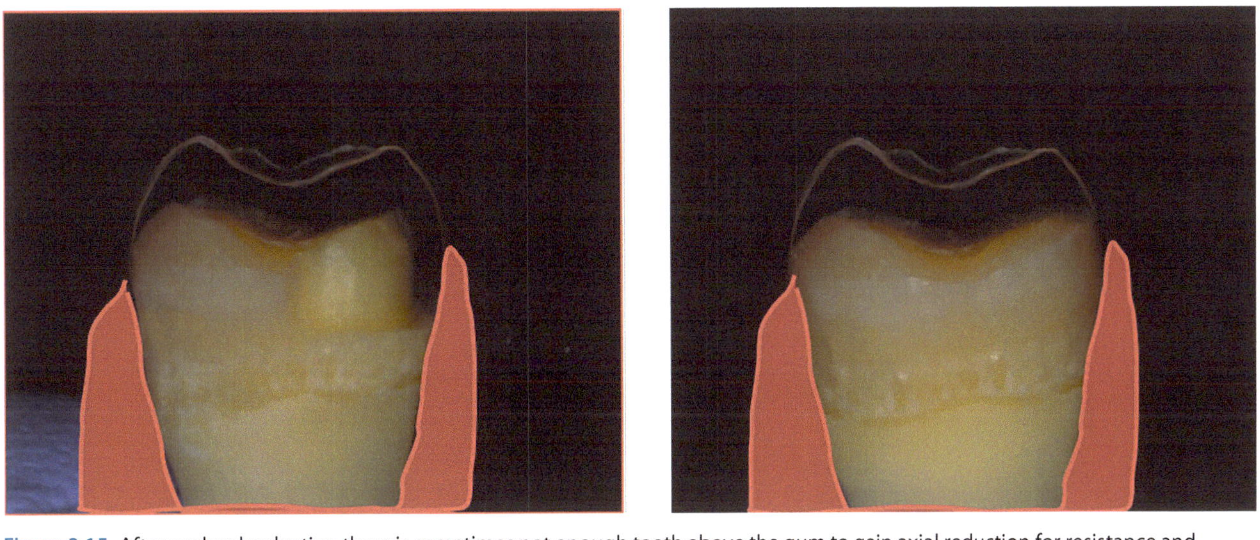

Figure 3.15 After occlusal reduction there is sometimes not enough tooth above the gum to gain axial reduction for resistance and retention forms. This will force the margins subgingivally.

Box 3.2 An alternative technique for substituting a proximal box in indirect restoration (Figure 3.18a–g)

1) If no box has been previously cut, do not cut a traditional box (Figure 3.18a).
2) Perform marginal ridge occlusal reduction of approximately 2–3 mm with a U-shaped motion. Sometimes it is necessary to reduce 3+ mm of the marginal ridge to go slightly below the contact point, but above the gingiva. It is desirable to use a safe wedge.
3) Soften internal line angles if an existing box is present.
4) Never attempt to create gingival clearance by dropping the gingival floor.

Cervical margin separation technique

1) Use a safe-sided metal strip, a finishing strip (such as Jiffy® Diamond Strip) or a "mosquito"-shaped bur (such as the Brasseler 8392-016) to perform the cervical margin separation, allowing for a clean impression and easy modeling work.
2) Attention must be paid to avoiding the creation of separation when the adjacent tooth is in heavy contact, as the separation will be very difficult and it will lead to a flat, unnatural long contact, which is hard to correct with a indirect restoration (Figure 3.18f). Again, it is important to reduce marginal ridge slightly below the contact point.

great importance, as it simplifies and increase predictability of every following procedure (Figure 3.19a–e). It is well documented that finishing a restoration on enamel increases the long-term seal of the restoration [18].

For direct restorations, this method of allowing the preparation cavosurface margin and restorative margin to remain supragingival will greatly simplify direct restorations. Supragingival margins are easier to isolate, it is easier to place matrix bands, seal the margin with a wedge, restore, and remove composite flash and finish, thus making direct restorations easier and more successful (Figure 3.20a,b). In indirect cases, after the enamel margin preservation procedure is finished, an impression will be performed with ease, and subsequently the adhesive procedure to bond an onlay or veneer will be greatly simplified

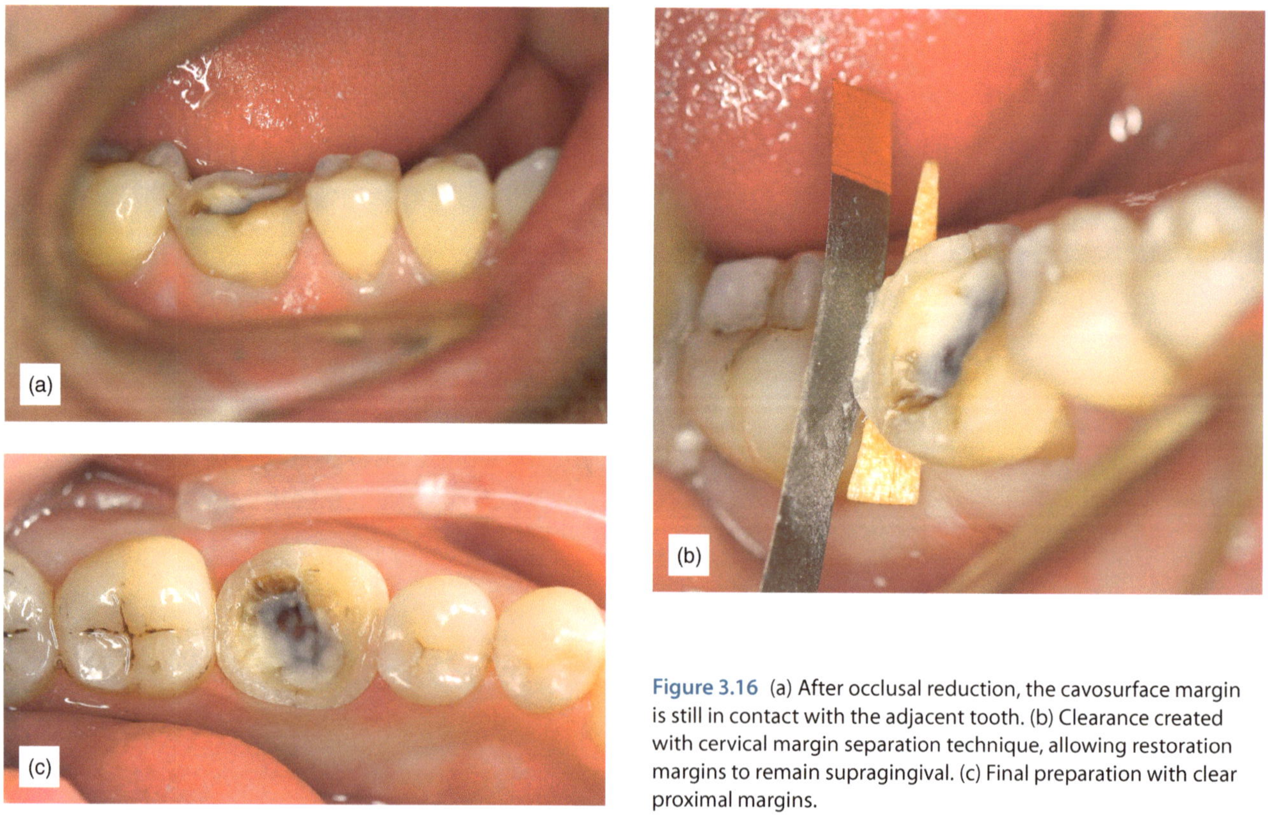

Figure 3.16 (a) After occlusal reduction, the cavosurface margin is still in contact with the adjacent tooth. (b) Clearance created with cervical margin separation technique, allowing restoration margins to remain supragingival. (c) Final preparation with clear proximal margins.

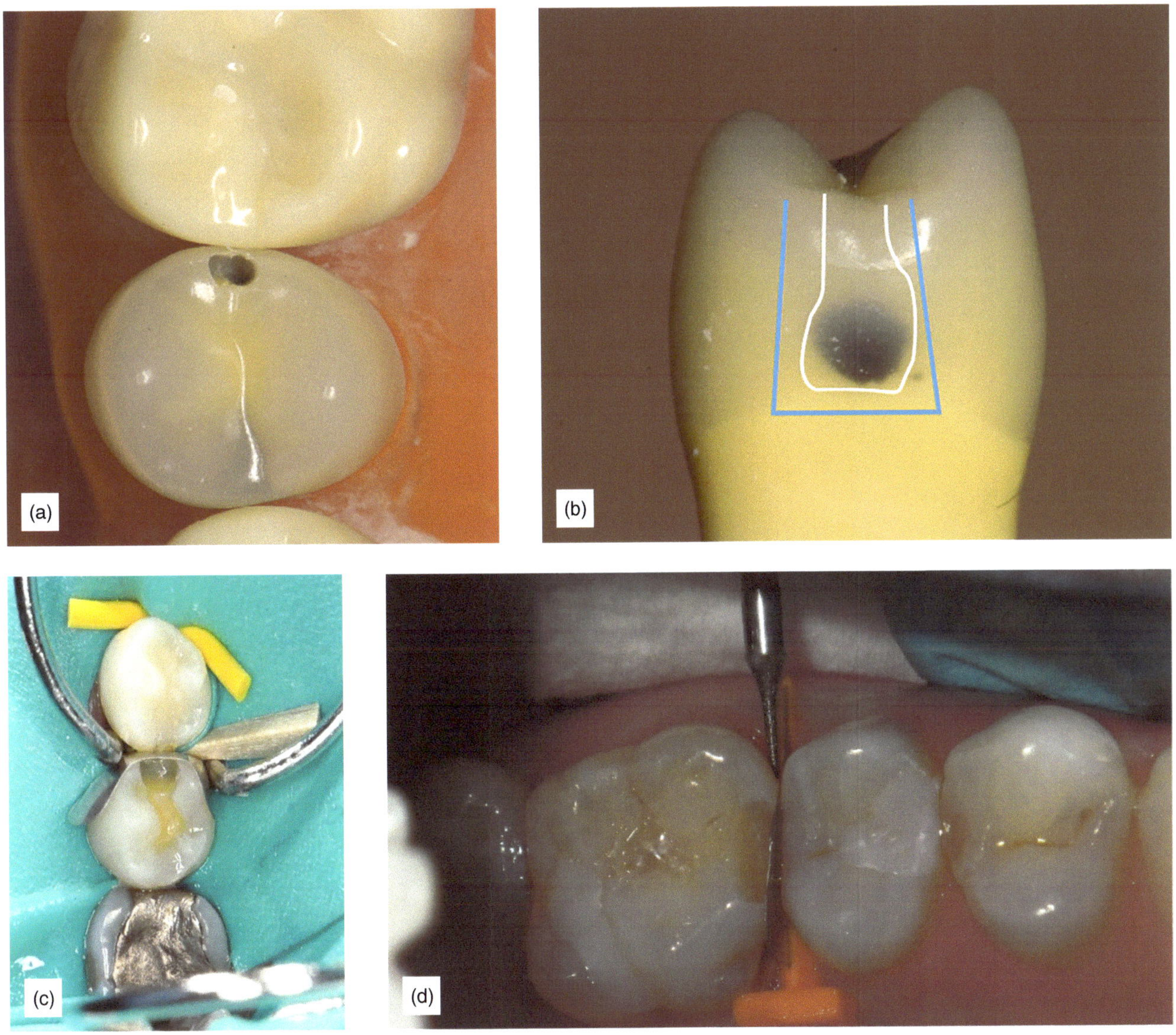

Figure 3.17 (a) Small occlusal access to cavity. (b) Proximal view showing undercuts during preparation (c) Showing wedge placed to fit matrix band. (d) With a wedge guard in place, using a "mosquito" bur to create slight separation to allow for matrix band placement..

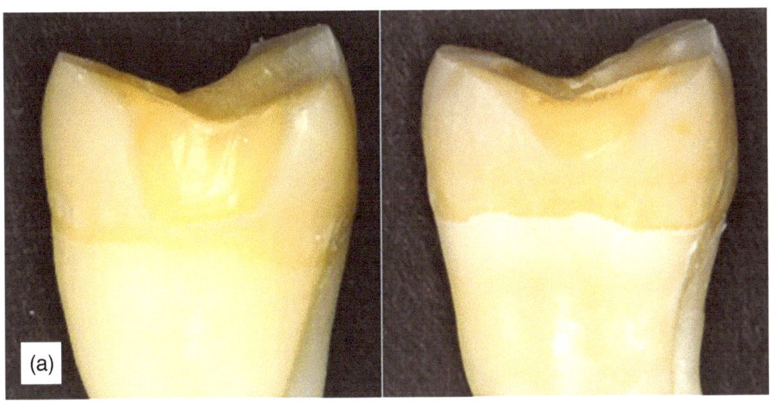

Figure 3.18 (a) Occlusal reduction of proximal tooth with a U-shape rather than a box. (*Continued*)

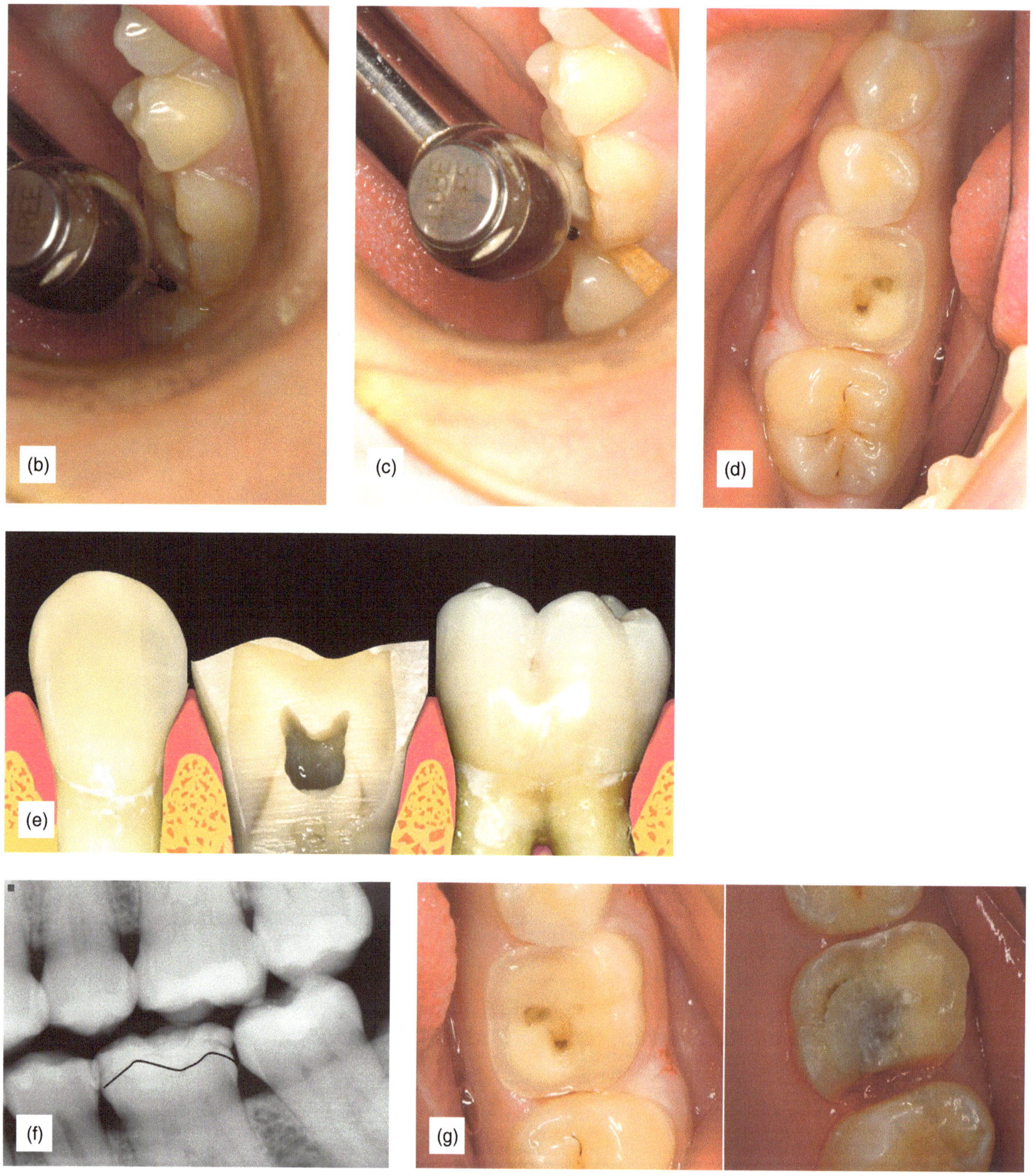

Figure 3.18 *(Continued)*
(b) Using an occlusal reduction bur with a U-shaped motion. (c) Using a wedge, create safe gingival clearance needed for easy clean impression and plaster die work. (d) Finished separation with supragingival results. (e) Attention must be paid to reducing the marginal ridge below the contact point, but above the gingiva. Mesial reduction is correct, permitting ideal margin separation. Distal reduction is insufficient. (f) X-ray showing an inappropriate example of margin separation; the black line shows where the margin should have been placed. (g) Compare the different outcomes using boxes for proximal clearance compared with margin separation technique, at the time of cementation.

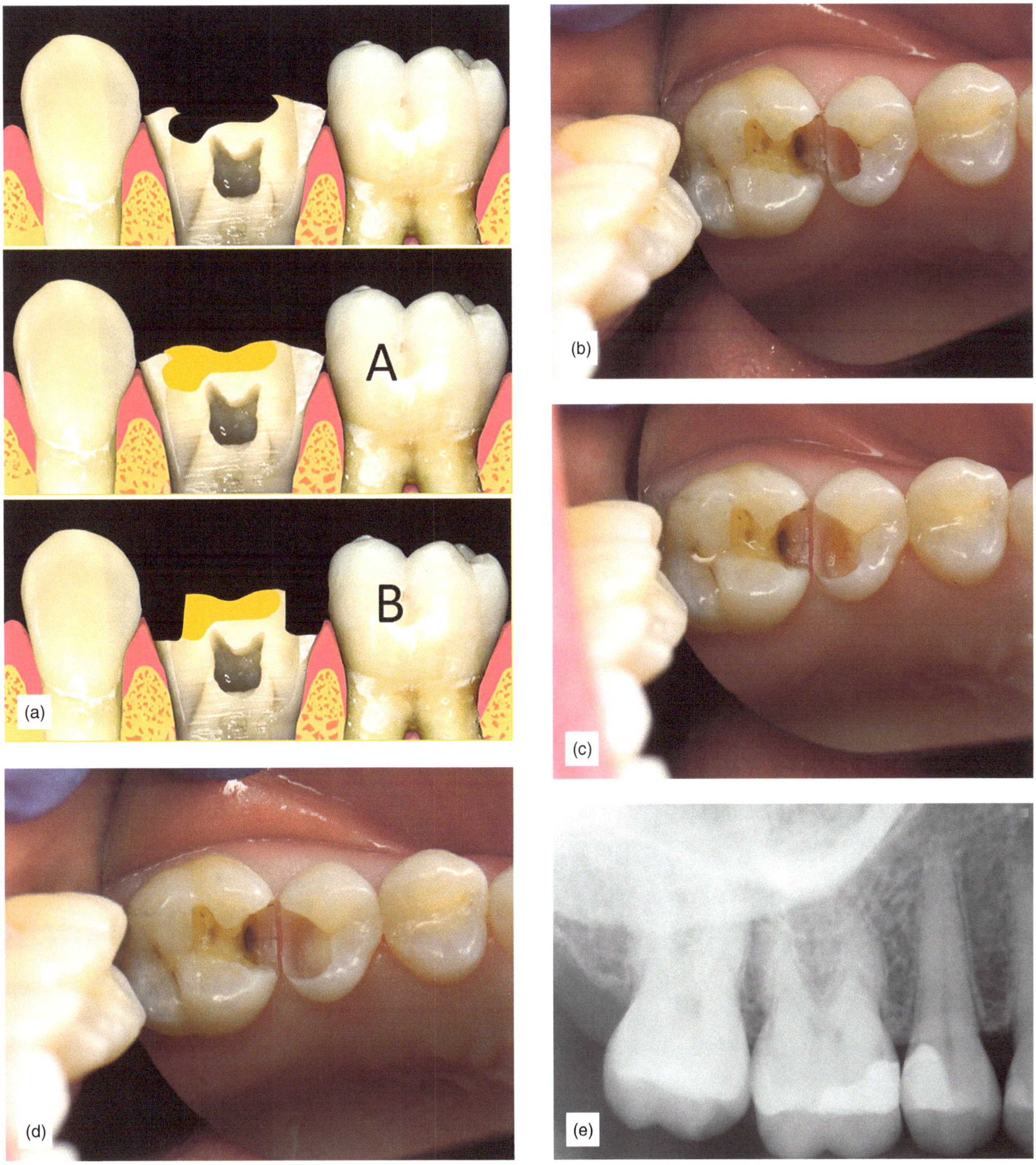

Figure 3.19 Outcome comparison: (a) A badly damaged tooth with unsupported enamel after a supragingival approach (A) or with traditional crown preparation approach (B). (b) Deep caries on bicuspid; enamel is healthy but there are much deeper caries on the dentin. (c) Dentin caries continues while healthy enamel is preserved supragingivally. (d) All caries have been removed, and an indirect pulp cap has been placed. (e) Final x-ray showing discrepancy between supragingival enamel level and dentin level; supragingival enamel made restoration much more simple.

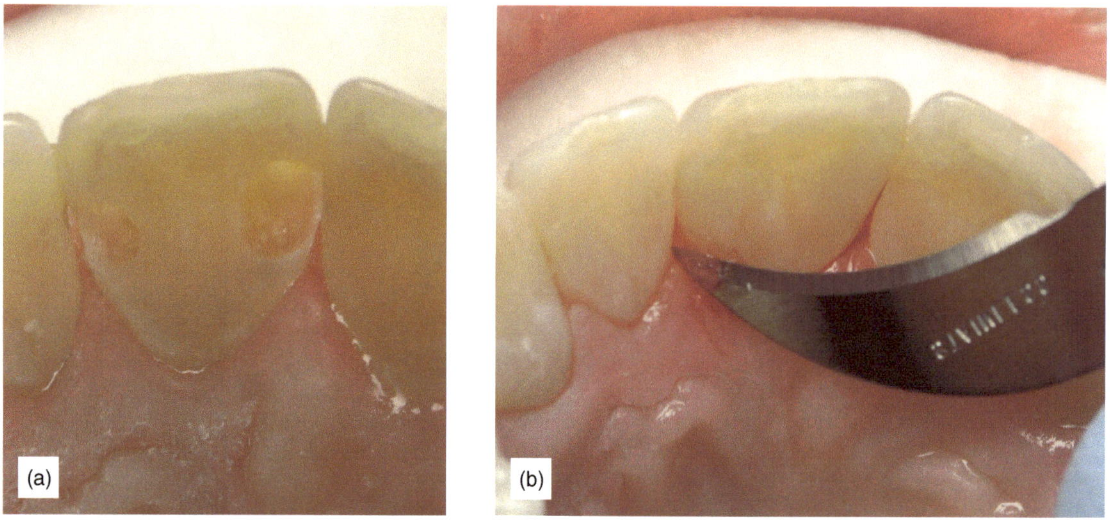

Figure 3.20 (a) Enamel preservation in a direct clinical case. (b) Supragingival margins allow for a much easier cleanup of composite flash and finishing.

by the easy isolation allowed by supragingival margins. The bonded restoration will further cover and protect the preserved enamel margin further reinforcing the area (Figure 21a–c). Extensive clinical success has been experience with this procedure by the author (Figure 3.22a–i).

Enamel margin preservation is used in cases with extensive cervical caries, where the enamel is healthy but the dentin is infected. The supragingival enamel is carefully preserved without dentin support, and the unsupported enamel is subsequently repaired with properly bonded composite. Based on evidence from the

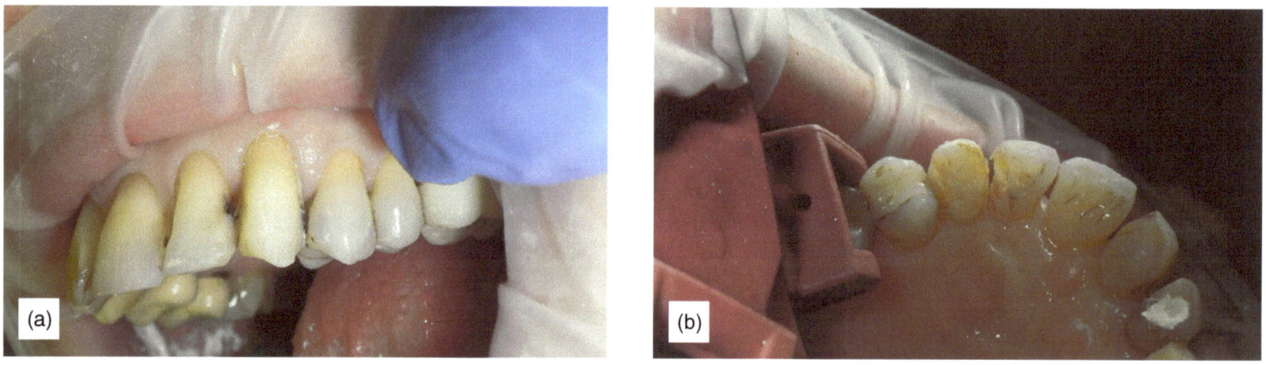

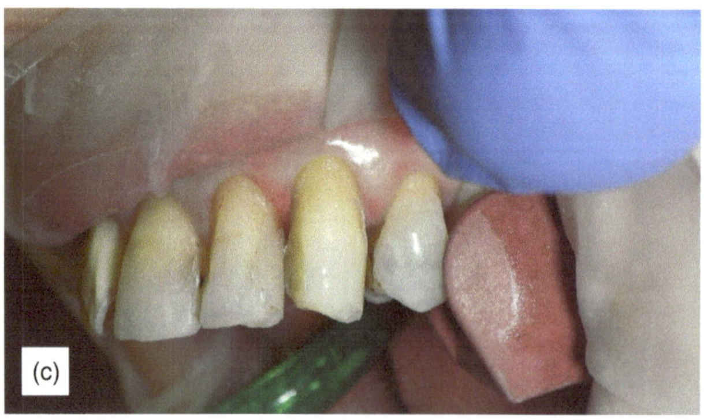

Figure 3.21 (a) Caries which appear to go deeply subgingival, after initial veneer preparation. (b) Lingual view of extreme caries and removal using enamel preservation technique preparation. (c) Finishing preparation, after repair with composite; the tooth looks natural.

literature, it is reasonable to expect that the enamel will regain a large part of its original strength [19,20,21]. It is well known that enamel without dentinal support is weak and, for that reason, a careful and well thought out protocol must be followed to protect such enamel during the repair procedure and to minimize polymerization forces which could cause cracks in the enamel. In an in vitro study, Ruiz and Finger demonstrated no enamel micro-cracks on unsupported enamel when using a technique for preserving enamel [22]. Improved

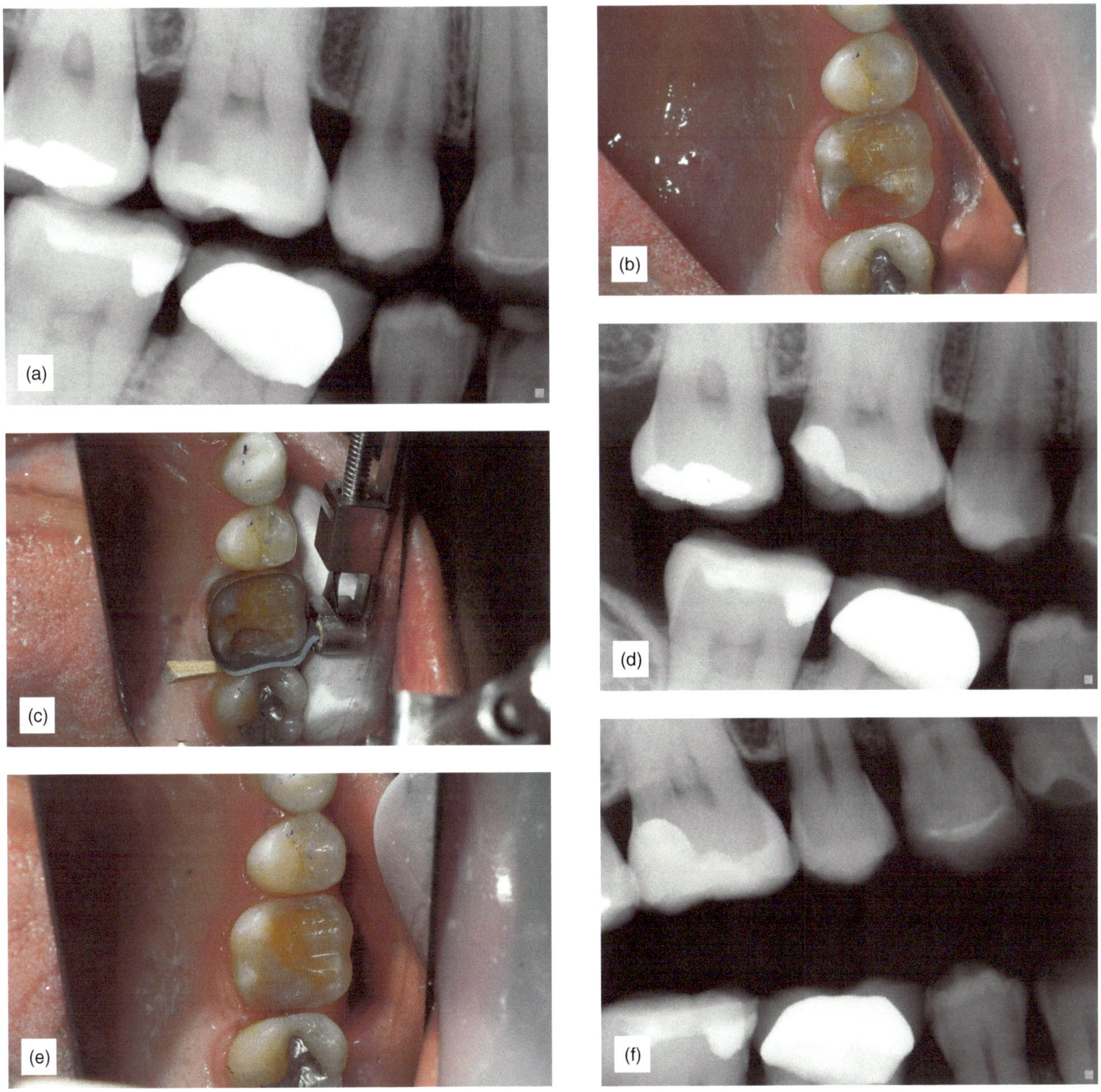

Figure 3.22 (a) Badly damaged tooth which appears to have a deep subgingival cavity on the distal side. (b) Careful removal of infected dentin using caries indicator, leaving a largely supragingival margin, with a very small slightly subgingival defect. (c) Enamel preservation and repair procedure using a matrix band and wedge for isolation and bleeding control. (d) Radiographic appearance of enamel repair and buildups. (e) Clinical appearance after enamel preservation and repair procedure. (f) Final x-ray confirming excellent marginal seal. *(Continued)*

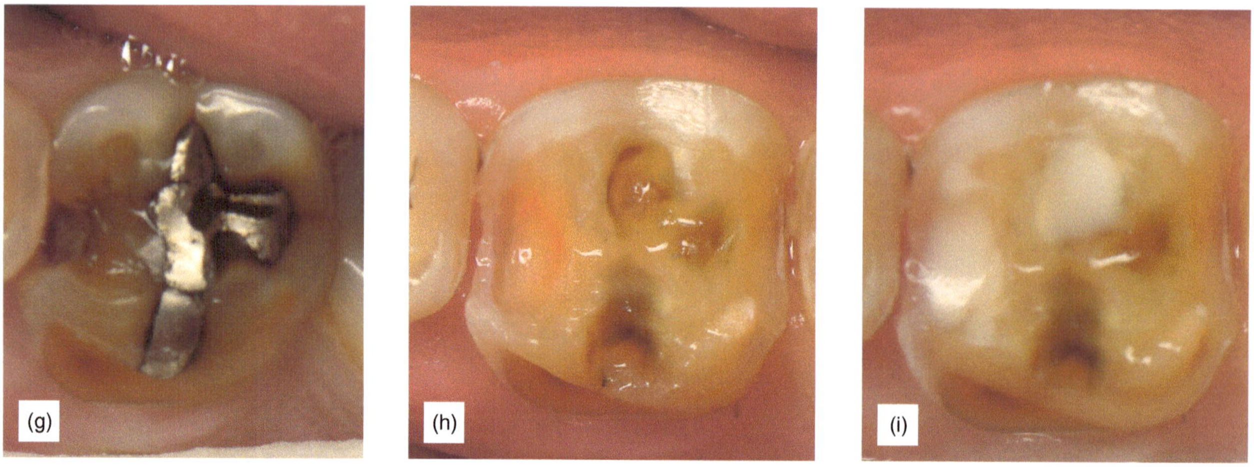

Figure 3.22 (*Continued*)
(g) Clinical appearance of a certain subgingival margin with traditional techniques. (h) After occlusal reduction and using caries indicator to remove only infected dentin. (i) After enamel repair using bonded composite; from here, the preparation can be finished with simplicity and supragingival margins.

results were obtained when the enamel thickness was greater than 1 mm (Figure 3.23a,b). The technique used is shown in Box 3.3.

The Fourth Principle: Technique for Margin Elevation

There are many cases in which caries or old restorative margins are already subgingival. Clinical experience shows that 0.5–1 mm of subgingival margin is usually easy to manage when limited to a small area. Isolation and good bonded cementation are possible. When the restorative margin is deeper than 1.5 mm below the gingiva, isolation during adhesive cementation may be compromised and may be less predictable and less successful. In such cases, a traditional mechanically retained full crown is usually indicated, which allows the use of resin-modified glass ionomer (RMGI) crown and bridge cement (such as Meron Plus AC, VOCO, or RelyX™ Luting Cement, 3M) which are less sensitive to contamination [23]. A more expensive, painful and complicated option would be crown lengthening, which also would be mandatory if the cavosurface margin will violate the biological width [24].

An alternative technique to a traditional crown or crown lengthening is a procedure called margin elevation (Figure 3.25a–e) [25,24,25,26,27]. This procedure has been shown to be successful and to increase simplicity and success with indirect restorations. It is used after the removal of caries and old restorative materials, when the margin is considerably subgingival. At

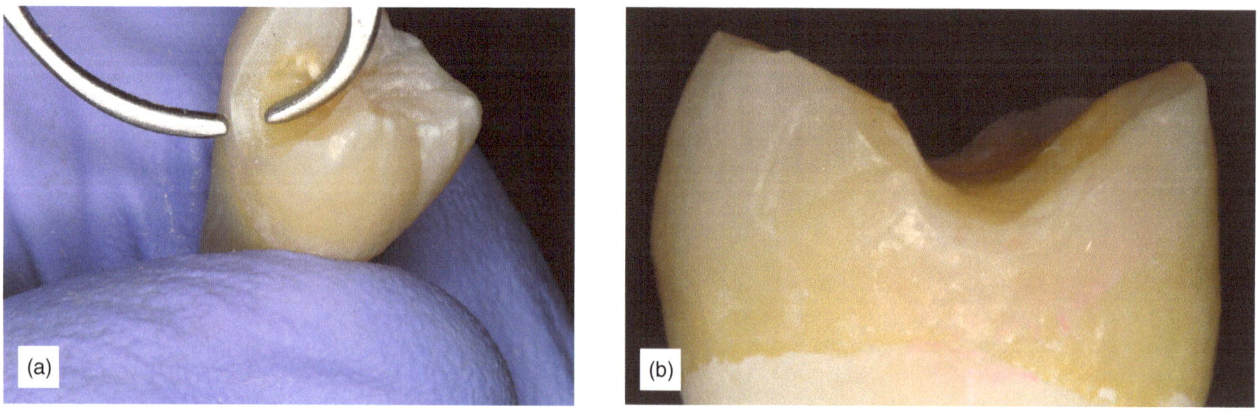

Figure 3.23 (a) Tooth prepared for enamel preservation study (1 mm thick enamel). (b) A close-up of non-stained margin on enamel preservation study.

Box 3.3 Clinical steps for preserving the enamel margin in direct and indirect procedures

1) Carefully remove cervical caries, using a caries indicator (Figure 3.24a).
2) Preserve the full thickness of healthy enamel, even in the absence of dentinal support, allowing the cavosurface margin to remain supragingival (Figure 3.24b).
3) Immediately after removing the caries, isolate with your choice of isolation system; avoid saliva touching the tooth.
4) If appropriate, carefully place matrix band and wedge.
5) Selectively etch enamel margin using phosphoric acid for 10 seconds using an etching fluid (such as SureEtch® Gel, Danville; Figure 3.24c).
6) Apply a self-etching bonding system (such as Clearfil™ SE Protect, Kuraray), using proper protocol and cure (Figure 3.24d) For a detailed bonding protocol, see Chapter 4.
7) Place a thin layer of flowable composite on the dentin alone, to minimize polymerization stress on the unsupported enamel, followed by an incremental cure (Figure 3.24e). For an explanation of incremental cures, see Chapter 10.

8a) For indirect restoration, place a second layer of restorative composite just to the level of the enamel, cure, finish preparation and take an impression (Figure 3.24f).

8b) For direct restoration, place additional increments of restorative composite to fill the cavity and finish (for a detailed protocol for incremental filling, see Chapter 10).

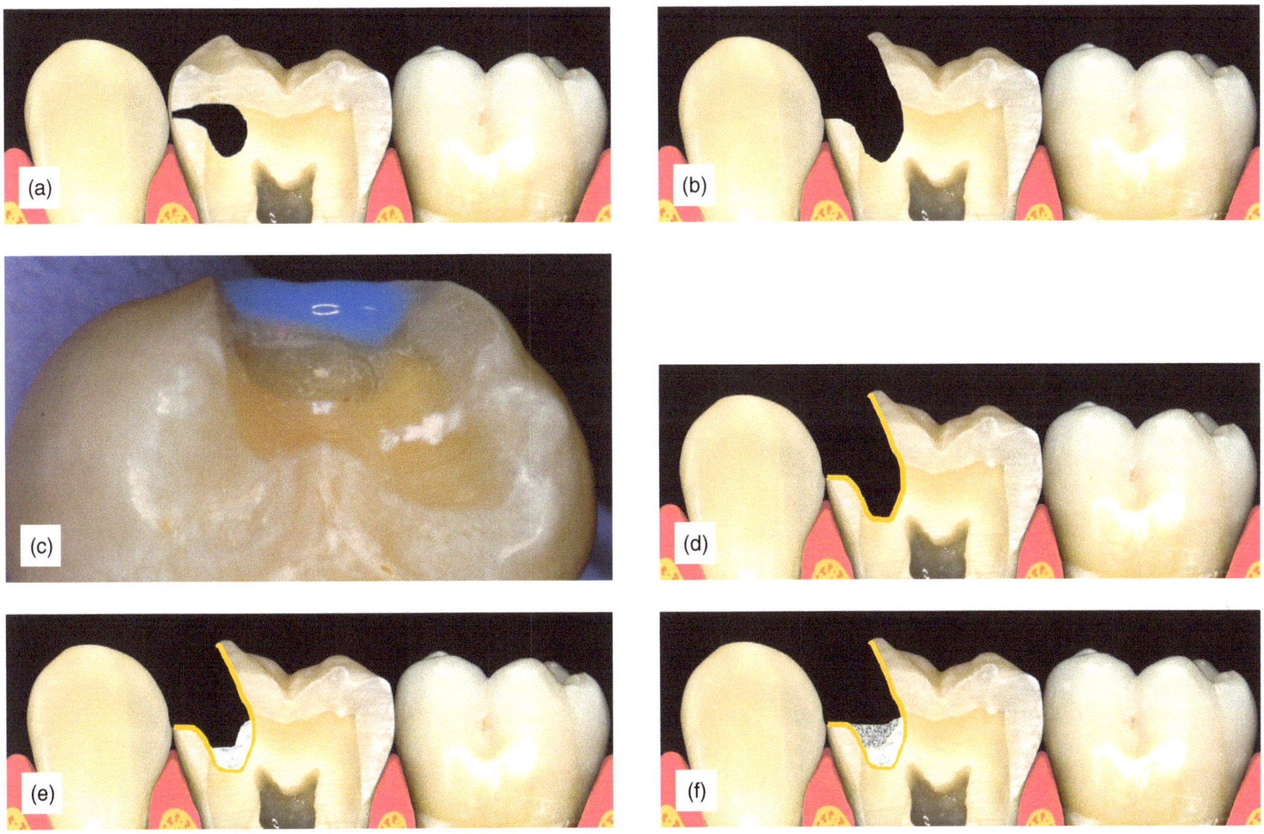

Figure 3.24 (a) Caries usually expand after entering enamel. (b) Supragingival enamel without dentin support. (c) Applying etch on enamel for 10 seconds (SureEtch® Gel, Danville). (d) Correct application of bonding system. (e) Correct incremental filling of cavity with initial layer of flowable composite only on enamel, to minimize the effects of polymerization shrinkage on weak enamel. (f) Second increment of restorative composite; final filling or final preparation will follow depending on whether it is a direct or indirect restoration.

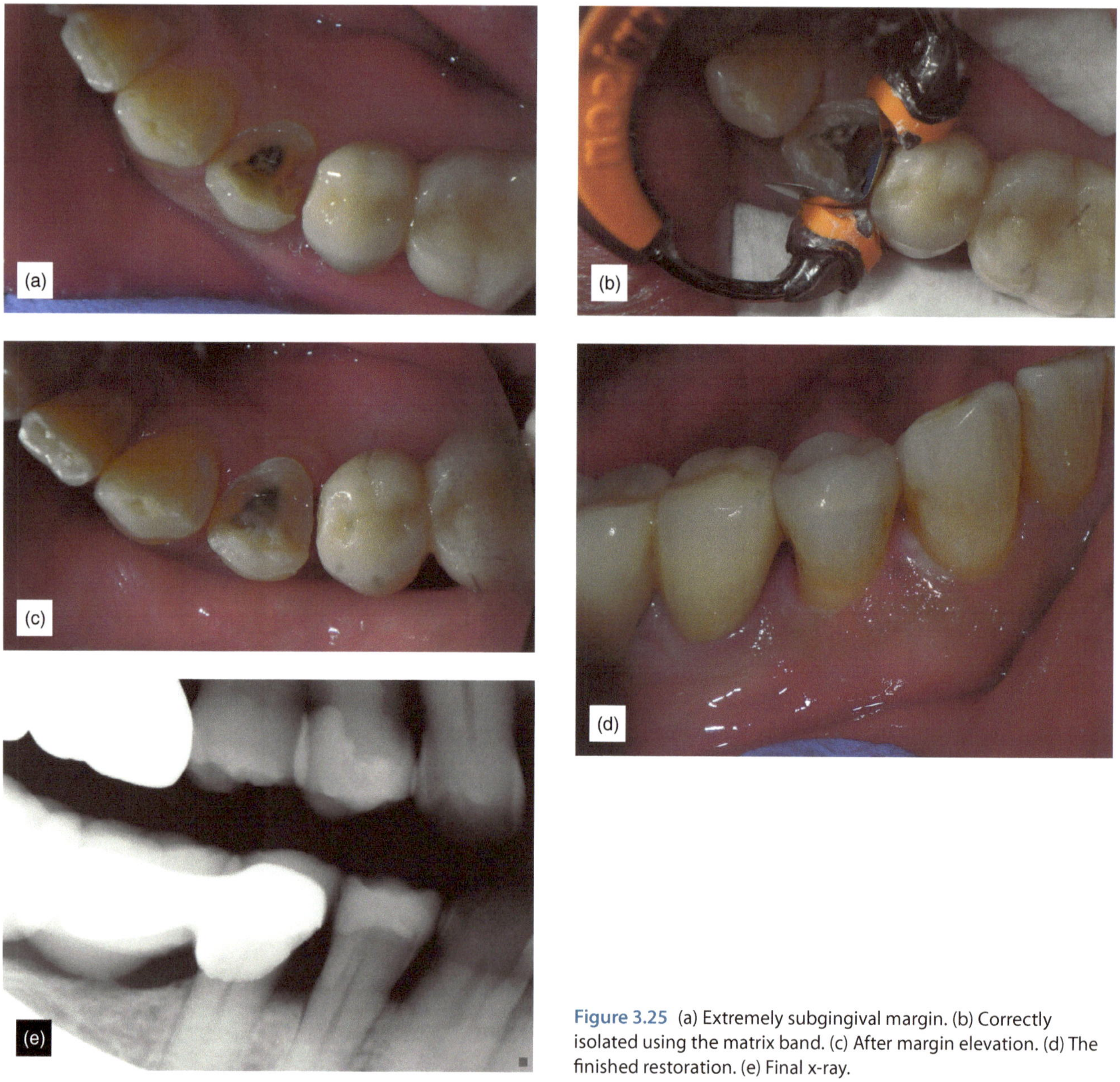

Figure 3.25 (a) Extremely subgingival margin. (b) Correctly isolated using the matrix band. (c) After margin elevation. (d) The finished restoration. (e) Final x-ray.

that point, a matrix band is placed and the buildup or elevation is performed, it could be considered to be a short class II restoration, without the need to achieve proximal contacts. One important advantage of this technique is that, when the correct technique is used, the polymerization shrinkage and stresses are favorable. A better cervical marginal seal can be achieved when the first increment is isolated on one bonded surface. The cervical floor and the polymerization shrinkage will pull the composite towards the bonded margin surface [28,29]. Care must be taken to perform a meticulous isolation, creating a well-sealed restoration. Confirmation with an x-ray is desirable, together with clinical confirmation of marginal seal (Figure 3.26a–g). Using a very highly radiopaque flowable composite will make x-ray verification easier. RMGI may be used for the margin elevation, although it is currently less popular. To avoid margins which mistakenly appear on the x-ray to be open, a very thin bonding agent is desirable, unless the bonding agent is radiopaque.

After the margin elevation, an impression will be taken and the tooth can be provisionalized. The bonded cementation will be easy and stress free, as all margins

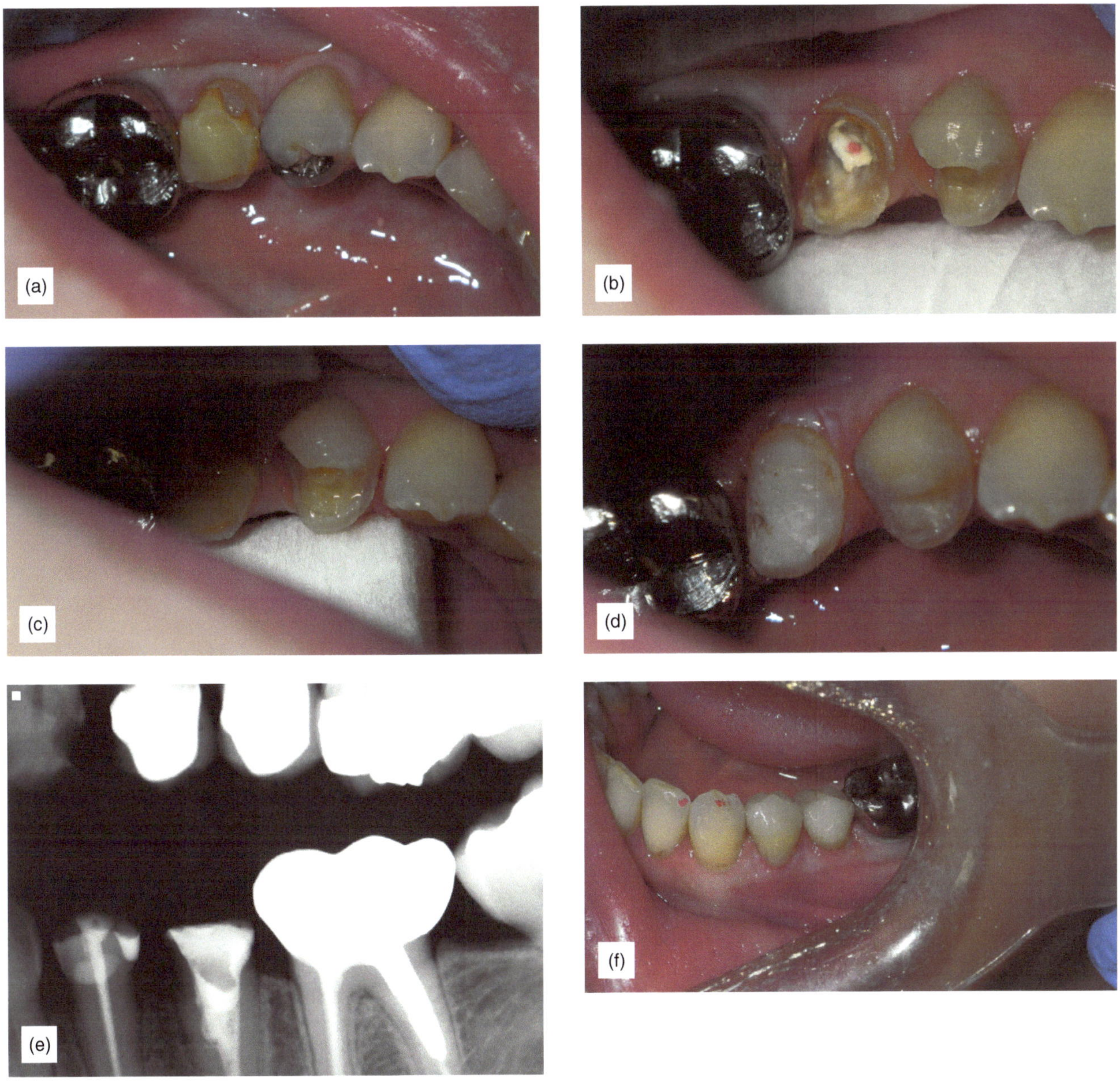

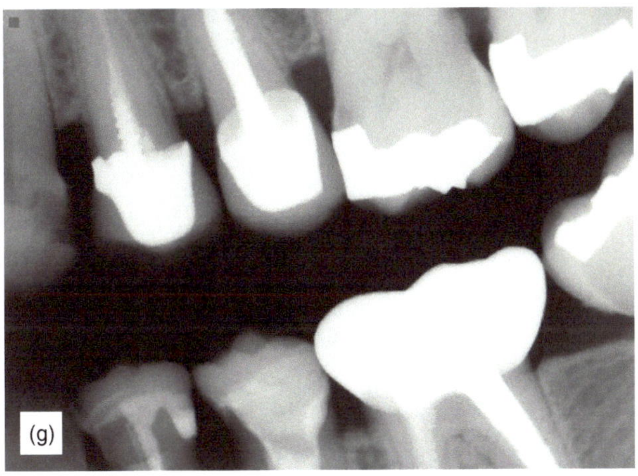

Figure 3.26 (a) This patient was informed of the poor prognosis of the second bicuspid. (b) Observe the extent of the damage to both teeth. (c) A different view to show how subgingival the margins are, and how difficult this would be if indirect bonded restorations were attempted with gingiva this deep. (d) After margin elevation. (e) X-ray confirming good margin elevation seal. (f) Immediately after cementation. (g) Two years postoperative x-ray.

Box 3.4 Clinical steps for margin elevation

1) Careful removal of caries and old restorative material, use caries indicator stain to avoid unnecessary removal of non-infected dentin (Figure 3.27a).
2) Immediately after the removal of the caries, isolate with your choice of isolation system.
3) Place matrix band and wedge.
4) Apply self-etching bonding system and cure (Figure 3.27b).
5) Place a thin layer of flowable composite on the gingival floor, avoiding contact with enamel axial walls, followed by incremental cure (Figure 3.27c,d). Remember to allow 2 minutes before the next cure to allow for polymerization stress reduction.
6) Place a second increment, which now will touch axial walls and gingival floor. Using a restorative composite, fill to 1–2 mm above the gingiva, and perform an incremental cure (Figure 3.27e).
7) Confirm a proper seal with an x-ray.
8) Perform a final cure, finish the preparation and take a final impression.

will be supragingival. The clinical steps for margin elevation are shown in Box 3.4.

The Fifth Principle: Proper Use of Translucency for Ideal Restorative Margin Blending and Esthetics

As explained in Chapters 1 and 2, the blending of the tooth and the restorations is dependent upon the amount of light allowed through to the tooth by the restorative material. It is desirable to create a "contact lens" effect for maximum blending of the restorative margin. Three factors are crucial to achieve the desirable blending. The first factor is the correct choice of restorative material, its level of translucency and thickness. The second factor is the translucency or opacity of the chosen cement, and the third is the underlying tooth color. A naturally translucent restoration, especially at the margin level, facilitates placing restorative margins supragingivally.

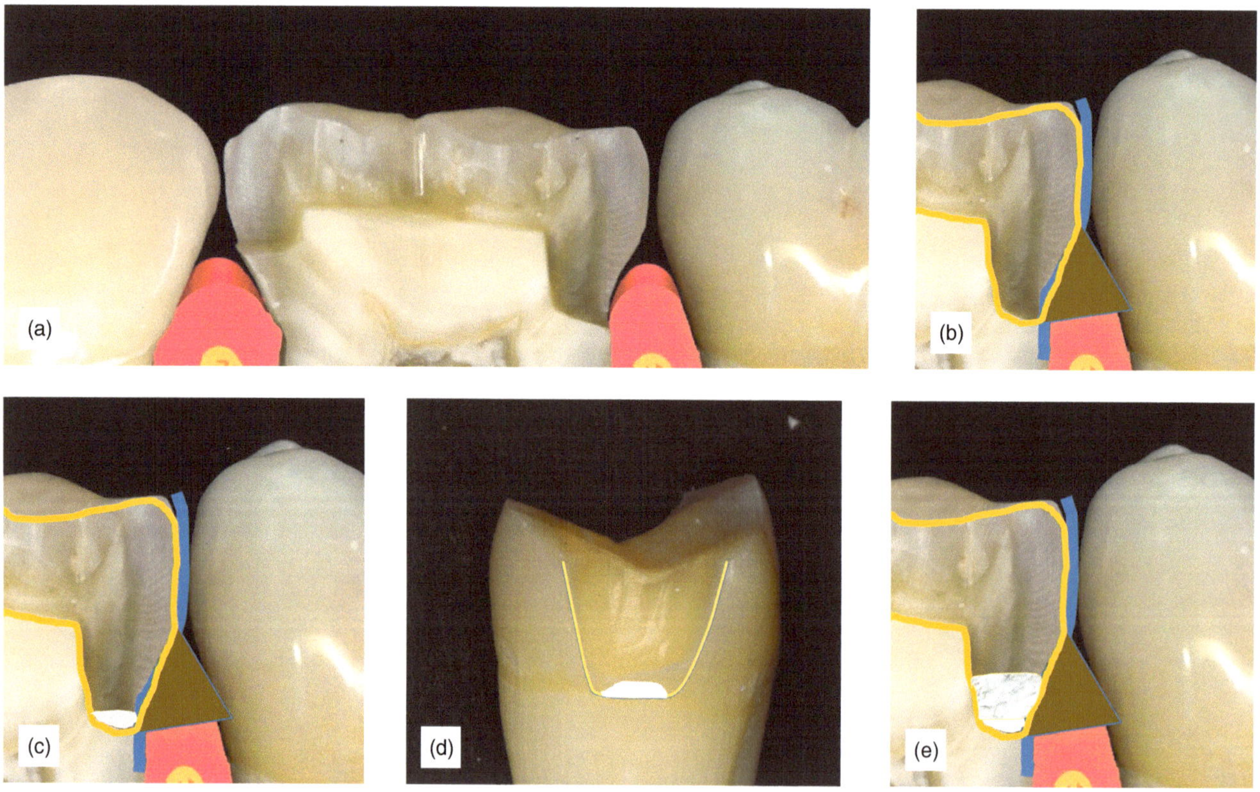

Figure 3.27 (a) Caries or old restoration is deeply subgingival on the distal side, so the cervical margin will be on dentin or cementum. (b) Matrix and wedge placed and proper bonding procedure performed. (c) Flowable increment on gingival floor to allow for favorable polymerization forces. (d) Distal view, showing that the increment is placed on contact with the dentin gingival margins and never in contact with the enamel walls, to avoid unfavorable polymerization shrinkage. (e) Second increment using restorative composite to 1–2 mm above the gingiva.

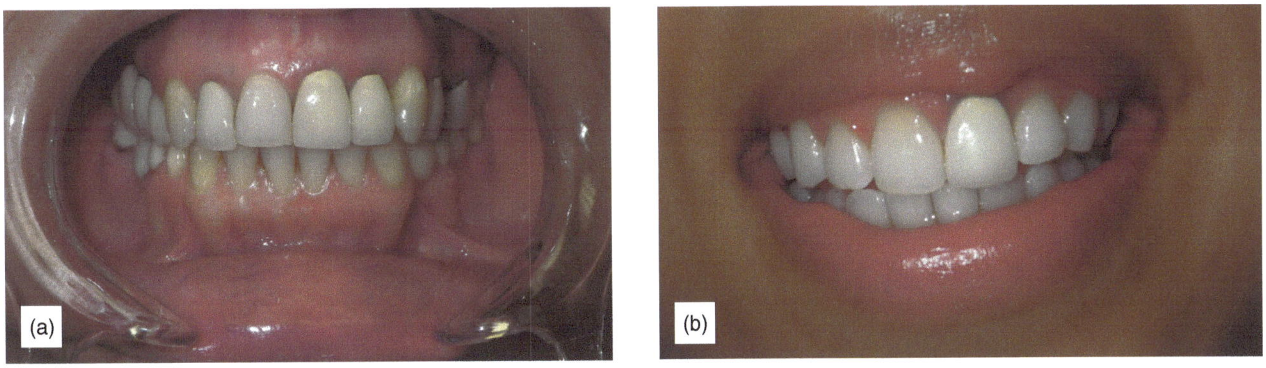

Figure 3.28 (a) Anterior crown with subgingival margins. (b) Extremely unesthetic opacious porcelain-fused-to-metal crown.

Lack of knowledge about how to manage translucency and lack of understanding of the disadvantages of subgingival margins have made the use of opacious materials popular, sometimes even intentionally avoiding more translucent options [30]. The use of opacious restorations makes subgingival margin placement a standard procedure (Figure 3.28a,b). Remedying a large difference in shade with the restorative materials (porcelain or composite) will require the use of opacious materials. Opacious materials are less esthetically pleasing, and often lead to final restorations which look opacious, and to poor restorative marginal blending, forcing a subgingival margin placement (Figure 3.29).

On the other hand, using translucent materials requires attention to the color of the tooth substrate, because this will affect the final shade of the restoration [31]. Thus, it is often desirable to whiten the teeth before the restorative procedure is performed, to obtain a shade closer to the desired final shade. This will allow for the use of a more translucent restorative material, with more natural results and better margin blending with supragingival margins (Figure 3.30).

In-office bleaching products such as Venus White® (Kulzer) are very successful (Figure 3.31a–e). In cases of dark endodontic treated teeth, it would be desirable to undertake internal bleaching to get a dark tooth to appear lighter and closer to the final desired shade (Figure 3.32a–d). Although there is a chance of color relapse (with good technique, the risks are small), the alternative would be to routinely place the crown margin subgingivally. As previously discussed, that alternative is short-lived and less healthy, because subgingival margins will cause inflammation, leading to gingival resection and ultimately exposure of the unsightly margin. Nevertheless, very dark teeth are problem cases and any solution is a compromise. Additional information on this topic is available in Chapter 7.

Understanding that anterior and posterior teeth have very different esthetic and occlusal requirements means that the material chosen will vary. The more anterior the teeth, the higher the esthetic requirements, and the lower the occlusal force, so layered feldspathic or pressed ceramics are often indicated. In the posterior region, the forces are higher, and the esthetic requirements are lower, so materials with complementary properties, such as lithium disilicate, layered or monolithic zirconia or Lava™ Ultimate Restorative (3M), would be desirable. It is interesting to note that, generally speaking, the more translucent the material the weaker it is, although this is not an absolute [32].

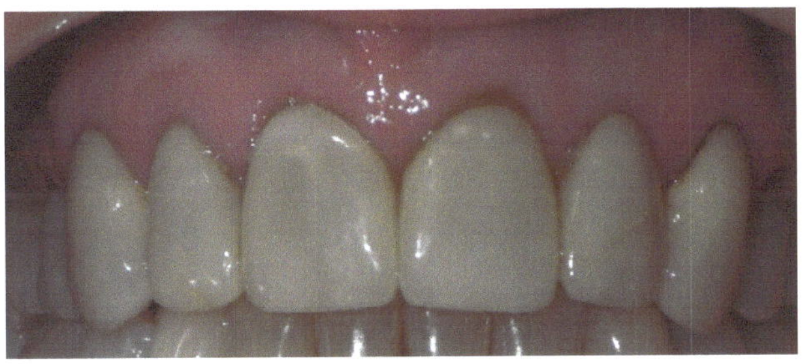

Figure 3.29 Opacious-looking restorations.

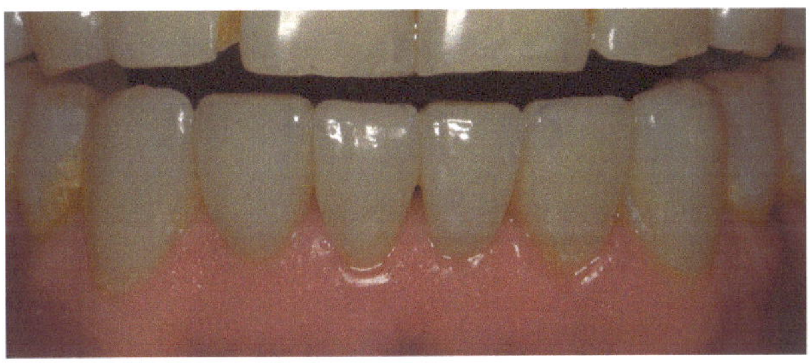

Figure 3.30 Almost 1 mm supragingival margins on six lower anterior veneers, 1 year postoperatively.

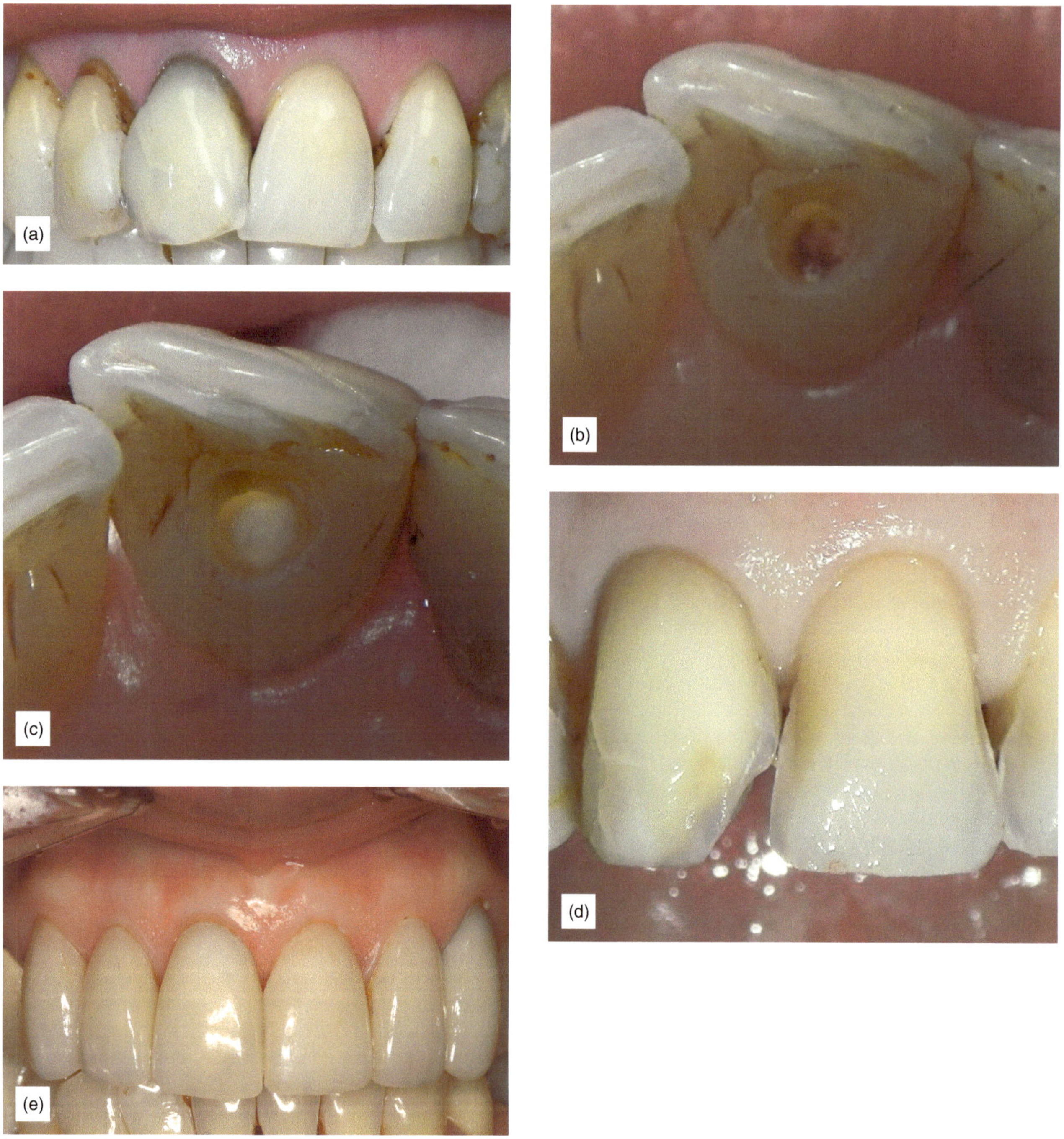

Figure 3.31 (a) Dark tooth before internal bleaching. (b) Open endodontic access and removal of pulp and cement debris. (c) Lingual view after one cycle of internal bleaching. (d) Veneer preparation procedure showing how much more simple this case is now. (e) The final restoration.

Finally, the science of translucency is complicated [33]. There is limited practical clinical knowledge of translucency and how to communicate it. For that reason, restorative dentists should simplify communication with laboratories and colleagues. Use translucency values equivalent to dental structures similar to those commonly employed with composites [34]. The thickness of the restorations and the use of the correct cement based on the requirements for translucency is of great importance and are discussed in Chapters 7 and 9 [35].

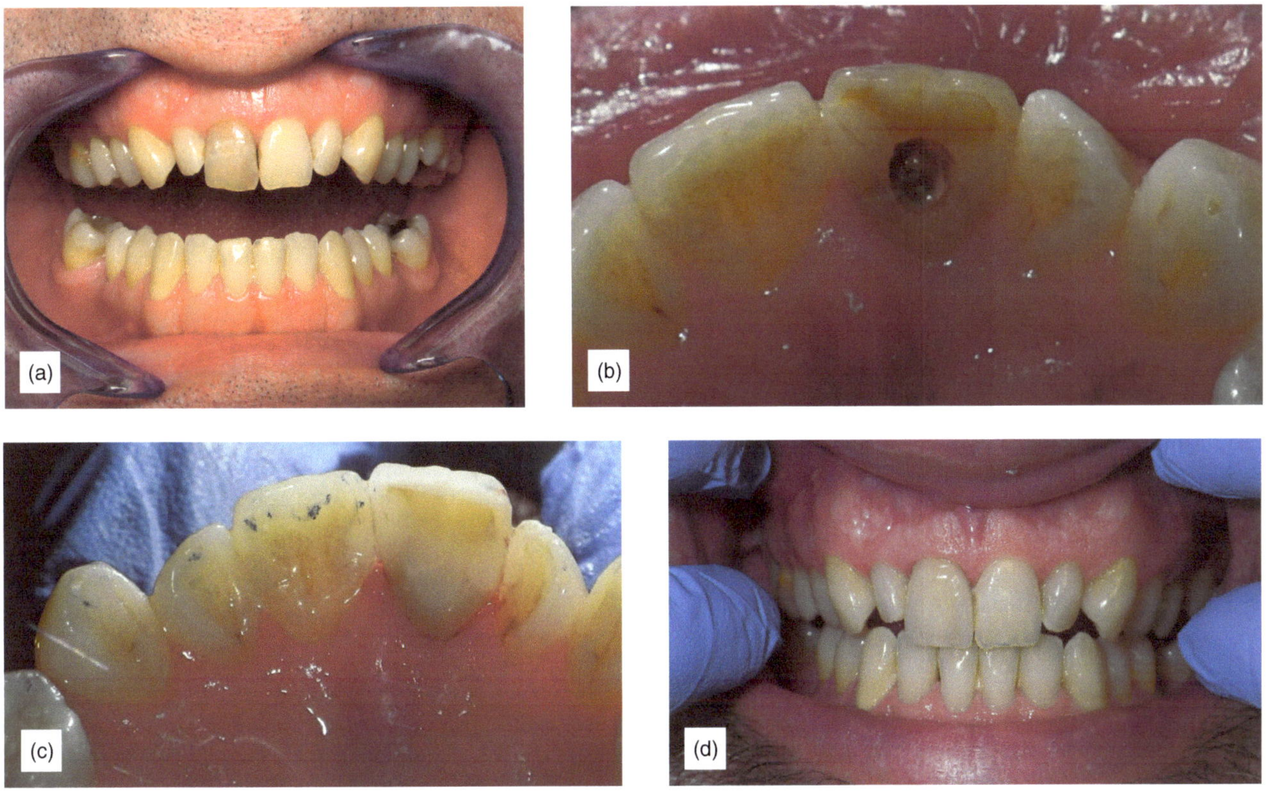

Figure 3.32 (a) Extremely dark central. (b) Lingual view before internal bleaching. (c) Internal view after bleaching and endodontic access filled. (d) Final veneer cemented with supragingival margins.

References

1 Hosoda H, Fusayama T. A tooth substance saving restorative technique. *Int Dent J*, 1984; 34(1): 1–12.
2 Bertolotti RL. Laboratory laminate veneers. *Oral Health*. 1989; 79(3): 11–16.
3 Santos MJMC, Bezerra RB. Fracture resistance of maxillary premolars restored with direct and indirect adhesive techniques. *J Can Dent Assoc*, 2005; 71(8): 585–590.
4 Shor A, Nicholls JI, Phillips KM, Libman WJ. Fatigue load of teeth restored with bonded direct composite and indirect ceramic inlays in MOD class II cavity preparations. *Int J Prosthodont*, 2003; 16(1): 64–69.
5 Christensen GJ. Are tooth color onlays viable alternatives to crowns? *Clin Rep*, 2012; 5(1): 1,3.
6 Bakeman EM, Kois JC. Posterior, all porcelain, adhesively retained restorations. *Inside Dentistry*, 2009; 5(5): 20–30.
7 Kois DE, Chaiyabutr Y, Kois JC. Comparison of load fatigue performance of posterior ceramic onlay restorations under different preparation designs. *Compend Contin Educ Dent*, 2012 ; 33(Spec No 2): 2–9.
8 Meyer A Jr, Cardoso LC, Araujo E, Baratieri LN. Ceramic inlays and onlays: clinical procedures for predictable results. *J Esthet Restor Dent*, 2003; 15(6): 338–352.
9 Barghi N, Berry TG. Clinical evaluation of etched porcelain onlays, a 4 year report. *Compend Contin Educ Dent*, 2002; 23(7): 657–674.
10 Heymann, HO, Swift EJ, Ritter AV. Indirect tooth color restorations, in *Sturdevant's Art and Science of Operative Dentistry*, 6th ed. Elsevier Mosby, 2013, pp. 280–295.
11 Ruiz JL. Supragingival dentistry using metal-free restorations. *Dent Today*, 2008; 27: 104–109.
12 Ruiz JL. Simplifying the cementation of porcelain onlays. *Dent Today*, 2004; 23(3): 76–79.
13 Alleman DS, Magne P. A systematic approach to deep caries removal end points: The peripheral seal concept in adhesive dentistry. *Quintessence Int*, 2012; 43(3): 197–208.
14 Black GV. *The Technical Procedures in Filling Teeth*. Chicago: HO Shepard Co. Printers; 1899, pp. 20–21.
15 Denehy GE, Torney DL. Internal enamel reinforcement through micromechanical bonding. *J Prosthet Dent*, 1976; 36(2): 171–175.
16 Hilton TJ, Broome JC. Direct posterior esthetic restorations, in *Summitt's Fundamentals of Operative Dentistry: A Contemporary Approach*, 4th ed. Chicago, IL: Quintessence Publishing, pp. 279–323.
17 Black GV. *Operative Dentistry*. Chicago, IL: Medico-Dental Publishing Company, 1908, p. 115.
18 Tredwin CJ, Stokes A, Moles DR. Influence of flowable liner and margin location on microleakage

of conventional and packable class ii resin composite. *Oper Dent*, 2005; 30(1): 32–38.
19 Ayad MF, Maghrabi AA, García-Godoy F. Resin composite polyethylene fiber reinforcement: effect on fracture resistance of weakened marginal ridges. *Am J Dent*, 2010; 23(3): 133–136.
20 Mirzaei M, Ghavam M, Rostamzadeh T. Reinforcement of unsupported enamel by restorative materials and dentin bonding agents: an in vitro study. *J Dent (Tehran)*, 2010; 7(2): 84–88.
21 Eidelman E. Composite resin support of undermined enamel in amalgam restorations. *Pediatr Dent*, 1999; 21(2): 118–120.
22 Ruiz JL, Finger WJ. Enamel margin preservation and repair technique. *J Dent Res*, 2016: 95(Spec Iss 5): abstract 2370749.
23 Lindquist TJ, Connolly J. In vitro microleakage of luting cements and crown foundation material. *J Prosthet Dent*, 2001; 85(3): 292–298.
24 Padbury A Jr. Interactions between gingiva and the margin of restorations. *J Clin Periodontol*, 2003; 30(5): 379–385.
25 Dietschi D, Olsburgh S, Krejci I, Davidson C. In vitro evaluation of marginal and internal adaptation after occlusal stressing of indirect class ii composite restoration with different resinous bases. *Eur J Oral Sci*, 2003; 111: 73–80.
26 Frankenberger R. Effect of proximal box elevation with resin composite on marginal quality of ceramic inlays in vitro. *Clin Oral Invest*, 2013; 17(1): 177–183.
27 Roggendorf MJ, Krämer N, Dippold C, Vosen VE, Naumann M, Jablonski-Momeni A, Frankenberger R. Effect of proximal box elevation with resin composite on marginal quality of resin composite inlays in vitro. *J Dent*, 2012; 40(12): 1068–1073.
28 Ferracane JL. Developing a more complete understanding of stresses produced in dental composites during polymerization. *Dent Mater*, 2005; 21(1): 36–42.
29 Braga RR, Hilton TJ, Ferracane JL. Contraction stress of flowable composite materials and their efficacy as stress-relieving layers. *J Am Dent Assoc*, 2003; 134(6): 721–728.
30 Chu FC, Chow TW, Chai J. Contrast ratios and masking ability of three types of ceramic veneers. *J Prosthet Dent*, 2007; 98(5): 359–364.
31 Azer SS, Rosenstiel SF, Seghi RR, Johnston WM. Effect of substrate shades on the color of ceramic laminate veneers. *J Prosthet Dent*, 2011; 106(3): 179–183.
32 Barizon KT, Bergeron C, Vargas MA, Qian F, Cobb DS, Gratton DG, Geraldeli S. Ceramic materials for porcelain veneers: Part II. Effect of material, shade, and thickness on translucency. *J Prosthet Dent*, 2014; 112(4): 864–870.
33 Johnston WM. Review of translucency determinations and applications to dental materials. *J Esthet Restor Dent*, 2014; 26(4): 217–223.
34 Kim DH, Park SH. Evaluation of resin composite translucency by two different methods. *Oper Dent*, 2013; 38(3): E1–15.
35 de Azevedo Cubas GB, Camacho GB, Demarco FF, Pereira-Cenci T. The effect of luting agents and ceramic thickness on the color variation of different ceramics against a chromatic background. *Eur J Dent*, 2011; 5(3): 245–252.

4

Should We Trust in Dental Adhesives and Adhesive Dentistry?

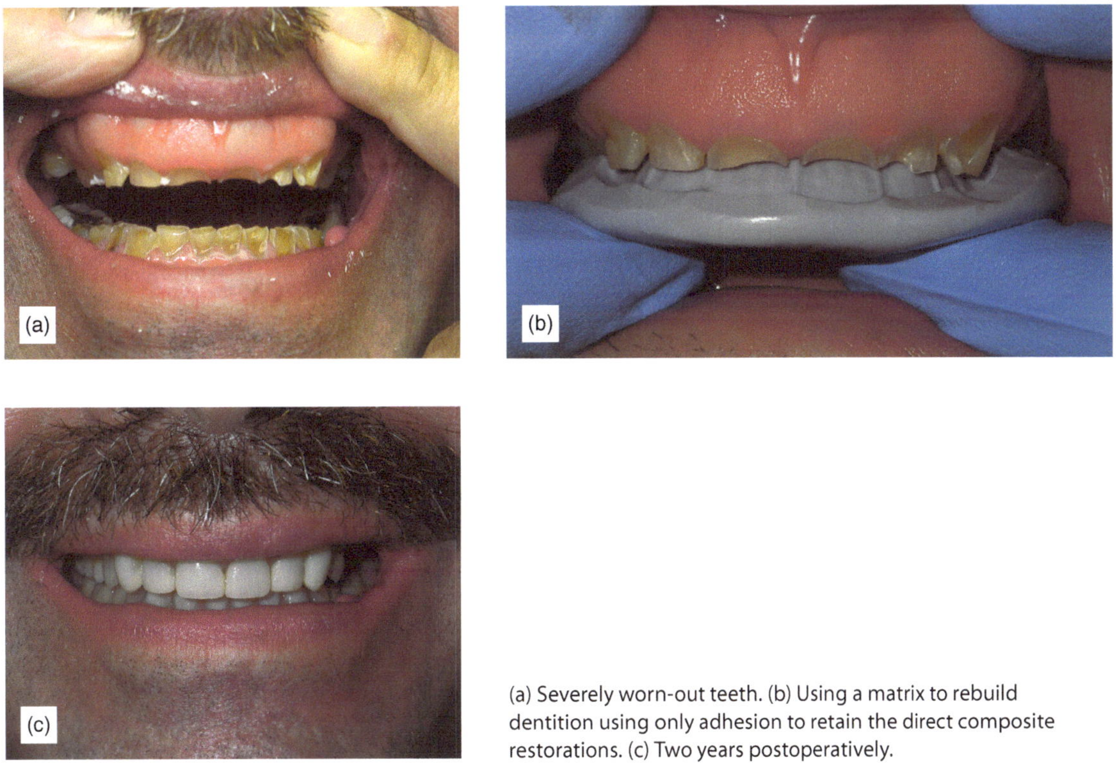

(a) Severely worn-out teeth. (b) Using a matrix to rebuild dentition using only adhesion to retain the direct composite restorations. (c) Two years postoperatively.

Introduction

Adhesion plays an indispensable role in modern dentistry. Much is owed to the pioneers of adhesive dentistry, who faced many obstacles in helping the profession accept these techniques [1,2,3]. When dentists fully trust adhesion, the need for mechanical retentive features, such as retention and resistance forms, is eliminated, and thus a more healthy tooth structure can be preserved. The health benefits do not end with tooth preservation. Through confidence in adhesion and bonding translucent restorative materials, clinicians can retain the restorative margins above the gum line by eliminating the need for traditional mechanical retentive features such as axial walls, boxes or ferrules, thus preserving periodontal health. Unfortunately, there is a current lack of trust that adhesion can truly replace retention and resistance mechanically retentive features. This lack of trust has prevented the widespread acceptance of partial coverage restorations retained solely by adhesion. Teeth continue to be drilled way past the point where caries has been fully removed, and often vital tooth structure is cut away for the purpose of traditional mechanical retention (Figures 4.1–4.3a,b).

Supra-Gingival Minimally Invasive Dentistry: A Healthier Approach to Esthetic Restorations, First Edition. By Jose-Luis Ruiz.

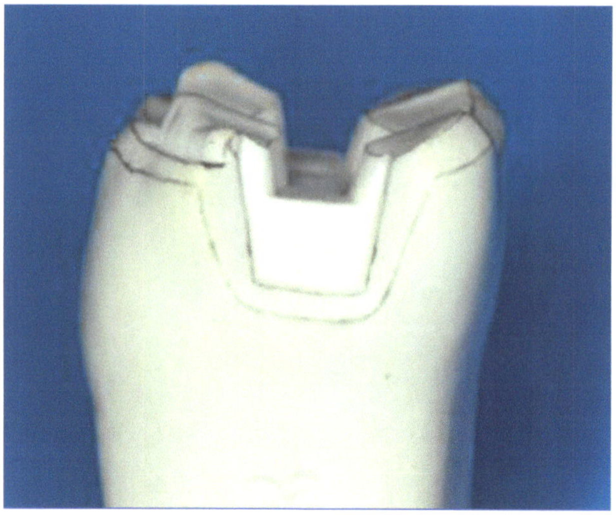

Figure 4.1 Extensive geometric mechanical features necessary for retention and resistance forms, requiring considerable healthy tooth removals (courtesy of Dr Boris Keselbrener).

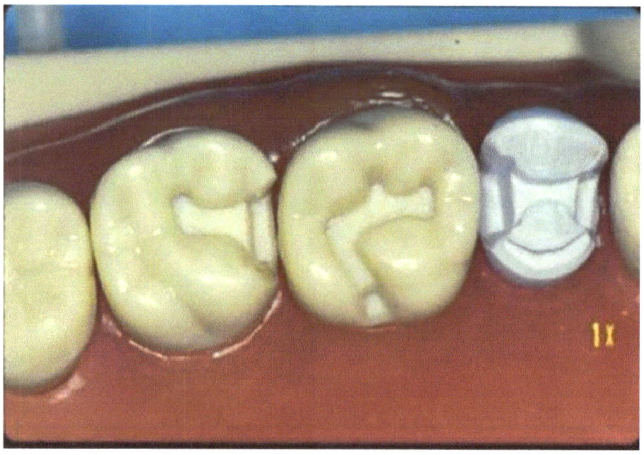

Figure 4.2 Traditional proximal box, requiring extensive healthy tooth removal to create form.

Trusting in Adhesion is Key To Success

Supragingival minimally invasive dentistry depends upon adhesion and trust in adhesion. Lack of trust in dental adhesives should be reconsidered in light of the advances in adhesive technology and the trust that other industries place in adhesion. In modern airplanes, newer cars and even building construction, adhesives are increasingly replacing conventional joining techniques such as welding, riveting or bolting. Modern industries are placing great trust in adhesion and allowing crucial components to be held together by this means [4,5]. Modern society as a whole depends on adhesion.

Lack of trust in adhesion as a full replacement for retention and resistance form in restorative dentistry has slowed the acceptance of supragingival partial-coverage, tooth-preserving, restorative dentistry. Lack of trust in adhesion while performing bonded restoration in fact decreases success with bonded restorations. Deep-rooted habits such as the need to have retention and resistance form and ferrule often leads restorative dentists to undertake axial wall preparation in planned bonded restorations. Margins are thus placed subgingivally, making adhesive cementation more difficult and more unpredictable (Figures 4.4, 4.5a,b). Supragingival margins with a good enamel periphery are ideal for achieving predictable success with adhesive dentistry [6], so there is a need for a supragingival protocol which depends fully on adhesive retention of the restoration. It is important to note that preserving as much enamel as possible increases durability and success. Nevertheless, this should not be understood to imply that a lack of a full enamel margin is a contraindication with bonded restorations. The lack of enamel margin in segments of the peripheral margin

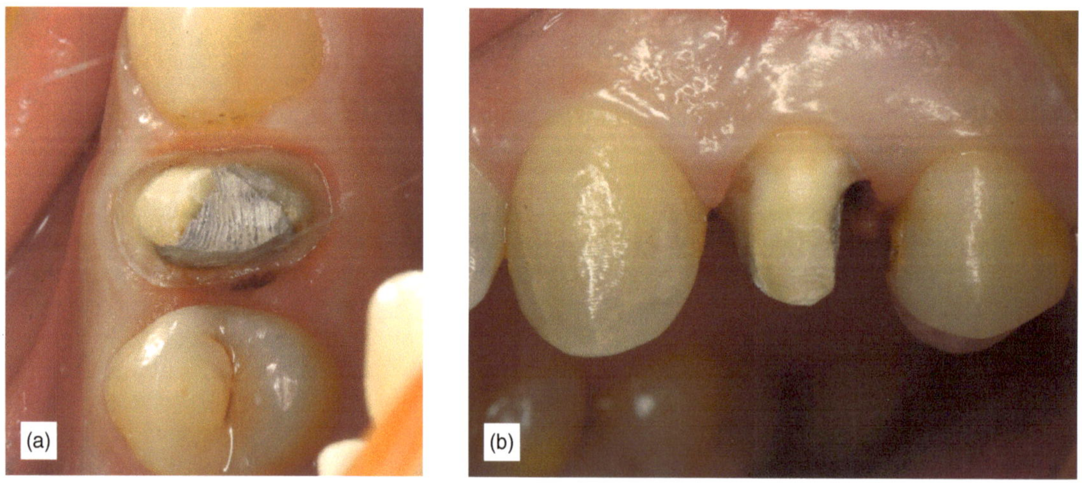

Figure 4.3 (a) Traditional crown preparation requiring extensive healthy tooth removal for axial walls and resistance and retention form. (b) Facial view showing the amount of tooth usually removed with a traditional full crown resistance form.

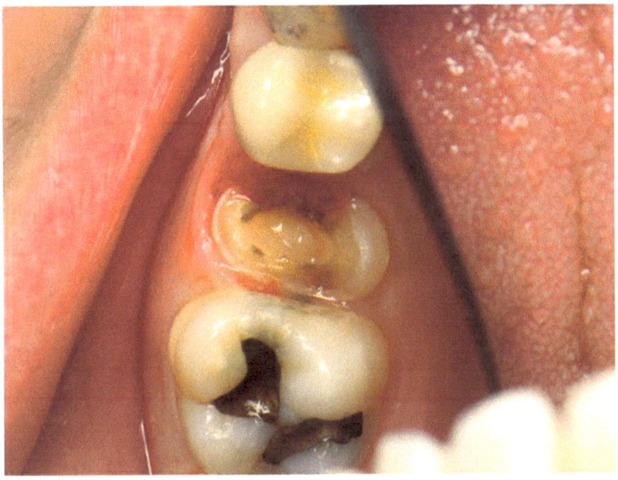

Figure 4.4 Onlay prepared with subgingival margin placement and bleeding.

is not a contraindication to bonded onlays and veneers, as clinical experience and current literature provides evidence that, with some bonding systems like Clearfil™ SE Protect (Kuraray) adhesion to dentin may in fact be reaching similar success as adhesion to enamel [7,8,9].

Restorations retained purely by adhesion, such as porcelain veneers, have shown some of the best longevity of any restoration, especially when the preparations have been left mostly on enamel [10,11,12,13]. Direct bonded composite restorations have rapidly replaced traditional mechanically retained amalgam with great predictability and success [14,15]. Other types of largely adhesively retained restorations, such as class V and posterior-bonded inlays and onlays, have been successful but have also encountered some complications, caused mainly by improper technique. Nevertheless, evidence from the literature and from clinical experience has shown that adhesion retention itself is not the primary reason for the failure of such restorations. In a retrospective clinical evaluation, Ruiz and colleagues [16] reported 100% inlay/onlay restoration success at 54 months, with no retention failures and only two small reparable fractures in 57 restorations recalled. Understanding the limited value of anecdote, in my personal experience in full-time private practice, placing approximately 10,000 bonded veneers (Figure 4.6a–c) and onlays, and many more thousands of direct composite restorations over the past 24 years, restoration failure due to loss of retention has been extremely rare and limited to a handful of cases. Evidence from the literature shows that, with bonded restorations, failure has most often been related to restorative material fracture and marginal leakage. Both problems are related to the failure of restorative materials, improper management of occlusion, complications caused by subgingival margins and difficulty in isolation, and improper technique, but not to lack of adhesive retention [8,17,18,19].

Adhesion to Enamel

As previously discussed, adhesion to enamel has been considered to be the ideal interface to which to bond because it is reliable and durable. In fact, not much has changed in 50 years since enamel etching was introduced by Michael Buonocore in 1955 [1] with a bond strength of 15–20 MPa. The only real change has been in etching time. While the original etching time with 85% acid was one full minute, currently enamel is only etched for 20–25 seconds with 35–37% phosphoric acid. It is now known that 37% acid is a more aggressive etchant than 85% acid. Even when using self-etch bonding systems, selective enamel etching enhances adhesion [20] and seal [21], both very important for long-term success (Figures 4.7a–c, 4.8a,b). Because enamel is the most predictable substrate on which to bond, success with bonded restorations improves greatly when enamel is preserved, which is one of the five principles of supragingival dentistry.

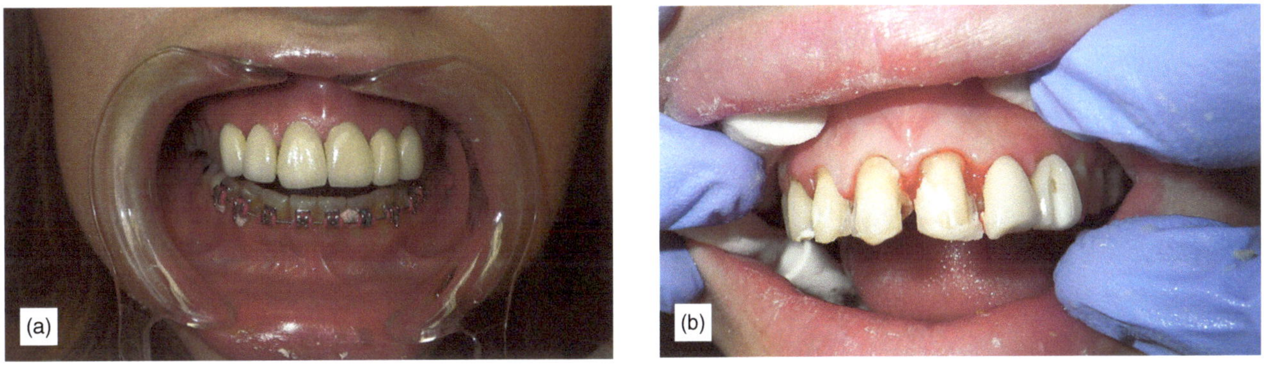

Figure 4.5 (a) This patient had severe sensitivity on leaky and anesthetic veneers. (b) The deep subgingival preparation was very difficult to isolate and was probably contaminated at cementation.

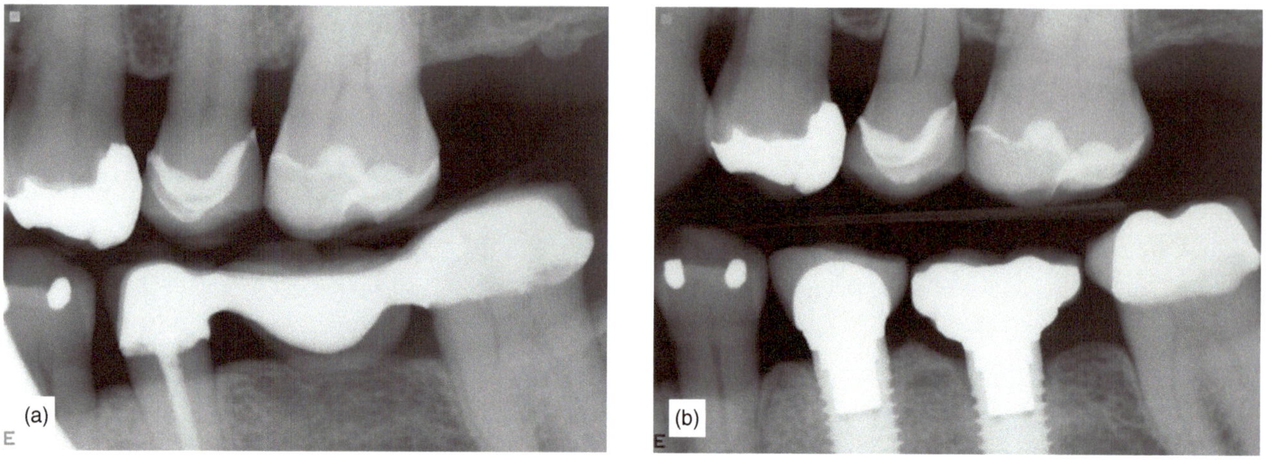

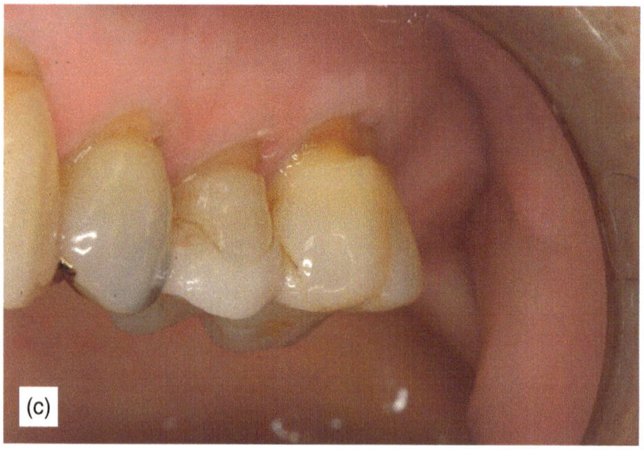

Figure 4.6 (a) X-ray of VenusCeram (Heraeus-Kulzer; pressable) onlays completed in 2000, in a heavy bruxer. (b) The same patient, 15 years later, showing the loss of bridge abutment LL bicuspid and implant replacement. (c) Fifteen-year recall onlay 13 and 14, showing no secondary caries and functional restorations.

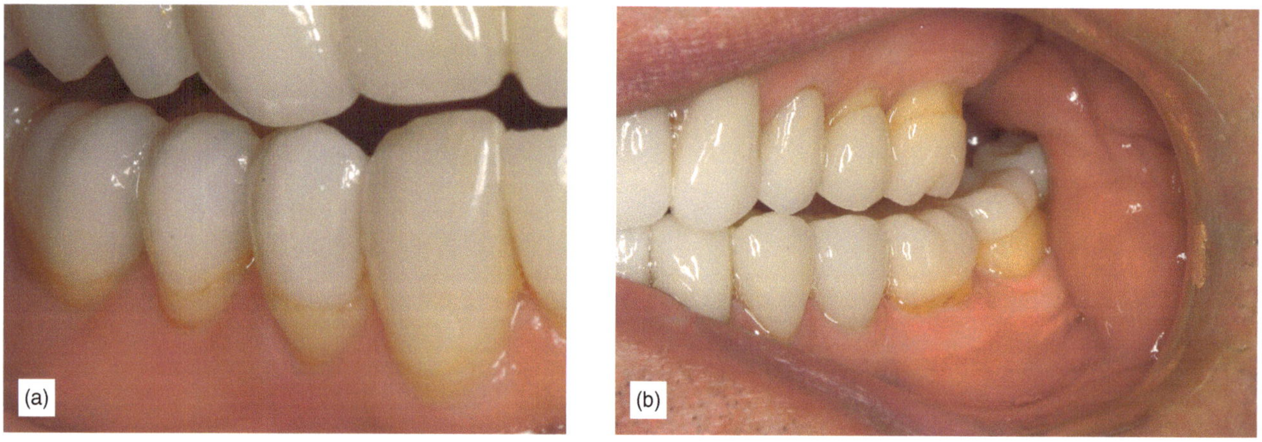

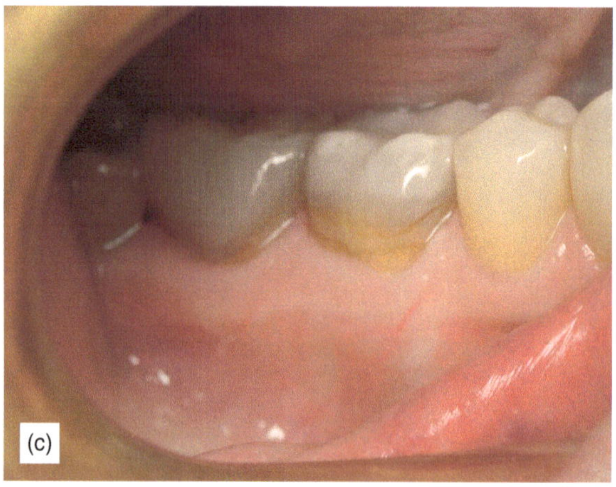

Figure 4.7 (a) 5-year postoperative onlays cemented with Clearfil™ LinerBond 2V without selective enamel etching, showing the traditional marginal staining. (b) Different 5-year postoperative onlays cemented with Clearfil LinerBond 2V without selective enamel etching, also showing margin staining. (c) One year postoperatively, showing margin staining, no selective enamel etching was done.

Figure 4.8 (a) Selective enamel etching of enamel for 10 seconds. (b) Seven years postoperatively, showing a stain-free margin using self etch bonding system and selective enamel etching.

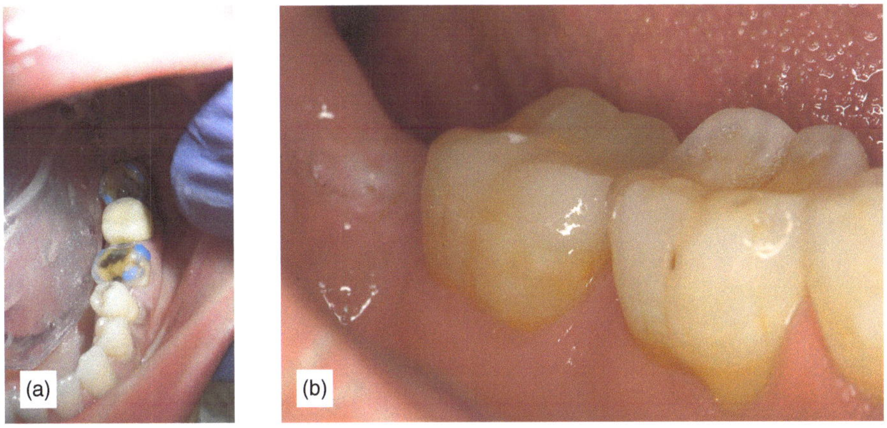

Adhesion to Dentin

Bonding to dentin has been less consistent or reliable, because dentin is a much more complex substrate to which to bond. It is 30% organic and 20% fluid (Figure 4.9). It was only after the introduction of hydrophilic resin infiltration [22] and the total etch concept [2], and subsequent improvements in the dentin bonding systems that true adhesion to dentin has become possible [3]. To define clinical success with dentin bonding, multiple factors must be taken into consideration. What makes for predictable clinical success bond strength is very important, but not the only factor to consider. What good is having amazing bond strength if postoperative sensitivity makes the restoration a failure from the patient's perspective or it ends up causing pulp damage? During early attempts to bond to dentin, the entire dental community suffered, as even the smallest direct composite restoration led to postoperative pain and much frustration. We now know that the shallowest class I restorations are the most prone to sensitivity to bite pressure. The reason for this is higher shrinkage stresses in these composites, described by configuration factors [23] (Figure 4.10). In addition to bond strength, other important characteristics are that adhesives should produce no postoperative sensitivity, should have a good marginal seal, should be easy to use, and should be durable. The issue of the durability of bond to dentin has been one of the major concerns, although newer bonding systems such as Clearfil SE Protect have improved this situation [8].

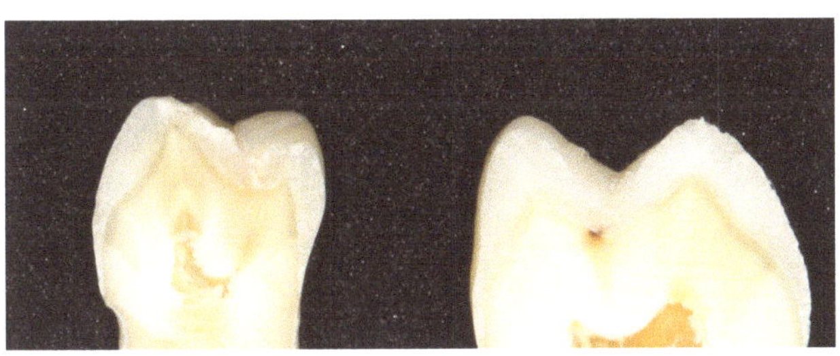

Figure 4.9 Dentin changes as it gets closer to the pulp.

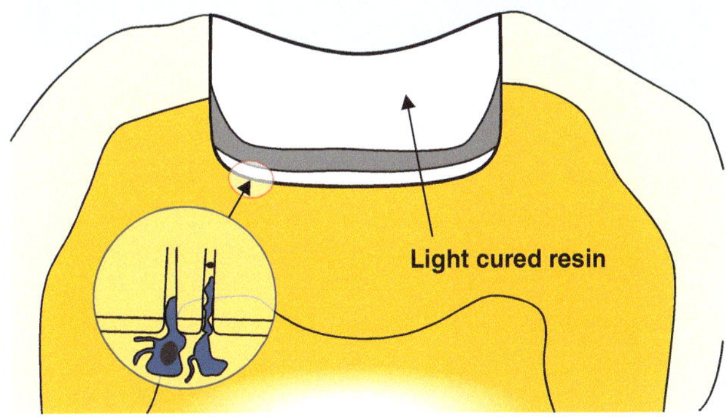

Figure 4.10 Shallow composite and micro-gap (courtesy of Dr Ray Bertolotti).

There have been different categories and names for the fourth to seventh generations of bonding systems. Regardless of the nomenclature, though, they can be divided into two families, the etch and rinse (also called "total etch") and the self-etch (Table 4.1).

Etch and Rinse Systems (Fourth and Fifth Generations)

The first generation of bonding systems to actually achieve good adhesion to dentin is the so-called fourth-generation, two-component system. This system was first introduced by Fusayama in 1979 and

Table 4.1 The bonding families.

Total Etch	Self-Etch
2 Bottles (4th generation)	2 Bottles (6th generation)
1 Bottle (5th generation)	1 Bottle (7th generation)

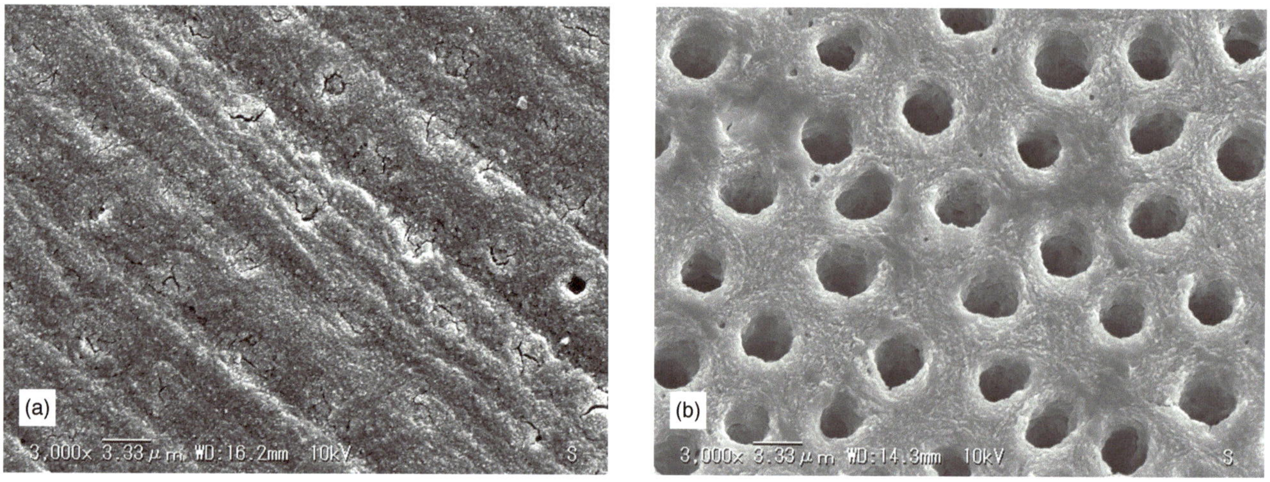

Figure 4.11 (a) Dentin before etching showing smear layer covering the tubules. (b) Scanning electron microscopy of open dentin tubules after etching (both courtesy of Dr Masafumi Kanehira).

Nakabayashi in 1982. These fourth-generation bonding systems have a long history of success.

Fourth-generation bonding systems work by acid etching the dentin and enamel with around 37% phosphoric or equivalent acid. Mineral components of both enamel and dentin dissolve. Enamel and dentin are then washed with water and the dissolved minerals are washed away, leaving the etched enamel, and the dentin with protein fibers and open exposed tubules (Figure 4.11a,b). On the now demineralized dentin and exposed tubules, a hydrophilic resin (such as hydroxyethyl methacrylate, HEMA), or dental primer, is applied. This resin goes down into the tubules, creates resin tags and infiltrates the demineralized dentin to create a hybrid layer (Figure 4.12). This mechanical/chemical adhesion is very strong. It is then reinforced by the third component, a slightly filled hydrophobic resin, making the entire complex thicker and less soluble.

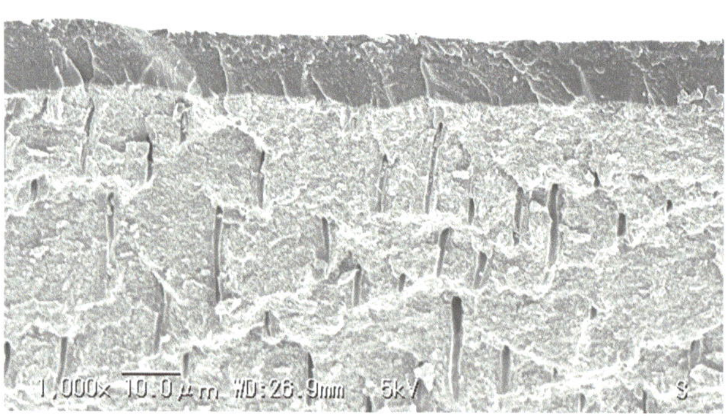

Figure 4.12 Scanning electron microscopy of hybrid layer of self-etching primer and bonding system (courtesy of Dr Masafumi Kanehira).

Fifth-generation bonding systems are contained in one bottle, which combines primer and bond in one single component. Some have questioned the benefits of mixing primer and bond. These bonding systems suffer from several problems such as shelf-life stability and transudation (Figure 4.13) [24,25].

The problems associated with total-etch bonding systems are that they can be very technique sensitive or difficult to use. One complication is that the dentin can be easily over-etched. Research shows that more than 15 seconds of etching dentin can "demineralize dentin to a depth greater than resin monomers can penetrate" [26], which will leave a layer of demineralized dentin that has not been filled with resin. This can lead to a weak bond, because this demineralized but uninfiltrated layer is subject to degradation over time, probably by the action of matrix metalloproteinases (MMPs) [27].

A second problem with total etch is that it is moisture sensitive. When minerals are removed from dentin, weak dentin fibers are supported by water or moisture (Figure 4.14) [28]. It is easy to over-dry the dentin after the phosphoric acid is washed off, allowing the fibers to collapse. It is then difficult to re-expand the collapsed fibers [29]. Additional materials have been used to revive the collapsed fibers, but this procedure adds a clinical step. Wet bonding to overcome such problems has had some limited success, but also has serious disadvantages [30]. Excessive humidity or water is undesirable, as hydrophobic resins (HEMA) only work with slight moisture. Too much is counterproductive, especially if not carefully evaporated, and remaining water

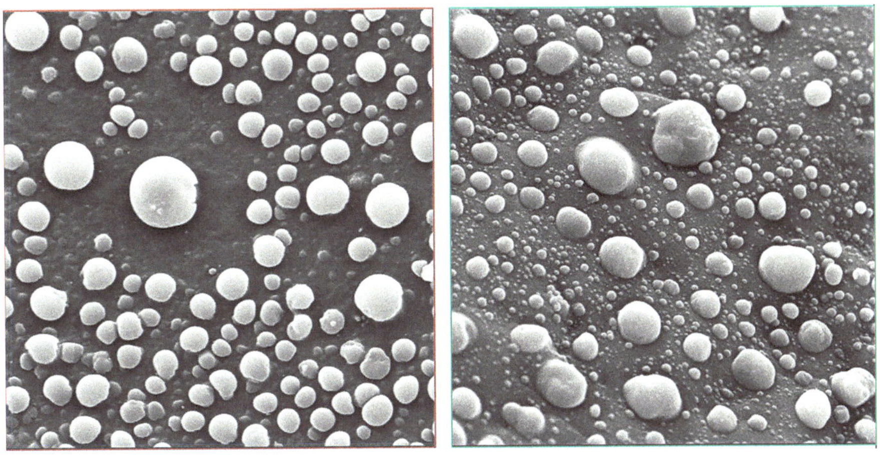

Figure 4.13 Transmission electron microscopy of transudation (contributed by Dr Franklyn Tay).

and solvents can shorten the life of the adhesion in the long term [31]. Minor errors during the total-etch procedure can also lead to postoperative sensitivity and weaker adhesion.

Total-etch systems have proven that they can be very effective adhesives, and it is possible to be very successful with such systems. Some clinicians have become masters at using them, with great success. The complexity of the total-etch technique can make it a struggle for some less-experienced clinicians and produce unsuccessful and discouraging results [32]. Reports show increased postoperative sensitivity. The results of a 2003 survey of 4,446 dentists are shown in Table 4.2 [33]. Literature is very clear that postoperative sensitivity has plagued the profession [34]. Looking at this from a realistic clinical perspective, postoperative sensitivity is one of the worst enemies of a happy dental practice.

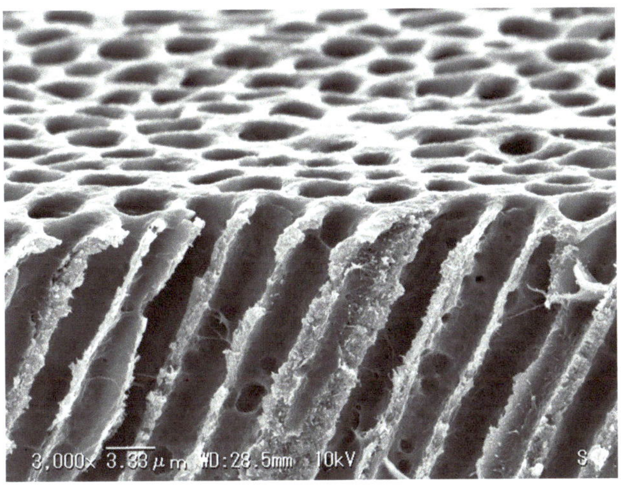

Figure 4.14 Scanning electron microscopy of vertical fractured dehydrated dentin tubules after etching (courtesy of Dr Masafumi Kanehira).

Table 4.2 Postoperative sensitivity in self-etch and total-etch systems.

Postoperative sensitivity	Self-etch (%)	Total-etch (%)
None	24	12
Severe	4	17

Source: Christensen G. Self-etch primer (SEP) adhesives update. *CRA Newsletter*, 2003; 27(11/12): 1–5.

For all of the above reasons, an entirely new category of dentin bonding systems has been developed, which may better fulfill the requirements of an ideal bonding system, the self-etch bonding systems.

Self-Etch Systems (Sixth and Seventh Generations)

Self-etch bonding systems originally comprised two components. These were called sixth-generation systems. The first component "primer" is an acidic resin, which replaces the need for phosphoric acid as a dentin etch. When the primer is applied to dentin, the smear layer dissolves, forming a hybrid layer, and the primer mixes with the smear plugs to reinforce them. At no time are the dentin tubules open. It is not necessary nor desirable to rinse with water after priming. The benefit of using an acidic resin as both the etching agent and primer is that, unlike in total-etch systems, there is no possibility for the etching agent to go deeper than the resin primer, because they are one and the same. The occluded dentinal tubules prevent fluid movement from the pulp, which prevents postoperative sensitivity to bite pressure.

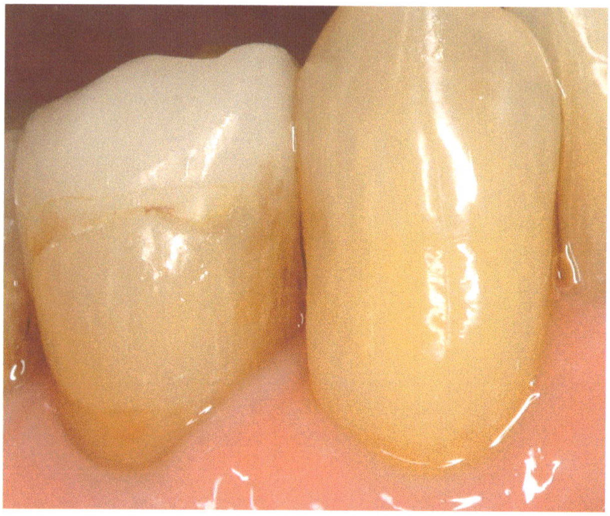

Figure 4.15 5-year yellow and brown margin on onlay cemented with self-etch bonding systems.

The second great benefit of self-etch dentin systems is that because dentin is never demineralized, rinsed and left unprotected, the issue of fiber collapse and the perfect level of moisture is nonexistent. Moisture level is not a concern, as there is no demineralization and thus no unprotected fibers. Warner Finger's research confirms insensitivity to moisture and suggests that because of such tolerance, a rubber dam is not compulsory, as it can often be with total-etch systems, because of the sensitivity to moisture of total-etch systems [35,36].

Once the solvents from the primer are removed, the second component, a lightly filled hydrophobic resin is applied. It serves to strengthen the layer and increase the hydrophobia and durability of the entire complex. The water-free second layer prevents "transudation" – the movement of pulpal fluid through water rich zones in the hybrid layer [24].

Clinical experience shows that one flaw of some self-etch systems is their inability to etch enamel ideally, especially uncut enamel. Etching success varies with the system being used. As many dentists have discovered, using some systems as the manufacturers recommend leaves the patient with yellow or brown margins (Figure 4.15) and the possibility of redeveloping caries on the same tooth. In 2004, I performed a study with Warner Finger, inventor of iBond® (Heraeus Kulzer), a seventh-generation system. This study compared the use of iBond only versus etching the enamel first with phosphoric acid and then using iBond (Figure 4.16a,b) [20]. The study concluded that bond strength is doubled when enamel is etched prior to placing the bonding system. Selective enamel etching also increases the marginal seal [21,37,38], significantly reducing the risk of recurrent caries and the hated brown and yellow margins [39]. I suggest a 10-second selective etch protocol, focusing specially on the uncut enamel (Figure 4.17). When selective etching enamel is used, it is important to avoid dentin etching. There is always the chance of human error, and some etch may touch the superficial dentin. One study demonstrated that there is no significant decrease in bond strength when dentin is accidentally etched for a short period of time, although it is important to avoid allowing the etch to get anywhere close to deep dentin [40]. Care must be taken to minimize etching of the dentin to avoid the possibility

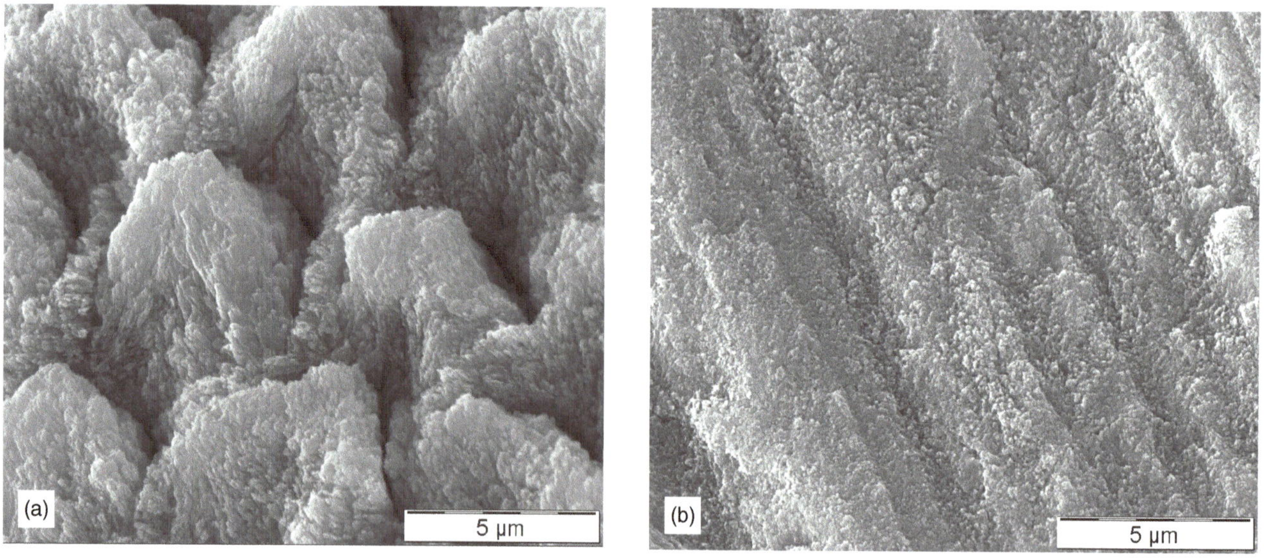

Figure 4.16 Enamel appearance: (a) With phosphoric acid etch, observe the nice micro-mechanical retentive features. (b) Appearance using a self-etch bonding system only.

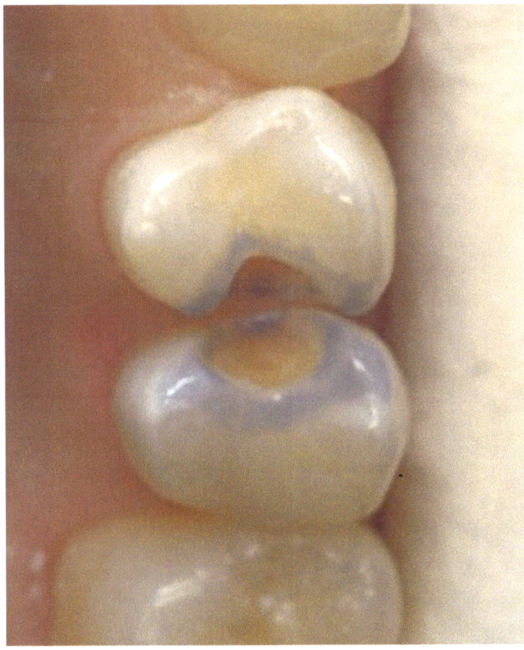

Figure 4.17 Selective etching focusing mostly on uncut enamel.

of sensitivity to bite pressure created by opening dentinal tubules, especially if the tubules of deeper dentin are opened.

An alternative technique for direct restorations, to eliminate the possibility of dentin etching and opening tubules, is to finish the preparation, perform the bonding procedure with both primer and bond, as previously described, and to follow this with correct curing and the first layer of flowable composite and cure. Then carefully clean the enamel with a diamond to remove the bonding layer, etch the enamel and bond with only the second component. Add a hydrophobic bond to the enamel. A primer is not necessary unless dentin is exposed. For indirect cases, sealing the dentin straight after tooth preparation is an option, often called immediate dentin sealing.

A huge benefit with self-etch systems is the increased durability of dentin bonding. Research and clinical experience shows that bonding to dentin with total-etch systems decreases over time. Studies show that total-etch systems require some moisture to be left behind, which can lead to long-term degradation of the dentin–adhesive union [41,42,43]. This can be caused by multiple factors, the risk of over-etching and improper resin infiltration, and some demineralized dentin left under-filled, which weakens the dentin in the long term. MMPs could also be a factor, and it is desirable to inhibit the activity of MMPs ether by the use of chlorhexidine [44] or a bonding system such as the antibacterial monomer 12-methacryloyloxydodecylpyridinium bromide and fluoride release, which have been shown to be MMP inhibitors [45]. Good quality self-etch bonding systems have shown improved durability [7,46]. Using Clearfil SE Protect, a modification of Clearfil SE Bond [47], Tagami has demonstrated the formation of a dentin layer that is more durable and resistant to acid, which he calls "super dentin" (Figure 4.18a,b). Another successful adhesive gaining in popularity is Prelude™ Self-Etch (Danville). This adhesive works in both self-etch and total-etch modes and additionally can work as dual curing.

Although many experts continue to suggest that total etch is the gold standard, the literature and clinical experience has shown that the best self-etch bonding systems can have many advantages over total etch. They can out-perform total etch in bond strength [48,49]. Self-etch

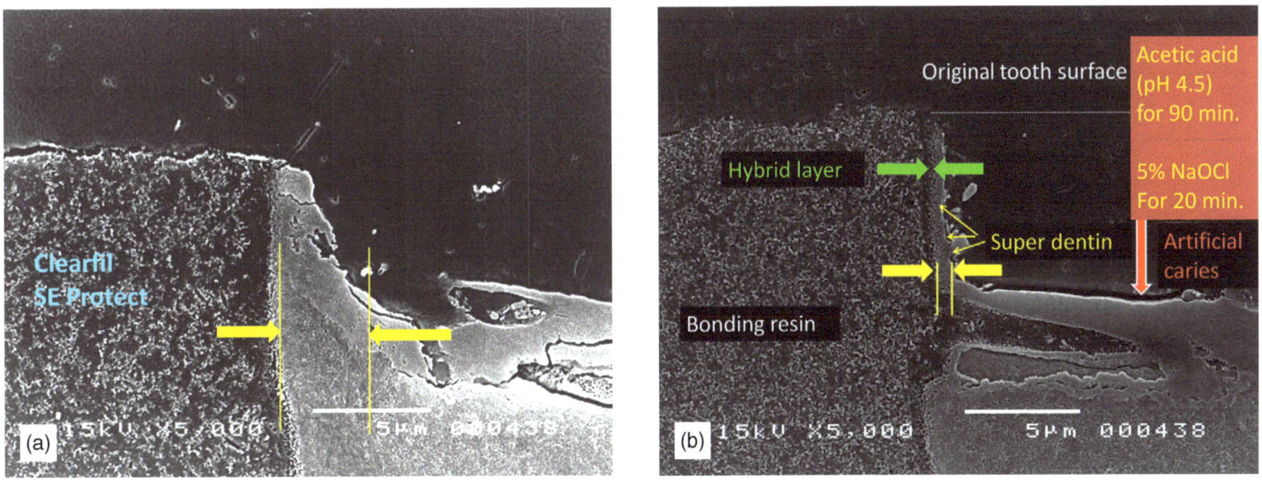

Figure 4.18 (a) and (b) Scanning electron microscopy of "super dentin" (acid-resistant dentin) (courtesy of Dr Jugi Tagami).

bonds are better designed to minimize or eliminate postoperative sensitivity. Optimal enamel adhesion and seal can be achieved with selective enamel etching. Adhesion to dentin is more durable when using self-etch systems. Self-etch systems are easier to use without the concern of over etching or moisture control. For all of these reasons, the best self-etch system should be considered the new gold standard for clinical dentistry.

Isolation and Adhesive Dentistry

It is clear that bonding of resin-based composites is completely intolerant of contamination. This reality may move many to consider that a rubber dam is mandatory when performing any adhesive procedures [50]. Clinical experience (Figure 4.19) and evidence from the literature does not support the superiority of the rubber dam and shows that, with correct technique, isolation can be achieved with cotton roll isolation or other isolation means with equally positive results [51,52]. While excellent isolation is mandatory, achieving such isolation depends on preference, practice style, and skill level with each isolation technique. Clinical reality shows that rubber dam isolation is used by less than 22% of practicing clinicians for restorative dentistry [53]. Suggesting that rubber dam isolation is mandatory for adhesive dentistry, also adds an undue burden to many practitioners and may discourage some from performing adhesive dentistry. I taught at the University of Southern California for close to a decade, and can attest that a large number of teeth isolated with a rubber dam were far from isolated (Figure 4.20). As with any procedure in dentistry, technique is crucial, and in many cases it is impossible to successfully use a rubber dam. The use of self-etch bonding systems, which are more tolerant of moisture levels [54] and following supragingival protocols makes achieving proper isolation easier with any isolation technique. Finally it must be emphasized that maximum isolation is mandatory.

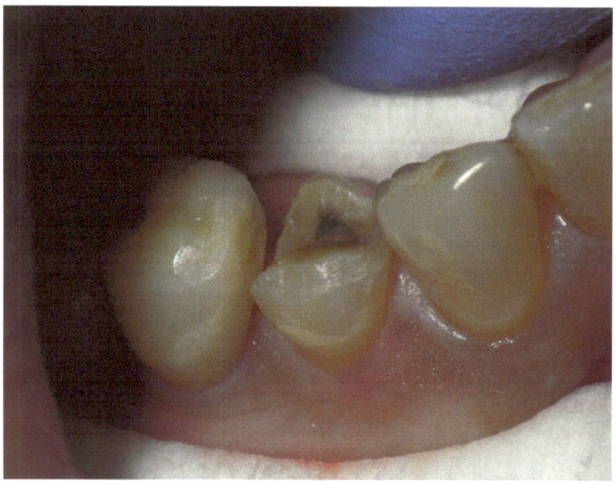

Figure 4.19 Non-rubber dam isolation showing excellent moisture control.

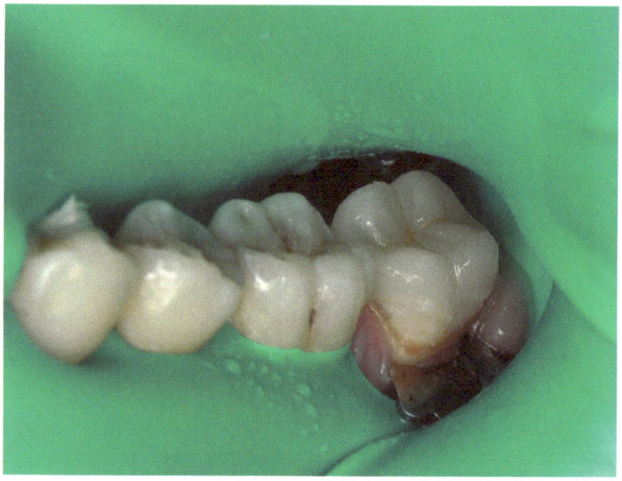

Figure 4.20 Rubber dam isolation showing leaks.

The Importance of Technique

The operator plays a leading role in the success of the procedure. The same materials and the same tooth in the hands of different clinicians can render considerably variable results [55,56,57]. Meticulous technique is needed for success. There are a few key steps required for optimal adhesion to occur with a self-etch bonding system.

Step-by-Step Bonding Procedure

Step 1

Remove infected dentin correctly using traditional instrumentation, and check with a caries indicator to avoid removing affected dentin, which can remineralize (Figure 4.21a). For further details of correct caries removal, see Chapter 10.

Step 2

Immediately after preparation, isolate the tooth, and do not allow saliva or any contaminant to touch it, to avoid unnecessary contamination. Excellent isolation is imperative.

Step 3

It is desirable to apply a selective enamel 35–37% phosphoric acid etch for 10 seconds, using a thick no-droop etchant (such as SureEtch® Gel, Danville), limiting the etch to the enamel and focusing primarily on the uncut enamel, avoiding dentin as much as possible. Careful

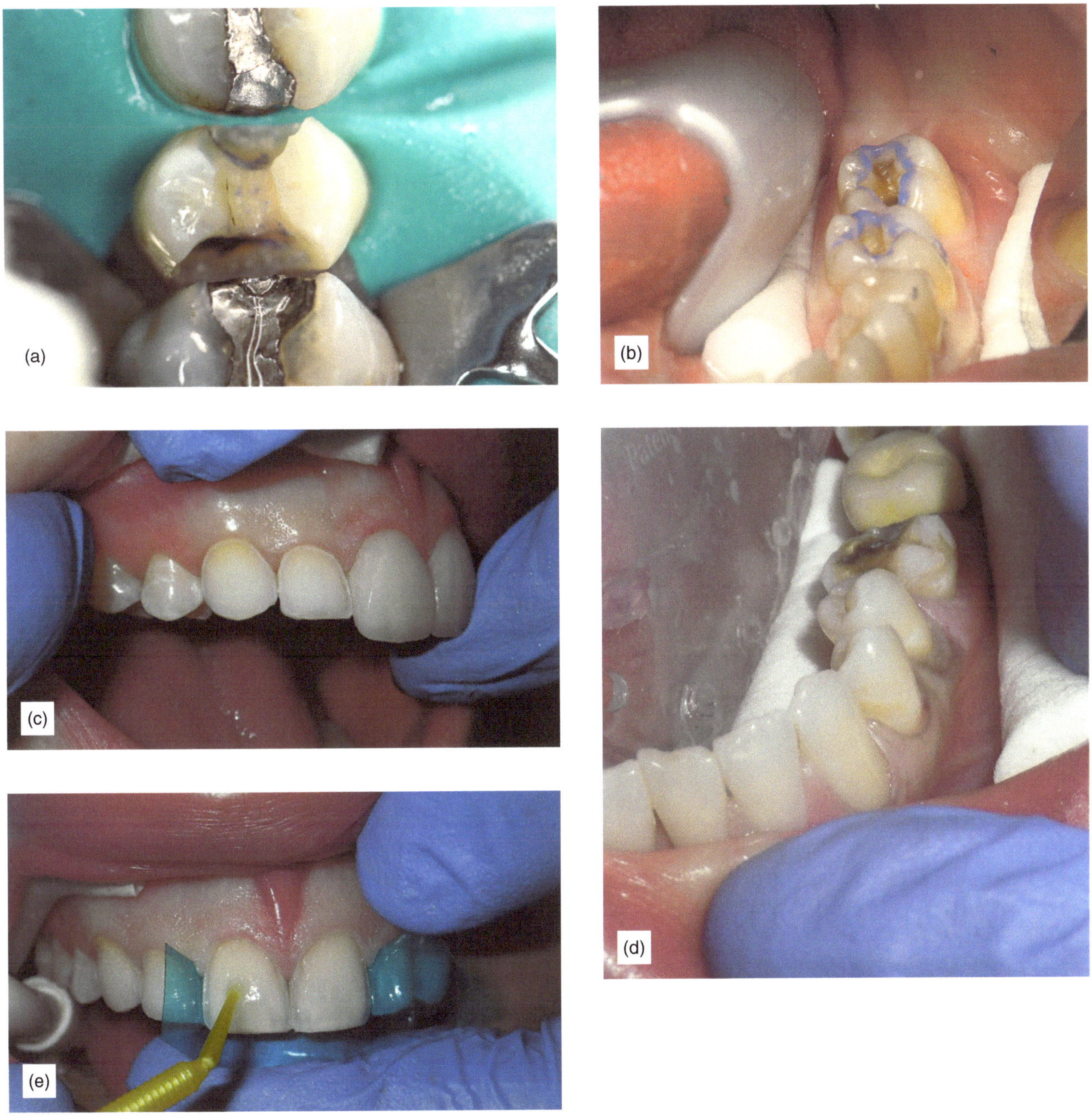

Figure 4.21 (a) Deep cavity showing the use of caries indicator. (b) PropGard® (Ultradent) isolation and selective enamel etching, focusing primarily on the uncut enamel. (c) Veneer preparations showing frosted appearance after etch and dry. (d) Posterior tooth onlay cementation showing dry enamel (frosty). (e) Primer applied for 20–25 seconds.

technique is important (Figure 4.21b). It may be unavoidable that a small amount of etchant comes into contact with the superficial dentin. This will produce only minor consequences, unless it reaches deeper dentin (close to the pulp), which is very undesirable. If such contact occurs, immediately rinse with water, and re-etch the enamel with more accuracy. If deep dentin is etched, the tubules will open. To minimize the possibility of postoperative sensitivity in such a scenario, apply GLUMA® (Kulzer GmbH) or Microprime™ G (Danville) desensitizer for 40 seconds to the dentin. This will minimize the consequences.

An alternative technique to the above, which is more time consuming but guarantees no accidental etching of the dentin, would be to apply self-etching bond to both enamel and dentin, and cure. Optionally apply a layer of flowable composite to the dentin, cure, and then clean the enamel margins and etch with phosphoric acid. Wash, dry (or leave damp, depending on the bond), then reapply the bond. When using Clearfil, both the primer and the bond need to be reapplied. If Prelude SE is being used, only the adhesive (#2) need be applied and cured.

Step 4

Wash and dry the etchant. Because the dentin has not been etched before priming, collapsing the dentin is not a concern, so drying can be accomplished safely with an air–water syringe. Drying is beneficial in self-etching systems. The enamel should look frosty and the dentin should not be shiny, but avoid desiccating the tooth (Figure 4.21c,d).

Step 5

Use a good quality two-component self-etching system, such as Clearfil SE Bond or Clearfil SE Protect, or Prelude SE. Newer one-component self-etching bonding systems are also a possibility, but most research shows that two components are better than one.

Step 5a

Apply a bonding system liberally with a microbrush to both dentin and enamel, agitating the dentin primer on the dentin for 20–25 seconds (Figure 4.21e).

Step 6

Removing the solvent in the primer is a major concern. More than 90% of the primer is solvent, and any solvent left on the tooth will have a counterproductive effect on the success of the bond and its longevity. The solvent can be evaporated by an air stream – and the only way to be sure that the solvent has been thoroughly evaporated is through visual confirmation. The air stream will move the liquid primer, and the motion of the liquid will decrease as the solvent evaporates, until it stops moving, at which time we will know that the solvent has evaporated. Incomplete drying of the solvent can lead to significant leakage, one of the most common errors in using these systems. It is simply impossible to over dry. Attention must be placed on the source of the air stream; the air should be uncontaminated and dry. The high-velocity vacuum should be used next to the tooth to evacuate the solvent pushed away from the tooth by the blast of air.

Step 7

Step 7a

When using a two-component system (sixth generation) such as Clearfil SE Protect, apply the second component then thin it. After applying the second layer, this "bond" layer should be thinned to prevent radiolucency of a thick layer. An effective method is to dry a microbrush, then wick the excess bond layer. The manufacturer's suggestion of air-blow thinning does not appear to be as effective as wicking. The second layer of Prelude SE is also air blown. It does not need thinning, since it is already very thin, but we do need to evaporate some solvent (which is present to thin the material).

Step 7b

For indirect restorations, mix the second component, the hydrophobic adhesive, with the dual cure catalyst. It should be applied thinly.

Step 8

Step 8a

Cure for a full cycle. Incorrect curing is a significant factor in the failure of bonded restorations. With direct procedures, the bonding system would be cured at this point.

Step 8b

With indirect procedures, the bond will be left uncured, and both bond and cement are cured at the same time [57]. If you are using Prelude SE, it is so thin that it may be cured at this time with no concern about affecting the restoration fit. A detailed technique for adhesive luting of indirect restorations is explained in Chapter 9.

Sealing Deep Dentin and Buildup for Indirect Procedures

The traditional bonding techniques presented above have decades of success, but in some indirect cases where caries is very deep, less than 2 mm to the pulp, pulp protection may be desirable (Figure 4.22). Traditionally, resin-reinforced glass ionomer liners have been successfully used for direct restorations with deep dentin [58], but for very deep indirect restorations "immediate dentin sealing" has shown excellent results. This method has additional advantages, such as enhanced adhesion to fresh dentin, pulp protection and decreased postoperative sensitivity [59,60,61]. In cases where reinforcement of one or more fractured cusps is necessary, or in badly

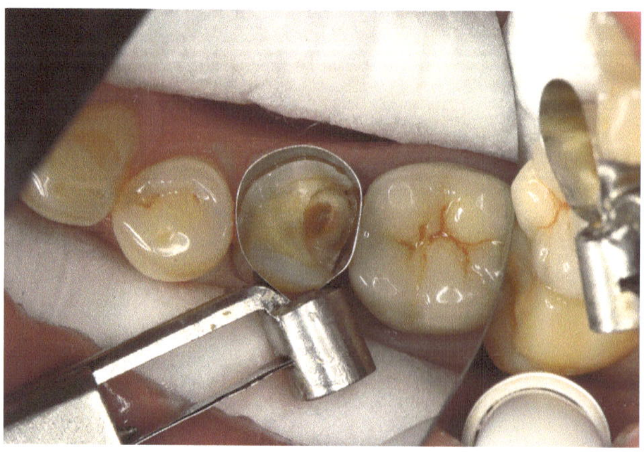

Figure 4.22 Very deep cavity needing buildup and dentin sealing.

damaged teeth, endodontically treated teeth needing buildup or where cervical margin will end up on dentin, immediate dentin sealing can enhance success. It is most practical to seal the deep dentin at the same time as building the tooth, reinforcing the damaged cusp, fixing large undercuts and elevating the margins on deep subgingival cavosurface margins, or any other desired buildup.

Sealing dentin is not necessary or desirable in every case, because there are also some disadvantages that must be considered. It is time consuming and it complicates provisionalization. For this reason, deep dentin sealing and buildup should be reserved for badly damaged teeth. Experience and a long history of using the traditional approach of tooth preparation and impression without sealing dentin, as described in the literature, suggests that it has been extremely successful and predictable (Figure 4.23). It is important to remember that to achieve good adhesion when the dentin is not sealed, it is necessary to thoroughly clean the dentin and the enamel before cementation. Using an intraoral sand blaster will provide excellent results. Proper selection of preimpression and cementation techniques are discussed in detail in Chapters 6 and 7.

Technique for Deep Dentin Sealing and Buildup

Step 1
Remove infected dentin correctly, using traditional instrumentation in addition to checking with a chemical caries indicator, to avoid removing affected dentin, which can remineralize.

Step 2
Immediately after preparation, isolate the tooth, and do not allow saliva or any contaminant to touch tooth, to avoid contamination. Excellent isolation is imperative.

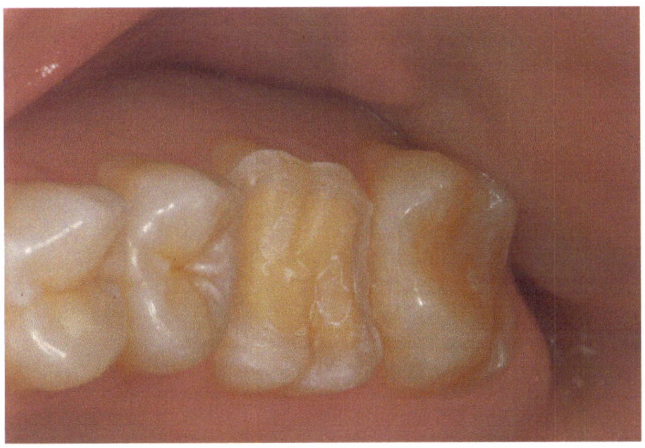

Figure 4.23 Regular preparation where dentin sealing was not necessary.

Step 3
Apply a selective enamel etch using phosphoric acid for 10 seconds, only if enamel margin preservation or enamel cusp reinforcement will be performed at this point. If no enamel is to be reinforced, go to step 5. It is preferable to have fresh enamel to bond final restoration.

Step 4
Wash and dry etchant, as described above. If no enamel is to be reinforced, go to step 5.

Step 5
Apply preferred bonding system liberally with a microbrush to the dentin (and the enamel if it is being reinforced), agitating the dentin primer on the dentin for 20–25 seconds.

Step 6
Remove the solvent as previously described.

Step 7
If a two-component system (sixth generation) material is being used, apply a thin layer of the second component, then wick the extra off the tooth with a dry microbrush.

Step 8
Cure, as previously described.

Step 9
Apply a thin layer, less than 1 mm, of a highly filled, highly radiopaque flowable material.

Step 10
If there is a great deal of damage or a large undercut, or margin elevation, build up as necessary with a restorative composite, and cure. A detailed description of the technique is given in Chapter 3.

Step 11
Use an oxygen inhibitor, to do a final cure. It is known that resin-based composite does not cure in the presence of oxygen. Using a layer of glycerin-based gel, which excludes oxygen, will ensure proper curing of the entire composite.

Step 12
Retouch the preparation, remove any composite or bonding system from the enamel and take a final impression with a high-quality impression material or make a digital impression.

Conclusion

Good Bonding System + Good Technique = Success

Adhesion has changed the face of restorative dentistry. Much is owed to the pioneers of adhesive dentistry, and advances are happening every day. Today, we have adhesives and the techniques necessary for success. The above formula sums up this chapter, and each factor it contains has been well-defined. Total-etch and self-etch systems have proved themselves to be successful, as they are the result of the dental profession overcoming the complexities of adhesion to human tissues. Currently, self-etch systems are clinically preferable to total-etch, for several reasons. The best bonding system is nothing without proper technique implemented by the clinician. Success has been defined as strong adhesion, no postoperative sensitivity, a proper seal, ease of use, and durability. All these elements are found when we couple a good bonding system with good technique.

References

1 Buonocore MG. A simple method of increasing the adhesion of acrylic filling materials to enamel surfaces. *J Dent Res*, 1955; 34(6): 849–853.
2 Fusayama T, Nakamura M, Kurosaki N, Iwaku M. Non-pressure adhesion of a new adhesive restorative resin. *J Dent Res*, 1979; 58(4): 1364–1370.
3 Bertolotti RL. Total etch: The rational dentin bonding protocol. *J Esthet Dent*, 1991; 3(1): 1–6.
4 Adhesives and Sealants: Transportation. Adhesives .org. http://www.adhesives.org/adhesives-sealants/market-overview-applications/transportation (accessed November 2016).
5 Structural Bonding of Aircraft Airframes and Components, 3M, 2016. http://solutions.3m.com/wps/portal/3M/en_EU/AerospaceSolutions/Home/Applications/StructuralBondingAircraftComponents (accessed November 2016).
6 Uludag B, Yucedag E, Sahin V. Microleakage of inlay ceramic systems luted with self-adhesive resin cements. *J Adhes Dent*, 2014; 16(6): 523–529.
7 Donmez N, Belli S, Pashley DH, Tay FR. Ultrastructural correlates of in vivo/in vitro bond degradation in self-etch adhesives. *J Dent Res*, 2005; 84(4): 355–359.
8 Kramer N, Frankenberger R. Clinical performance of bonded leucite-reinforced glass ceramic inlays and onlays after 8 years. *Dent Mater*, 2005; 21: 267–271.
9 Lacy AM, Wada C, Du W, Watanabe L. In vitro microleakage at the gingival margin of porcelain and resin veneers. *J Prosthet Dent*, 1992; 67(1): 7–10.
10 Gurel, G. Influence of enamel preservation on failure rates of porcelain laminate veneers. *Int J Restor Dent*, 2013; 33(1): 31–39.
11 Burke, J. Survival rates for porcelain laminate veneers with special reference to the effect of preparation in dentin: a literature review. *J Esthet Restor Dent*, 2012; 24(4): 257–265.
12 Gurel, G. Clinical performance of porcelain laminate veneers: outcomes of the aesthetic pre-evaluative temporary (APT) technique. *Int J Periodont Restor Dent*, 2012; 32(6): 625–635.
13 Gresnigt, M. Esthetic rehabilitation of anterior teeth with porcelain laminates and sectional veneers. *J Can Dent Assoc*, 2011; 77: b143.
14 Opdam NJ, Bronkhorst EM, Roeters JM, Loomans BA. A retrospective clinical study on longevity of posterior composite and amalgam restorations. *Dent Mater*, 2007; 23(1): 2–8.
15 Gaengler P, Hoyer I Montag R, Gaebler P. Micromorphological evaluation of posterior composites: A 10 year report. *J Oral Rehab*, 2004; 31(10): 991–1000.
16 Ruiz JL, Christensen GJ, Sameni A, Vargas L. Clinical performance of bonded ceramic and resin based composite inlays and onlays using self-etch bonding system: a 51-month report. *Inside Dent*, 2007; 3(5): 62–65.
17 Beier, US. Clinical long-term evaluation and failure characteristics of 1,335 all-ceramic restorations. *Int J Prosthodont*, 2012; 25(1): 70–78.
18 Fasbinder DJ. Clinical performance of chairside CAD/CAM restorations. *J Am Dent Assoc*, 2006; 137; 25s–31s.
19 Barghi N, Barry TG. Clinical evaluation of etched porcelain onlays: a 4-year report. *Compend Contin Educ Dent*, 2002; 23(7): 657–664.
20 Finger W, Endo T, Ruiz JL. Conventional and self-etching adhesive effects on retention of luting resins. *J Dent Res*, 2005; 84(A): Abstract 2672.
21 Perdigão J, Dutra-Corrêa M, Anauate-Netto C, Castilhos N, Carmo AR, Lewgoy HR, Amore R, Cordeiro HJ. Two-year clinical evaluation of self-etch adhesives in posterior restorations. *J Adhes Dent*, 11(2): 129–159.
22 Nakabayashi N, Kojima K, Masuhara E. The promotion of adhesion by the infiltration of monomers into tooth substrates. *J Biomed Mater Res*, 1982; 16(3): 265–273.
23 Yoshikawa T, Burrow MF, Tagami J. The effects of bonding system and light curing method on reducing stress of different C-factor cavities. *J Adhes Dent*, 2001; 3(2): 177–183.
24 Tay FR, Frankenberger R, Krejci I, Bouillaguet S, Pashley DH, Carvalho RM, Lai CN. Single-bottle adhesives behave as permeable membranes after polymerization. I. In vivo evidence. *J Dent*, 2004; 32(8): 611–621.
25 Sauro S, Watson TF, Tay FR, Chersoni S, Breschi L, Bernardi F, Prati C. Water uptake of bonding systems applied on root dentin surfaces: a SEM and confocal microscopic study. *Dent Mater*, 2006; 22(7): 671–680.
26 Abu-Hanna A, Gordan VV, Mjor I. The effect of variation in etching times on dentin bonding. *Gen Dent*, 2004; 52(1): 28–33.

27 Brackett MG, Li N, Brackett WW, Sword RJ, Qi YP, Niu LN, Pucci CR, Dib A, Pashley DH, Tay FR. The critical barrier to progress in dentine bonding with the etch-and-rinse technique. *J Dent*, 2011; 39(3): 238–248.

28 Carvalho RM, Yoshiyama M, Pashley EL, Pashley DM. In vitro study on the dimensional change of human dentin after demineralization. *Arch Oral Biol*, 1996; 41(4): 369–377.

29 Carvalho RM, Mendonça JS, Santiago SL, Silveira RR, Garcia FC, Tay FR, Pashley DH. Effect of HEMA/Solvent combination on bond strength to dentin. *J Dent Res*, 2003; 82(8): 597–601.

30 Kanca J III. Improving bond strength through acid etching of dentin and bonding to wet dentin surfaces. *J Am Dent Assoc*, 1992; 123(9): 35–43.

31 Tay F, Pashley D. Water treeing—a potential mechanism for degradation of dentin adhesives. *Am J Dent*, 2003; 16: 6–12.

32 Perdigão J, Geraldeli S, Hodges JS. Total etch versus self etch adhesives, effects on postoperative sensitivity. *J Am Dent Assoc*, 2003; 134(12): 1621–1629.

33 Christensen G. Self-etch primer (SEP) adhesives update. *CRA Newsletter*, 2003; 27(11/12): 1–5.

34 Berkowitz G, Horowitz A et al. Postoperative hypersensitivity in class I resin-based composite restorations in general practice: Interim Results. *Compend Contin Educ Dent*, 2009; 30(6): 356–363.

35 Werner JF, Tani C. Effect of relative humidity on bond strength of self-etching adhesives to dentin. *J Adhes Dent*, 2002; 4(4): 277–282.

36 Armstrong SR, Vargas MA, Chung I, Pashley DH, Campbell JA, Laffoon JE, Quin F. Resin–dentin interfacial ultrastructure and microtensile dentin bond strength after five-year water storage. *Operative Dent*, 2004; 29(6); 705–712.

37 Peumans M, De Munck J, Van Landuyt K, Lambrechts P, Van Meerbeek B. Five-year clinical effectiveness of a two-step self-etching adhesive. *J Adhes Dent*, 2007; 9(1): 7–10.

38 Perdigao J, Monteiro P II, Gomes G. Enamel sealing ability of self-etch adhesives. American Association of Dental Research, 37th Annual Meeting and Exhibition, Dallas, Texas. Abstract no. 0360.

39 Fabianelli A, Kugel G, Ferrari M. Efficacy of self-etching primer on sealing margins of class II restorations. *Am J Dent*, 2003; 16(1): 37–41.

40 Ruiz JL, Kobashigawa A. Bond strength of SE adhesives with phosphoric acid etching. *J Dent Res*, 2007; 87(A): Abstract 0827.

41 Burrow MF, Harada N, Kitasako Y, Nikaido T, Tagami J. Seven-year dentin bond strength of a total- and self-etch system. *Eur J Oral Sci*, 2005; 113(3): 265–270.

42 Yamauti M, Hashimoto M, Sano H, Ohno H, Carvalho RM, Kaga M, Tagami J, Oguchi H, Kubota M. Degradation of resin-dentin bonds using NaOCI storage. *Dent Mater*, 2003; 19(5): 399–405.

43 Braem M. Microshear fatigue testing of tooth adhesives interface. *J Adhes Dent*, 2001; 9(Suppl 2): 249–253.

44 Breschi L, Mazzoni A, Nato F, Carrilho M, Visintini E, Tjäderhane L, Ruggeri A Jr, Tay FR, Dorigo Ede S, Pashley DH. Chlorhexidine stabilizes the adhesive interface: a 2-year in vitro study. *Dent Mater*, 2010; 26(4): 320–325.

45 Pashley DH, Tay FR, Imazato S. How to increase the durability of resin-dentin bonds. *Compend Contin Educ Dent*, 2011; 32(7): 60–66.

46 Waldyasekera K, Nikaido T, Weerasinghe DS, Ichinose S, Tagami J. Reinforcement of dentin in self-etch adhesive technology: a new concept. *J Dent*, 2009; 37: 604–609.

47 Imazato S, Kinomoto Y, Tarumi H, Torii M, Russell RR, McCabe JF. Incorporation of antibacterial monomer MDPB into dentin primer. *J Dent Res*, 1997;76(3): 768–772.

48 Cura C, Saraçoglu A, Cötert HS. Effect of different bonding agents on sheer bond strengths of composite-bonded porcelain to enamel. *J Prosthet Dent*, 2003: 89(4): 394–399.

49 Türkun LS. The clinical performance of one and two step self-etch adhesive systems at one year. *J Am Dent Assoc*, 2005; 136(5): 656–664.

50 Magne P, Belser U. Try-in and adhesive luting procedures, in *Bonded Porcelain Restorations in the Anterior Dentition: A Biomimetic Approach*. Chicago: Quintessence Publishing, 2002, pp. 335–370.

51 Reich S, Wichmann M, Rinne H, Shortall A. Clinical performance of large all ceramic CA-CAM generated restorations. *J Am Dent Assoc*, 2004; 135(5): 605–612.

52 Thordrup M, Isidor F, Horsted-Bindslev P. A 5 year study of direct and indirect resin composite and ceramic inlays. *Quintessence Int*, 2001; 32(3): 199–205.

53 Christensen GJ. Real world moisture control, to dam or not to dam. *Clin Rep*, 2015; 8(5): 1, 3.

54 Peumans M, Kanumilli P. Clinical effectiveness of contemporary adhesives: a systematic review of current clinical trials. *Dent Mater*, 2005; 21(9): 864–881.

55 Sensi LG, Lopes GC, Monteiro S Jr, Baratieri LN. Dentin bond strength of self-etching primers/adhesives. *Oper Dent*, 2005; 30(1): 63–68.

56 Soderholm KJ, Soares F. Shear bond strength of one etch-and-rinse and five self-etching dental adhesives when used by six operators. *Acta Odontol Scand*, 2008; 66(4): 243–249.

57 Ruiz JL, Powers J, Yapp R. Bond Strength of Resin Cements to Dentin. *J Dent Res*, 2008; 87(A): abstract no. 1816.

58 Ruiz JL, Mitra S. Using cavity liners with direct posterior composite restorations. *Compend Contin Educ Dent*, 2006; 27(6): 347–351.

59 Magne P. Immediate dentin sealing; a fundamental procedure for indirect bonded restorations. *J Esthet Restor Dent*, 2005; 17(3): 144–155.

60 Cohen RG, Razzano MV. Immediate dentin sealing using an antibacterial self-etching bonding system. *Pract Proceed Aesthet Dent*, 2006; 18(9): 561–565.

61 Magne P, So WS, Cascione D. Immediate dentin sealing supports delayed restoration placement. *J Prosthet Dent*, 2007; 98(3): 165–174.

Part II

Supragingival Minimally Invasive Indirect Posterior Restorations: A Replacement for Full Crowns

5

Supragingival Minimally Invasive Bonded Onlays: The Replacement for Full Crowns

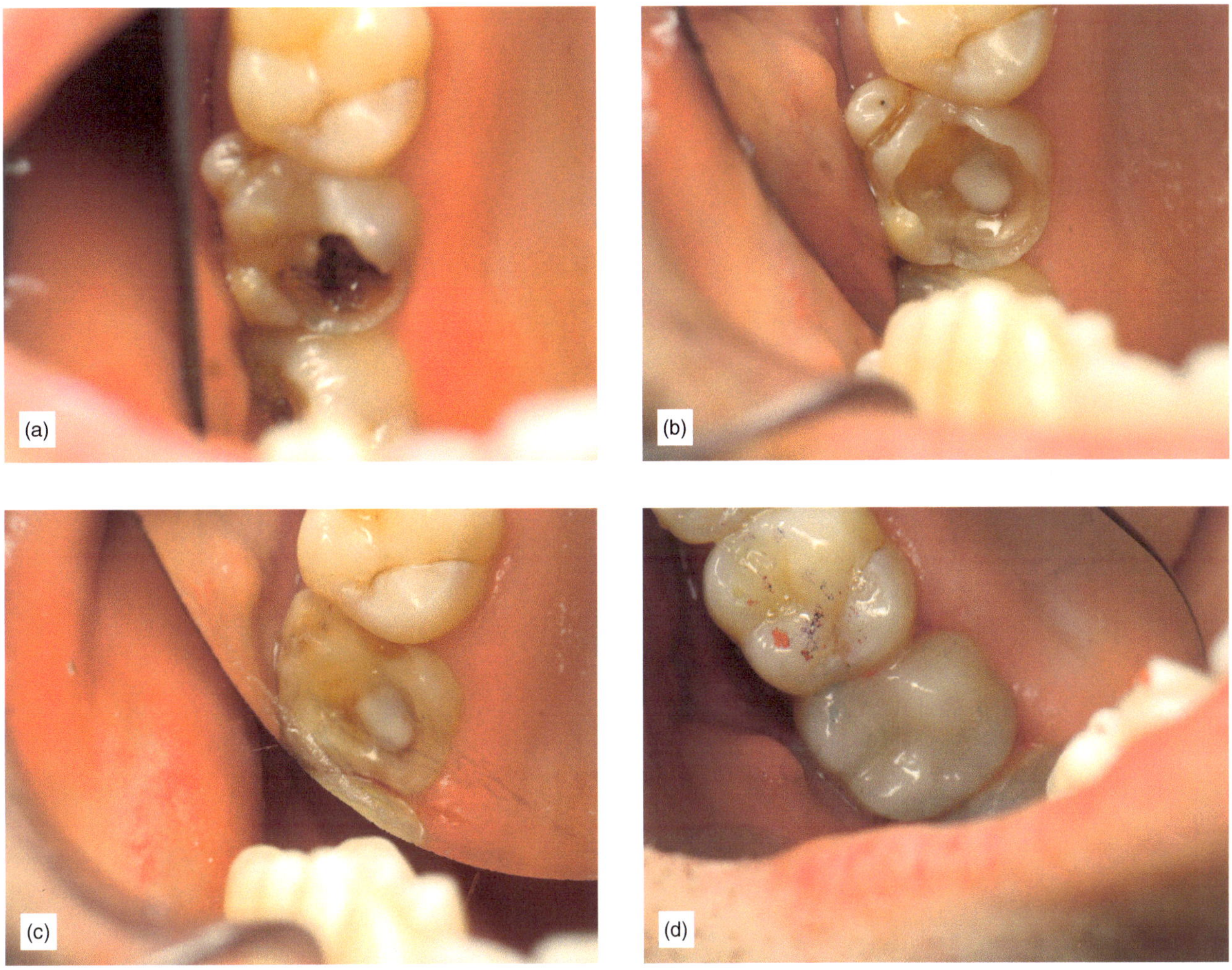

Badly broken down tooth restored with a supragingival bonded onlay.

Indications For Bonded Onlays

The indication for supragingival minimally invasive bonded onlays is simple: Any situation where the need for a full crown would have been identified and the tooth has not yet been cut for a crown. It is always preferable to make restorative dentistry healthier by retaining a supragingival margin and preserving tooth structure. Nevertheless, this is a departure from the popular view and traditional recommendations for bonded onlays. Bonded onlays have been indicated for simple cases that fulfill strict requirements, such as sufficient tooth structure available (Figure 5.1a–c), acceptable tooth color (Figure 5.2a–c), ideal location in the arch

Supra-Gingival Minimally Invasive Dentistry: A Healthier Approach to Esthetic Restorations, First Edition. By Jose-Luis Ruiz.

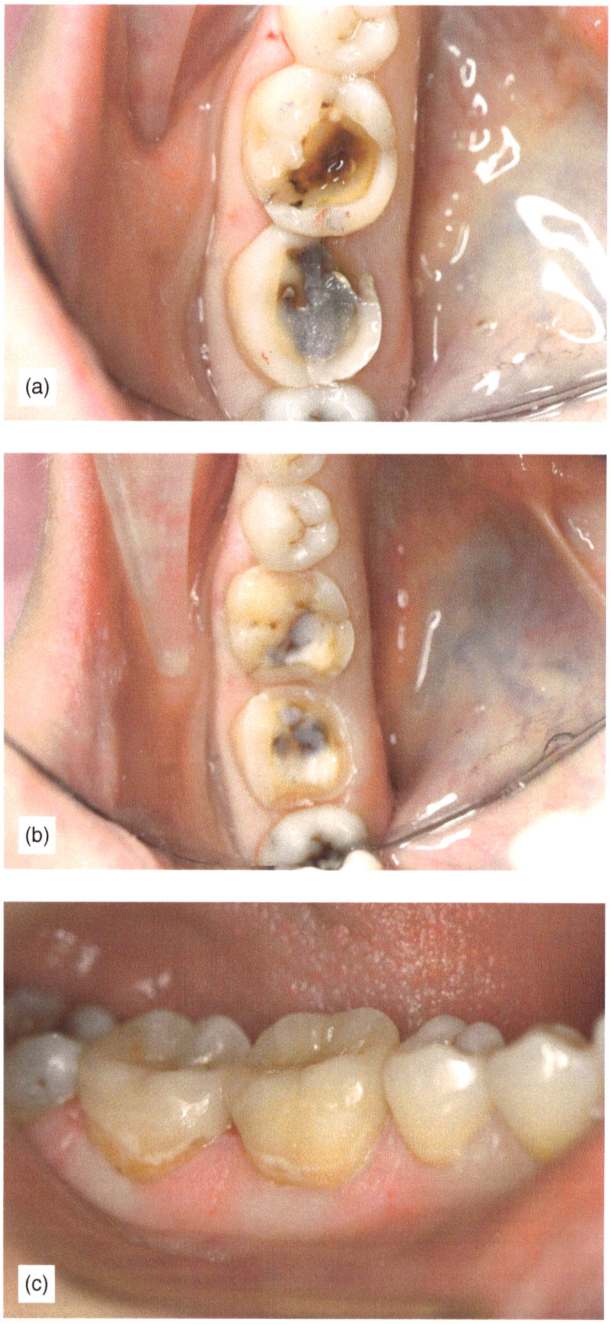

Figure 5.1 (a) Severe tooth structure loss, first and second molars. (b) Preparation for bonded onlay, no mechanical retention. (c) Postoperative view.

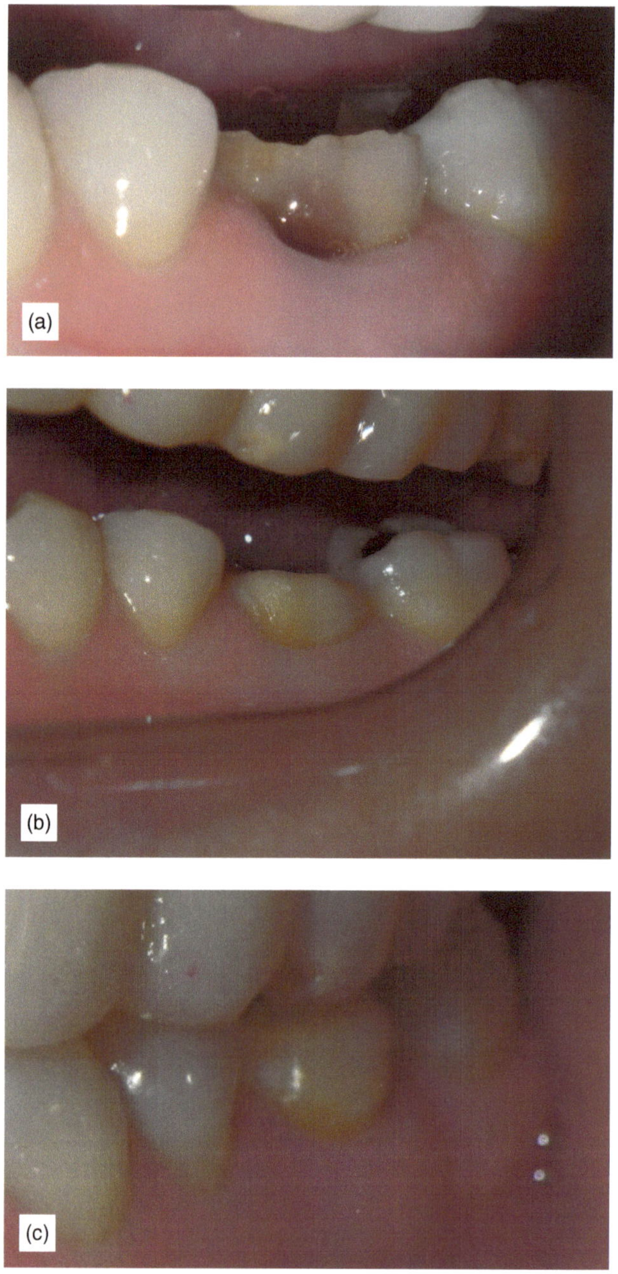

Figure 5.2 (a) Molar with internal discoloration. (b) After internal bleaching. (c) Finished onlay.

(Figure 5.3a–d), existing supragingival margin (Figure 5.4a–d), ideal occlusion (Figure 5.5a–g) [1,2,3,4,5]. When these requirements are not fulfilled, traditional full crowns have been indicated. With such strict recommendations, it is not surprising that well over 95% of teeth needing an indirect restoration end up being prepared for full crowns [6].

Indirect restoration should be reserved for badly damaged and weakened teeth. Less damaged teeth should be repaired with direct composite restorations. Direct composites can serve the patient very well. They allow for tooth structure preservation, are less costly for the patient and have excellent durability (Figure 5.6) [7]. Additionally, experience and clinical studies show that direct composites can perform as well as or may outperform indirect inlays [8]. For this reason, I do not recommend the use of indirect inlays. Only when the tooth is badly damaged, including badly weakened or missing

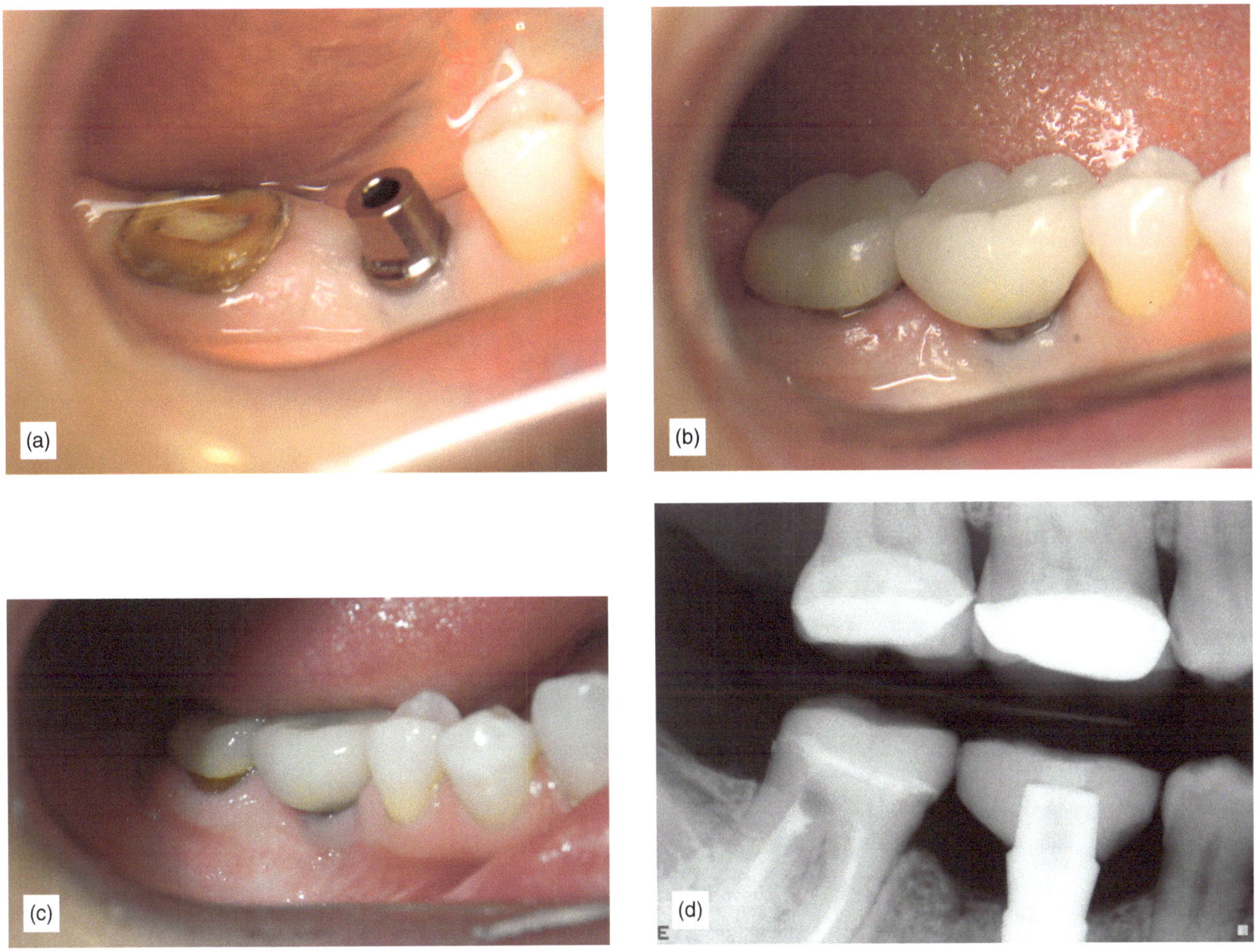

Figure 5.3 (a) Root-canal treated second molar in a bruxer, zero crown structure left. (b) Immediately following bonding with e-Max onlay. (c) Five years postoperatively. (d) X-ray of molar 5 years postoperatively.

cusp or cusps, or in the case of a fracture, is the option of an indirect onlay preferred to a direct composite. While it is possible to restore such teeth with a direct technique, it is more difficult and time consuming to perform a free-hand reconstruction of the morphology of a tooth's occlusal surface, and the results are usually less than ideal. Additionally, some degree of fracture resistance is added by constructing the occlusal surface with a higher-modulus, strong, restorative material, such as porcelain. Very large composites, as in the case with very large amalgams, are less durable and predictable [9,10,11]. Endodontically treated posterior teeth should have full occlusal coverage [12] but are ideal for supragingival minimally invasive onlays, which preserve more of the already badly compromised tooth (Figure 5. 7a,b) [13].

Clinical experience and the literature show that different outcomes can be expected from restoration, depending on the amount of remaining tooth, extension of the caries, old restorative material or fracture, as well as other circumstances. For these reasons, modifications and different types of preparation and restoration should be considered [14]. Posterior teeth requiring an indirect restoration can be divided into three major categories:

- simple partial and full coverage on vital teeth;
- complex partial and full occlusal coverage requiring buildups on vital teeth; and
- complex full coverage on endodontically treated teeth or teeth with vertical fractures.

Simple Partial and Full Coverage on Vital Teeth

In cases where one or more of the cusps are undermined, fractured or missing, and must be onlayed (Figure 5.8a–d), a direct restoration would not be indicated. Simple cases have ideal, natural, tooth color, and the amount of remaining tooth structure, especially the periphery of the enamel, is sufficient, the final preparation

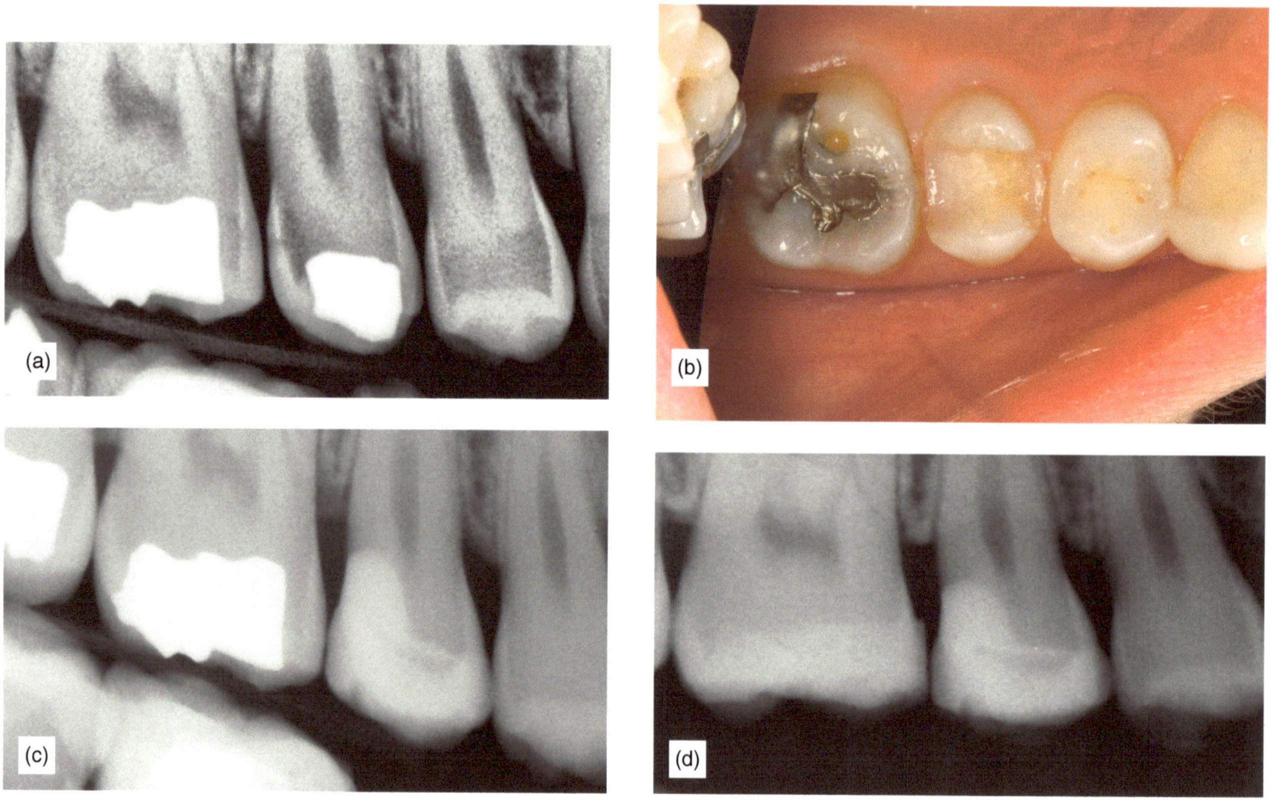

Figure 5.4 (a) Tooth with deep subgingival caries treated with an onlay. (b) Finished margin elevation and enamel preservation. (c) X-ray taken immediate postoperatively. (d) Three years postoperatively.

is more than 2 mm from the pulp, and the existing margins are supragingival. Using a supragingival protocol would allow the margins to remain supragingival, without the need for dentin sealing or buildups. These are the cases that most experts recommend for bonded onlays. Currently, however, these cases are usually treated with full crowns (Figure 5.9a–e) [15]. Full-mouth rehabilitation is also well suited for simple onlay preparation. Many of these cases are in patients with severe occlusal wear, and, although some experts consider severe occlusal wear a contraindication to bonded onlays [2], condemning these patients to a mouth full of crowns, much experience shows that bonded onlays cases have excellent results in such patients (Figure 5.10a–e).

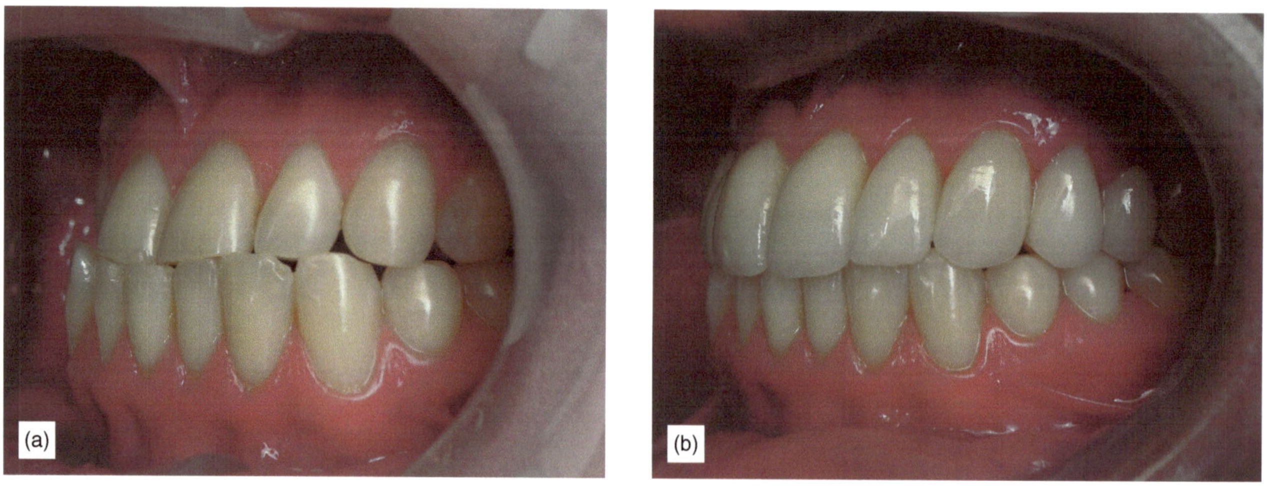

Figure 5.5 (a) Severe bruxer. (b) After full upper arch with 2 mm vertical dimension of occlusion opening using VenusCeram™ Pressable. (*Continued*)

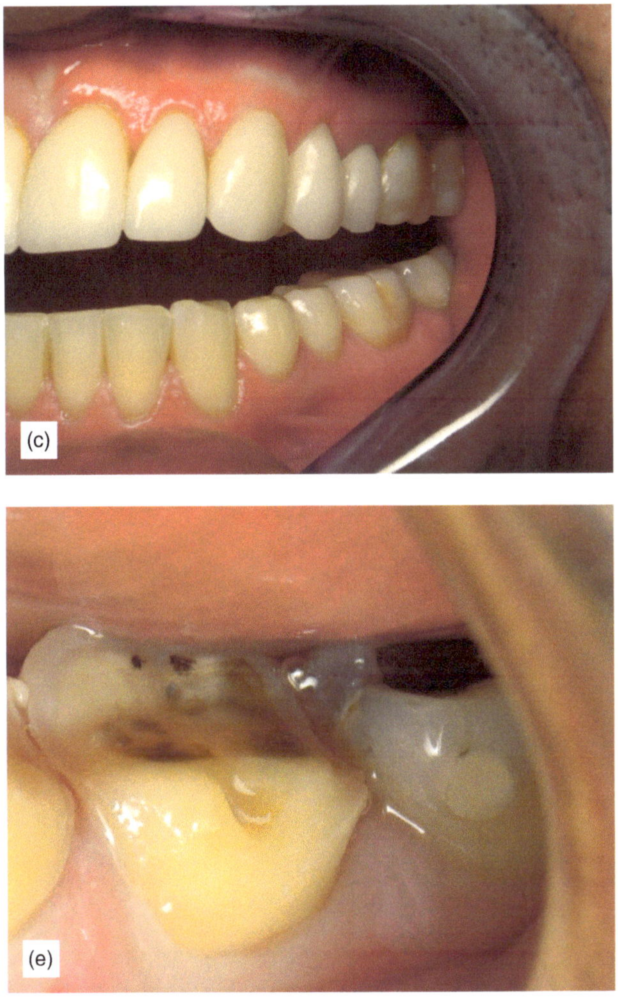

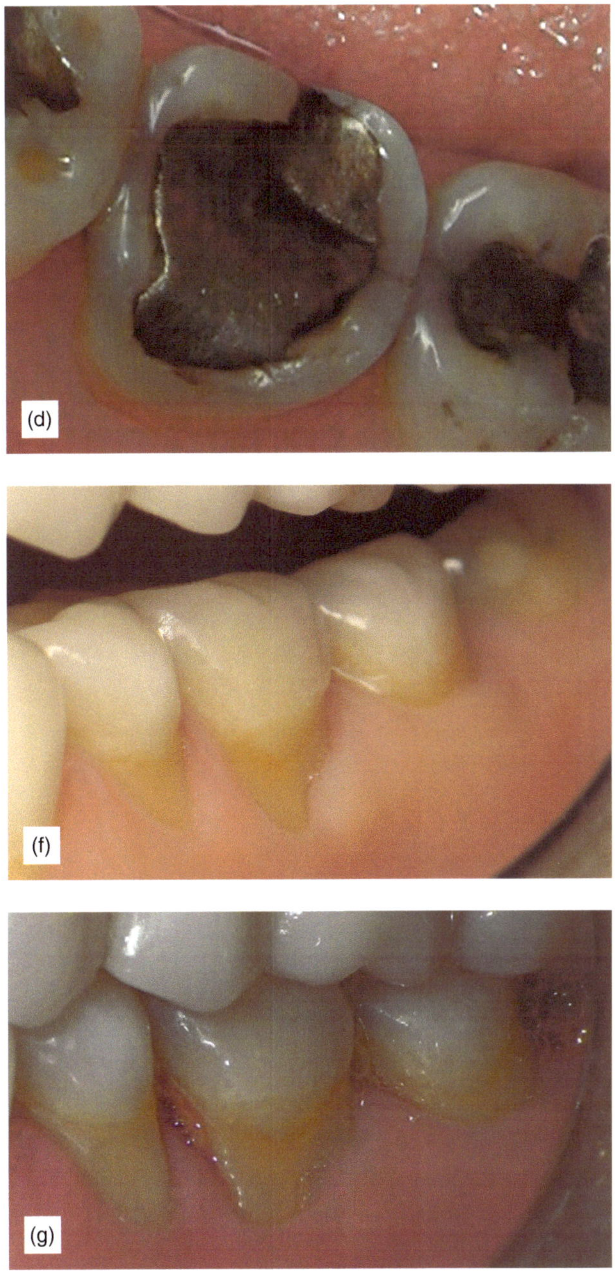

Figure 5.5 (*Continued*)
(c) Ten years postoperatively, all posterior onlays are functional. (d) A second severe bruxer. (e) Onlay preparations. (f) Cemented restorations. (g) Eight years postoperatively.

Complex Partial and Full Occlusal Coverage Requiring Buildup on Vital Teeth

Badly damaged vital teeth require dentin sealing and some type of buildup, such as where the caries is very close to the pulp, where large undercuts and a weak cusp or cusps need to be reinforced, and cases where the caries is deep at the cervical margin area, and where enamel margin preservation techniques or margin elevation technique must be performed (Figures 5.11a–c, 5.12a–d). As these teeth are vital, color is usually not generally an issue. Traditionally, these cases have been recommended for crowns. Nevertheless, with the advances in adhesion, and materials, and by implementing a supragingival protocol, these cases can be very successful with partial coverage supragingival restorations.

Complex Full-Coverage Endodontically Treated Teeth or Teeth With Vertical Fractures

Teeth with vertical fractures, cracked-tooth syndrome and endodontically treated teeth can and should be treated with partial coverage bonded onlays [16]. The literature shows an increased risk of failure [17,18], restoration of these teeth requires some modification to the preparation. They may require buildups or "margin elevation". Depending on the location in the arch and the

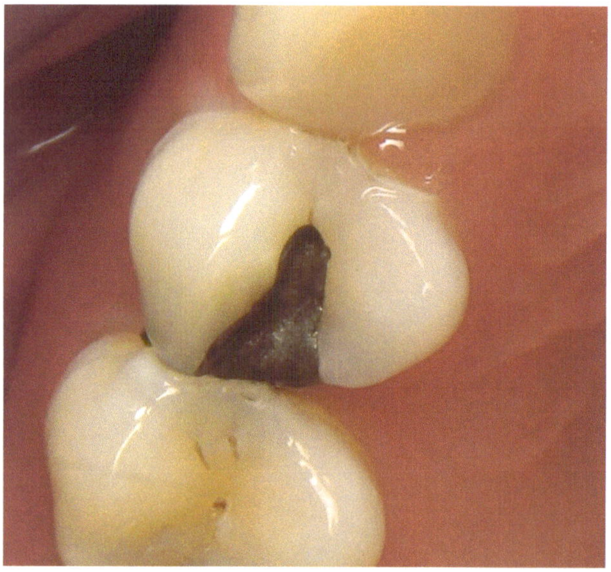

Figure 5.6 Direct composite restoration, indirect inlay not needed.

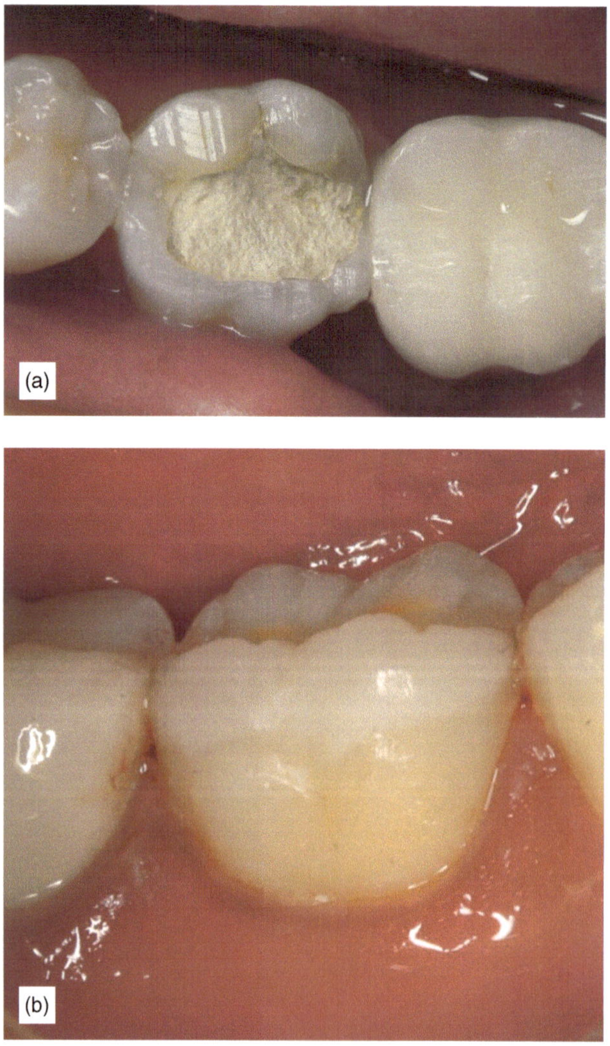

Figure 5.7 Weak tooth prone to fracture: (a) Only the periphery of the tooth is left. (b) After full-coverage onlay.

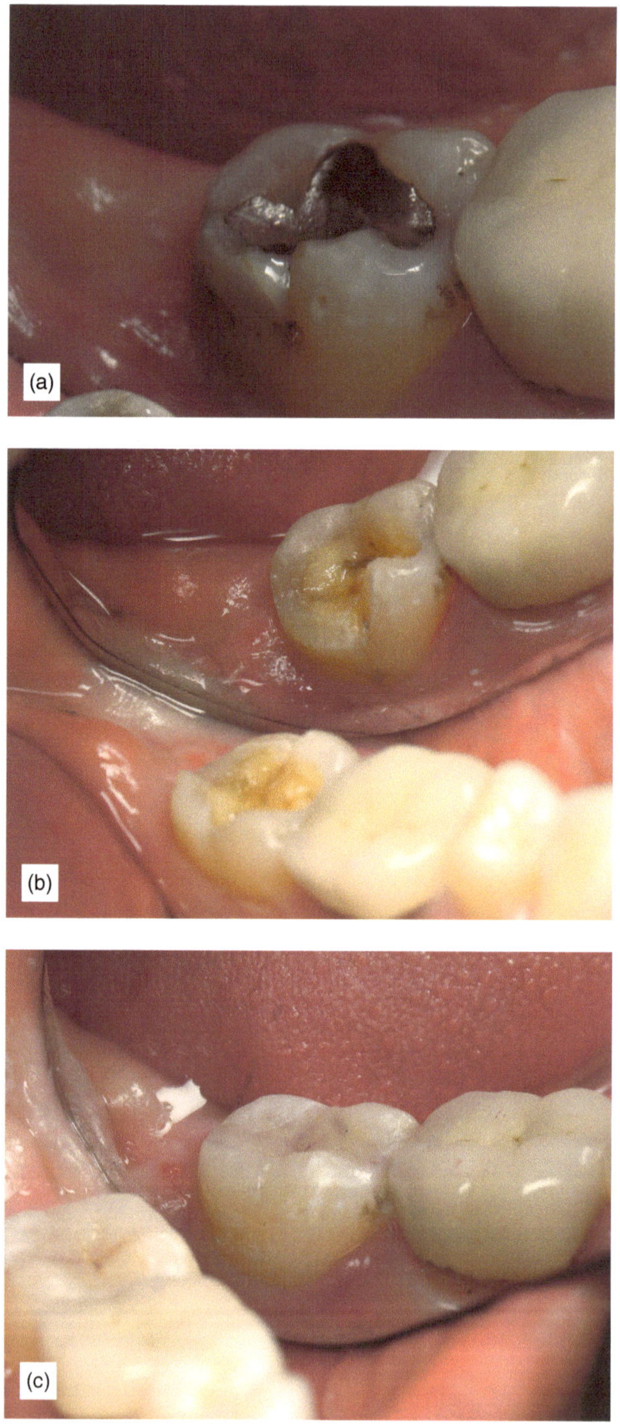

Figure 5.8 (a) Fractured distobuccal cusp. (b) Supragingival preparation. (c) The finished restoration.

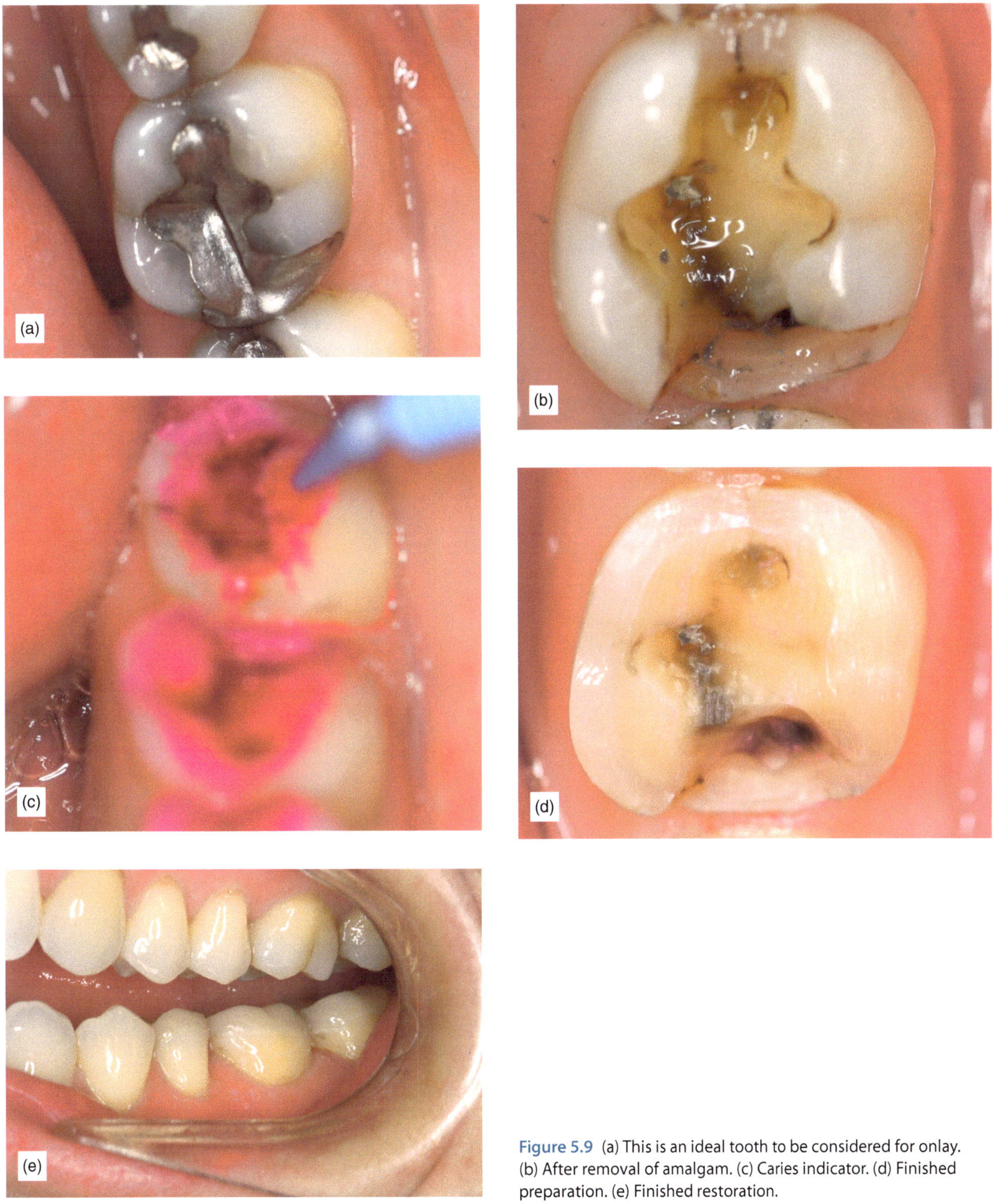

Figure 5.9 (a) This is an ideal tooth to be considered for onlay. (b) After removal of amalgam. (c) Caries indicator. (d) Finished preparation. (e) Finished restoration.

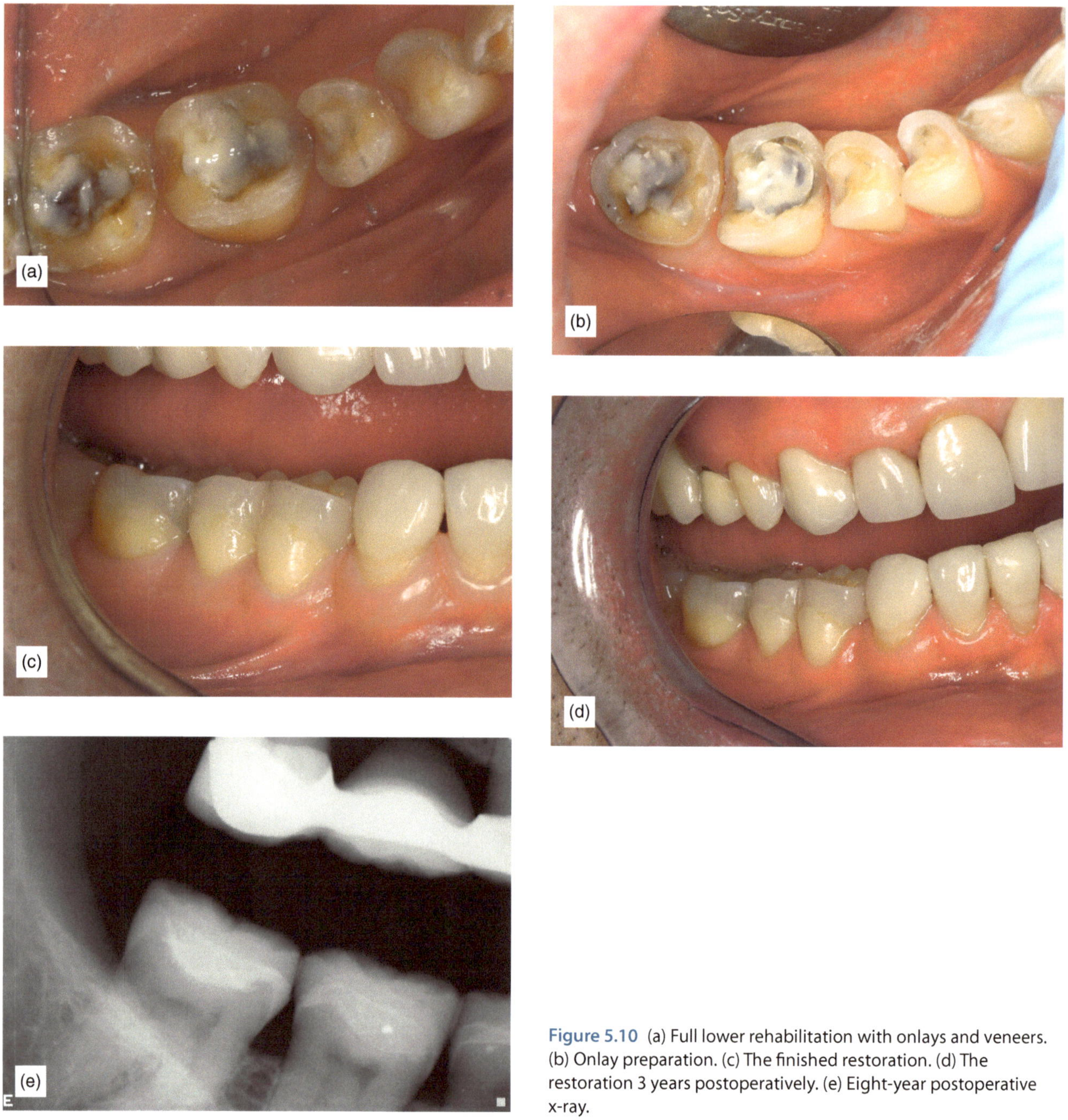

Figure 5.10 (a) Full lower rehabilitation with onlays and veneers. (b) Onlay preparation. (c) The finished restoration. (d) The restoration 3 years postoperatively. (e) Eight-year postoperative x-ray.

anticipated forces, stronger restorative materials such as zirconia may be indicated (Figures 5.13, 5.14a–c). To ensure sufficient strength of the restorative material, a slight increase in occlusal reduction is required. Reduction should be a minimum of 2.5 mm final occlusal thickness for lithium disilicate, which is ideal for the more esthetic demanding premolars, and 2 mm minimum final occlusal thickness for zirconia, which is ideal for teeth which must resist higher forces and have lower esthetic demands, such as second molars.

Clinical and finite-element studies have shown that increased thickness of the restorative material decreases the risk of fracture [19,20]. As the tooth is devitalized, there may be concerns as to its final shade, so the application of principle 5 is desirable. Traditionally, such teeth have been indicated for traditional full crowns. It is important to realize that, most of the time, these teeth already have large amounts of tooth missing. It is counterintuitive to remove further large amounts of the tooth to prepare the axial walls for mechanical retention in teeth

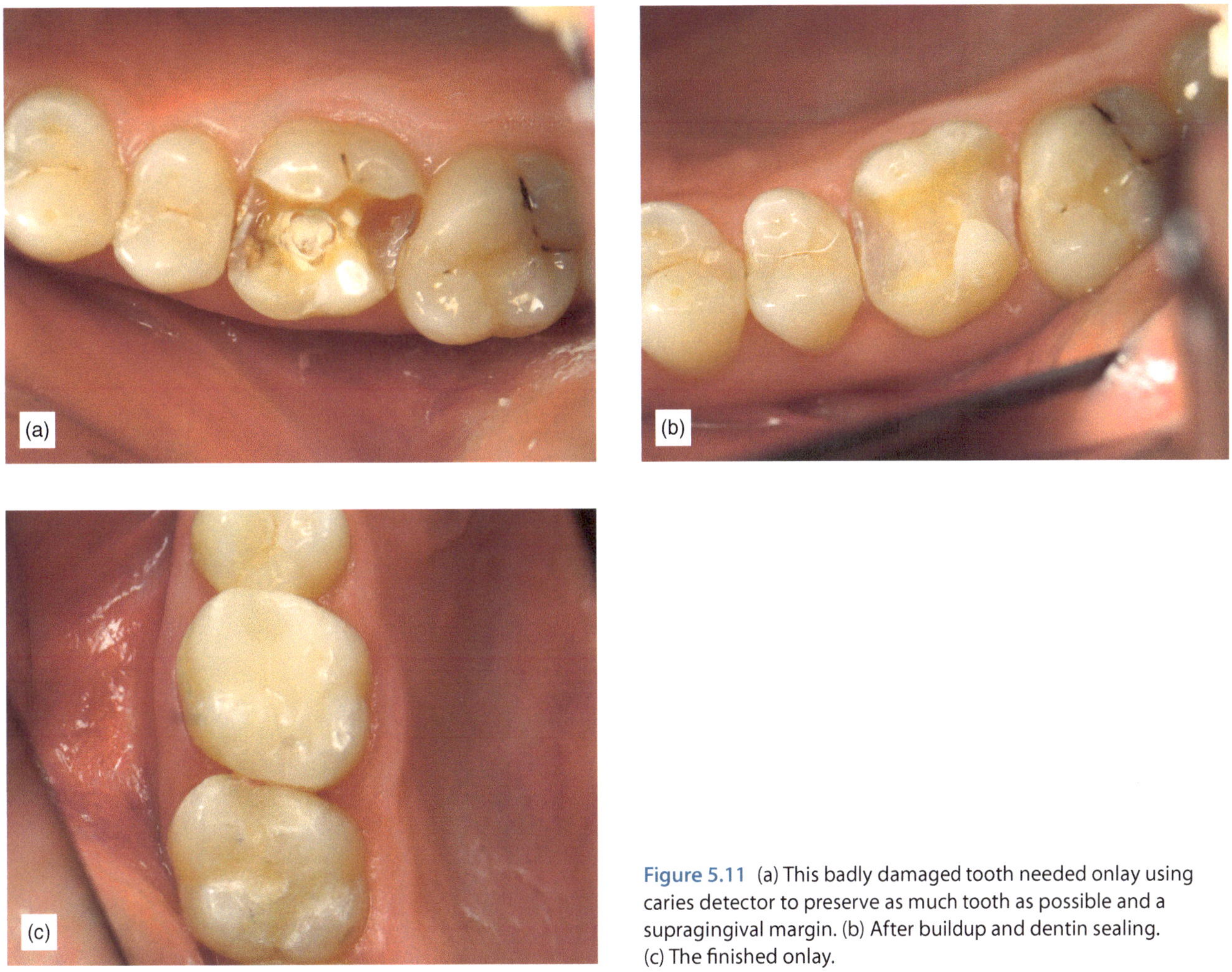

Figure 5.11 (a) This badly damaged tooth needed onlay using caries detector to preserve as much tooth as possible and a supragingival margin. (b) After buildup and dentin sealing. (c) The finished onlay.

that are already in a very weak state (Figure 5.15a–c). For this reason, supragingival minimally invasive bonded onlay restoration is the best option.

Restorative Material Options Specific to Bonded Onlays

The choice of restorative materials for partial or full coverage supragingival minimally invasive onlays or partial crowns is of paramount importance. Patient satisfaction and the success and longevity of the restoration depend on this choice. There are many restorative materials for partial coverage onlays, including gold. Bertolotti has outlined techniques for bonding gold to a tooth [21]. Currently, gold has diminished in popularity because it is not esthetic and is expensive. However, it should be considered for non-visible short teeth such as maxillary second molars. Gold does not fracture, so the restoration can be made thinner than ceramics, which is ideal for short teeth. Bonded partial coverage onlays or overlays can be made of different types of non-metal materials: Laboratory composite, leucite-reinforced pressed feldspathic porcelain, lithium disilicate and zirconia. Bonding with zirconia has been questioned, probably because it cannot be etched with hydrofluoric acid like most other ceramics. However, with the appropriate technique, zirconia can be bonded reasonably well [22,23]. Although not currently a popular material, alumina (aluminum oxide, Al_2O_3) can be bonded using the same methods as for zirconia.

Composite

Composite material can be divided into intraoral composite used for semi-direct onlays or laboratory composite used for indirect onlays and computer-aided design and milled (CAD-CAM) composite. The benefits of composite onlays are that they can be easy to fabricate, intrinsically polychromatic, highly esthetic, initially, less expensive, and easy to repair. Although they may lose luster and look dull over time (Figure 5.16), composite onlays show good fracture strength, similar to strong

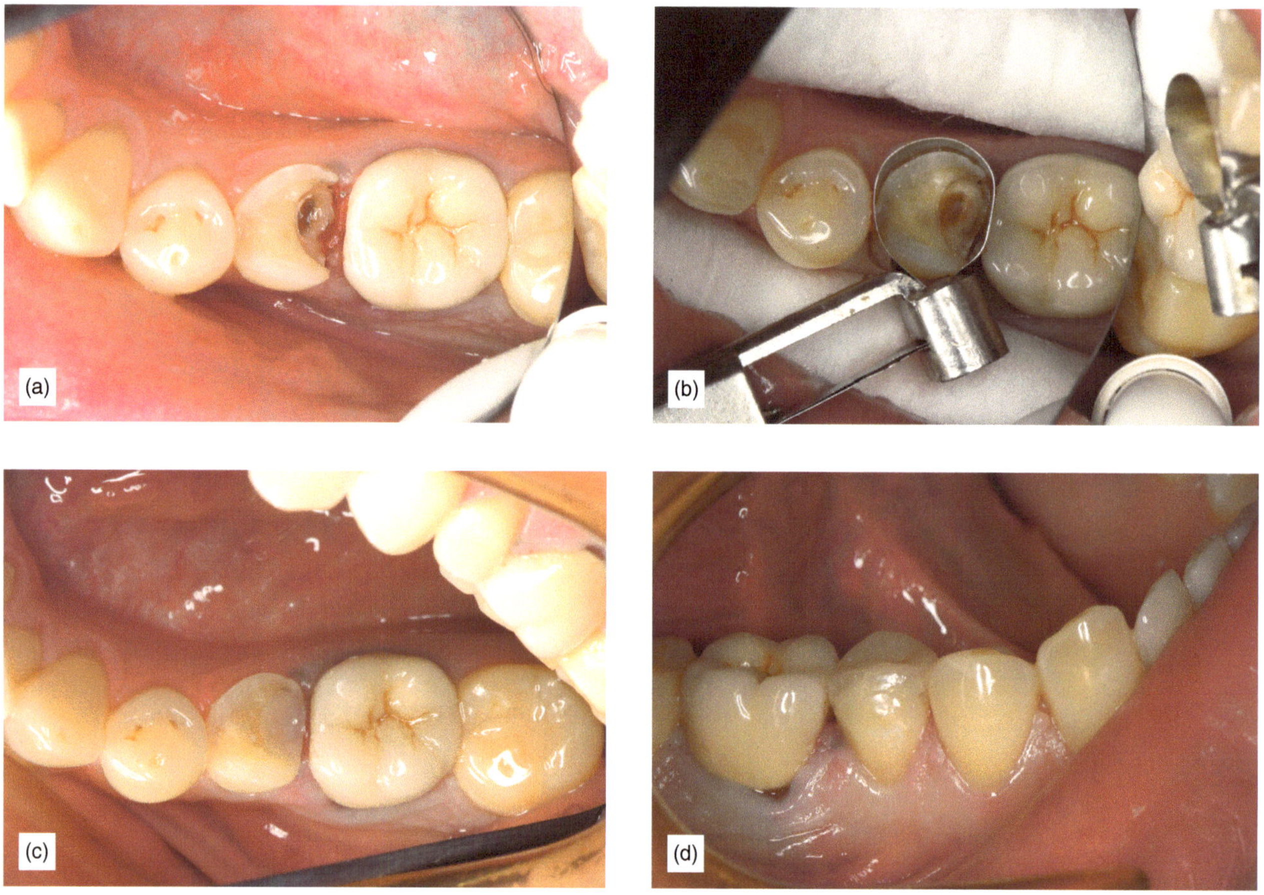

Figure 5.12 (a) A deep subgingival margin. (b) Elevation procedure. (c) After buildup. (d) The finished restoration.

ceramic [24]. The disadvantage of composite is its lack of rigidity, which may lead to an increased risk of bond failure and possibly shorter durability [21,25]. Clinical experience and research indicates that composite wears faster than tooth over the long term [26]. Super-thin composite occlusal veneers, while very strong in relation to fracture, will have a shorter clinical life because of the poor wear resistance of composite (Figure 5.17a,b) [27]. New hybrid nanocomposites, such as Lava™ Ultimate (no longer indicated for crowns by 3M but still suitable for bonded onlays) and Z Nano, which combine ceramics and silica nanoparticles, have been shown to be very strong, but only time will tell whether they wear as well as or better than more conventional composites.

Leucite-Reinforced Pressed Feldspathic Porcelain

Leucite-reinforced pressed feldspathic porcelain can be layered, pressed (Figure 5.18) or milled in a CAD-CAM machine. Leucite-reinforced feldspathic pressed restorations have a long history of success for bonded onlays. Millions of successful restorations have been done with these materials and the literature is replete with the excellent results achieved with them [28,29]. This material has the capacity to provide the best esthetics and blending of the restorative margin and the tooth because it has ideal translucency. When bonded to a rigid tooth structure, it can be as strong as lithium disilicate in compressive strength [6]. Its shear strength is low and much attention must be paid to occlusion to avoid lateral interferences, which can cause fractures. The primary form of failure for restorations made from this material is bulk fracture (Figure 5.19a,b) [30,31]. Nevertheless, with sufficient remaining tooth structure, proper adhesion and good attention to occlusion, these materials have performed very well, and I have placed several thousands with overwhelming success (Figure 5.20).

Lithium disilicate

Lithium disilicate can be pressed or milled in a CAD-CAM machine. For a multitude of reasons, this material has quickly become the most ideal for bonded onlays. When strength is a priority [32,33], the pressed version appears to be a little stronger and provides a better fit [34]. Lithium disilicate strength can exceed 500 MPa,

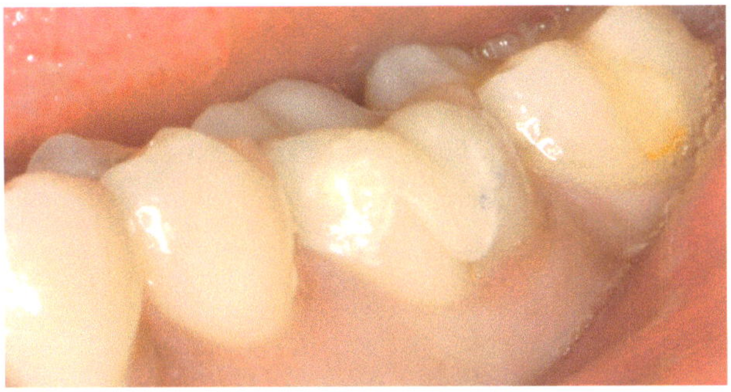

Figure 5.13 Zirconia for a fracture.

and is much stronger when bonded than when cemented (Figure 5.21). When largely bonded to rigid tooth structure such as enamel, its strength can be close to that of zirconia. When bonded to a less rigid structure such as dentin, it becomes considerably weaker than zirconia [35]. There are two version: high and low translucency. High translucency is preferable for most cases of partial coverage onlays where the cavosurface margin is considerably coronal to the gingival line and good blending is important (Figure 5.22a–c) Low translucency may be preferred if the color of the tooth needs to be hidden, but the disadvantage is that the union of the tooth and restoration will be very visible and will often need to be placed equi- or subgingivally (Figure 5.23). There are techniques that will allow the color to be corrected first, thus allowing supragingival techniques to be used. As with anything in life, exceptions exist when no other option will be available other than a subgingival margin.

Zirconia

Zirconia has a long history of success in dentistry [36,37,38]. Its intrinsic strength is remarkable, exceeding 1,000 MPa. It can be milled to a thin coping, then layered or pressed veneer ceramics can cover the coping, creating a layered restoration, porcelain fused to zirconia (PFZ), similar to the porcelain fused to metal of old. It is

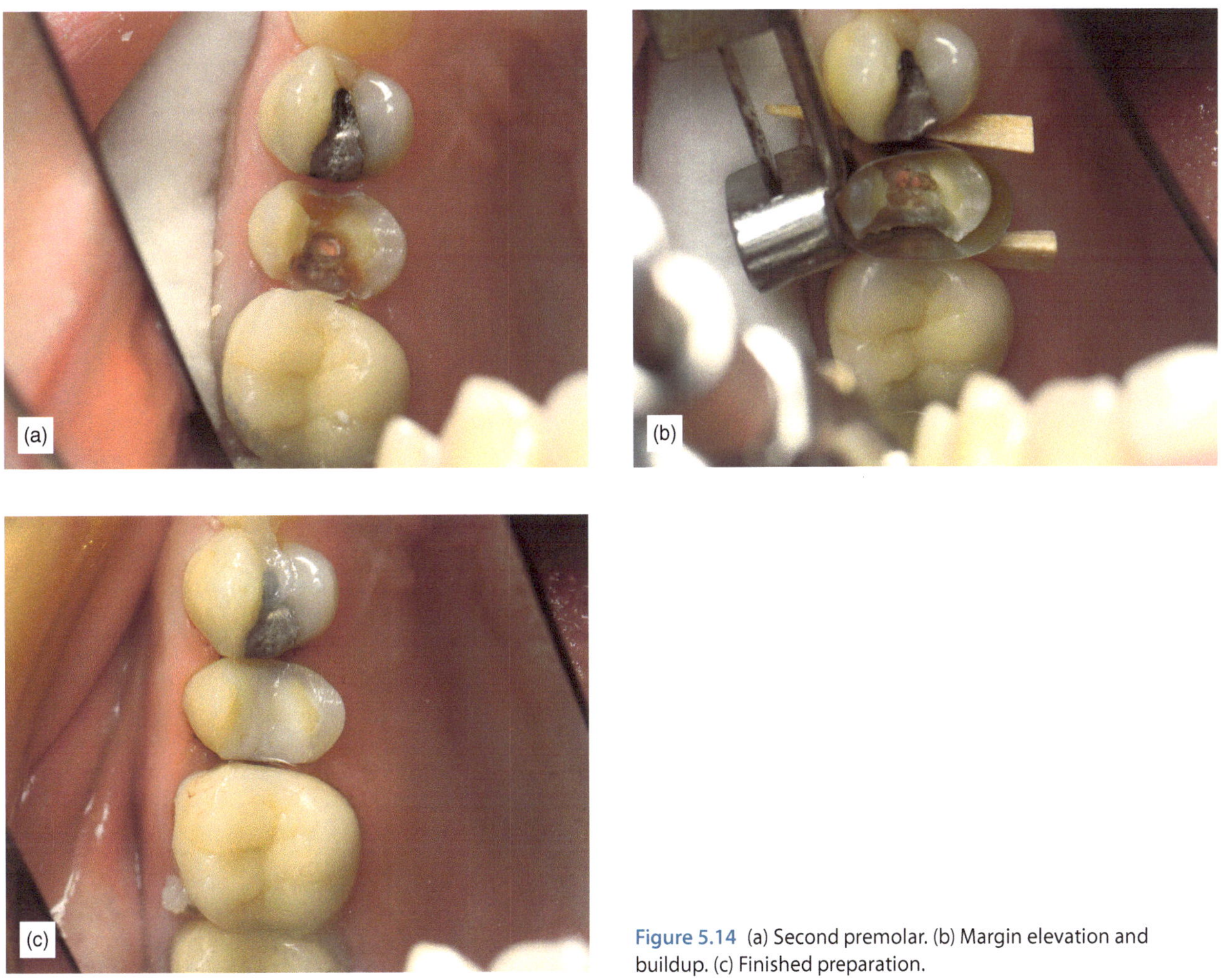

Figure 5.14 (a) Second premolar. (b) Margin elevation and buildup. (c) Finished preparation.

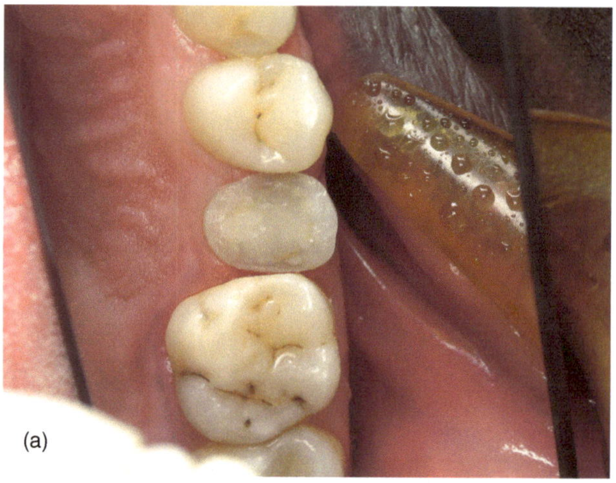

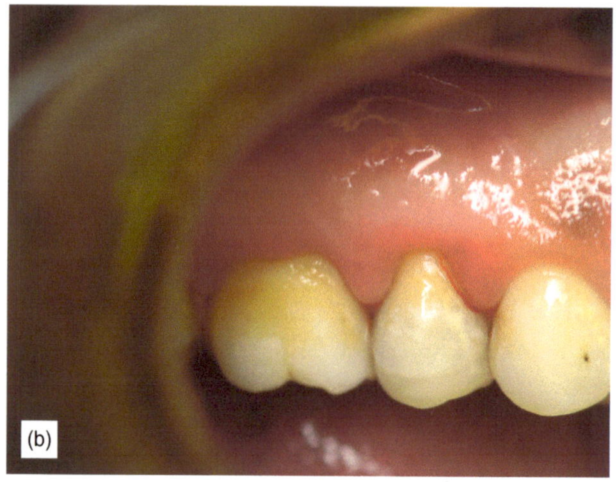

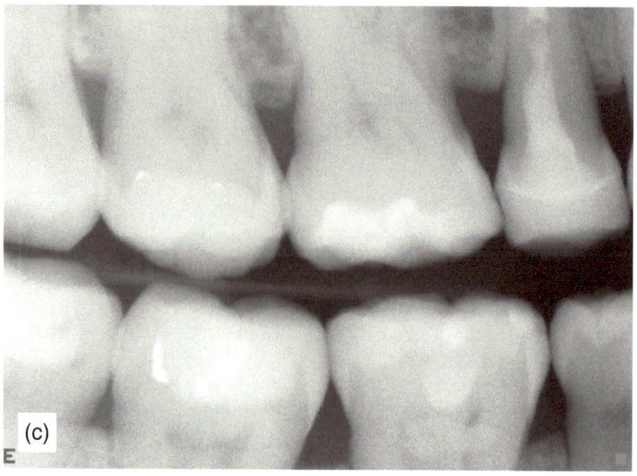

Figure 5.15 (a) Root canal treated after buildup. (b) Immediately after cementation. (c) Successful onlay 7 years postoperatively.

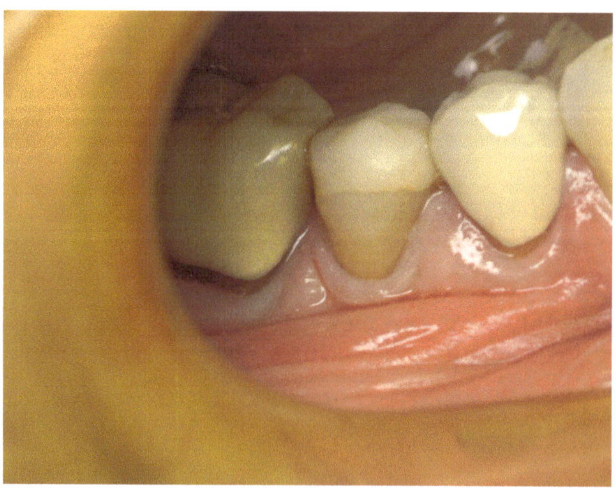

Figure 5.16 Dull belleGlass composite onlay.

opacious (Figure 5.24) unless very thin. Zirconia can also be made monolithic; that is, a full-contour zirconia without a veneer. This material is more ideally indicated for full crowns and bridge frameworks. Zirconia onlays are usually monolithic and are indicated in cases with lower esthetic requirements, in cases with a high risk of fracture, and in teeth which have lost their rigidity, such as endodontically treated teeth, especially first and second molars. For most onlays, the monolithic option is usually more desirable, as it requires less reduction of the tooth. Because of its poor translucency and lack of ability to blend with the tooth, zirconia onlay preparations require extension of the restorative margin closer to the gingiva, but ideally not subgingivally. Correct adhesion to zirconia is not as well known, but excellent results can be achieved using a bonding enhancement air abrasive powder [39] (see Chapter 9 for details of adhesion techniques).

Longevity of Onlays Compared with Crowns

It would be impossible to compare the long-term durability of onlays with that of crowns, as crowns in different

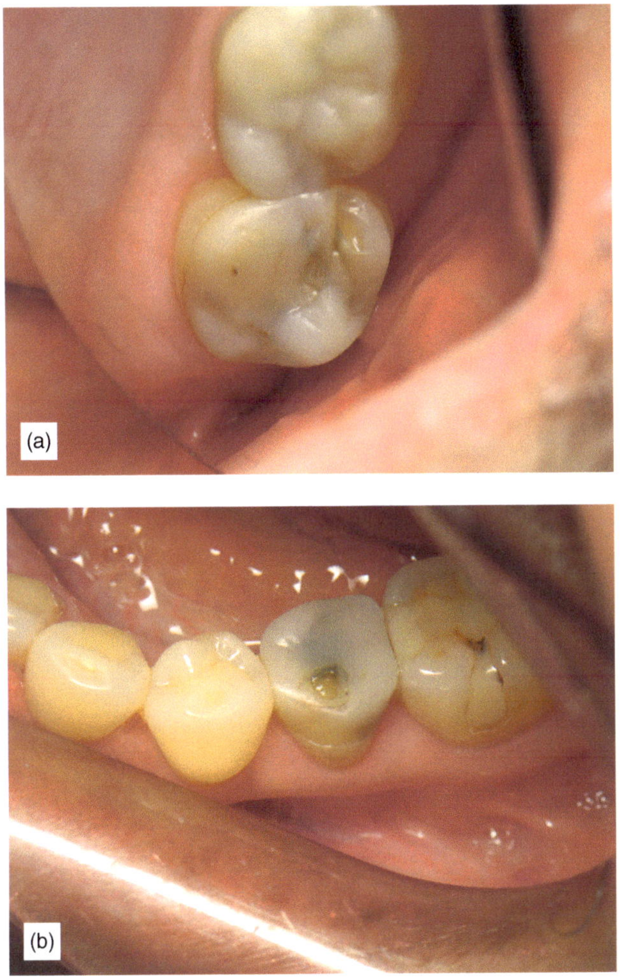

Figure 5.17 (a) Ten-year onlay recall, both belleGlass onlays damaged owing to excessive composite wear. (b) Nine-year recall showing excessive wear and necessity for replacing a composite onlay due to wear.

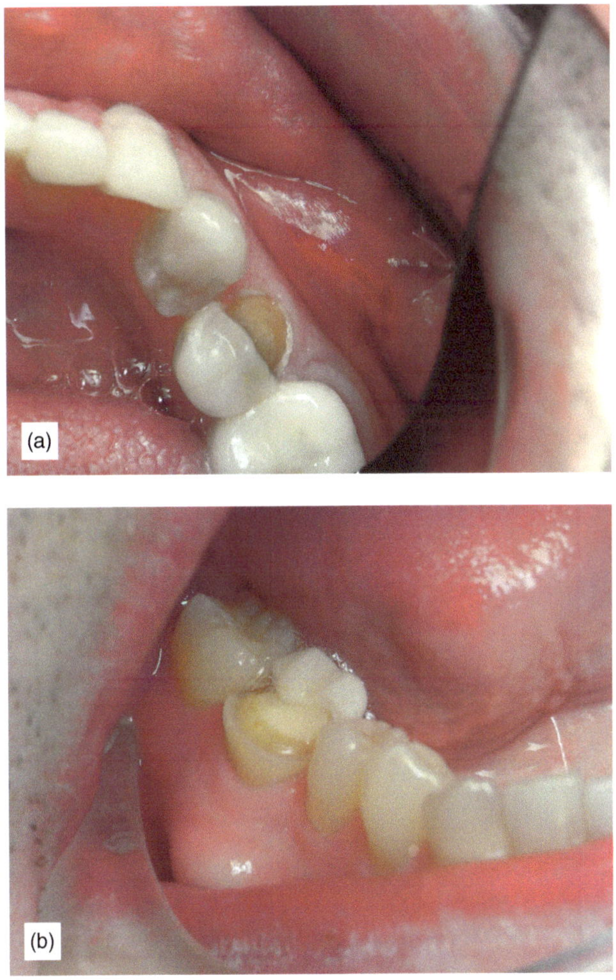

Figure 5.19 (a) Many bulk fractures of pressable onlay are related to adhesive failure; the restoration came clean off the tooth. (b) Bulk fracture of pressable onlay, also showing a clean separation of the restoration, showing that this was an adhesive failure.

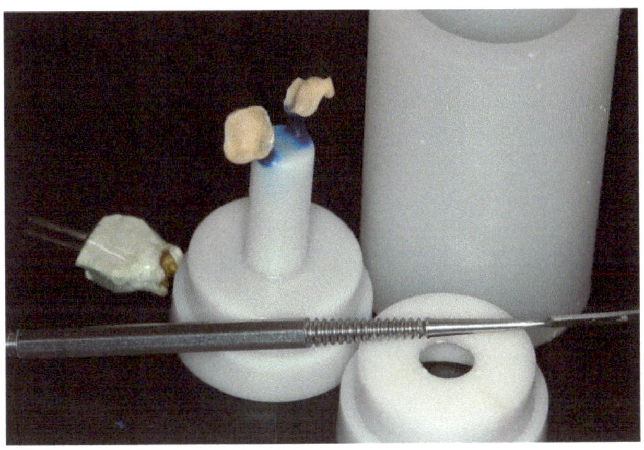

Figure 5.18 Waxed onlays being invested.

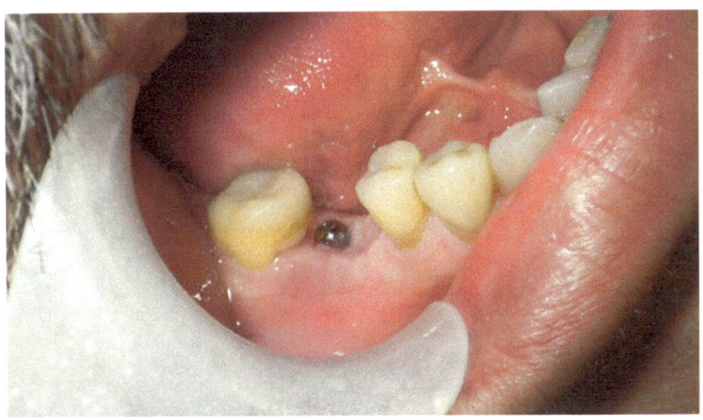

Figure 5.20 Three 14-year-old VenusCeram pressed onlays in good condition.

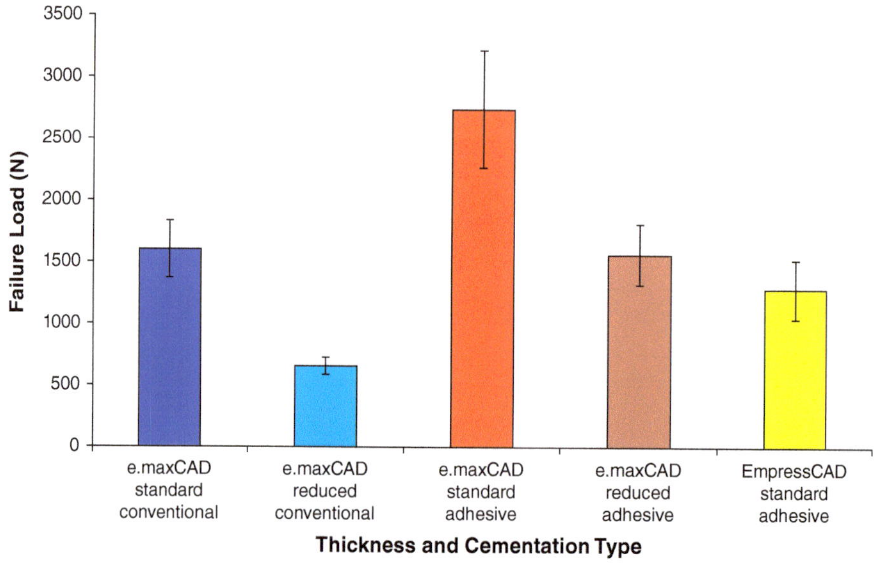

Figure 5.21 Ivoclar graph of strength of bond compared with cement.

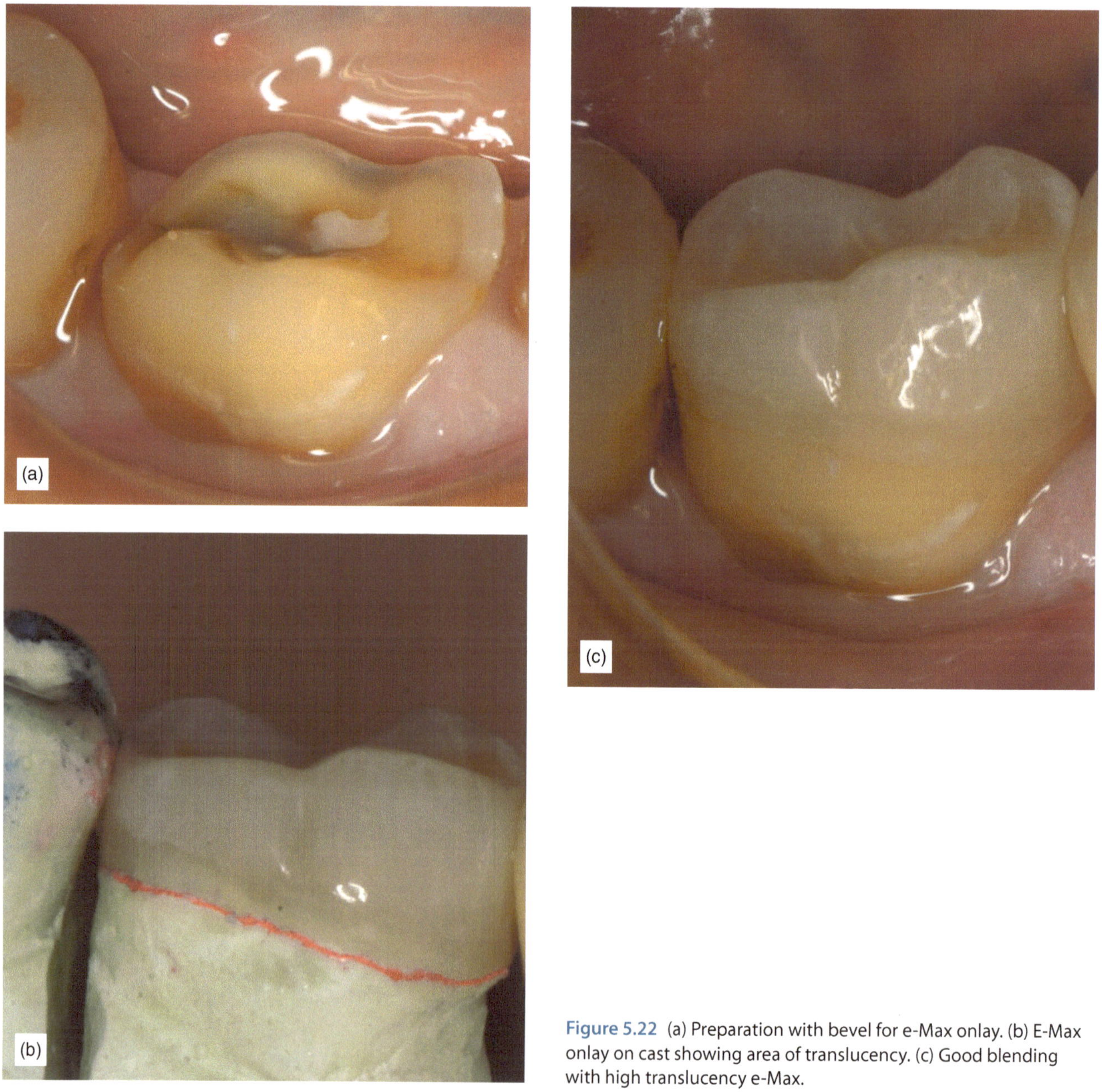

Figure 5.22 (a) Preparation with bevel for e-Max onlay. (b) E-Max onlay on cast showing area of translucency. (c) Good blending with high translucency e-Max.

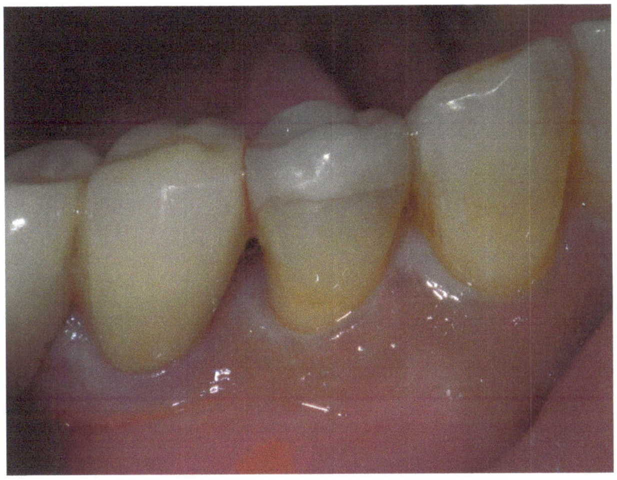

Figure 5.23 Opacious low translucency e-Max will not allow good blending of restorative margins.

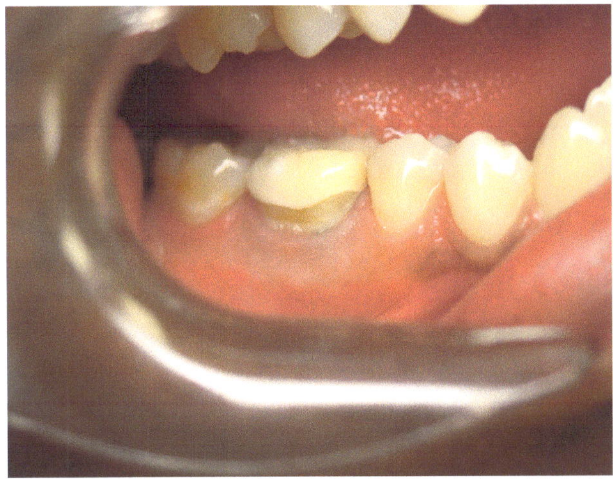

Figure 5.24 Very ugly zirconia margin.

forms and materials have been around for over 100 years, while bonded onlays have only been successfully performed for around 20 years. Great advances in restorative materials and adhesion are now at a point where it is reasonable to predict that bonded onlays may well outperform traditional crowns, which are plagued with complications, leading to a shorter clinical life [40]. Gold, because it does not break, has had an unmatched record of durability, but as with any other indirect restorative procedure, correct technique influences durability.

Thus, supragingival minimally invasive bonded onlays are the most healthy restorations ever performed. With current materials and techniques, they can have a very long clinical life. It must be remembered that because the pulp is less traumatized by the tooth preparation procedure, and the periodontium is left unharmed, the ultimate longevity of the tooth itself is undoubtedly going to benefit from this approach. When supragingival minimally invasive onlays fail, it is rarely catastrophic and correction is easier (Figure 5.25a–c).

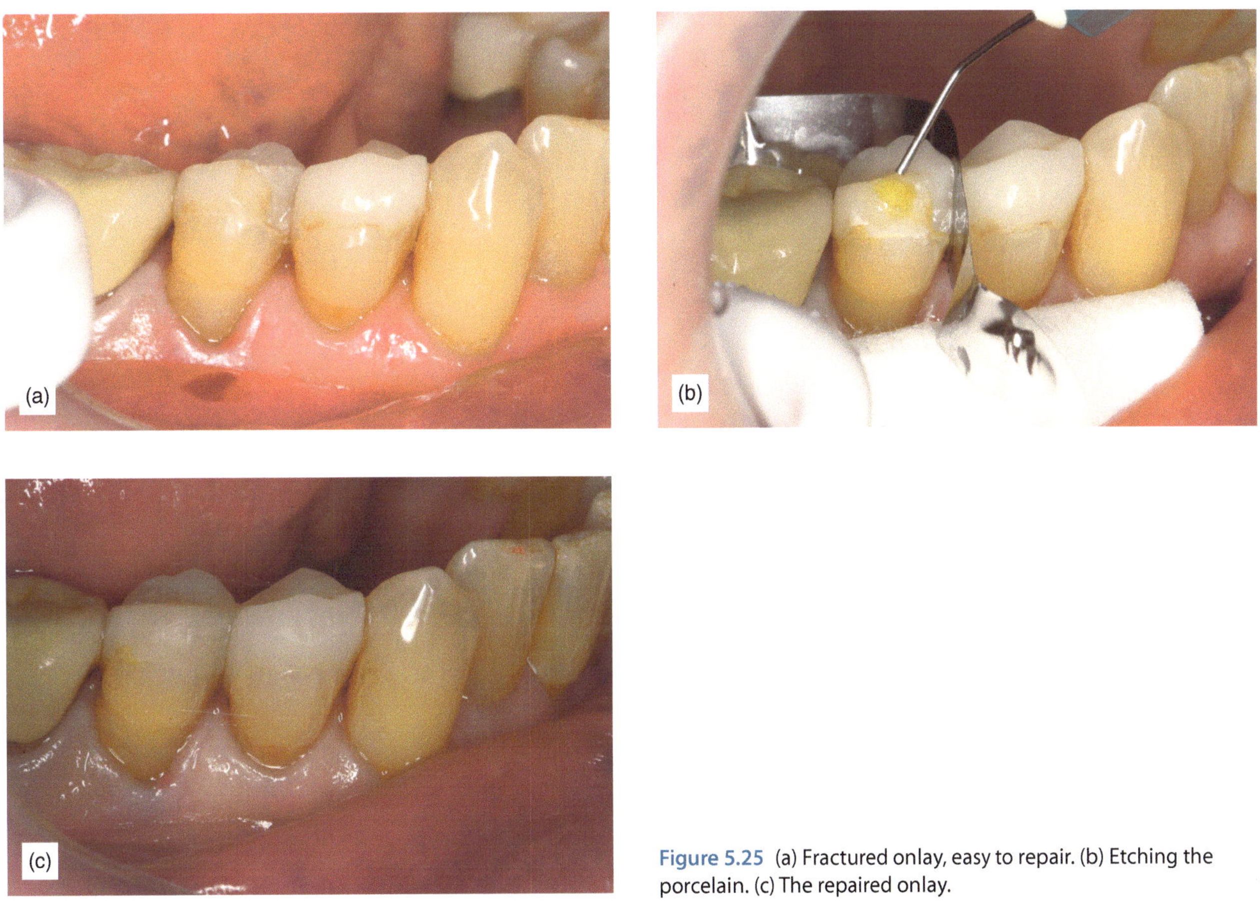

Figure 5.25 (a) Fractured onlay, easy to repair. (b) Etching the porcelain. (c) The repaired onlay.

References

1 Bakeman EM, Kois JC. Posterior, all porcelain, adhesively retained restorations. *Inside Dentistry*, 2009; 5(5): 20–30.

2 Kois DE, Chaiyabutr Y, Kois JC. Comparison of load fatigue performance of posterior ceramic onlay restorations under different preparation designs. *Compend Contin Educ Dent*, 2012; 33(Spec No 2): 2–9.

3 Meyer A Jr, Cardoso LC, Araujo E, Baratieri LN. Ceramic inlays and onlays: clinical procedures for predictable results. *J Esthet Restor Dent*, 2003; 15(6): 338–352.

4 Barghi N, Berry TG. Clinical evaluation of etched porcelain onlays, a 4 year report. *Compend Contin Educ Dent*, 2002; 23(7): 657–674.

5 Heymann H, Swift E, Ritter A. Indirect tooth color restorations, in *Sturdevant's Art and Science of Operative Dentistry*, 6th ed. Elsevier Mosby, 2013, pp. 280–295.

6 Christensen GJ. Are tooth color onlays viable alternatives to crowns? *Clin Rep*, 2012; 5(1): 1,3.

7 Opdam NJ, Bronkhorst EM, Roeters JM, Loomans BA. A retrospective clinical study on longevity of posterior composite and amalgam restorations. *Dent Mater*, 2007; 23(1): 2–8.

8 Pallesen U, Qvist V. Composite resin fillings and inlays: An 11 year evaluation. *Clin Oral Invest*, 2003; 7: 71–79.

9 Kolker J. Teeth with large amalgam restorations and crowns: Factors affecting the receipt of subsequent treatment after 10 years. *J Am Dent Assoc*, 2005; 136: 738–748.

10 Wahl M. Prevalence of cusp fractures in teeth restored with amalgam and with resin-based composite. *J Am Dent Assoc*, 2004; 135: 1127–1132.

11 da Rosa Rodolpho PA, Cenci MS, Donassollo TA, Loguércio AD, Demarco FF. A clinical evaluation of posterior composite restorations: 17-year findings. *J Dent*, 2006; 34(7): 427–435.

12 Panitvisai P, Messer H. Cuspal deflection in molars in relation to endodontic and restorative procedures. *J Endod*, 1995; 21: 57–61.

13 Linn J, Messer HH. Effect of restorative procedures on the strength of endodontically treated molars. *J Endod*, 1994; 20(10): 479–485.

14 Land MF, Hopp CD. Survival rates of all-ceramic systems differ by clinical indication and fabrication method. *J Evid Based Dent Pract*, 2010; 10(1): 37–38.

15 Christensen GJ. Are tooth-colored onlays viable alternatives to crowns? *Clin Rep* 2012; 5(1): 1, 3.

16 Ozyoney G, Yan Koğlu F, Tağtekin D, Hayran O. The efficacy of glass-ceramic onlays in the restoration of morphologically compromised and endodontically treated molars. *Int J Prosthodont*, 2013; 26(3): 230–234.

17 Dietschi D, Duc O, Krejci I, Sadan A. Biomechanical considerations for the restoration of endodontically treated teeth: A systematic review of the literature, Part II (Evaluation of fatigue behavior, interfaces, and in vivo studies). *Quintessence Int*, 2008; 39(2): 117–129.

18 van Dijken JW, Hasselrot L. A prospective 15-year evaluation of extensive dentin-enamel-bonded pressed ceramic coverages. *Dent Mater*, 2010; 26(9): 929–939.

19 Murgueitio R, Bernal G. Three-year clinical follow-up of posterior teeth restored with leucite-reinforced IPS Empress onlays and partial veneer crowns. *J Prosthodont*, 2012; 21(5): 340–345.

20 Magne P, Belser UC. Porcelain versus composite inlays/onlays: effects of mechanical loads on stress distribution, adhesion, and crown flexure. *Int J Periodontics Restorative Dent*, 2003; 23(6): 543–555.

21 Bertolotti RL. Adhesion to porcelain and metal. *Dent Clinics North Am*, 2007; 51: 433–451.

22 Kern M. Bonding to oxide ceramics: Laboratory testing versus clinical outcome. *Dent Mater*, 2015; 31(1): 8–14.

23 Yang B, Wolfart S, Scharnberg M, Ludwig K, Adelung R, Kern M. Influence of contamination on zirconia ceramic bonding. *J Dent Res*, 2007; 86(8): 749–753.

24 Belli, R. Mechanical fatigue degradation of ceramics versus resin composites for dental restorations. *Dent Mater*, 2014; 30(4): 424–432.

25 Hopp C, Land MF. Considerations for ceramic inlays in posterior teeth: a review. *Clin Cosmet Investig Dent*, 2013; 5: 21–32.

26 Yesil ZD, Alapati S, Johnston W, Seghi RR. Evaluation of the wear resistance of new nanocomposite resin restorative materials. *J Prosthet Dent* 2008; 99(6): 435–443.

27 Magne P, Stanley K, Schlichting LH. Modeling of ultrathin occlusal veneers. *Dent Mater*, 2012; 28(7): 777–782.

28 Frankenberger R, Taschner M, Garcia-Godoy F, Petschelt A, Krämer N. Leucite-reinforced glass ceramic inlays and onlays after 12 years. *J Adhes Dent*, 2008; 10(5): 393–398.

29 Ruiz JL, Christensen GJ, Sameni A, Vargas L. Clinical performance of bonded ceramic and resin-based composite inlays and onlays using a self-etch bonding system; a 51-month report. *Inside Dentistry*, 2007; 3(5):62–65.

30 El-Mowafy O, Brochu JF. Longevity and clinical performance of IPS-Empress ceramic restorations: a literature review. *J Can Dent Assoc*, 2002; 68: 233–237.

31 Lehner C, Studer S, Brodbeck U, Schärer P. Six-year clinical results of leucite-reinforced glass ceramic inlays and onlays. *Acta Med Dent Helv*, 1998; 3: 137–146.

32 Culp L, McLaren EA. Lithium disilicate: the restorative material of multiple options. *Compend Contin Educ Dent*, 2010; 31(9): 716–725.

33 Fasbinder DJ, Dennison JB, Heys D, Neiva G. A clinical evaluation of chairside lithium disilicate CAD/CAM crowns: A two year report. *J Am Dent Assoc*, 2010; 141(6 Suppl): 10s–14s.

34 Anadioti E, Aquilino SA, Gratton DG, Holloway JA, Denry IL, Thomas GW, Qian F. Internal fit of pressed and computer-aided design/computer-aided manufacturing ceramic crowns made from digital and conventional impressions. *J Prosthet Dent*, 2015; 113(4): 304–309.

35 Ma, L. Load-bearing properties of minimal-invasive monolithic lithium disilicate and zirconia occlusal onlays: finite element and theoretical analyses. *Dent Mater*, 2013; 29(7): 742–751.

36 Christensen RP, Ploeger BJ, A clinical comparison of zirconia, metal and alumina fixed-prosthesis frameworks veneered with layered or pressed ceramic: a 3 year report. *J Am Dent Assoc*, 2010; 141(11); 1317–1329.

37 Keough BE, Kay HB, Sage RD, Keen E. Clinical performance of scientifically designed, hot isostatic-pressed (HIP'd) zirconia cores in a bilayered all-ceramic system. *Compend Contin Educ Dent*, 2011; 32(6): 58–68.

38 Albashaireh ZS, Ghazal M, Kern M. Two body wear of different ceramic materials opposed to zirconia ceramics. *J Prosthet Dent*, 2010; 104(2): 105–113.

39 Wolfart M, Lehmann F, Wolfart S, Kern M. Durability of the resin bond strength to zirconia ceramic after using different surface conditioning methods. *Dent Mater*, 2007; 23(1): 45–50.

40 Crispin BJ. Conservative alternative to full esthetic crowns. *J Prosthet Dent*, 1979; 42(4): 392–397.

6

Supragingival Simple and Complex Onlay Preparation

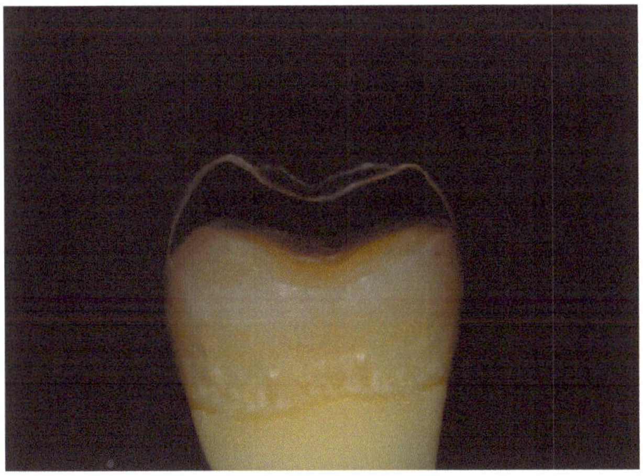

An ideal onlay preparation relies on adhesion for retention; resistance and retention form are unnecessary.

Introduction

Correct preparation is crucial to the success of bonded onlays and partial crowns. In many cases, less than ideal results occur because clinicians have followed habits created by traditional school training and years of working in the same way. Crown preparation and gold onlay preparation require tooth preparation with exacting geometric features, retention and resistance form (Figure 6.1) Thus, when presented with a preparation for partial or full coverage porcelain onlay, instinctively it is assumed that this preparation will have similar mechanical features and only minor variations will be made to the preparation, as experience and the literature attest [1,2,3]. Additionally, lack of trust in the long-term success of adhesion continues to encourage clinicians to use mechanical retention during bonded onlay preparation. There is great variation in what is suggested to be the "ideal" onlay preparation. Some suggest modifications to geometric preparations, with time-consuming routine buildups to soften boxes, and other geometric features [4]. Others recommend flat preparations with limited features, and unbroken contacts, which some call flat-top design. This type of preparation has the disadvantage of the lack of indexing during fabrication and the inability to find a positive seating at cementation. Some consider that badly worn or damaged teeth are contraindicated for bonded onlays, and thus encourage full coverage (Figure 6.2a–d) [3,5]. While others suggest super-thin composite or ceramic occlusal veneers for severely worn teeth, which could easily lead to a short clinical life, as occlusion will wear through the restoration (Figure 6.3) [6,7]. Etemadi and colleagues determined that, in prosthodontic practice, the variation in tooth preparation design for all ceramic posterior restorations is quite large, and suggested that more needs to be known about the consequences of such variation [8]. Adhesively retained, partial-coverage bonded porcelain onlays do not require exacting tapers on axial walls, internal angles, offsets, grooves, and other retention and resistance features used in mechanically

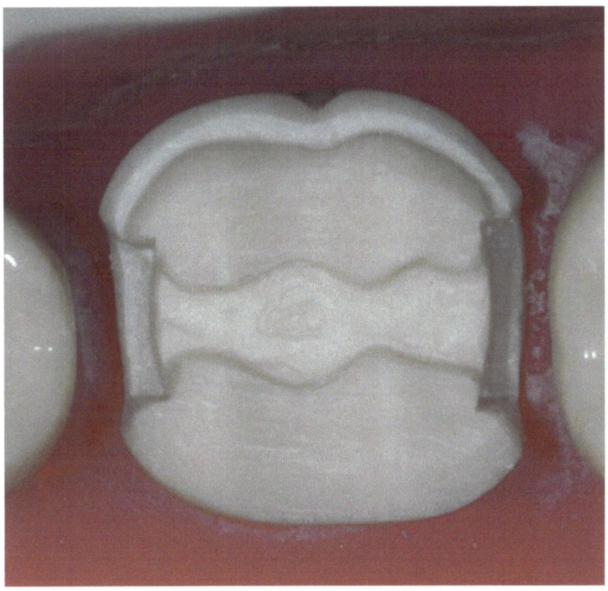

Figure 6.1 Geometric gold onlay preparation.

Supra-Gingival Minimally Invasive Dentistry: A Healthier Approach to Esthetic Restorations, First Edition. By Jose-Luis Ruiz.

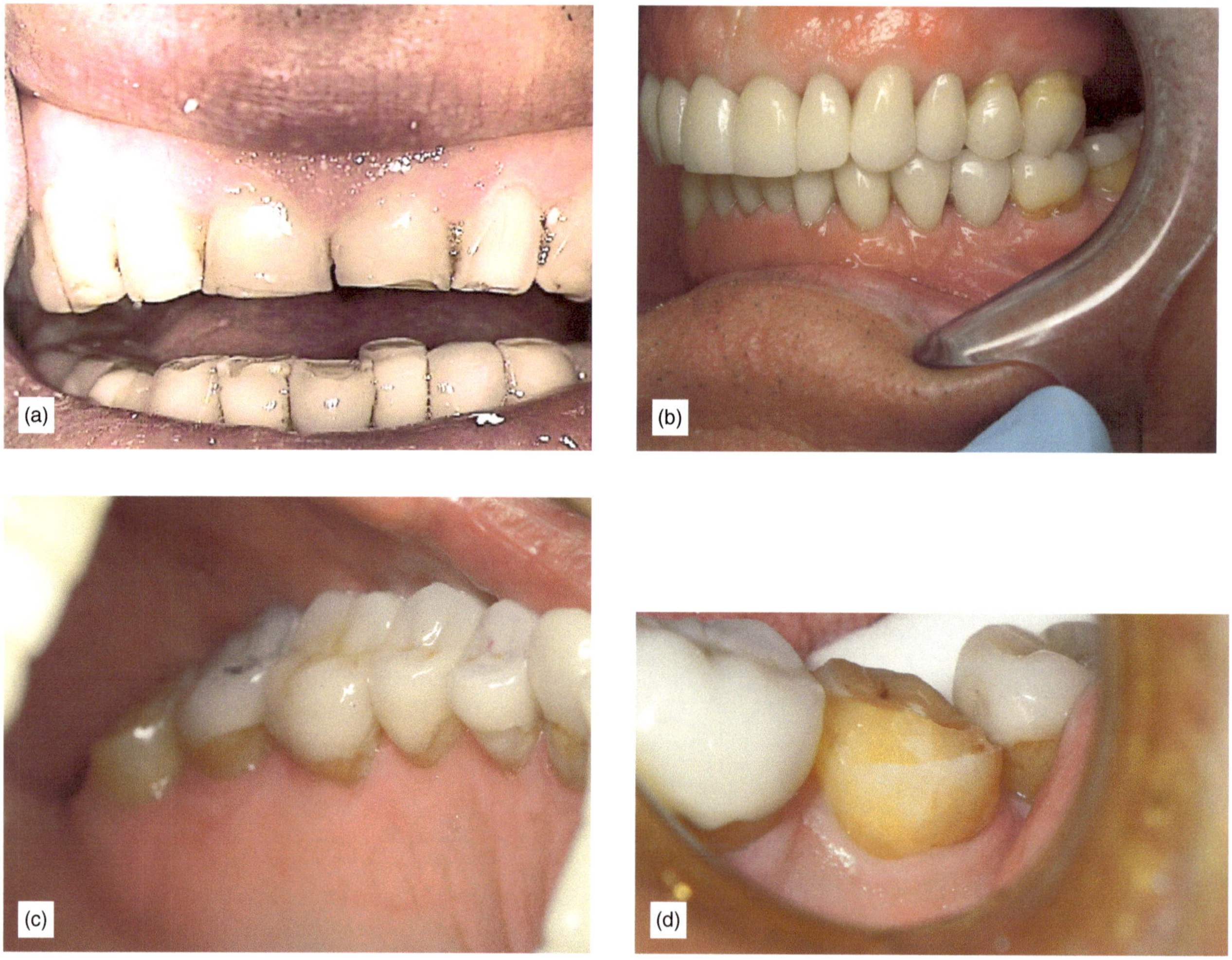

Figure 6.2 (a) This severe bruxer had a full mouth rehabilitation with feldspathic bonded onlays and veneers. (b) Fifteen-year postoperative facial view. (c) Fifteen-year postoperative lingual view. (d) The same patient 16 years postoperatively; the patient had fractures on the lower first molar onlay, showing minimal preparation, no catastrophic failures for the tooth, replacement onlay with e-max was simple.

retained restorations. Adhesion is sufficient to retain the final restoration.

Procedures which employ adhesive retention and have no need for mechanical retentive features have many advantages. Many years of experience and thousands of restorations have shown that bonded onlays can be used successfully in cases when the tooth is only missing a limited amount of structure (for example, one or two cusps, and for badly damaged endodontically treated teeth (Figure 6.4a–d). Clearly, the preparation required for a simple tooth should be different from the preparation for a complex, badly damaged tooth. Correct use and a proper understanding of adhesion and new restorative materials should allow the restorative dentist to select a material that best fits the condition of the tooth.

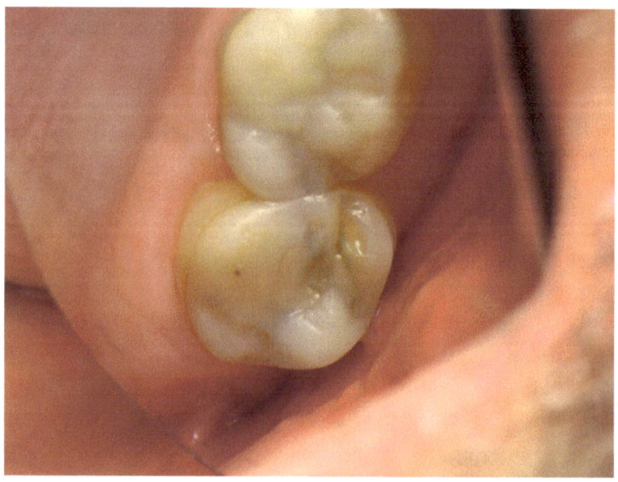

Figure 6.3 Partial coverage composite onlay at 10-year recall.

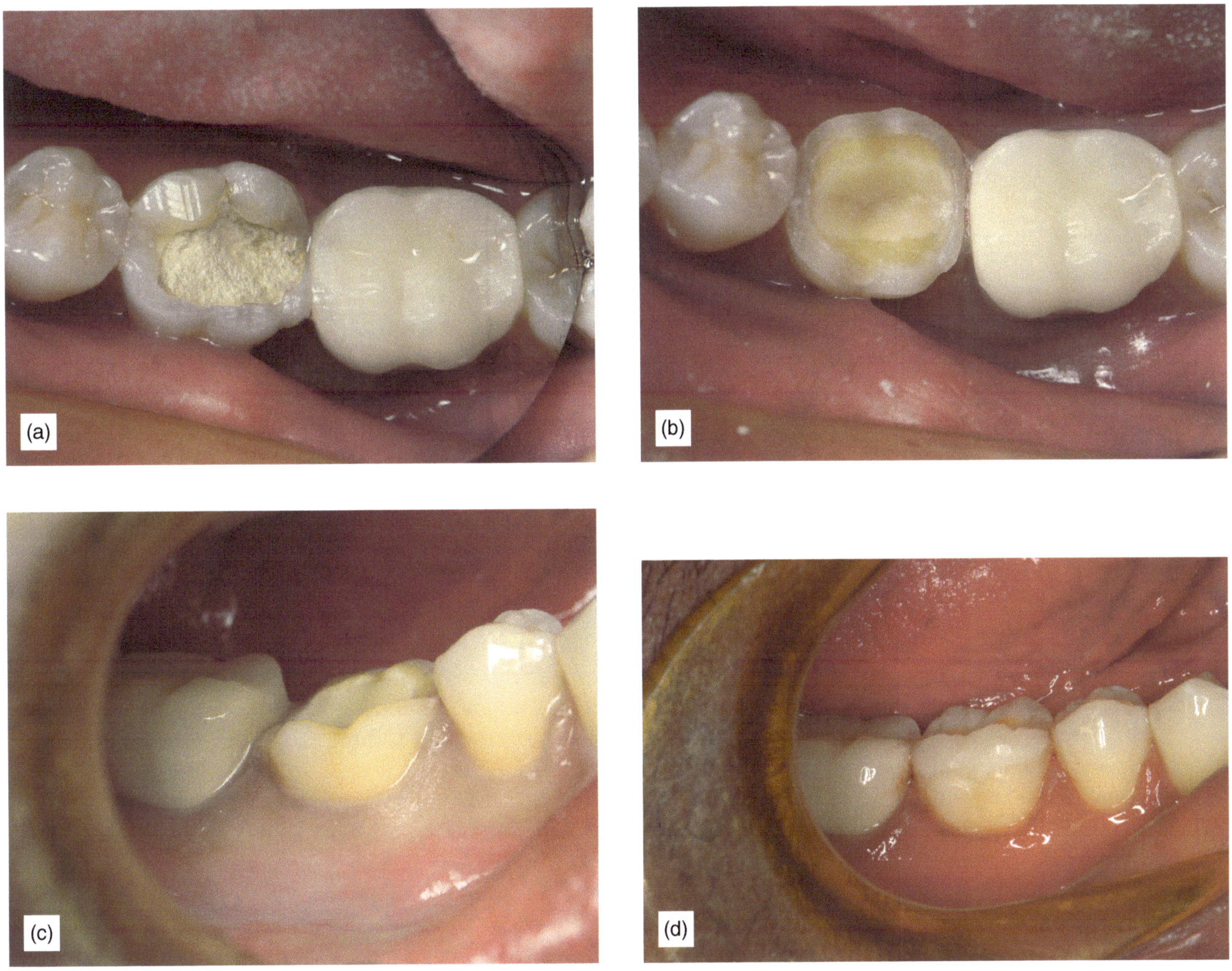

Figure 6.4 (a) Very weak root canal treated tooth. (b) Preparation and buildup. (c) Side view. (d) Completed restoration.

Purpose of Tooth Preparation and Universal Principles

The purpose of tooth preparation is first to remove the damaged and carious tooth structure, and then to create space for the restorative material. Tooth preparation should also include retention and resistance forms (for traditional mechanically retained restorations), creating a design that facilitates laboratory fabrication of the restoration, simplifies cementation or adhesive bonding of the restoration. An additional preparation requirement, unique to the supragingival approach, is the use of a protocol which avoids or greatly limits the risk of placing the restorative material subgingivally. Clearly, retention and resistance forms are unnecessary when we use adhesion. Supragingival minimally invasive bonded restoration requires a preparation that preserves more of the tooth. It is tissue protective and is, in fact, simpler to perform than traditional crown and bridge work. To achieve the above requirements, there are some universal rules that should be applied to all bonded onlay preparations. While some principles are widely agreed upon, some are open to the interpretation of the available literature [9,10] mixed with clinical experience.

Basic Universal Principles for Onlay Preparations

A minimum thickness of 2 mm is desirable for the restorative material [11]. Some studies suggest that very thin restorative material becomes weaker and more likely to fracture [3], although other studies show that strong materials such as lithium disilicate and zirconia can perform well when thinner, or when bonded with resin cement [12,13]. Thus a 2 mm space or reduction should be the goal, on the understanding that sometimes,

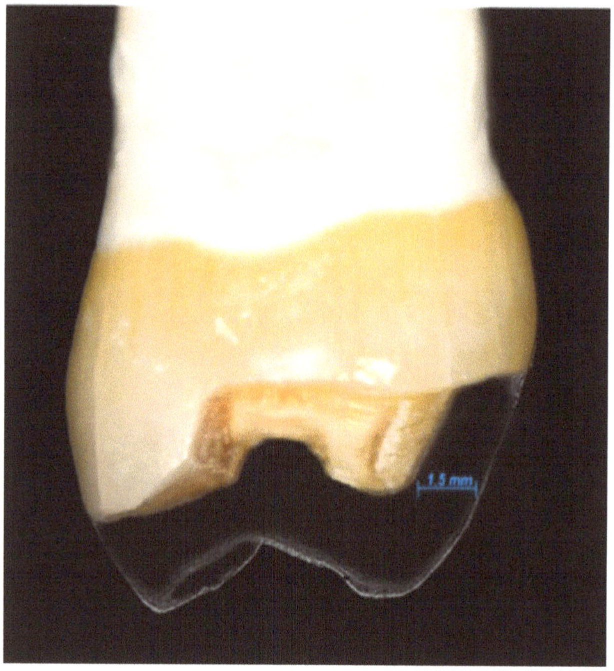

Figure 6.5 Occlusal reduction compared with axial reduction.

during occlusal adjustment, porcelain will be removed and the final thickness will be less.

It is reassuring to realize that the pulp is farther away from the occlusal surface of the tooth. Thus, occlusal reduction will cause the least trauma to the pulp, compared with other surface reductions, especially axial reduction (Figure 6.5). Sufficient reduction is important so it is desirable to confirm the space using an occlusal reduction ring of the clinician's choice or a flexible clearance tab, to ensure an accurate 2 mm reduction (Figure 6.6). A thermoplastic tab may be used, on which the patient bites down after it has been

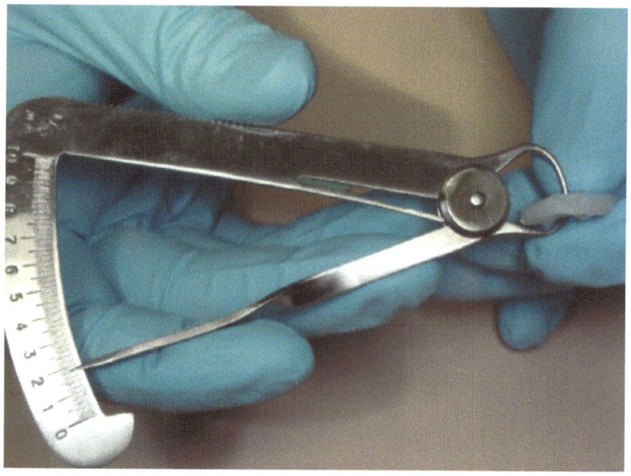

Figure 6.7 Measuring thermoplastic tab with calipers.

softened by hot water. The space is then measured with calipers (Figure 6.7).

A flatter preparation is desirable, as it preserves more tooth structure. Geometrical preparations can prevent full seating of a restoration, owing to the film thickness of the adhesive cement (Figure 6.8). The occlusal reduction should follow the same morphology of the natural tooth, and not be a full flat-top reduction. If the condition of the tooth is such that, after occlusal reduction and caries removal, the preparation is flat, it is unnecessary to reduce it further to create grooves of isthmus – a flat preparation will be well retained by the adhesive. Proximal ridge areas are prepared to be more concave, but not as a box (Figure 6.9). Reduction follows the inclination of the cusp and grooves. The result is a wavy preparation which resembles the initial natural occlusal surface. A nicely sloped and anatomical occlusal reduction preserves

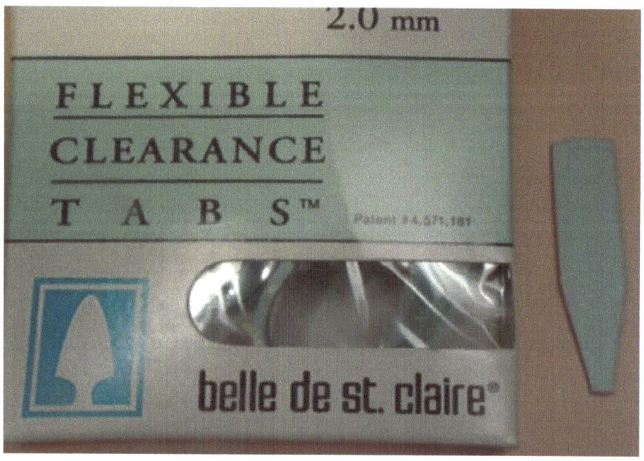

Figure 6.6 An easy way to confirm sufficient occlusal clearance is the use of Clearance Tab (Kerr).

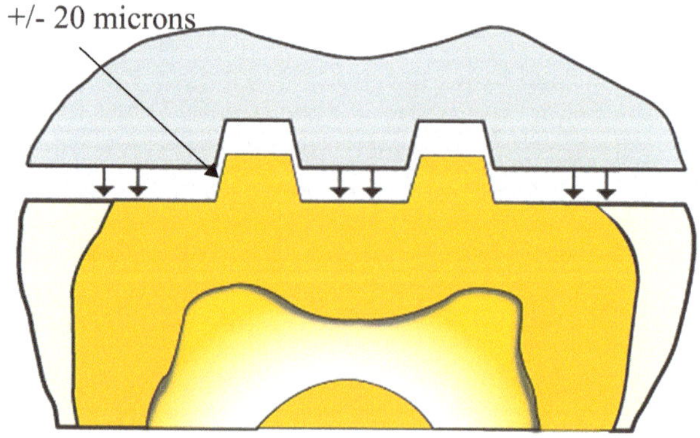

Figure 6.8 Internal boxes and retention line angles create areas where the cement film thickness interferes with full seating of the restoration. Increasing cement thickness has a negative effect on cement polymerization shrinkage. Courtesy of Dr Raymond L. Bertolotti.

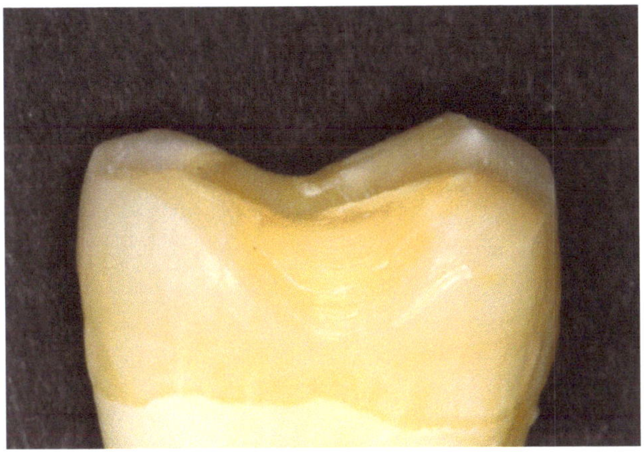

Figure 6.9 U-shaped proximal reduction.

more tooth structure and also serves for indexing when seating the restoration: the onlay should only fit one way (Figure 6.10).

In partial occlusal coverage inlay/onlay combination, the preparation must always ensure a minimum of 2 mm in the transitional areas (Figure 6.11). The prepared tooth should have internal rounded angles.

Great effort should be taken to maintain supragingival, or at least equigingival margins. This can be achieved by the implementation of the five rules of supragingival dentistry previously discussed in Chapter 3. Ideally, enamel margins should be retained if at all possible. However, if this is not possible, it is not a contraindication. Procedures to ensure preservation of enamel margins should be used [14].

Use compressive force on porcelain, whenever possible, and avoid shear force. This generally means avoiding axial reduction, as in traditional mechanically retained crowns. Axial reduction increases shear forces on the final restoration (Figure 6.12).

After occlusal reduction of the lingual cusps, when indicated, create a shallow 1 mm bevel, fully within the enamel, to ensure better enamel rod direction. Avoid

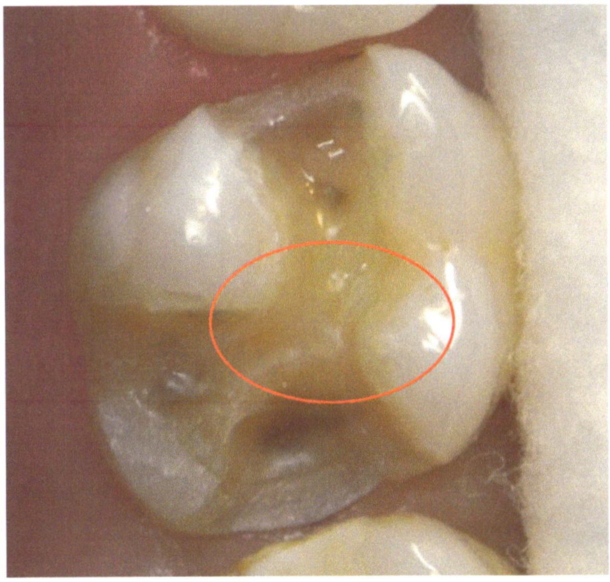

Figure 6.11 Transition area (red circle) must be 2 mm minimum thickness in any direction.

this step if you are in danger of getting too close to the gingiva or the subgingival margin. It is acceptable to leave a lingual butt margin.

Facial bevel for esthetic blending of the onlay restoration is ideal. The bevel should be entirely within the enamel, at approximately 45 degrees (Figures 6.13 a–c, 6.14a,b). The thin, knife-edge porcelain at the end of the bevel will provide for maximum blending capacity. Knife-edge margins can be easily fabricated with pressable lithium disilicate. Fabricating this type of thin margin with a computer-aided designed and manufactured (CAD-CAM) restoration may be more challenging, overbulking the margins at CAD design and after adhesive cementation. Finishing the restoration to the thin design is a way of circumventing the limitations of CAD-CAM design. While some consider thin porcelain margins to be contraindicated [15], other studies may suggest equal success with bevelled and

Figure 6.10 Finish occlusal reduction correctly following cusp inclinations and ondulations.

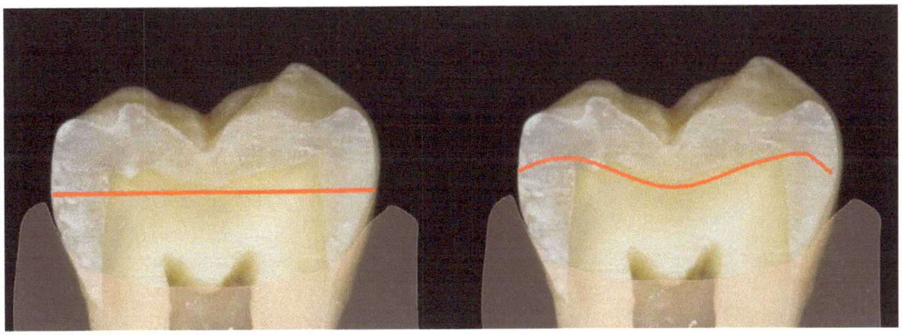

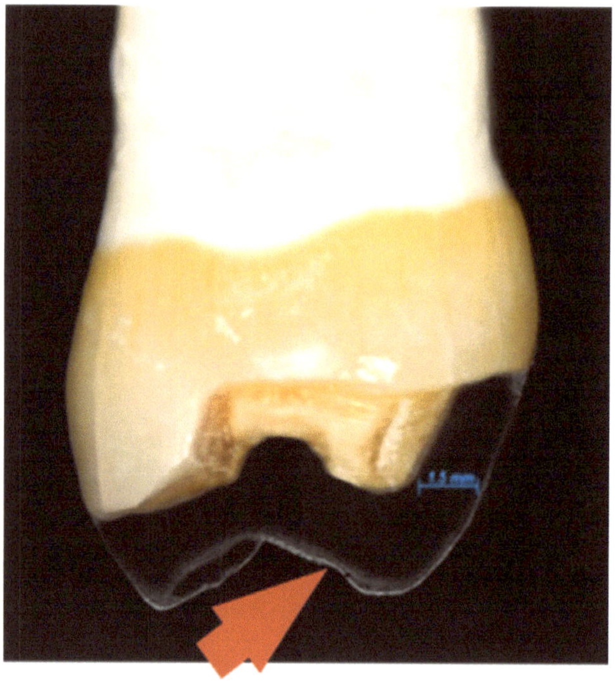

Figure 6.12 Axial reduction enhances the effect of shear forces.

unbevelled onlays [16]. My own extensive clinical experience of thousands of restorations, with not one fracture at the margin, shows that clinical reality sometimes does not follow “supposed truths” or even in-vitro testing.

Slight interproximal separation, while not absolutely necessary [15], is desirable, to allow the laboratory or the scanner to easily view the restoration margins and to provide clean margins. Unclear margins lead to defective margins (Figure 6.15).

Three Variations Based on Tooth Damage

Teeth requiring bonded onlay will have different amounts of damage and, for that reason, the complexity of the preparation will be different. It is very successful and time efficient to prepare teeth with simple problems using a simple approach, while reserving buildups and other time-consuming techniques for more complex cases. There are three variations to the preparation, based on the amount of tooth damage: simple partial and full coverage for vital teeth, complex full

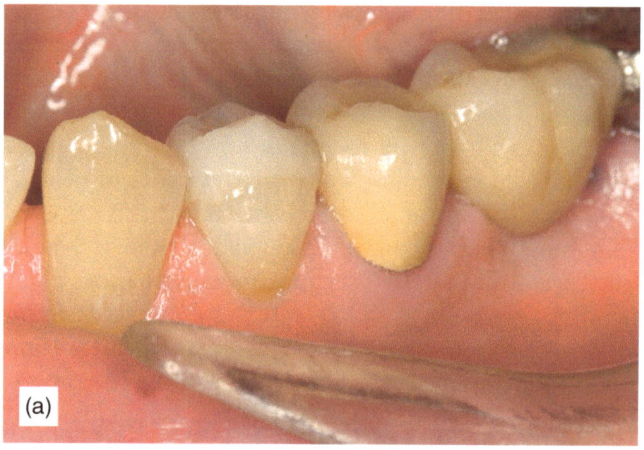

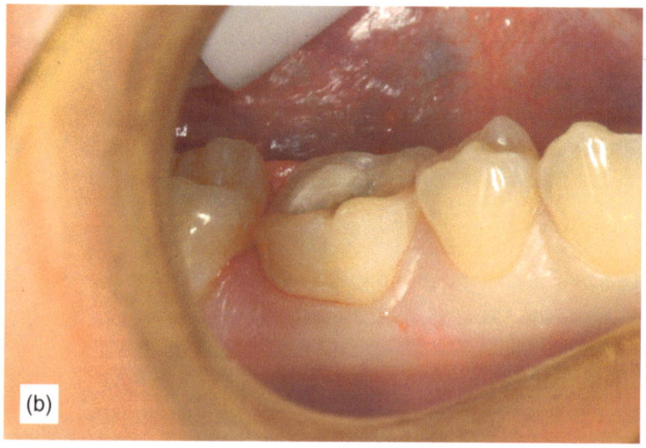

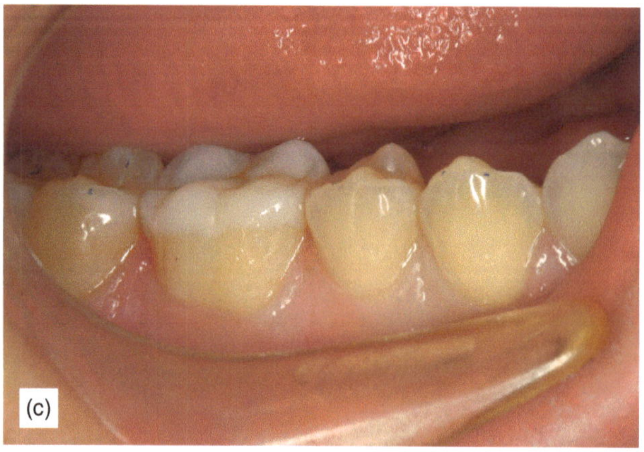

Figure 6.13 (a) Onlay without a bevel but with a margin, allowing for poor marginal blending and less than desirable esthetic results. (b) Too small a bevel for transition will affect the transition blending. (c) Poor margin blending as a result of lack of sufficient bevel and opacious material.

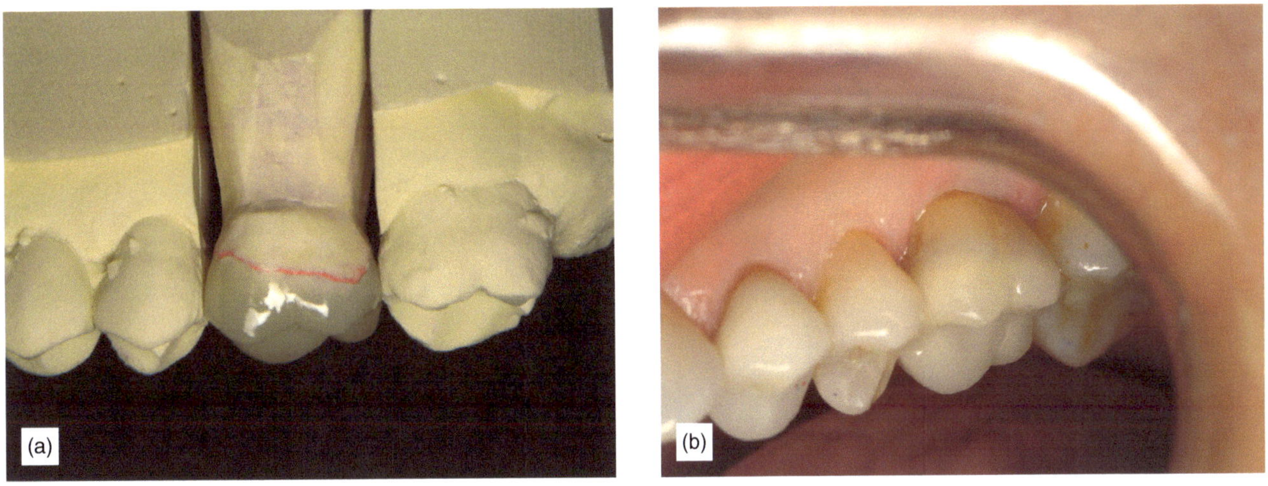

Figure 6.14 (a) A 2–3 mm facial bevel on enamel for maximum blending, visible on the cast; (b) good blending with a high-translucency onlay.

occlusal coverage requiring buildup on vital teeth, and finally complex full coverage for endodontically treated teeth or vertical fractures. Each one has variation based on the tooth condition, but they all fulfill the above general guidelines. In real clinical practice, all the above preparations use the simplified bur and diamond armamentarium, which help to keep things uncomplicated (Figure 6.16).

Simple Partial and Full Coverage for Vital Teeth

Preparations are simple because the tooth condition is ideal. The remaining tooth structure is sufficient to support the restoration without buildup, and the cervical margin placement will end up supragingival, with an enamel periphery, or a supragingival dentin margin, without the need for buildup, using careful caries removal techniques (using the first principle, as outlined in Chapter 3). If the existing old restoration or caries goes up to the equigingival margin or to 1 mm subgingivally in a small segment of the tooth (e.g., distal box), the preparation can be finished without the need to elevate the margin. Experience shows that these margins should

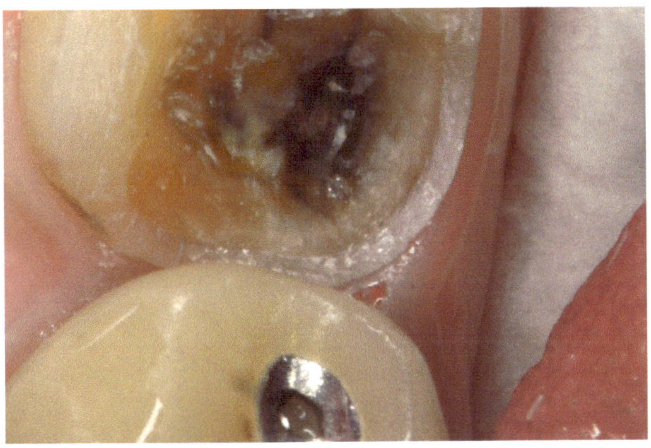

Figure 6.15 Taking impression with tooth in contact will increase difficulty for the laboratory to give accurate restorative margins.

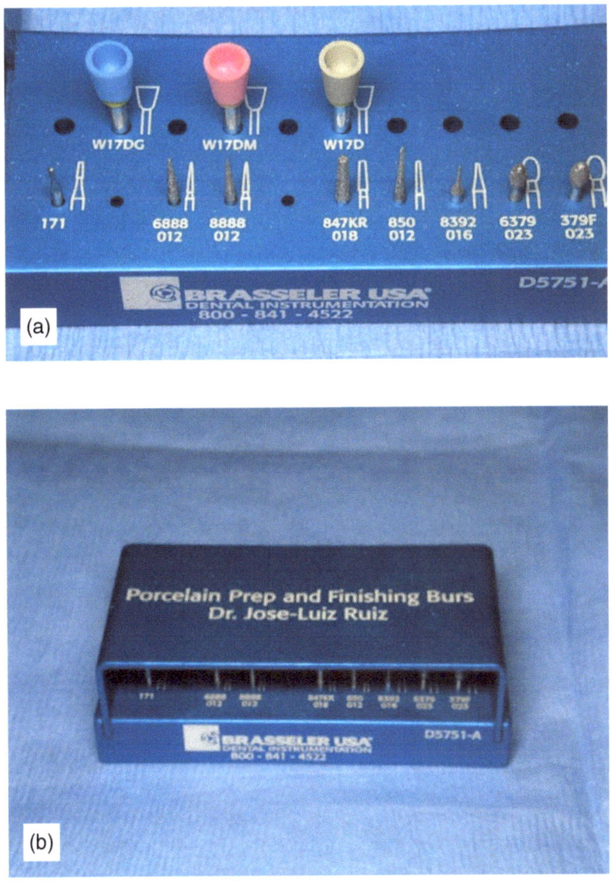

Figure 6.16 Bur block designed by the author to perform all supragingival restorations (Brasseler): (a) Closed. (b) Open.

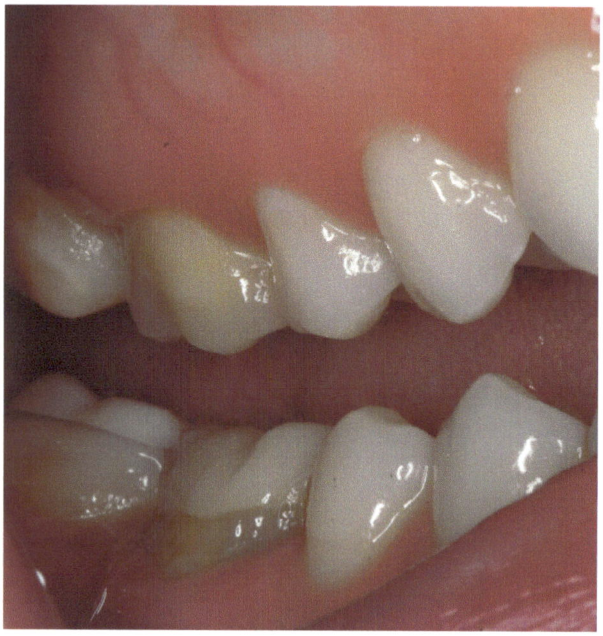

Figure 6.17 Maxillary molar immediately after cementation, showing good esthetics blending with supragingival margins, compared with the improperly managed esthetics of the lower molar.

be easy to control during bonded cementation. The distance to the pulp is sufficient to not require dentin sealing. The vital tooth shade is acceptable, allowing for very supragingival margin placement, as good blending of the restoration and the tooth can be achieved with a translucent material (Figure 6.17).

Simple Partial Coverage Step by Step

Step 1: Using a 2 mm taper occlusal reduction with proper inclination and a Brasseler 6826-025 diamond bur, perform occlusal reduction. Dipping the bur fully to create multiple depth cuts, and then joining them together helps to achieve this rapidly and accurately (Figure 6.18a). Avoid subgingival margins or unnecessary axial reduction.

Step 2: Carefully remove all other existing caries and old restorative material, using principle 1. Remember to be extra careful around cervical margin areas to prevent unnecessary subgingival margins; use a caries indicator. When partial coverage is required, ensure that all isthmus and transitional areas have a minimum thickness of 2.5 mm, as these tend to be the areas where restoration fracture can occur. The isthmus should have a slight taper of 10 degrees or greater (Figure 6.18b).

Step 3: If a box is not present when removing proximal caries and preparing the tooth for appropriate restorative material thickness in the proximal areas, avoid making a traditional box (the third principle). Instead, use proximal margin separation to avoid creating subgingival margin placement unnecessarily. Use a diamond bur at the proximal area, using a U-shaped motion, create the 2 mm reduction. An interproximal tooth shield can prevent unnecessary damage to the adjacent tooth. Only after viewing 2 mm of the adjacent proximal tooth should the margin separation procedure be performed, using a safe-side metal strip or a "mosquito" bur. Use an interproximal tooth shield to avoid touching the adjacent tooth. If the adjacent tooth is still in heavy contact, it is better to perform a more proximal reduction, as long as it does not go subgingival, to allow for easier margin separation (Figure 6.18c). There will often be existing boxes present, which should be carefully cleaned, and any sharp internal angles softened.

Step 4: Check that all margins flow, with no major sharp-angled transitions between proximal and facial lingual margins.

Step 5: If medium to small undercuts are present, remove them with a bur, including them in the preparation to avoid the need for buildups. Very small undercuts can be left, as the laboratory can block those out. If undercuts are larger and it is necessary to undertake buildup with bonded composite, the preparation will be more complex (if this is the case, see the section on complex preparation below).

Step 6: If any facial cusp was included, make a 2–3 mm bevel of the facial surface for improved blending of the restoration (Figure 6.18d). The ideal restorative material for these cases and bevel design would be lithium disilicate (e-Max, Ivoclar), or pressable leucite-reinforced porcelain (such as ZCR Press, Noritake, or EmPress, Ivoclar) for highly esthetic cases in a maxillary first premolar.

Step 7: Finalize the preparation by creating a shallow 1 mm bevel on the lingual margin to ensure better enamel rod direction. Avoid this step if it might lead to getting too close to the gingiva or subgingival margin (Figure 6.18e).

Step 8: Take a final impression and provisionalize.

Simple Full Coverage for a Vital Tooth, Step by Step

Step 1: Using a 2 mm taper occlusal reduction with proper inclination and a Brasseler 6826-025 diamond bur, perform an occlusal reduction. Dipping the bur fully to create multiple depth cuts, and then joining them together helps to achieve this rapidly and accurately (Figure 6.19a),

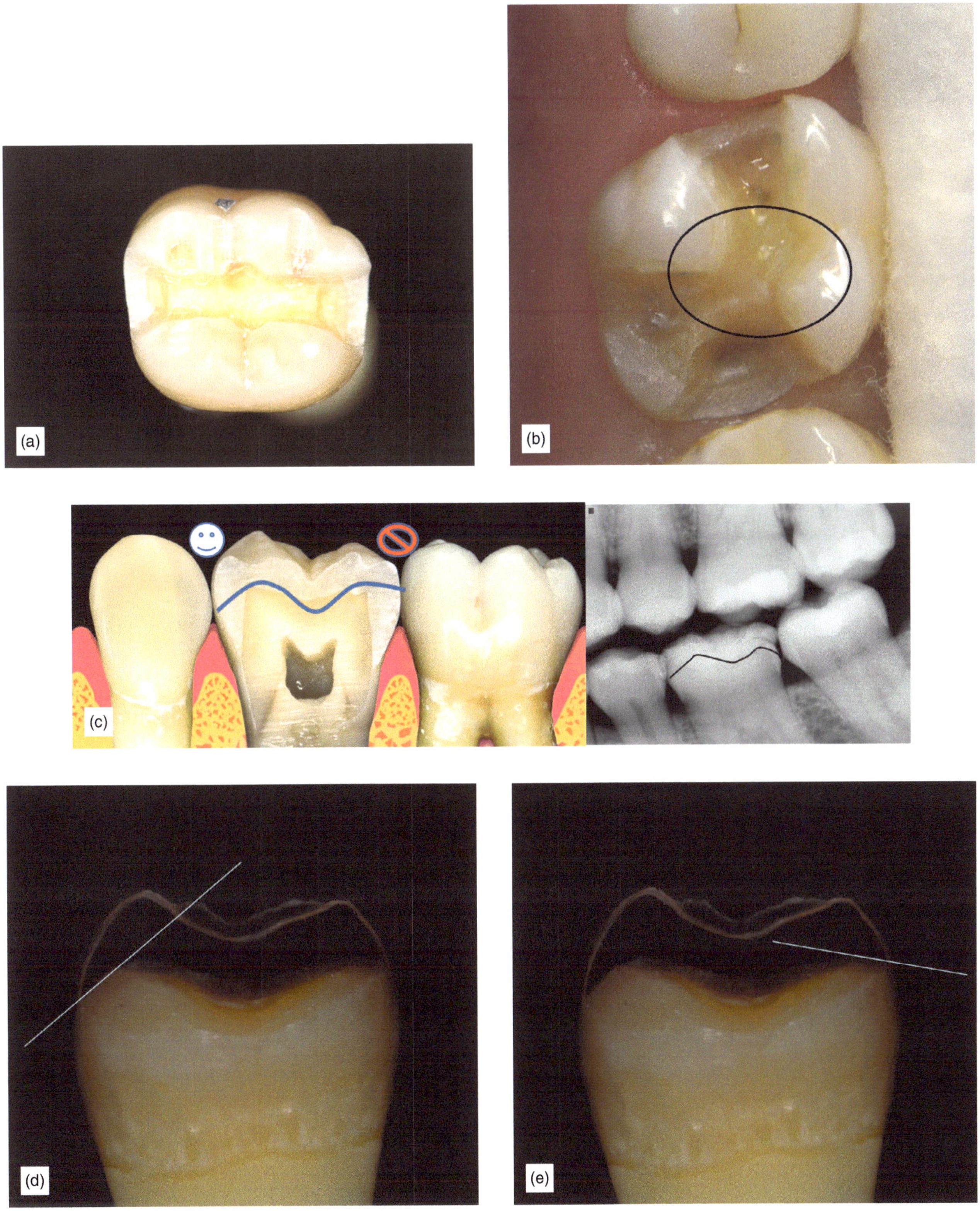

Figure 6.18 (a) Two-millimeter occlusal reduction depth cuts. (b) Two-millimeter minimum isthmus and transitional areas. (c) Correct margin separation procedure requires that the marginal ridge reduction is at least 2 mm and comes close to breaking contact to avoid long incorrect proximal separation. (d) Facial bevel of approximately 45 degrees. (e) Shallow lingual bevel.

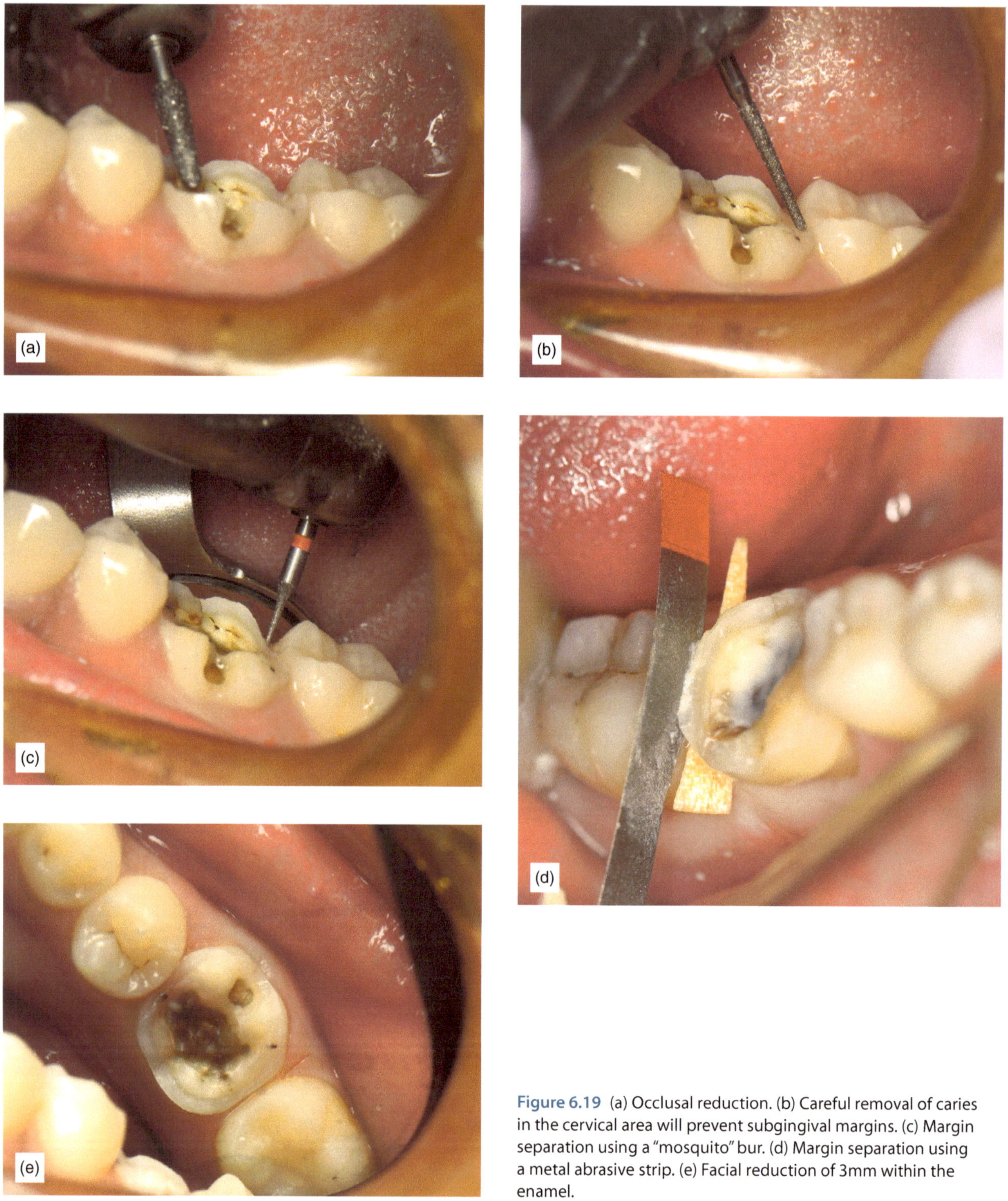

Figure 6.19 (a) Occlusal reduction. (b) Careful removal of caries in the cervical area will prevent subgingival margins. (c) Margin separation using a "mosquito" bur. (d) Margin separation using a metal abrasive strip. (e) Facial reduction of 3mm within the enamel.

avoiding subgingival margins and unnecessary axial reduction.

Step 2: Carefully remove all other existing caries and old restorative material (Figure 6.19b). Remembering the first principle, be extra careful around cervical margin areas to prevent unnecessary subgingival margin placement, and use a caries indicator (Figure 6.19c).

Step 3: When removing proximal caries and preparing the tooth for appropriate restorative material thickness in the proximal areas, if a box is not present, avoid making a traditional box (third principle), and use proximal margin separation, to avoid creating subgingival margins unnecessarily. Use a Brasseler 6826-025 diamond bur at the proximal area, with a U-shaped motion, to create the 2 mm reduction. An interproximal tooth shield can prevent unnecessary damage to adjacent tooth. Only after viewing 2 mm of the adjacent proximal tooth should the margin separation procedure be performed, using a safe-side metal strip or a "mosquito" bur. Use an interproximal tooth shield such as FenderWedge (Garrison) to avoid touching the adjacent tooth. If the adjacent tooth is still in heavy contact, it is better to perform a more proximal reduction, as long as it does not go subgingival, to allow for easier margin separation (Figure 6.19d). If boxes are present, carefully clean them, and soften any sharp internal angles.

Step 4: Check that all margins flow, with no major sharp-angled transitions between proximal and facial–lingual margins.

Step 5: If medium to small undercuts are present, remove them with a bur, including them in the preparation to avoid the need for buildups. Very small undercuts can be left, as the laboratory can block those out. Blocking undercuts out with bonded flowable composite is an option, but the time involved doing a buildup, plus the additional complication to provisionalize, make this option less desirable (Figure 6.19e).

Step 6: On the facial cusp, make a 2–3 mm bevel of the facial surface for improved blending of the restoration. Ideal restorative material for these cases and bevel design would be lithium disilicate, or pressable leucite-reinforced porcelain for highly esthetic cases in a maxillary first premolar.

Step 7: Finalize the preparation by creating a shallow 1 mm bevel on the lingual margin to ensure better enamel rod direction. Avoid this step if it might lead to getting too close to the gingiva or subgingival margin.

Step 8: Take a final impression and provisionalize.

Complex Full Occlusal Coverage Requiring Buildup in Vital Teeth

Complex onlay preparations in vital teeth are complicated by the excessive damage to the existing tooth. These cases will require one or more of the following processes:

- Dentin sealing may be required to avoid pulp irritation if the distance to the pulp became less than 2 mm during preparation and caries removal.
- Buildup may be necessary if large undercuts are present due to extensive caries.
- Enamel margin preservation may be necessary because gingival caries is extensive and the remaining healthy enamel can be preserved allowing the cavosurface margin to remain supragingival.
- Margin elevation may be necessary because caries or old restorative material is in fact subgingival to more than 1.5 mm and it is expected that, without margin elevation, bonded cementation will be unpredictable. The tooth is vital, so the margin can be placed anywhere and a good restoration blend can be anticipated (Figure 6.20a–c).

Complex Partial or Full Occlusal Coverage Step by Step

Step 1: Using a 2 mm taper occlusal reduction with proper inclination and a diamond bur, perform an occlusal reduction. Dipping the bur fully to create multiple depth cuts, and then joining them together helps to achieve this rapidly and accurately (Figure 6.21a), avoiding subgingival margins or unnecessary axial reduction.

Step 2: Carefully remove all other existing caries and old restorative material. With the first principle in mind, remember to be extra careful around cervical margin areas to avoid unnecessary subgingival margins, and use caries indicator (Figure 6.21b). When partial coverage is required, ensure that all isthmus and transitional areas have a minimum thickness of 2.5 mm, as these tend to be areas where restoration fractures can occur. The isthmus should have a slight taper 10 degrees or greater.

Step 3: After caries removal, assess what type of buildup will be required, whether there is a need for dentin sealing, whether there is a large undercut or weak cusp repair, if there is a need for enamel margin preservation or elevation. Perform all repairs and buildups at the same time. Pay attention to correct bonding and repair techniques (discussed in Chapters 3, 4 and 9), as well as minimizing polymerization shrinking while building up the tooth (discussed in detail in Chapters 3 and 9). Use an oxygen inhibitor to do the final cure of the buildups (Figure 6.21c).

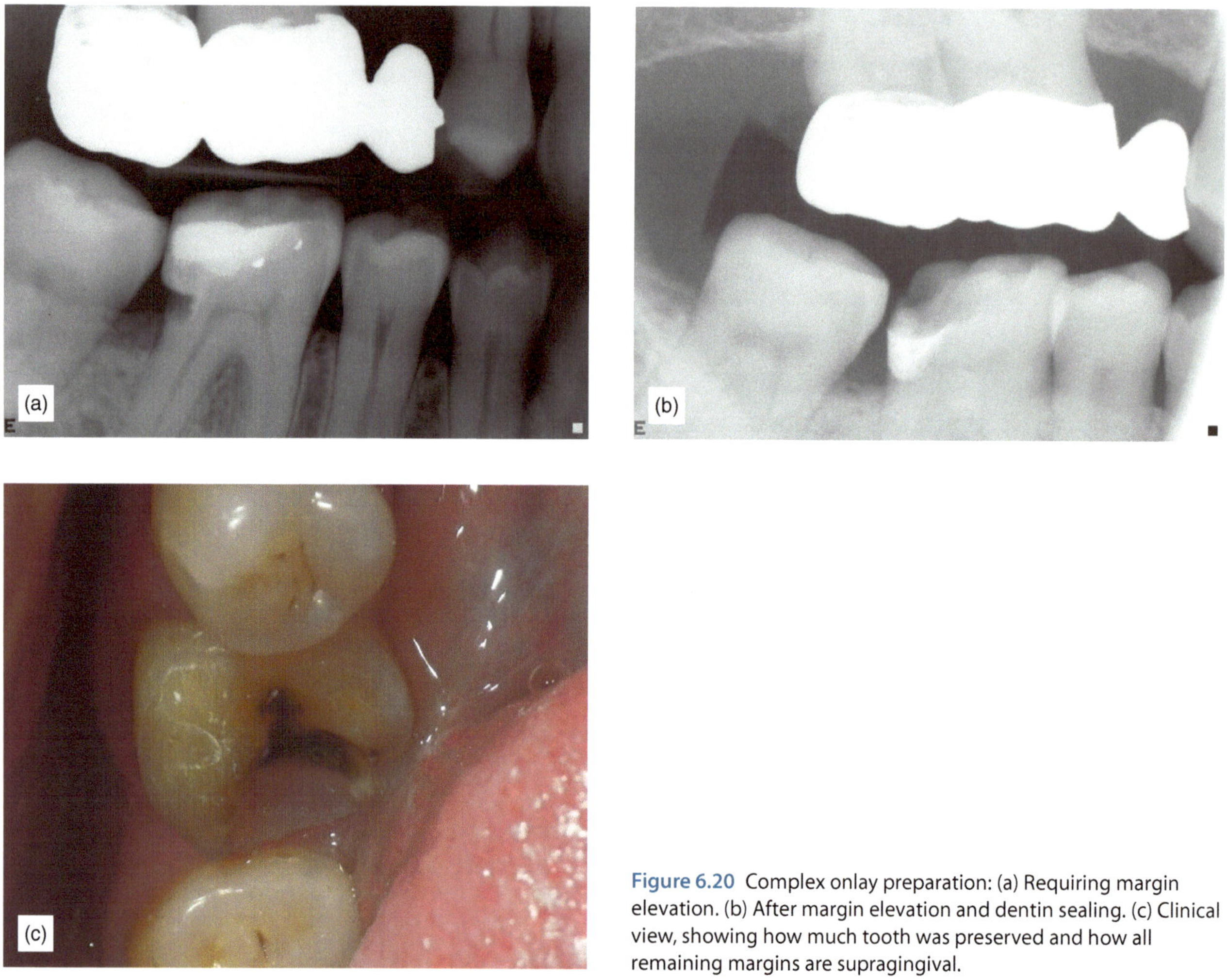

Figure 6.20 Complex onlay preparation: (a) Requiring margin elevation. (b) After margin elevation and dentin sealing. (c) Clinical view, showing how much tooth was preserved and how all remaining margins are supragingival.

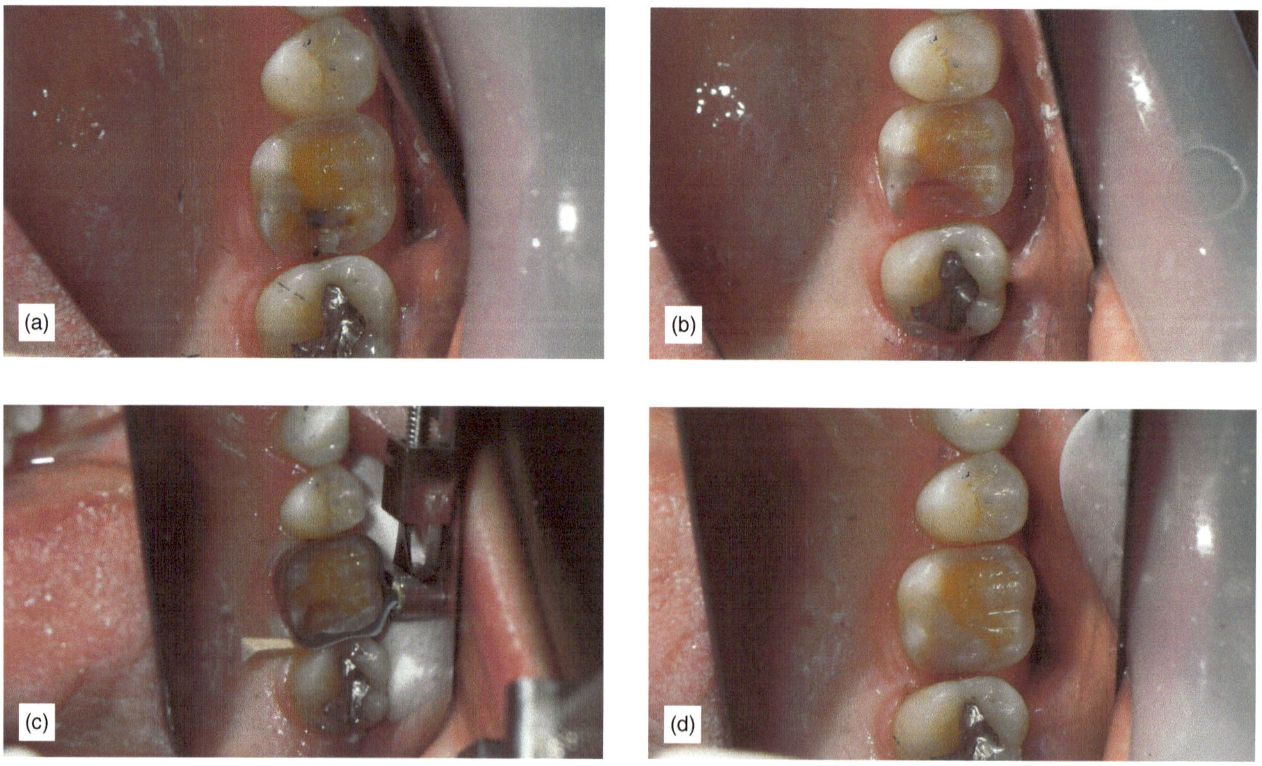

Figure 6.21 (a) After occlusal reduction. (b) Careful cervical caries removal using caries indicator. (c) Enamel preservation and buildup. (d) Ready for simple impression.

Step 4: Finish the preparation, treating the composite buildup as for a tooth.

Step 5: If a box is not present when removing proximal caries and preparing the tooth for appropriate restorative material thickness in the proximal areas, avoid making a traditional box (third principle). Instead, use a U-shaped reduction and proximal margin separation, to avoid creating subgingival margins unnecessarily (Figure 6.21d). Use a diamond bur at the proximal area, with a U-shaped motion, to create the 2 mm reduction. An interproximal tooth shield can prevent unnecessary damage to the adjacent tooth. Only after viewing 2 mm of the adjacent proximal tooth should the margin separation procedure be performed, using a safe-side metal strip or a "mosquito" bur. Use an interproximal tooth shield to avoid touching the adjacent tooth. If the adjacent tooth is still in heavy contact, it is better to perform a more proximal reduction, as long as it does not go subgingival, to allow for easier margin separation. There will often be existing boxes present. Carefully clean them, and soften any sharp internal angles.

Step 6: Check that all margins flow, with no major sharp-angled transitions between proximal and facial–lingual margins. Create a shallow 1 mm bevel on the lingual margin to ensure a better direction for the enamel rod. Avoid this step if it may lead to getting too close to the gingiva or the subgingival margin.

Step 7: Make an esthetic bevel of 2–3 mm in the facial surface for improved blending of the translucent restoration. Make a lingual bevel. Ideal restorative materials for these cases and bevel design would be lithium disilicate, or pressable leucite-reinforced porcelain for highly esthetic cases.

Step 8: Take a final impression and provisionalize.

Complex Full Coverage for Endodontically Treated or Vital Teeth with Vertical Fractures

The literature suggests that if the marginal ridges are intact and there are no fractures present on endodontically treated molars, the stiffness of the tooth may not be compromised [17] and full coverage may not be necessary. However, an endodontically treated tooth fracture is usually a catastrophic event resulting in the loss of the tooth, and in view of some studies showing up to a sixfold increase of tooth loss for endodontically treated teeth without a full-coverage crown [18], it would be wise to consider full coverage on endodontically treated posterior teeth. Tooth protection can be better achieved with a more tooth-preserving procedure such as a full-occlusal coverage bonded onlay, rather than the more tooth-destroying option of a full-coverage crown. Reducing the axial wall makes no sense, as it further weakens the tooth [19].

These are badly damaged teeth, which have lost their intrinsic rigidity, and they often have a history of vertical fractures or fracture syndrome. The literature and clinical experience show that this category of bonded onlay restoration has a higher rate of failure (Figure 6.22a–c) [20,21,22] and some modification in the preparation and choice of restorative material is necessary. These teeth will require proper buildup to repair the pulp chamber, endodontic access will be needed, and they will often also require enamel margin preservation; margin elevation may also be required. Because these restorations are more prone to fractures, ensuring an increase in thickness of the restorative material is desirable, as well as using a restorative material with increased strength. The minimum thickness of the restorative material must be ensured, as the weaker, less rigid tooth is not a reliably strong substrate to support the bonded onlay. In these cases, the strength of the restorative material is necessary to ensure durability and strength; thicker restorative material will increase stiffness and strength [23]. Occlusal reduction for lithium disilicate should be 2.5 mm to account for the usually necessary occlusal adjustment, and to ensure a minimum final thickness of 2 mm. When zirconia is used, a 2 mm occlusal reduction or space must be achieved, also accounting for some occlusal adjustment, which should leave a restoration of no less than 1.5 mm occlusal thickness. Additionally, some minor internal mechanical retentive features are desirable with bonded zirconia onlays. It should be mentioned that bonded gold is a very good alternative in cases where the tooth is not visible or the patient is willing to pay the extra laboratory costs and is not concerned with esthetics.

Complex Endodontically Treated or Vital Teeth with Vertical Fractures Step By Step

Step 1: Endodontically treated or vital teeth with vertical fractures require extra material thickness for strength. If lithium disilicate is being used, a 2.5 mm reduction or space is the minimum desirable; if zirconia is used, 2 mm is necessary, avoiding subgingival margins or unnecessary axial reduction.

Step 2: Carefully remove all other existing caries and old restorative material. Using the first principle, remember to be extra careful around cervical margin areas to avoid unnecessary subgingival margins.

Step 3: After caries removal, assess what buildup, endodontic access repair, large undercut or weak cusp repair, enamel margin preservation, or margin

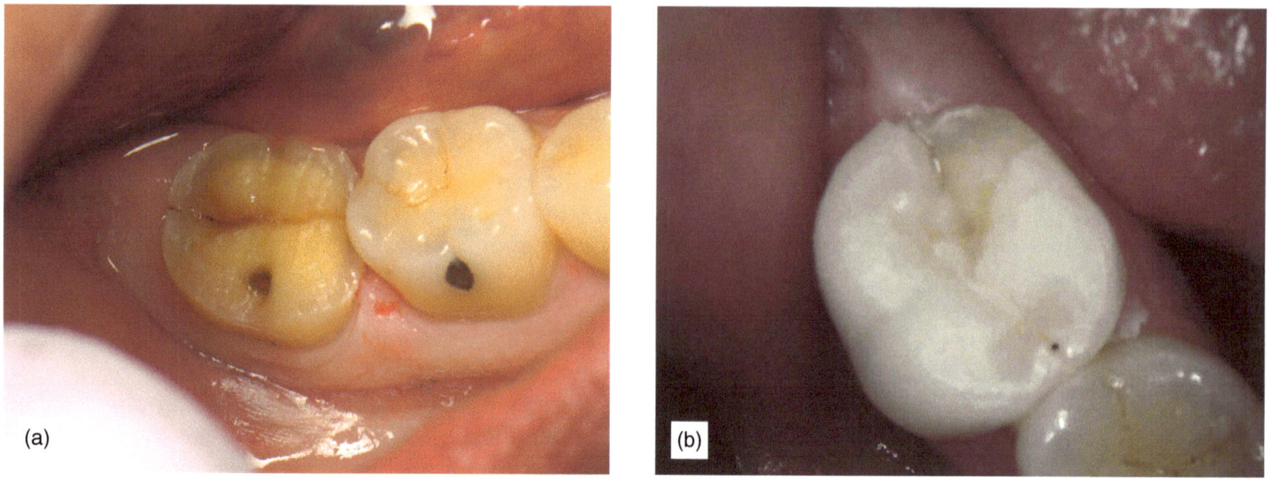

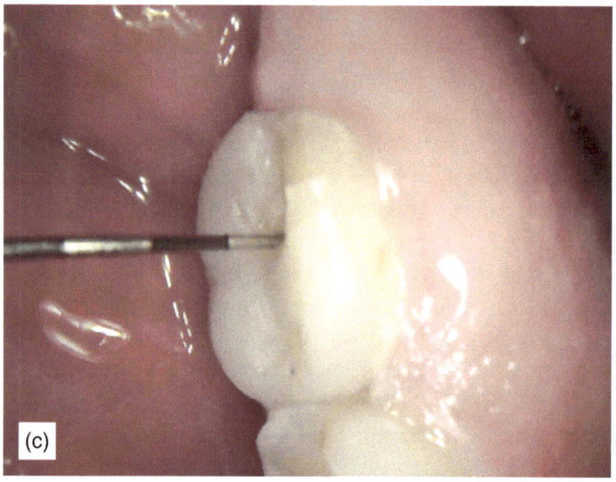

Figure 6.22 (a) Fractured tooth. (b) Failure in fractured tooth. (c) Thin e-Max onlay; these cases are better treated with thick e-Max or zirconia.

elevation will be required. Perform all the repairs and buildups at the same time. Endodontic access should be filled to 1 mm above the level of the top of the pulp chamber, with bonded composite. Pay attention to correct bonding and repair techniques (discussed in Chapters 3, 4 and 9) and minimize polymerization shrinking while building up the tooth (discussed in detail in Chapters 3 and 9). Use an oxygen inhibitor to do final cure of buildups.

Step 4: Finish the preparation, treating the composite buildup as if it were a tooth.

Step 5: If a box is not present when removing proximal caries and preparing the tooth for appropriate restorative material thickness in the proximal areas, avoid making a traditional box (third principle), and use proximal margin separation to avoid creating subgingival margins unnecessarily. Use a diamond bur at the proximal area, with a U-shaped motion, to create the 2 mm reduction. An interproximal tooth shield can prevent unnecessary damage to adjacent tooth. Only after viewing 2 mm of the adjacent proximal tooth, should the margin separation procedure be performed, using a safe-side metal strip or a "mosquito" bur. Use an interproximal tooth shield to avoid touching the adjacent tooth. If the adjacent tooth is still in heavy contact, it is better to perform a more proximal reduction, as long as it does not go subgingival, to allow for easier margin separation. There will often be existing boxes present. Carefully clean them, and soften any sharp internal angles.

Step 6: Check that all margins flow, with no major sharp-angled transitions between proximal and facial–lingual margins. For endodontically treated teeth, it is better to create a deep 2 mm bevel in the enamel on the lingual margin to

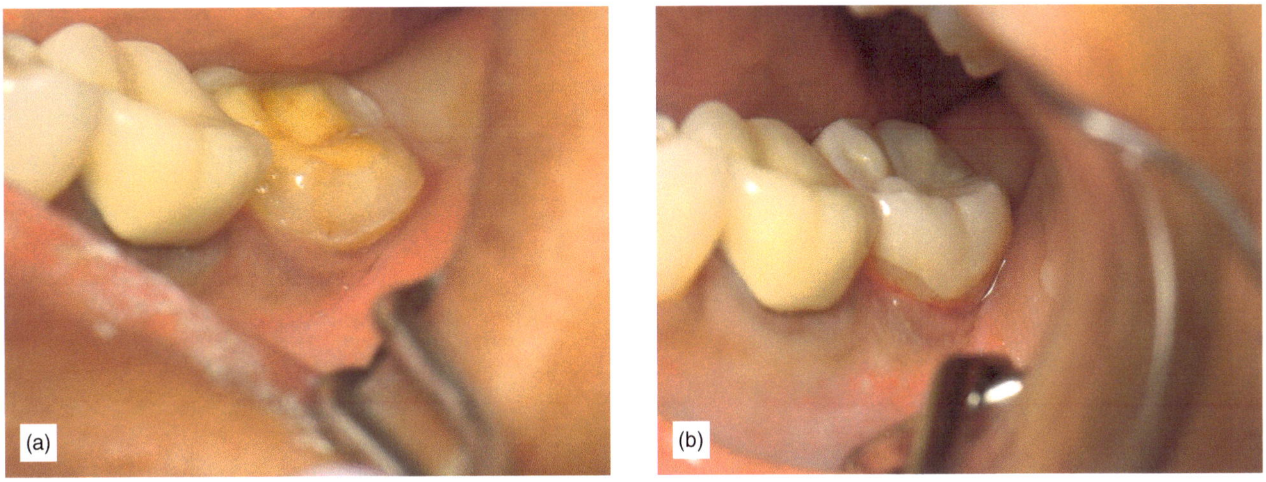

Figure 6.23 (a) Occlusal reduction and extended facial bevel to avoid the undesirable esthetic with zirconia. (b) Final restoration cemented.

ensure better protection of tooth and a better direction for the enamel rod. A smaller bevel is desirable if this step might lead to getting too close to the gingiva or subgingival margin.

Step 7: Bevel the facial surface and color match. If the color of the tooth is ideal, a translucent material such as lithium disilicate can be used. Make a 2–3 mm bevel of the facial surface for improved blending of the restoration and a 2 mm lingual bevel to ensure good splinting of the tooth and better enamel rod exposure. In areas of high force, zirconia maybe a better choice. The trade-off with zirconia is a lack of translucency and poor blending. It is desirable to carry the facial bevel to 1 mm above the gingival margin, ending with a light 0.5 mm chamfer. A 1–1.5 mm lingual bevel should be added to the lingual butt margin, as long as this does not create a subgingival margin (Figure 6.23a,b).

Step 8: Take a final impression and provisionalize.

Step 9: The restoration should be fabricated with thicker lithium disilicate or zirconia.

Impression

The impression process can easily be argued as one of the most unpredictable and often the least successful part of the indirect restorative preparation visit (Figures 6.24, 6.25) [24]. The primary reason for this stress is because, when restorative margins are placed subgingivally, the possibilities of lacerating the gingiva with the drill, or difficult cord packing make tissue management very difficult, as any experienced clinician can attest. Conversely, when a supragingival minimally invasive protocol is in place, the restorative margins will most likely end up above the gums, and these problems become nonexistent. The wonderful news is that, since this is supragingival dentistry, taking an impression is easy. A triple tray combined with a hydrophilic impression material (such as Panasil, Kettenbach) will lead to great results with extremely rare retakes. Digital impressions will also benefit greatly from keeping the margins supragingival.

Materials and Techniques for Temporary Restorations

A significant reason why dentists have been opposed to onlays is the aspect of temporization. The assumption that onlay temporaries have more difficulty in

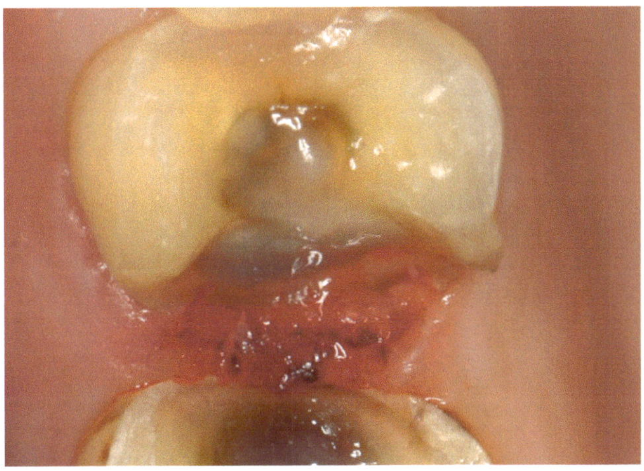

Figure 6.24 Even with a double cord technique, a good impression of the distal margin will be a challenge; a margin elevation would simplify this a great deal.

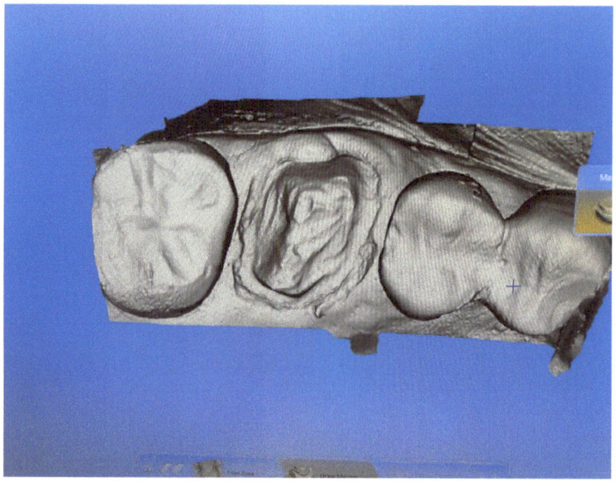

Figure 6.25 Computer-aided designed and manufactured digital impressions have the same challenges as when subgingival margins are present (courtesy of Dr Renee Kurts).

maintaining adhesive integrity owing to a lack of mechanical retention is a reality, but with correct modification of the technique, the problem can be predictably overcome. The technique is very similar to a full crown provisionalization.

1) A preimpression is taken with a hydrophilic alginate substitute silicone impression material, using a small segmental impression tray or triple tray using minimal material (Figure 6.26a). A good impression is always of paramount importance.
2) After preparation, fill the tooth with a good bis-acryl provisional material, like Structure 3 (VOCO) or a non-bis-acryl, like Bisylis (Kettenbach). Make sure to avoid catching bubbles during the filling procedure (Figure 6.26b).
3) Allow approximately 1 minute for full initial setting, the remove the impression and the temporary from the tooth; the material should be firm but slightly flexible.
4) Re-seat the provisional in the mouth for an additional 3 minutes, to allow for final setting and to avoid polymerization shrinkage outside of the mouth, which may deform the temporary and end up affecting correct fit.
5) Trim and polish (Figure 6.26c).
6) A critical decision is the cementation material to be used:
   a) If the provisional is being made on a tooth with no buildup or dentin sealing, any resin-based temporary cement can be used, allowing some extra

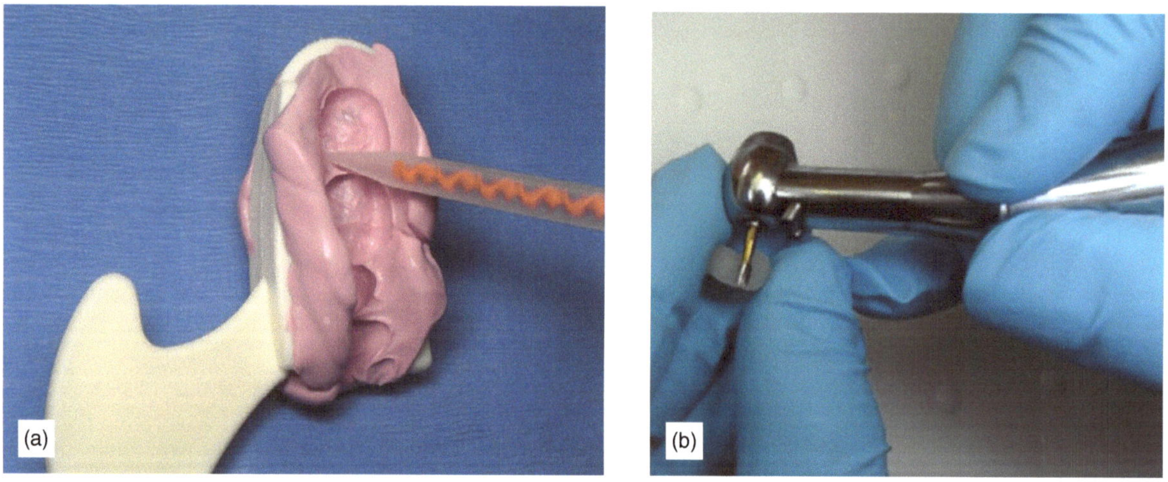

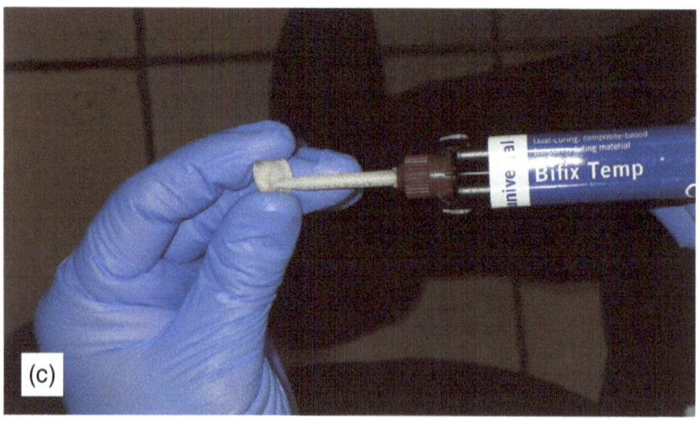

Figure 6.26 (a) A preoperative impression was taken with silginate and the tooth filled with Visalys® (Kettenbach). (b) Trimming the provisional restoration; (c) cement temporary with Bifix Temp (VOCO).

cement to go over the facial and lingual cavosurface margin, allowing that after setting the temporary will lock into place, and no excess should be left interproximally.

b) If the provisional is being made on a tooth with buildup or dentin sealing, the tooth should be coated with a micro-brush with a traditional crown and bridge non-eugenol temporary cement, leaving a small island in the center of the tooth with no cement. A small amount of resin temporary cement should be injected in that island and the provisional seated, followed by correct removal of the excess.

References

1 Edelhoff D. Tooth structure removal associated with various preparation designs for posterior teeth. *Int J Periodont Restorative Dent*, 2002; 22: 241–249.
2 Stappert C. Fracture resistance of different partial-coverage ceramic molar restorations: An in vitro investigation. *J Am Dent Assoc*, 2006; 137(4): 514–522.
3 Heymann H, Swift E, Ritter A. Indirect tooth color restorations, in *Sturdevant's Art and Science of Operative Dentistry*, 6th ed. Elsevier Mosby, 2013, pp. 280–295.
4 Dietschi D, Spreafico R. *Adhesive Metal Free Restorations, Current Concepts for Esthetic Treatment of Posterior Teeth*. Chicago: Quintessence Publishing, 1997, pp. 79–100.
5 Kois DE, Chaiyabutr Y, Kois JC. Comparison of load-fatigue performance of posterior ceramic onlay restorations under different preparation designs. *Compend Contin Educ Dent*, 2012; 33(Spec No 2): 2–9.
6 Magne P, Stanley K, Schlichting LH. Modeling of ultrathin occlusal veneers. *Dent Mater*, 2012; 28(7): 777–782.
7 Schlichting LH, Maia HP, Baratieri LN, Magne P. Novel-design ultra-thin CAD/CAM composite resin and ceramic occlusal veneers for the treatment of severe dental erosion. *J Prosthet Dent*, 2011; 105(4): 217–226.
8 Etemadi S, Smales RJ, Drummond PW, Goodhart JR. Assessment of tooth preparation designs for posterior resin-bonded porcelain restorations. *J Oral Rehabil*, 1999; 26(9): 691–697.
9 Beier U, Kapferer I, Dumfahrt H. Clinical long-term evaluation and failure characteristics of 1,335 all-ceramic restorations. *Int J Prosthodont*, 2012; 25: 70–78.
10 Ahlers MO, Mörig G, Blunck U, Hajt J, Pröbster L, Frankenberger R. Guidelines for the preparation of CAD/CAM ceramic inlays and partial crowns. *Int J Comput Dent*, 200; 12(4): 30–25.
11 Stappert CFJ, Guess PC, Gerds T, Strub JR. All ceramic partial coverage restorations: Cavity preparation design reliability, and fracture resistance after fatigue. *Am J Dent*, 2005; 18: 275–280.
12 Holberg C, Rudzki-Janson I, Wichelhaus A, Winterhalder P. Ceramic inlays: is the inlay thickness an important factor influencing the fracture risk? *J Dent*, 2013; 41(7): 628–635.
13 Bakeman E, Rego N, Chaiyabutr Y, Kois J. Influence of ceramic thickness and ceramic materials on fracture resistance of posterior partial coverage restorations. *Oper Dent*, 2015; 40(2): 211–217.
14 Ruiz JL, Finger WJ. Enamel margin preservation and repair technique. *J Dent Res*, 2016; 95(Spec Iss 5): abstract no. 2370749.
15 Bakeman, E, Kois J. Posterior, all-porcelain, adhesively retained restorations. *Inside Dentistry*, 2009; 5(5): 20–30.
16 Kois DE, Chaiyabutr Y, Kois JC. Comparison of load-fatigue performance of posterior ceramic onlay restorations under different preparation designs. *Compend Contin Educ Dent*, 2012; 33(Spec No 2): 2–9.
17 Reeh ES, Douglas WH, Messer HH. Stiffness of endodontically treated teeth related to restoration technique. *J Dent Res*, 1989; 68: 1540–1544.
18 Aquilino SA, Caplan DJ. Relationship between crown placement and the survival of endodontically treated teeth. *J Prosthet Dent*, 2002; 87: 256–263.
19 Cheung W. A review of the management of endodontically treated teeth. Post, core and the final restoration. *J Am Dent Assoc*, 2005; 136(5): 611–619.
20 Beier US, Kapferer I, Burtscher D, Giesinger JM, Dumfahrt H. Clinical performance of all-ceramic inlay and onlay restorations in posterior teeth. *Int J Prosthodont*, 2012; 25(4): 395–402.
21 van Dijken JW, Hasselrot L. A prospective 15-year evaluation of extensive dentin-enamel-bonded pressed ceramic coverages. *Dent Mater*, 2010; 26(9): 929–939.
22 Dietschi D, Duc O, Krejci I, Sadan A. Biomechanical considerations for the restoration of endodontically treated teeth: a systematic review of the literature, Part II (Evaluation of fatigue behavior, interfaces, and in vivo studies). *Quintessence Int*, 2008; 39(2): 117–129.
23 Ma L. Load-bearing properties of minimal-invasive monolithic lithium disilicate and zirconia occlusal onlays: finite element and theoretical analyses. *Dent Mater*, 2013; 29(7): 742–751.
24 Christensen GJ. The state of fixed prosthodontic impressions: room for improvement. *J Am Dent Assoc* 2005; 136(3): 343–346.

Part III

Supragingival Minimally Invasive Porcelain Veneers: A Replacement for Full Crowns

7

Indication, Preparation and Restorative Material for Supragingival Minimally Invasive Porcelain Veneers

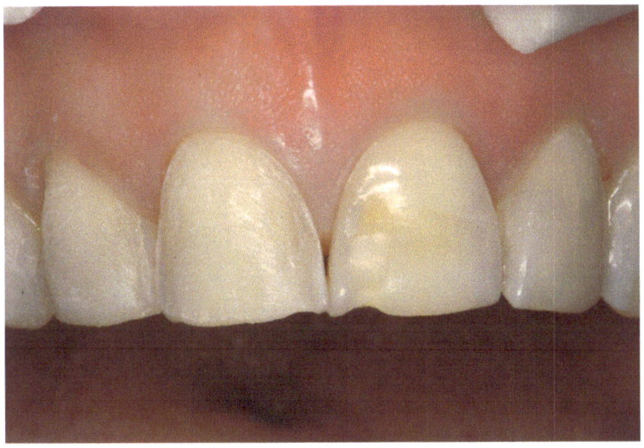

Prepared and unprepared veneer centrals.

Introduction

The indications for porcelain veneers should be expanded. Porcelain veneers can be used for the traditional esthetic rehabilitation of a tooth or teeth (Figure 7.1a–c, 7.2a,b). Porcelain veneers are the ideal material for restoration when teeth are badly damaged by fractures, large caries or old restorations, and when teeth have undergone endodontic procedures. Fractured teeth are great candidates for porcelain veneers to replace the damaged or missing incisal edge. Some in-vitro studies suggest that teeth with an extensive incisal edge missing could be at a higher risk of fracture or failure with veneers [1,2]. This may lead to the assumption that large fracture cases should be treated with more aggressive procedures, such as full crowns. This approach is counterintuitive, as it suggests that the solution to a large fracture or damage on a tooth would be to cut further large amounts of tooth for a full crown (Figure 7.3a,b). Fortunately, extensive clinical experience and the literature reports the success and durability of this restoration, even when several millimeters of incisal length are replaced (Figures 7.4a–c, 7.5a,b, 7.6a–e) [3,4].

Veneers can also be used for an occlusal rehabilitation to regain lost anterior guidance, although many experts have suggested that veneers are contraindicated for restorations of teeth with severe wear and when

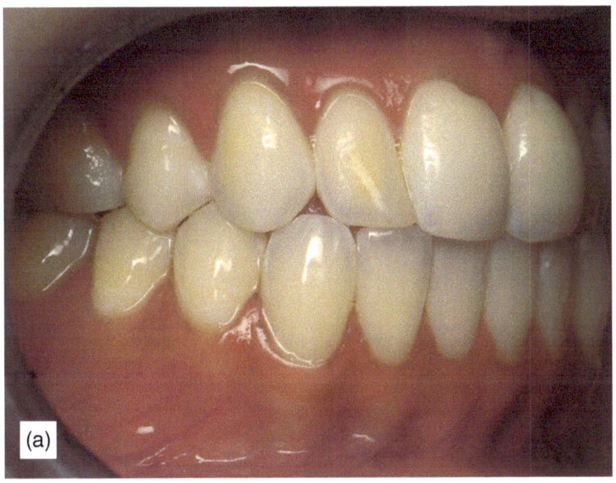

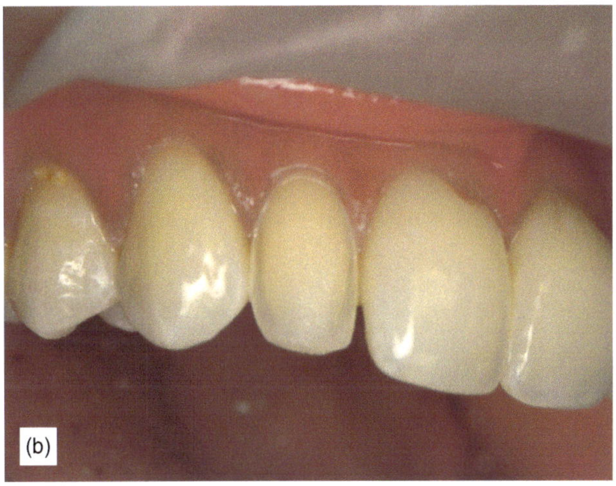

Figure 7.1 (a) A dentist's daughter with a peg lateral corrected with bonding. (b) Supragingival minimally invasive preparation. *(Continued)*

Supra-Gingival Minimally Invasive Dentistry: A Healthier Approach to Esthetic Restorations, First Edition. By Jose-Luis Ruiz.

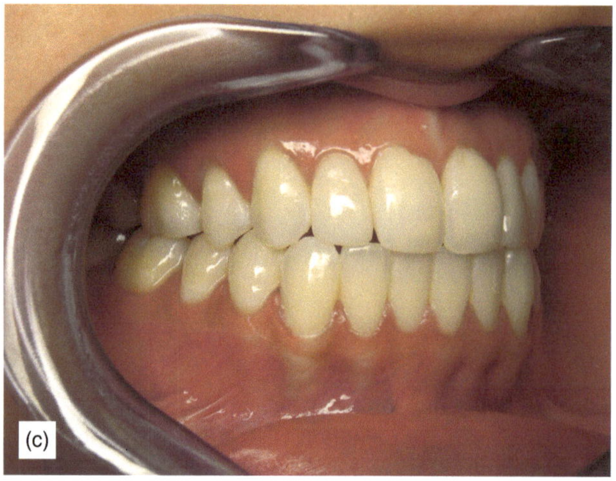

Figure 7.1 (*Continued*)
(c) Finished restoration.

occlusal problems are present [5,6] fearing a decrease in durability. In fact, these fears lead to the promotion of full-coverage crowns as the ideal treatment for worn-out teeth [7,8]. Nevertheless, porcelain veneers are the ideal restoration to repair occlusal trauma. They can help to regain lost tooth structure, and the necessary anterior guidance and posterior disclusion, without the need to grind away more of the already ground-down teeth (Figure 7.7a–e). Clinical experience and the literature also show that the durability of ceramo-metal crowns used in occlusally affected patients is equally compromised [9,10], with all the added disadvantages of a full crown. The success of porcelain veneers increases dramatically when the occlusion is managed, using good occlusal principles, such as the three golden rules of occlusion (Figure 7.8a–e). In other words, any time that a tooth requires an indirect restoration, a supragingival minimally invasive adhesively retained porcelain veneer should be the procedure of choice, because it will be as successful at restoring a damaged tooth as a full crown [11], with the benefit of less tooth preparation, decreased pulp irritation and supragingival margins, especially when margins are kept on the enamel.

Consequences of Unnecessary Tooth Removal

The aggressive tooth preparation required for full crowns of the anterior teeth has the disadvantage of further weakening badly damaged teeth [12,13]. The fact that anterior teeth are small and thin further amplifies the need to conserve as much of the remaining healthy structure as possible (Figure 7.9). Partial coverage bonded porcelain

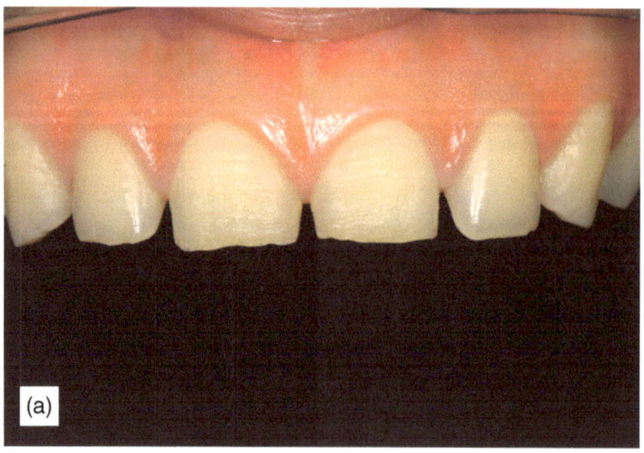

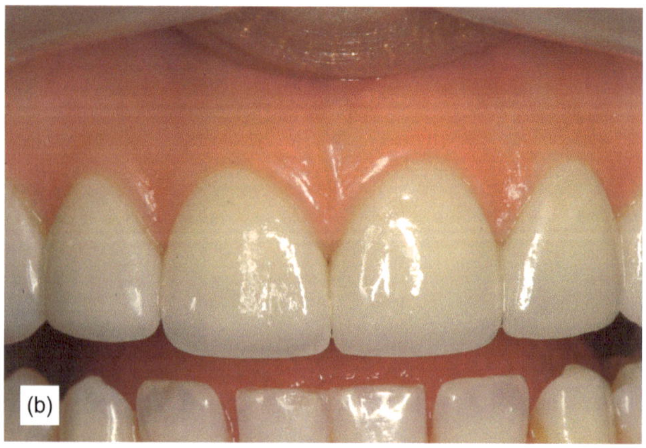

Figure 7.2 (a) Simple restoration in largely undamaged teeth. (b) Finished restoration.

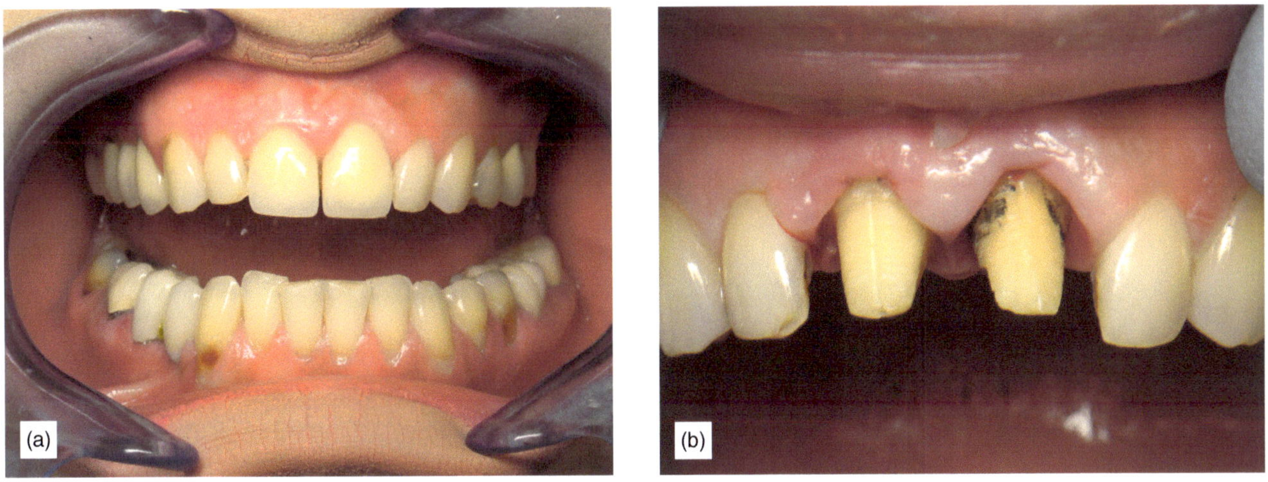

Figure 7.3 (a) Fractured front teeth, treated with a crown; the patient complained of a bad taste coming from the crowns. (b) Preparation performed to correct the fracture.

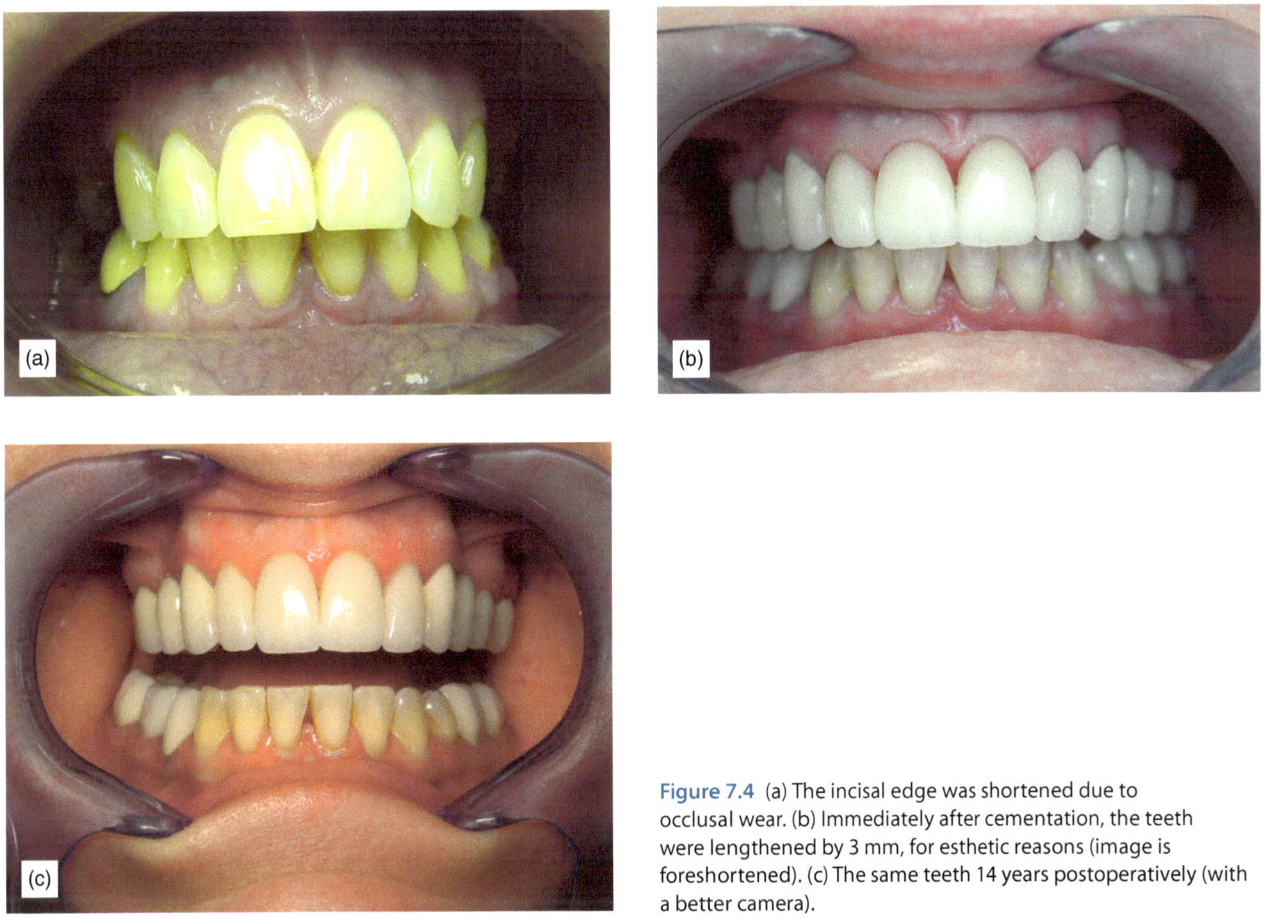

Figure 7.4 (a) The incisal edge was shortened due to occlusal wear. (b) Immediately after cementation, the teeth were lengthened by 3 mm, for esthetic reasons (image is foreshortened). (c) The same teeth 14 years postoperatively (with a better camera).

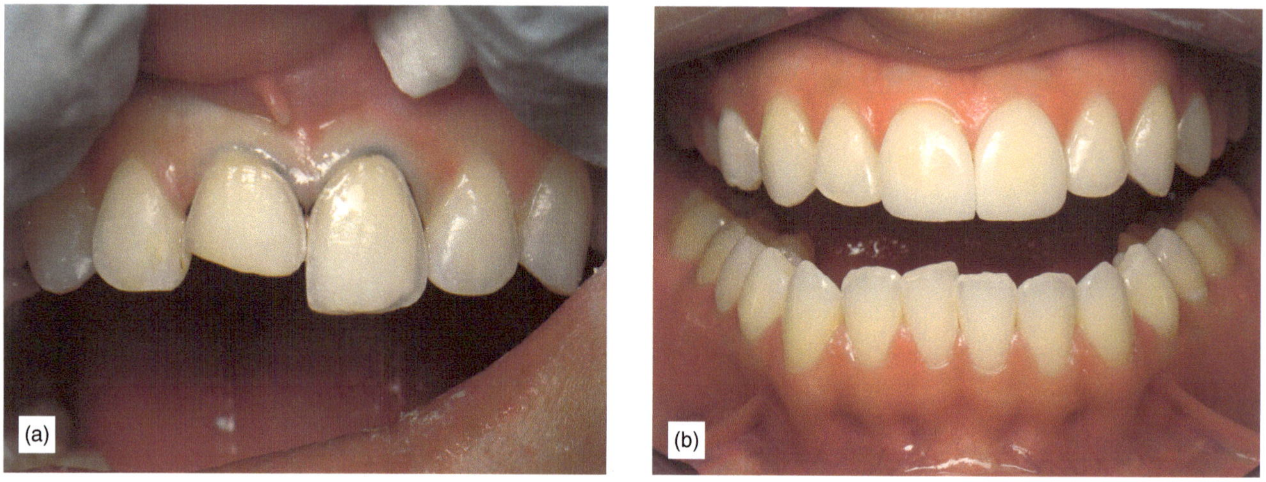

Figure 7.5 (a) Fractured right central; the patient requested a perfect color match, so two veneers were recommended and prepared. (b) One week postoperatively.

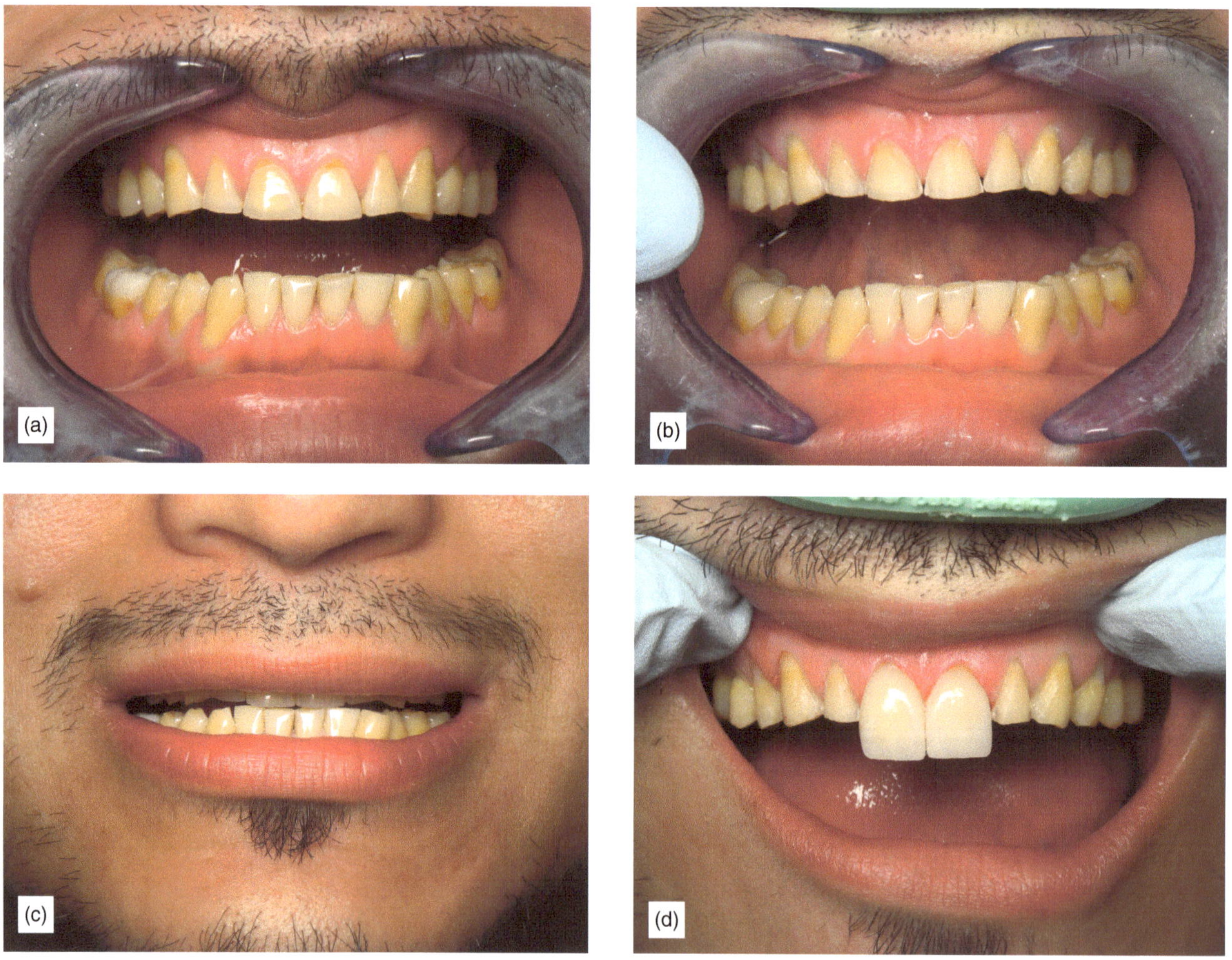

Figure 7.6 (a) Patient with severe occlusal disease and severe wear, needing esthetic rehabilitation. (b) The same teeth after supragingival veneer and onlay preparation. Compare with unprepared view (a) to see how little tooth was removed. (c) Observe the extreme lack of tooth showing in a very young man. (d) Five millimeters of unsupported feldspathic porcelain veneers. (*Continued*)

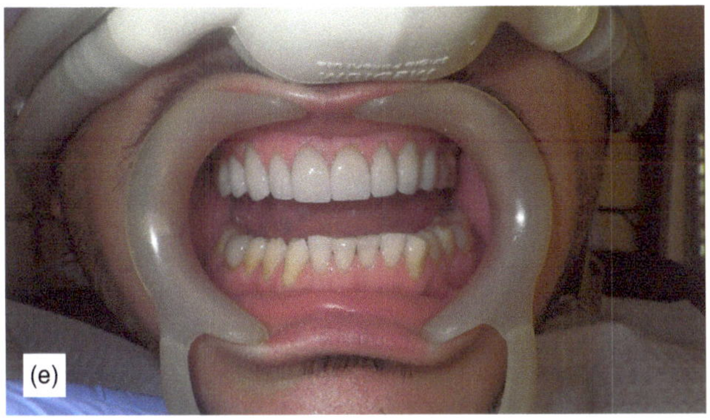

Figure 7.6 (*Continued*)
(e) The same teeth 5 years postoperatively, showing no chipping or fractures.

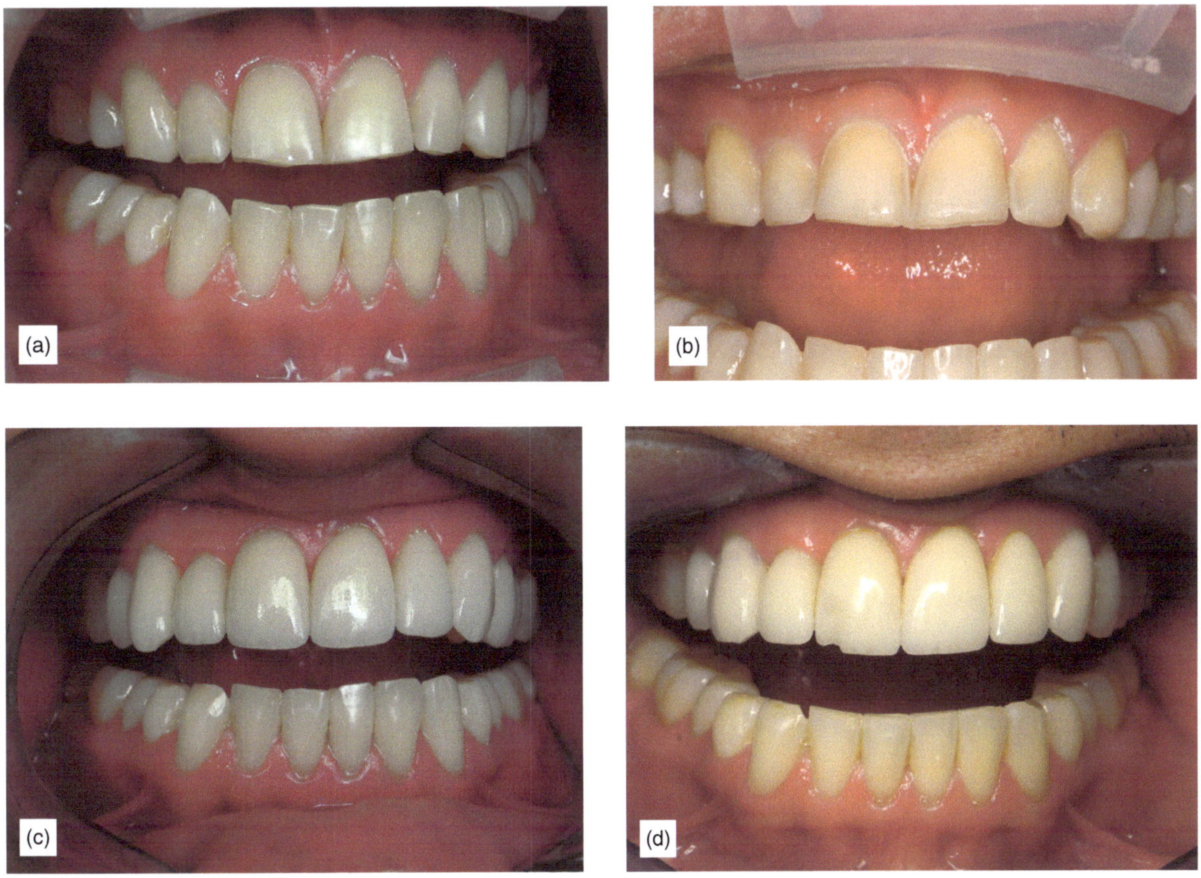

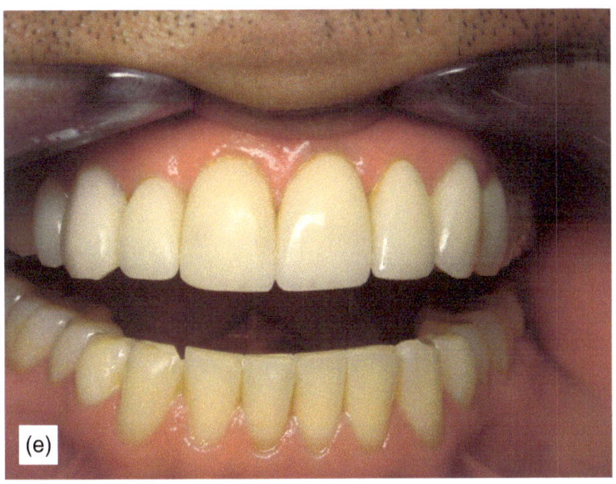

Figure 7.7 (a) Severe anterior wear on a bruxer. (b) Supragingival minimally invasive preparation. (c) Immediately after cementation. (d) Ten years postoperatively, the patient reported chipping the veneer while biting on a bone. (e) After composite repair.

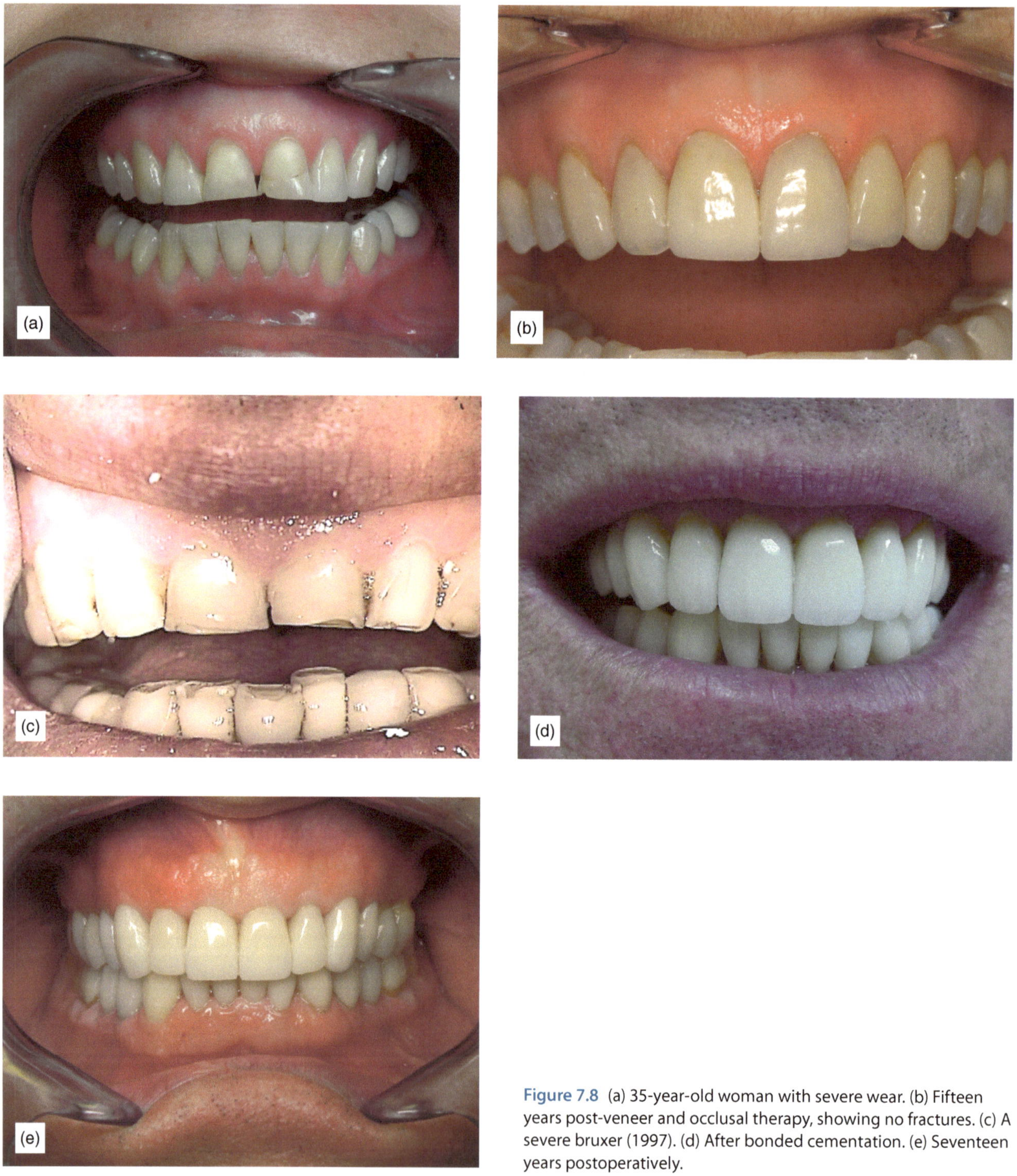

Figure 7.8 (a) 35-year-old woman with severe wear. (b) Fifteen years post-veneer and occlusal therapy, showing no fractures. (c) A severe bruxer (1997). (d) After bonded cementation. (e) Seventeen years postoperatively.

veneers in particular can be of great value to badly damaged teeth, as they allow the teeth to regain their optimal strength and rigidity. Full crown preparation weakens the tooth structure. Porcelain veneers should be considered as a complete substitute for full crowns. Porcelain veneers are an especially desirable option, even when the tooth has been treated with an endodontic procedure. As the literature shows, when the cingulum is preserved, the tooth maintains its rigidity better than when it is cut for a full crown and the cingulum is removed [14]. Enamel gives the thin anterior teeth their necessary rigidity.

The original veneer preparation was minimally invasive [15], as described by Bertolotti, a pioneer in this technique (Figure 7.10). Over the years, more

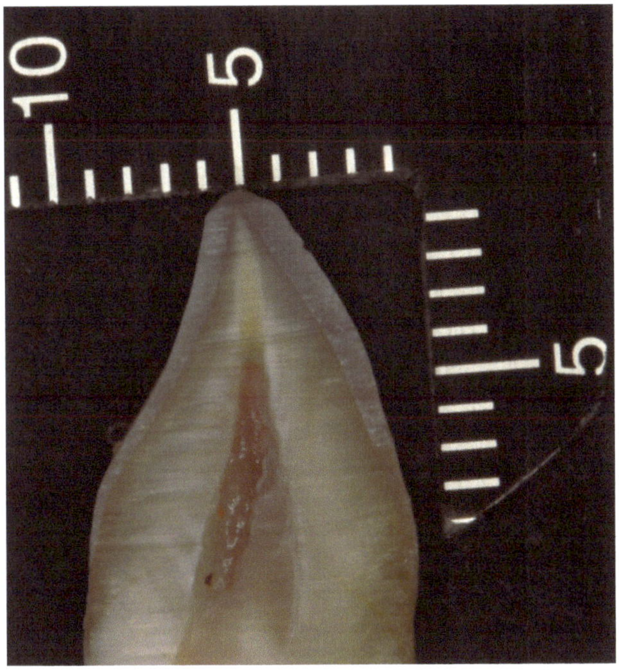

Figure 7.9 The proximity to the pulp on most anterior teeth; the 1.5 mm axial reduction necessary for a crown would leave the preparation fully without enamel and dangerously close to the pulp.

aggressive preparation has become more popular, for multiple reasons, including laboratory demands for more space, as thinner veneers are more difficult to do than thick veneers, and the choice of certain restorative materials which require more space [16,17]. The literature suggests that aggressive tooth preparation is detrimental when using bonded porcelain veneers; the more tooth is removed, the lower the survival rate and higher the rate of fracture [18]. Conversely, the more tooth-conserving is the preparation, the more durable the results can be expected to be [19,20]. Durability studies show a decrease in longevity with veneers

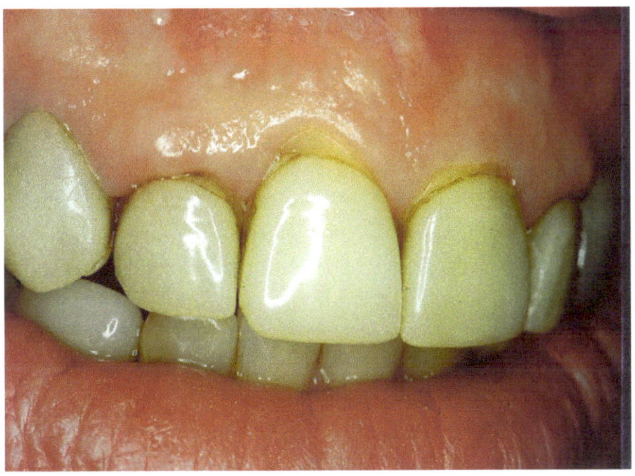

Figure 7.10 Veneers shown 27 years postoperatively (courtesy of Dr Raymond L. Bertolotti).

bonded largely to dentin [21]. Removing the enamel layer and bonding to dentin increases unpredictability, can lead to an increased risk of postoperative sensitivity and pulp damage, and may decrease longevity of adhesion, as dentin is a less predictable bonding substrate. Nevertheless, with the impressive performance of modern self-etching bonding systems for dentin, the long-term success of veneers bonding to dentin may dramatically increase [22,23].

Improper or incomplete diagnosis also leads to unnecessary tooth removal. The space needed for the restorative material should always be visualized from the final external outline of the finished restoration, using the “blueprint” wax-ups, not the current position of the tooth. This approach can help to save a considerable amount of enamel and increase long-term durability (Figure 7.11). This approach is explained in more detail in Chapter 8.

When patients are confronted with a decision of what is more important: a visible metal margin in the esthetic zone and healthy gums, or an invisible subgingival margin, risking the health of the gums, 63% of patients would choose healthier gums [24]. Additionally, Crispin found that gingival margins in the esthetic zone are not visible in approximately 50% of the population, making the need for subgingival margins additionally unnecessary [25]. When the appropriate level of translucency is used, the optimum blending of the veneers at the cervical margin can be achieved, making subgingival margin placement unnecessary (Figure 7.12). Preparation with subgingival margins will always complicate successfully bonded cementation. Isolation is so difficult to achieve when the clinician must fight with inflamed gingiva and blood (Figure 7.13). Using a supragingival protocol, such as the five principles of supragingival dentistry,

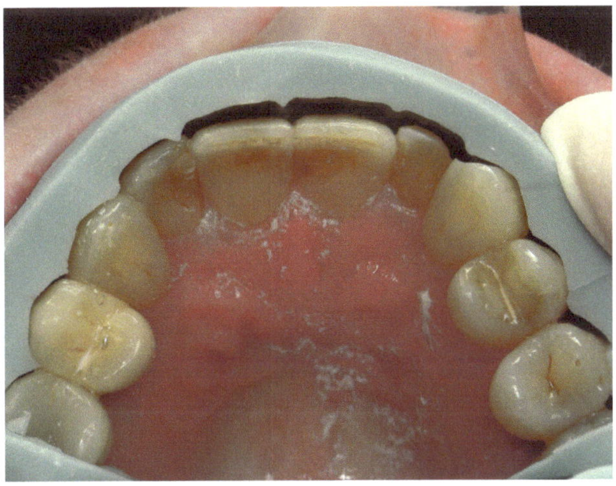

Figure 7.11 Using a reduction matrix (guide) from the wax-up allows a view of areas which may not need any reduction, and is more accurate.

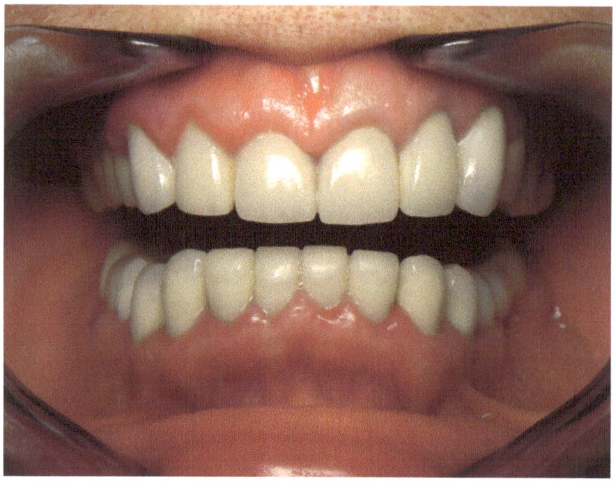

Figure 7.12 Recently completed porcelain veneers placed subgingivally, showing gingival inflammation.

which include enamel margin preservation techniques, margin elevation and other techniques geared towards minimizing the need for subgingival margins for restorative reasons, will permit the goal of completing the restoration with supragingival margin placement, making the entire procedure more simple and the outcome more predictable.

Tooth Preparation for Supragingival Minimally Invasive Porcelain Veneers

While the goal of the facial preparation for porcelain veneers is always to remain supragingival and within the enamel, creating a window in preparation for porcelain veneers, some buildups and other special techniques must be used in cases of badly damaged teeth. The simple preparation is the basic preparation for a mostly intact tooth, to create the space required by the restorative material of choice, to outline requirements for esthetic needs and requirements to simplify fabrication by the laboratory technician. It is desirable to be as minimally invasive as possible, preserving the healthy enamel, and always keeping a supragingival margin placement (Figure 7.14a–d). Studies evaluating the current literature in regards to preparation design point to window preparation with a butt lingual–incisal margin as the least invasive, with the most durable results, as this technique allows for maximum enamel retention [26]. Simple veneer preparation may need to be varied for esthetic needs, such as excessive proclination or misalignment, which may require a more aggressive tooth reduction, leading to heavy dentin exposure. In such cases, immediate dentin sealing is desirable (Figure 7.15a–c) [27].

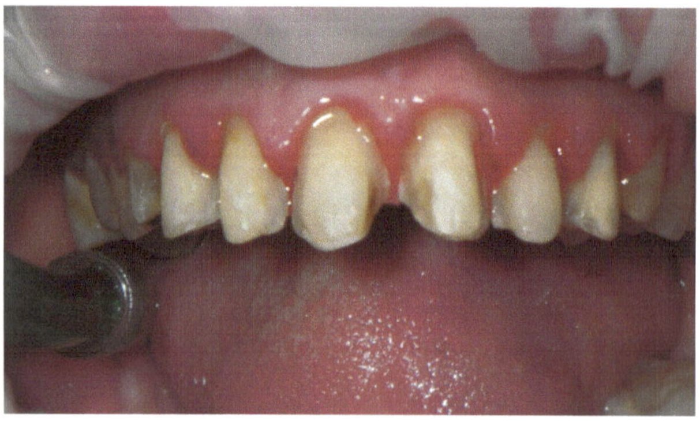

Figure 7.13 Inflamed and bleeding gums greatly complicate technique and predictability in bonded cementation.

The same preparation for a badly damaged vital tooth can be used for a single damaged tooth or as part of an esthetic rehabilitation. There are special considerations, which may include the repair of heavy interproximal caries, old failing restorations or large fractures, and will require extensive repairs and buildup. The literature shows that bonding porcelain veneers to teeth with composite restorations yields similar adhesion and marginal seal as bonding to natural tooth (Figure 7.16a–d). [28,29].

The preparation for an endodontically treated tooth can be used for a single damaged tooth as part of an esthetic rehabilitation. This use also requires special considerations, such as extensive buildups and in some situations a bonded post. Regardless of how damaged the tooth is, a supragingival minimally invasive adhesively retained porcelain veneer maintains the goal of restoring the damaged tooth back to its ideal esthetics and functional state. In the most minimally invasive way, preservation of the majority of the remaining healthy enamel and dentin, and avoiding the unnecessary invasion of the periodontium, is the goal.

Restorative Material for Supragingival Minimally Invasive Porcelain Veneers

Supragingival minimally invasive preparation, as the name suggests, means that the restorative margin will remain above the gum and the preparation will preserve as much healthy tooth structure as possible. This requires choosing a restorative material with the appropriate characteristics. The restoration should be able to be made very thin but still provide a natural polychromatic appearance and have maximum margin blending abilities to allow for a supragingival margin placement (Figures 7.17a,b, 7.18). The material of choice which fulfills these characteristics is layered feldspathic porcelain. A master technician can predictably fabricate a feldspathic layered porcelain veneer. In the cervical area, a higher chroma with more translucency can be used, with a slightly higher value in the middle third, and creating the incisal edge effects in the incisal third, all within the desired thickness (Figure 7.19a–c). The literature is

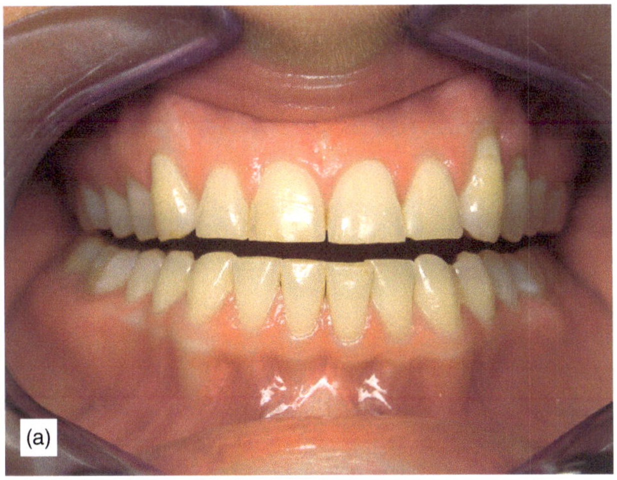

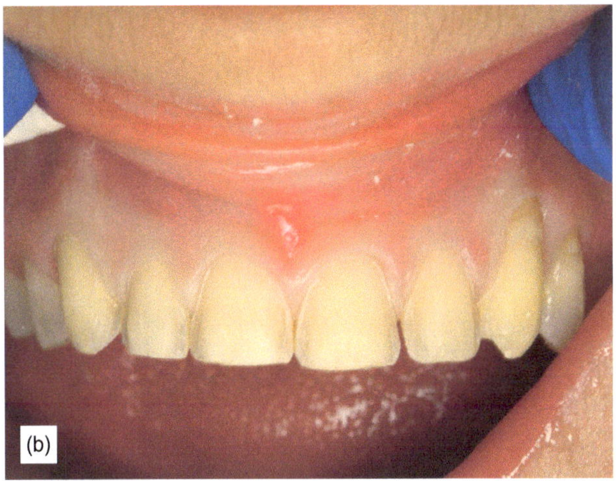

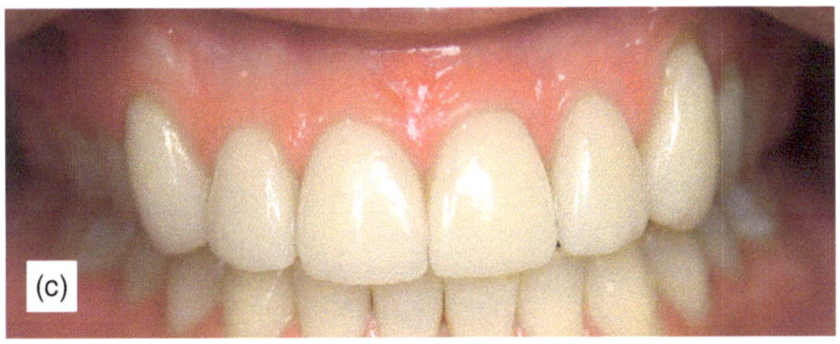

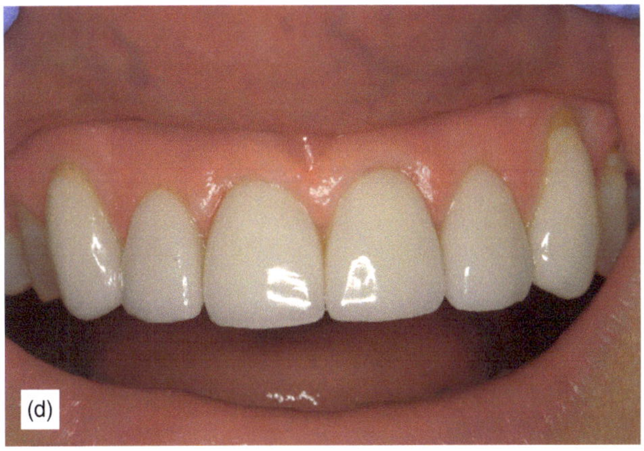

Figure 7.14 (a) Worn dentition treated with porcelain veneers. (b) Supragingival minimal preparation. (c) Final results. (d) Six-year post-veneers showing some cervical margins, but continuing to be esthetic.

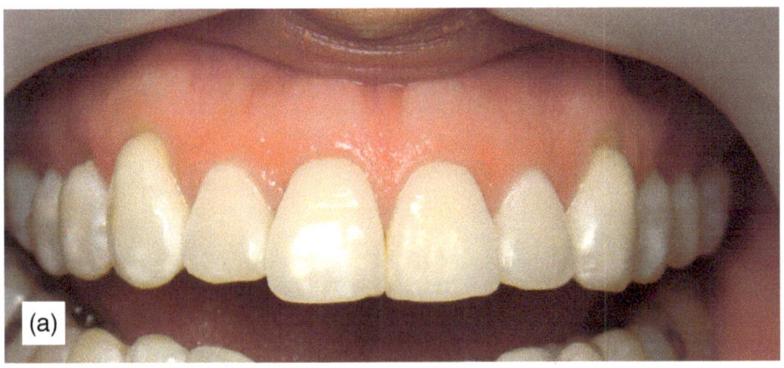

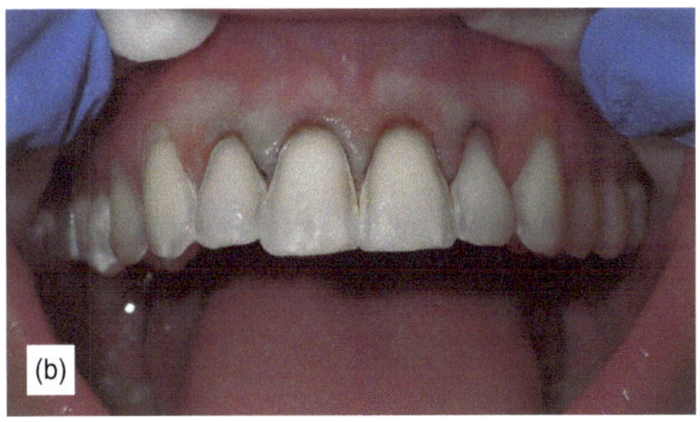

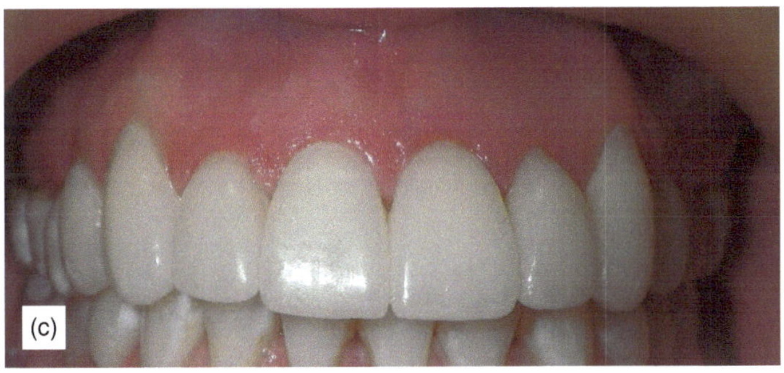

Figure 7.15 (a) This patient did not like the bulbous teeth and proclination. (b) Preparation requiring a more aggressive reduction, and dentin sealing. Also evident is the gingivectomy, performed to enhance gingival symmetry. (c) Immediately after bonded cementation, showing flatter less bulbous contours.

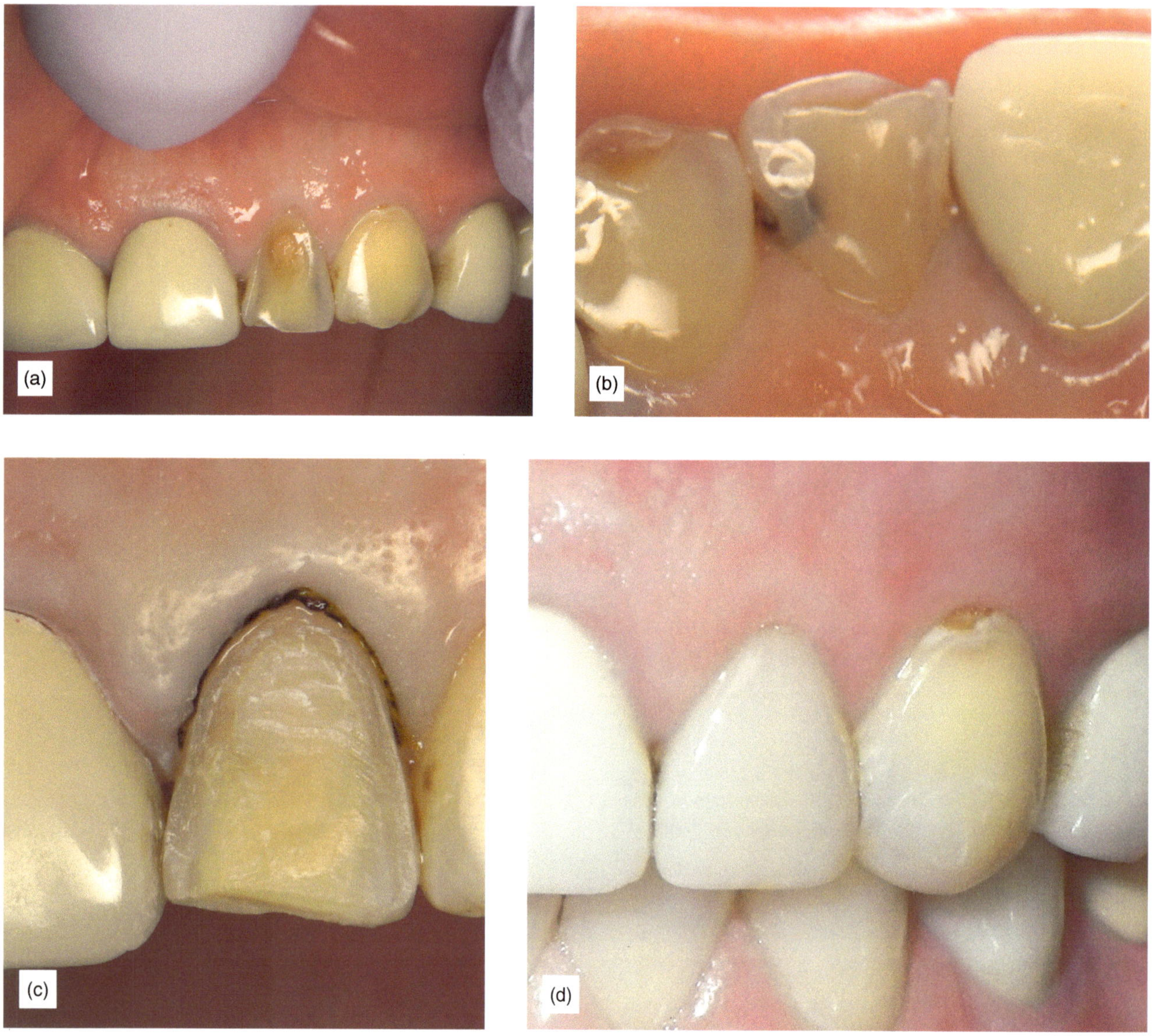

Figure 7.16 (a) This patient was expecting to have a crown on a badly damaged tooth. (b) Subgingival caries on the lingual aspect. (c) After facial and lingual caries repair, and before impression. (d) The same patient 2 years postoperatively.

replete with data showing the overwhelming success of restorations fabricated with feldspathic porcelain. With the above being said, the minimum space required for a feldspathic porcelain veneer is approximately 0.3–0.4 mm in the cervical margin, 0.6 mm in the middle third of the tooth and 1 mm for the incisal edge. Attention should be placed on the term "space required"; this does not necessarily mean "tooth reduction". In many cases, the final outline of the restoration may be longer or fuller than the current tooth, so no actual tooth reduction may be necessary to the final outline (Figure 20a,b). The final outline is dictated by proper diagnosis and smile design.

While thin feldspathic porcelain will provide the most esthetic results, more recently the use of lithium disilicate has been strongly advocated by many for porcelain veneers. While the benefits are clear (increased strength and much simplicity of fabrication) lithium disilicate has the strong disadvantage of not having enough translucency naturally, at least in the currently available version. While thick lithium disilicate can be layered and can achieve great beauty, experience shows that the opacity of the restoration will lead to poor marginal blending and the need to place the margins subgingivally (Figure 7.21). The only way of using this material and still achieving acceptable supragingival margin blending is to use it extremely thinly, thus increasing its translucency [30]. A maximum of 0.3–0.4 mm [31] in the cervical third and 0.5 mm in the facial third should be used, while the incisal edge can be 1 mm or more (Figure 7.22a–c). Very thin e-Max has the esthetic disadvantage of being gray, with low value.

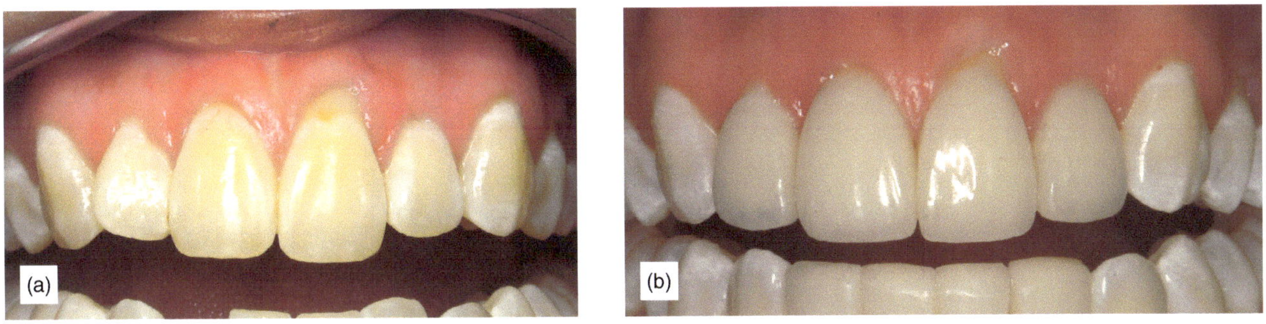

Figure 7.17 (a) This patient was unwilling to have root coverage surgery; she was informed that veneer would not cover the root. (b) Two weeks after bonded cementation, showing supragingival margins and good blending of the restoration.

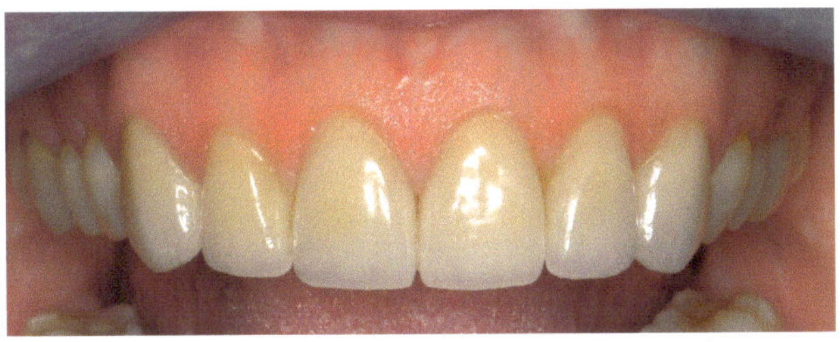

Figure 7.18 15-year recall showing supragingival margins with good blending and excellent esthetics.

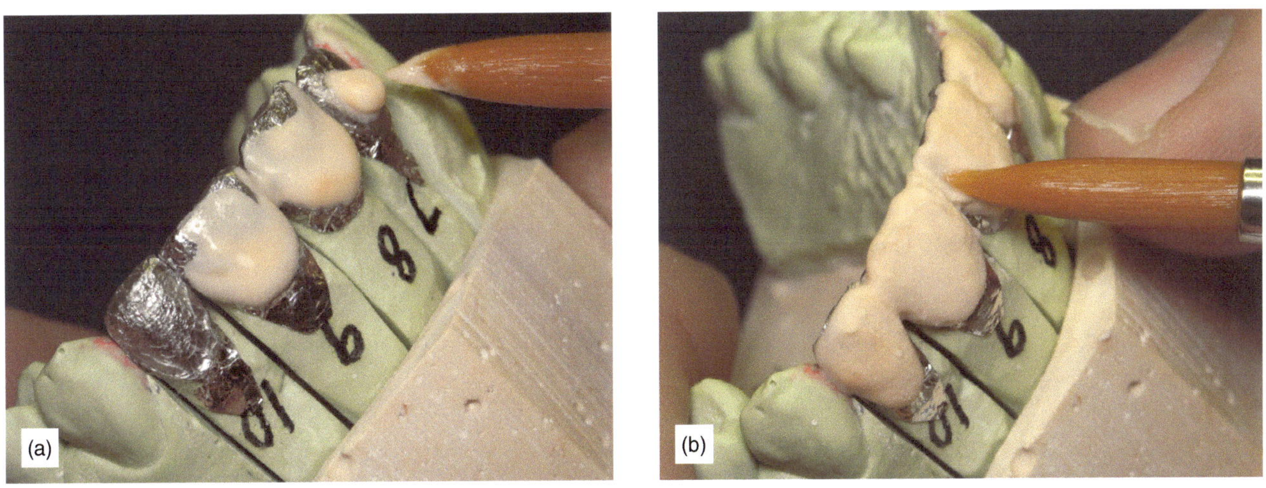

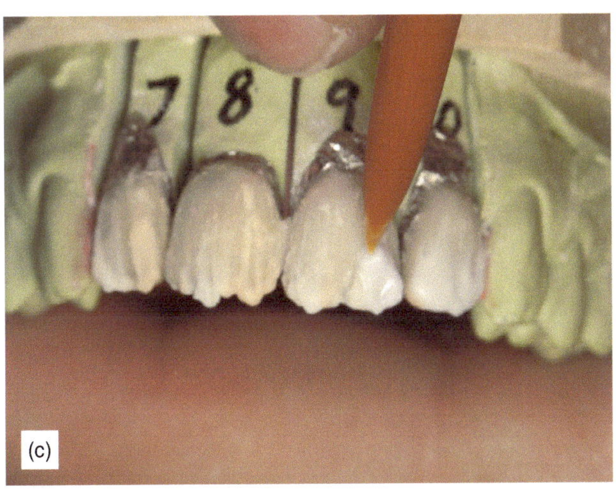

Figure 7.19 (a) Layered feldspathic cervical increment, higher chroma, higher translucency. (b) Middle third higher value. (c) Incisal effects including translucency.

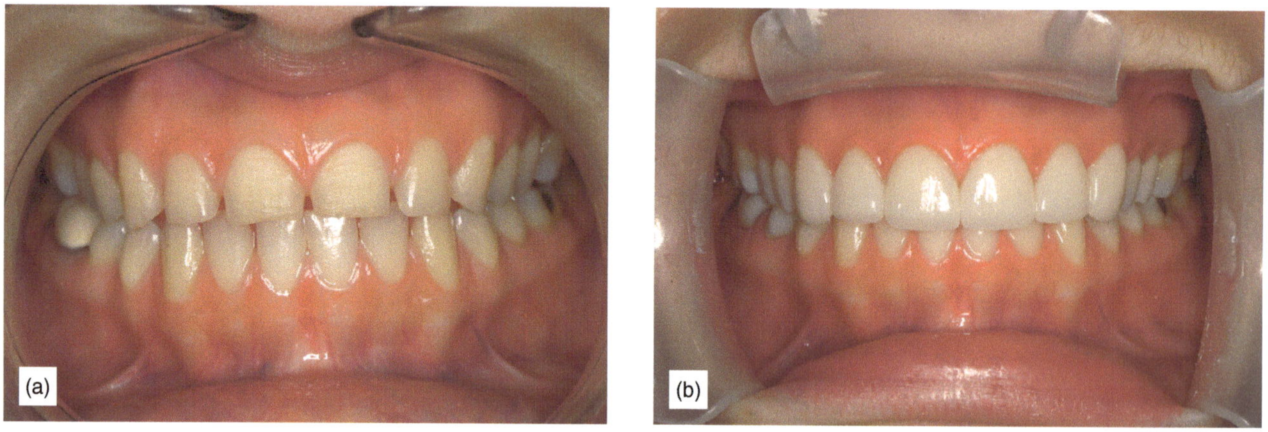

Figure 7.20 (a) Female patient with small acid damaged teeth, needing fuller, longer teeth; minimum preparation necessary. (b) Final thick veneers, showing fuller, longer teeth.

Experience shows that once lithium exceeds 0.5 mm, it becomes too opacious and this will increase the difficulty in achieving good margin blending. Even in cases when space is not an issue, a thin cervical third is desirable for translucency. Experience and the literature show that decreased thickness does not make veneers more fracture prone [32]. Very thin lithium disilicate will then be monochromatic, but the thinness of the material will allow some of the undelaying color to show through. Lithium disilicate may be a good choice of material for occlusally driven rehabilitations with lesser esthetic needs.

Simple Preparations

The basic facial preparation for porcelain veneers is usually done in mostly intact teeth. Sometimes a small class III cavity or filling may be present, which may need to be repaired or replaced and will then be treated as an intact tooth.

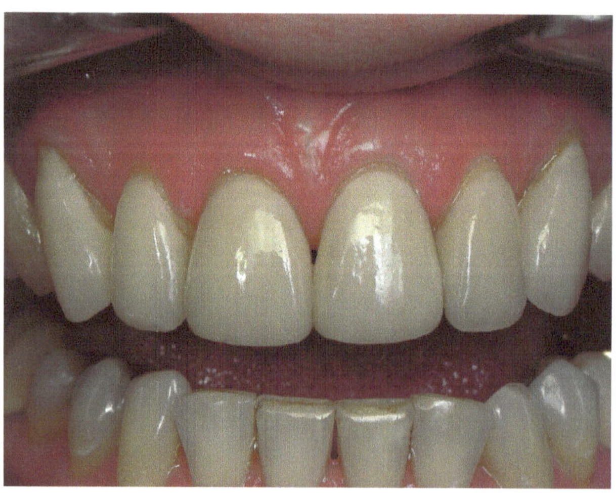

Figure 7.21 Because e-Max is more opacious, the margins can easily be poorly blended; when the gingiva recedes, it looks unattractive.

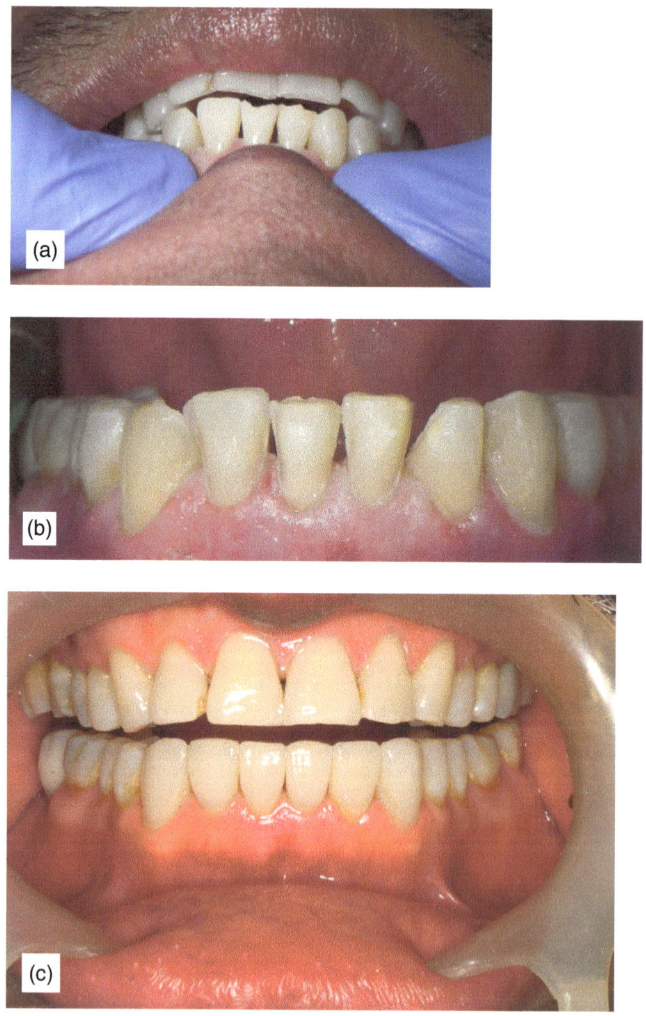

Figure 7.22 (a) Severe bruxer male patient, wanting veneers for esthetic and functional reasons. (b) After supragingival minimally invasive preparation, which required very thin veneers. (c) Very thin 0.3–0.4 mm cervical e-Max veneers showing excellent blending and allowing supragingival margin placement.

Step by Step Simple Preparation

Step 1: Supragingival veneer margins should be above the gums. In most cases, the preparations should be as close to the gingiva as possible without touching it (Figure 7.23a). This allows for optimal periodontal health at cementation, as well as for the life of the restoration and the tooth. Ideally, a silicone matrix should be used to assess how much of the tooth structure must be removed. The use of a silicon matrix is the best way of assessing the amount of space currently available, based on the desired final external outline, and thus being able to decide how much, if any, of the tooth needs to be prepared or removed (Figure 7.23b). The silicon matrix is made from the correctly designed "blueprint" waxup (Figure 7.23c), which will be made after proper smile design and occlusal analysis (discussed in Chapter 13). The matrix is then cut in an L-shape, allowing for an incisal and facial reduction assessment (Figure 7.23d). A second matrix is later used to fabricate the prototype provisionals.

Step 2: The amount of space or tooth reduction needed for the incisal edge is 1–1.5 mm. If the space is already available due to wear or fracture, there is no need for additional reduction. Simply flatten the incisal edge to 100 degrees from the cervical plane. The 1–1.5 mm reduction can be accomplished using a diamond bur which is 1 mm in the middle of the cutting surface and 1.5 mm on the base of the cutting surface (Figure 7.23e). Sinking the diamond to its full thickness in multiple places along the incisal edge provides depth cuts. The incisal reduction should be at 90 degrees or greater from the gingival plane, to ensure a facial path or insertion, and end in an incisal–lingual butt, as this has been shown to be preferable than a wrap-in to lingual surface (Figure 7.23f) [33,34,35]. The facial–incisal transition should be gently rounded (Figure 7.23g), then all the depth cuts can be joined together, giving a nearly consistent 1 mm reduction.

Step 3: The cervical margin reduction is the one that will be done in all cases, regardless of space. The purpose

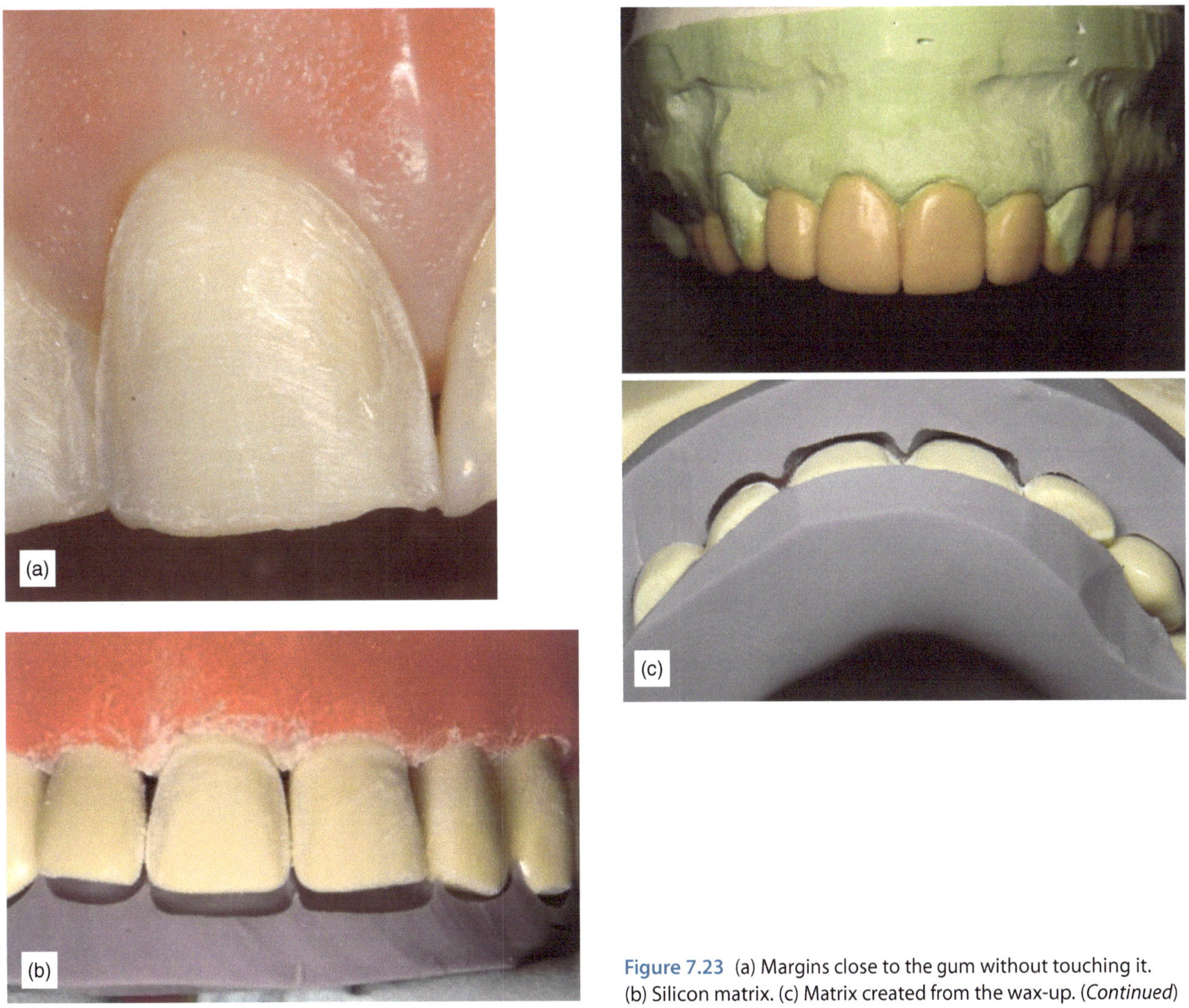

Figure 7.23 (a) Margins close to the gum without touching it. (b) Silicon matrix. (c) Matrix created from the wax-up. (*Continued*)

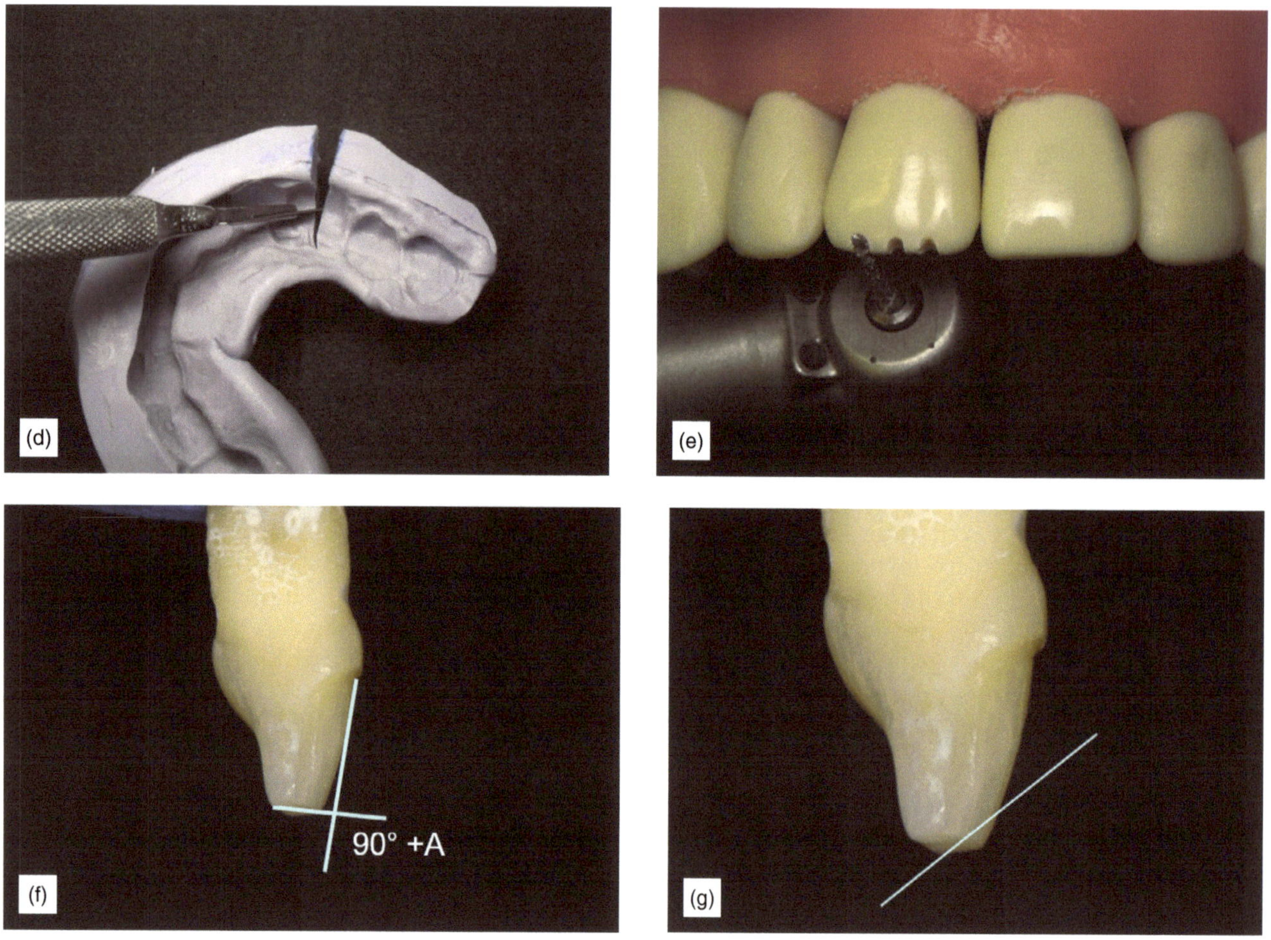

Figure 7.23 *(Continued)*
(d) Cut silicon matrix. (e) Incisal edge depth cuts. (f) Incisal reduction 90 degrees for cervical aspect. (g) Incisal reduction gently rounded.

is to create sufficient room for the thin porcelain to be seated without creating "steps" between the porcelain and the tooth. It also serves to index the restoration for easier orientation while undertaking the bonded cementation. Ideally, the preparation should remain on the enamel, but the cervical area is thinnest at the enamel so sometimes dentin will be exposed. Creating a thin feldspathic porcelain margin requires much skill. It is virtually impossible to make a porcelain margin of less than 0.3 mm; realistically, the best we can hope for is about 0.4–0.5 mm. For this reason, a 0.4 mm cervical reduction and margin is the goal. The same chamfer diamond bur will be used to create 0.3–0.4 mm depth cuts (Figure 7.23h). The diamond should be aligned parallel to the cervical plane, and sunk approximately halfway into the tooth, or approximately 0.4 mm depth, as the diamond is 0.8 mm in thickness at the tip (Figure 7.23i). A trick to gain even reduction after the depth cuts is to mark the depth of the cut with a sharp pencil (Figure 7.23j). Then, change the angulation of the diamond and join the depth cuts together (Figure 7.23k). When the marks disappear, there should be a consistent 0.4 mm reduction.

Step 4: The mid-tooth facial reduction should be about 0.6 mm of reduction or space and parallel to the facial plane of the tooth. Just as with the cervical area, complete several depth cuts, mark them with a pencil, then blend them together (Figure 7.23l). By the time the pencil marks are erased, the 0.6 mm reduction will be achieved.

Step 5: Sink the margins halfway in the interproximal region. It is important to note that this type of preparation never breaks contact. The goal is to just bring the repair halfway to the contact (Figure 7.23m). The tooth must be looked at from both sides to ensure that the cavosurface margin is not exposed. The purpose of this is to not be able to detect the cavosurface margin when looking at the mesial or distal areas. If the color is ideal, the proximal margin can be in full contact

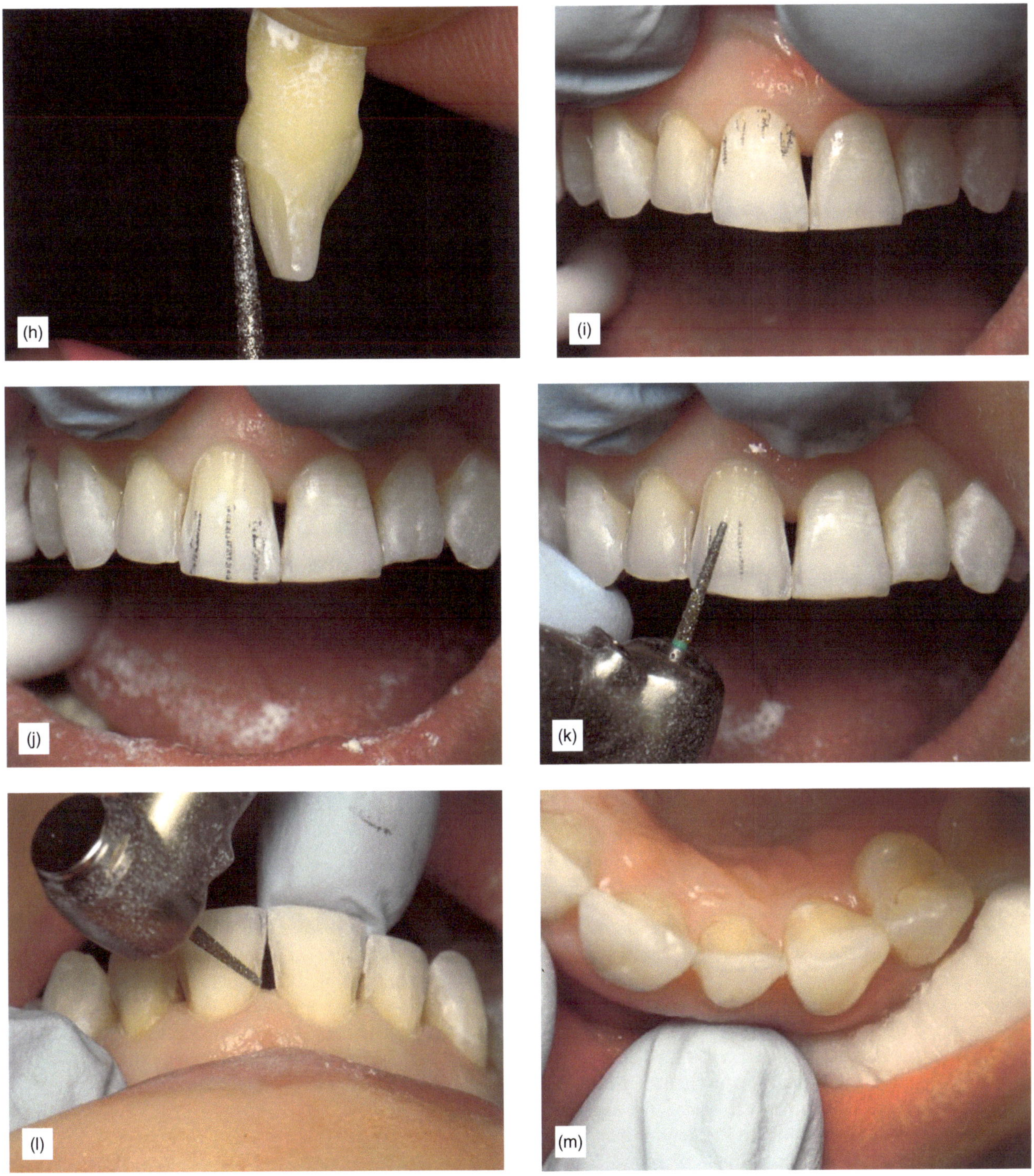

Figure 7.23 (*Continued*)
(h) Half of the 0.8 mm bur (Brasseler 6850-014). (i) Gingival depth cuts marked with a pencil. (j) Facial reduction depth cuts. (k) Facial reduction changing angulation to avoid depth cuts. (l) Proximal cut. (m) Proximal cut, incisal view.

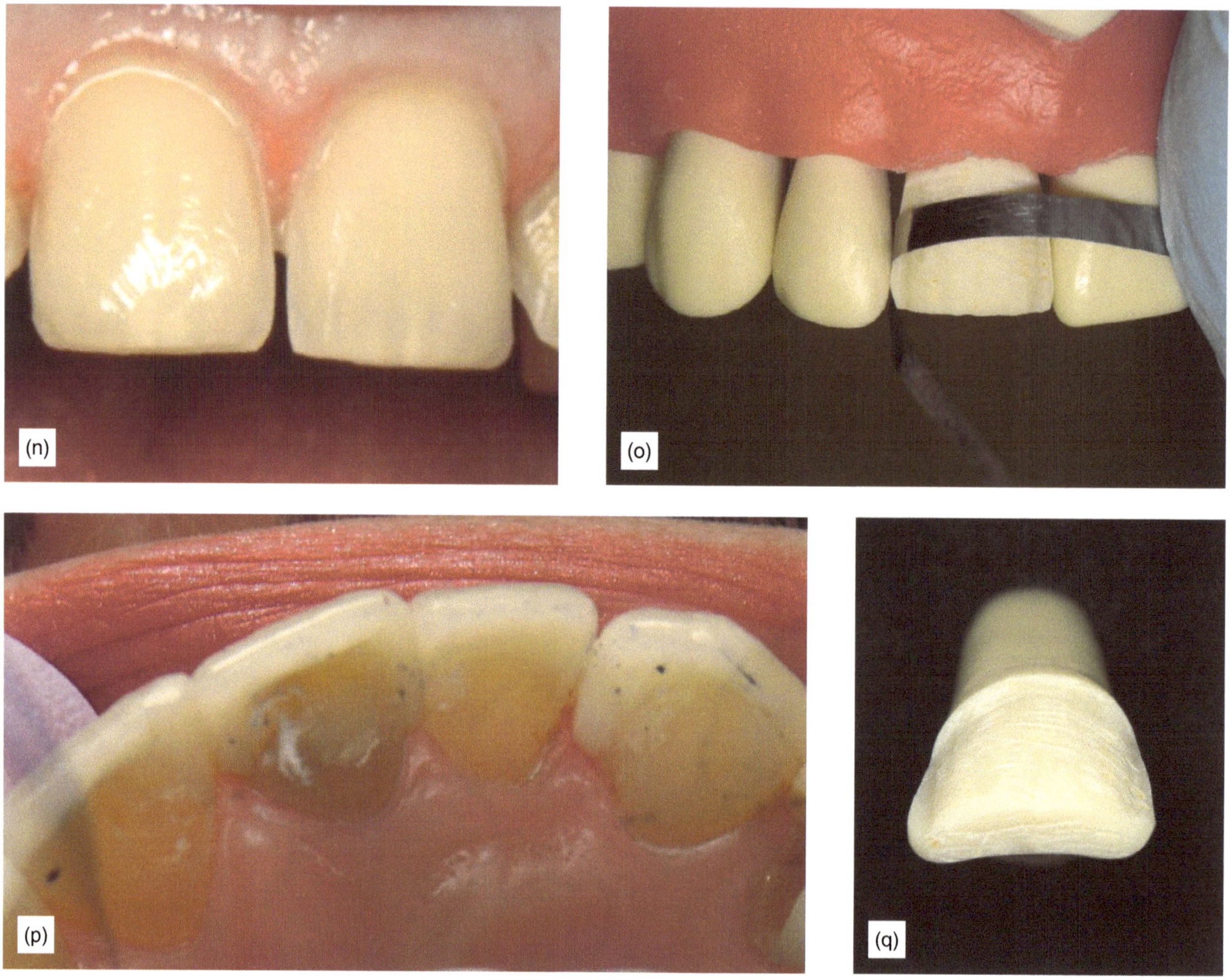

Figure 7.23 (*Continued*)
(n) Proximal with need to break contact, when teeth overlap or to change midline. (o) Using a metal strip. (p) Lingually exposed porcelain. (q) Finished simple preparation.

and cavosurface margins more superficial (Figure 7.23n).

Step 6: In some cases, the contact will be placed deeper interproximally and will require a step to break contact very slightly (Figure 7.23o), which can be done using a metal strip (Figure 7.23p). This perfects the interproximal surface. Remove any J margin and create a slight separation to allow the laboratory to see the margins and produce a restoration that is properly adapted. Unless dictated by already open contact, it would be a disadvantage to intentionally and unnecessarily fully break contact and have porcelain in lingual contact. As the bite changes over the life of the patient, the porcelain on the lingual side will break more easily when in contact with the opposing teeth. Figure 7.23q shows an example of a patient who keeps breaking the lingual side of his anterior restorations.

Step 7: Place a triple "0" retraction cord and take a full arch final impression with a highly hydrophilic impression material, such as Panasil (Kettenbach).

Step 8: Provisionalize using a silicon matrix of the wax up. Spot bonding will enhance retention.

Special Considerations

A Badly Damaged Vital Tooth

Badly damaged teeth with fractures, caries, or failing old restoration will often require a procedure to preserve the enamel margin, elevation, or other type of buildup. After the tooth is repaired, the preparation can be finished as a simple preparation.

- Start by performing steps 1–7 of Simple Preparation (above) developing the ideal preparation outline (Figure 7.24).

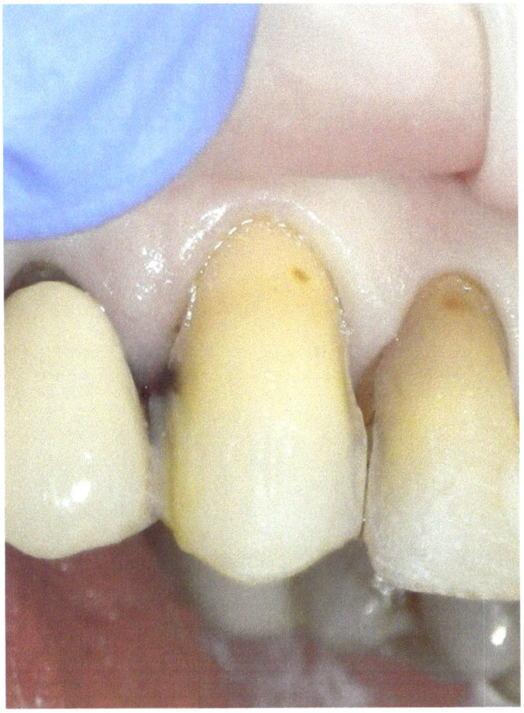

Figure 7.24 Basic preparation and outline before caries removal and buildup.

- When a large class III cavity or old restoration is present, repair as a normal class III direct restoration and refinish that section of the tooth, treating the composite filling as if it were tooth (Figure 25a–e).
- When a class IV caries or failing restoration is present, repair the lingual portion of the damage. There is no need to rebuild the entire lingual surface or the incisal edge, as the veneer will replace whatever part of the tooth is missing. The purpose of repairing the lingual surface is to avoid unnecessary removal of the facial enamel, further weakening the tooth, and losing more support for the restoration.
- When fractures are present, the incisal border of the fracture will be treated as the new incisal edge, and the preparation will be finished at that point (see Figures 7.5a and 7.6a). When lingual damage is present, the fracture should be treated similarly to class IV. Repair to preserve as much of the facial tooth structure and enamel as possible.
- When caries approach the cervical margin and threaten to go subgingival, the supragingival protocol (five principles) should be activated. Preventing a subgingival margin is the ideal approach. When prevention is not possible because the caries and/or old restoration are subgingival to a depth greater than 1.5 mm, elevate the margin to simplify and make cementation more predictable (Figure 7.26a–e). See Chapter 3 for full details.
- All necessary buildups should be performed with one application of adhesive and in one procedure for efficiency, followed by taking an impression and temporization.

An Endodontically Treated Tooth

The literature suggests that endodontically treated anterior teeth with minimal loss of structure do not require a full coverage restoration. Here, a simple bonded composite repair of the endodontic access would be sufficient [36,37]. Traditionally, full crowns are used when endodontically treated teeth are badly damaged, requiring extensive buildups and post, followed by cutting a full crown, which often removes most of the remaining natural tooth structure, leaving the post and buildup to be the main support for the crown. This approach requires long ferrules to increase strength and decrease fractures [38], with the

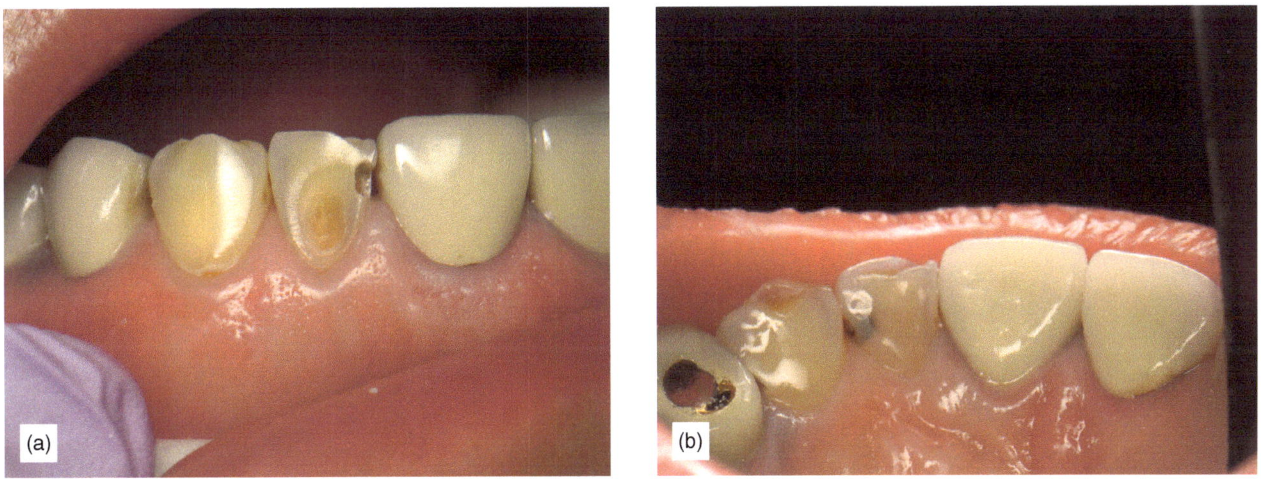

Figure 7.25 (a) Facial and proximal large caries on a tooth intended for a porcelain veneer. (b) Lingual view of the caries. (*Continued*)

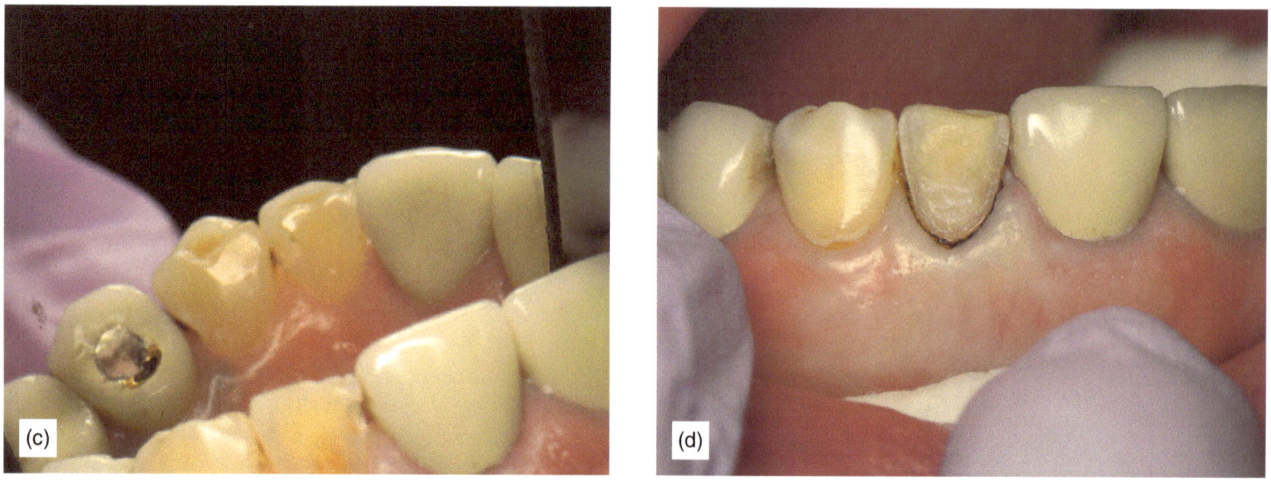

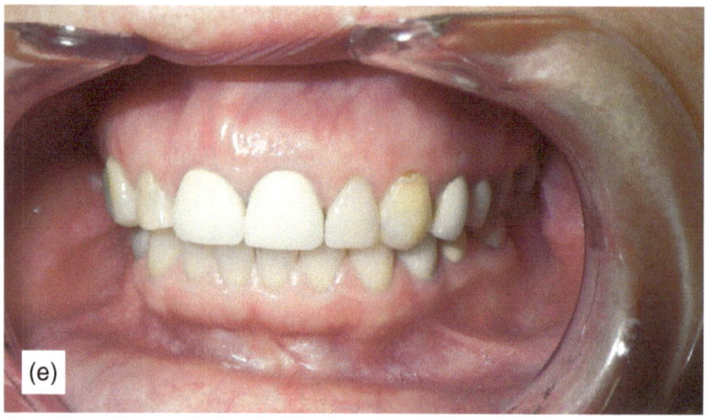

Figure 7.25 (*Continued*)
(c) After caries removal. (d) After composite repair. (e) After supragingival minimally invasive preparation.

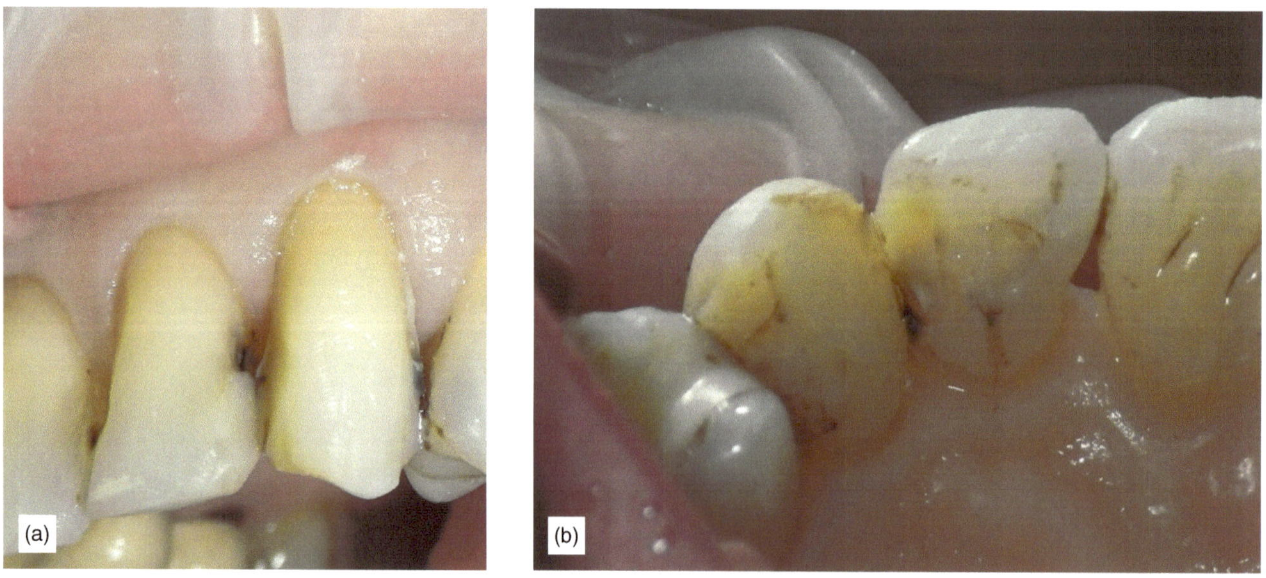

Figure 7.26 (a–e) Enamel margin preservation. (*Continued*)

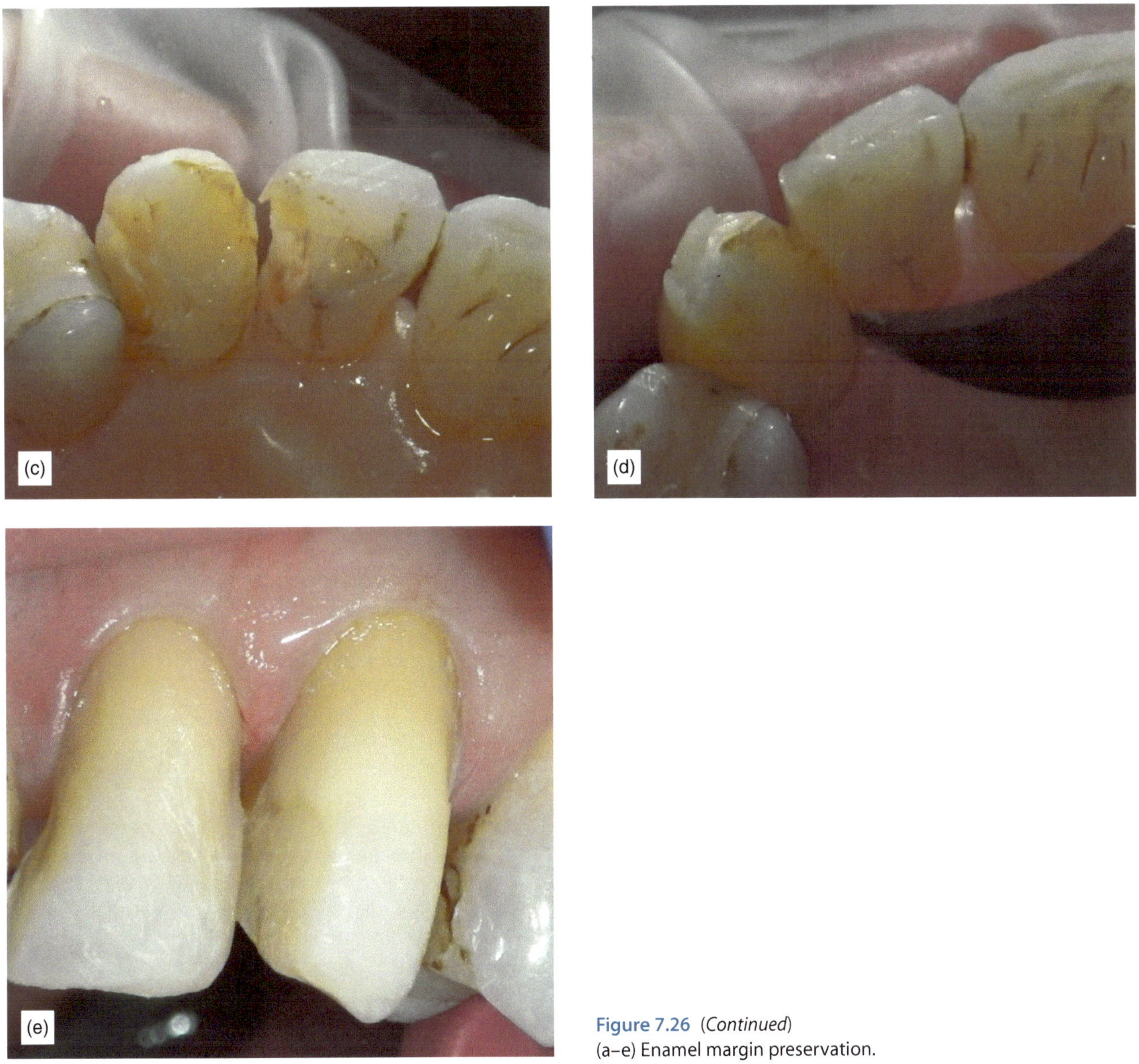

Figure 7.26 (*Continued*)
(a–e) Enamel margin preservation.

added disadvantage of forcing restorative margins to be placed subgingivally.

Porcelain veneers are the ideal means to restore endodontically treated teeth, to regain ideal esthetics and the best possible function, with the healthiest possible outcome. When past damage and endodontic procedures are responsible for a severe loss of tooth structure and rigidity of the anterior teeth [39], to successfully restore these teeth an effort must be made to regain rigidity. Porcelain veneers help to regain original crown rigidity and stiffness [40]. When much of the coronal structure is missing or very weak, a correctly bonded fiber-reinforced post has been shown to have an important effect on fracture resistance [41]. A post is also desirable when the neck of the tooth is narrow [42].

A minimally invasive porcelain veneer will preserve as much of the healthy coronal tooth structure as possible, and will increase the overall strength. It is assumed that a porcelain veneer on a non-vital tooth may have a shorter durability than porcelain veneers on a vital tooth [43]. Logic and clinical experience suggest that full crowns placed on badly damaged endodontically treated teeth will also have considerable complications and shorter durability than crowns placed on more ideal vital teeth.

Some endodontically treated teeth may be considerably darker than the adjacent teeth. The traditional approach is to deal with this issue by placing an opacious full-coverage crown with subgingival margin placement to hide the color difference, with all the disadvantages previously discussed. Internal bleaching, or

Box 7.1 Rotstein's walking bleaching technique

1) Familiarize the patient with the possible causes of discoloration, the procedure to be followed, the expected outcome, and the possibility of future further discoloration.
2) Radiographically assess the status of the periapical tissues and the quality of endodontic obturation. Endodontic failure or questionable obturation should always be retreated prior to bleaching.
3) Assess the quality and shade of any restoration present and replace it if defective. Tooth discoloration is frequently the result of leaking or discolored restorations. In such cases, cleaning the pulp chamber and replacing the defective restorations will usually suffice.
4) Evaluate tooth color with a shade guide and, if possible, take clinical photographs at the beginning of and throughout the procedure. These provide a point of reference for future comparison.
5) Isolate the tooth with a rubber dam. The dam must fit tightly at the cervical margin of the tooth to prevent possible leakage of the bleaching agent onto the gingival tissue. Interproximal wedges and ligatures may also be used for better isolation.
6) Remove all restorative materials from the access cavity, expose the dentin, and refine the access. Verify that the pulp horns and other areas containing the pulp tissue are clean.
7) Remove all materials to a level just below the labial–gingival margin (Figure 7.27a).
8) To cover the endodontic obturation, apply a sufficiently thick layer, at least 2 mm, of a protective white cement barrier. The coronal height of the barrier should protect the dentinal tubules and conform to the external epithelial attachment (Figure 7.27b).
9) Prepare the walking bleach paste by mixing sodium perborate and an inert liquid, such as water, saline, or anesthetic solution, to a thick consistency of wet sand. Although sodium perborate plus 30% H_2O_2 mixture may bleach faster, in most cases, long-term results are similar to those with sodium perborate and water alone, and therefore need not be used routinely. With a plastic instrument, pack the pulp chamber with the paste. Remove excess liquid by tamping with a cotton pellet. This also compresses and pushes the paste into all areas of the pulp chamber.
10) Remove the excess bleaching paste from undercuts in the pulp horn and gingival area and apply a thick well-sealed temporary filling, directly against the paste and into the undercuts. To ensure a good seal, carefully pack the temporary filling, at least 3 mm thick.
11) Remove the rubber dam and inform the patient that bleaching agents work slowly and that significant lightening may not be evident for several days.
12) Evaluate the patient 2 weeks later and, if necessary, repeat the procedure several times. Repeat treatments are similar to the first one.
13) As an optional procedure, and in limited cases, if initial bleaching is not satisfactory, strengthen the walking bleach paste by mixing sodium perborate with gradually increasing concentrations of H_2O_2 (3–30%) instead of water. Start with low concentrations, as low as possible and practical. The more potent oxidizers may have an enhanced bleaching effect but should not be used routinely because of the possibility of permeation into the tubules and damage to the cervical periodontium by these more caustic agents. In such cases, a protective cream, such as Orabase or Vaseline, must be applied to the surrounding gingival tissues prior to dam placement. In most cases, discoloration will improve after one to two treatments. If after three attempts there is no significant improvement, reassess the case for correct diagnosis of the etiology of discoloration and treatment plan.

(Reproduced courtesy of Dr I Rotstein.)

walking bleaching, is a desirable alternative to the more destructive crown option. Internal bleaching has been shown to be successful, durable and safe [44,45]. Rotstein and others have shown that sodium perborate has been found to be as effective as hydrogen peroxide, with a suggested decrease in the risk of oxidative irritation and root resorption (Box 7.1) [46,47]. Because endodontically treated teeth may have a tendency to darken over time, more tooth-preserving techniques such as porcelain veneers are not performed, to avoid this possibility. Tooth color changes can be minimized by correctly cleaning the pulp chamber of pulp remnants and endodontic filling materials [48]. In cases where the teeth become darker over time, internal bleaching can also be performed, even years after porcelain veneer is placed.

The V-Shaped Veneer

In patients with severely worn dentition, porcelain veneers can be a great tool to restore esthetics and function and to regain proper anterior guidance. Good results have been described in the literature using bonded porcelain veneers [49]. I have been performing this type of rehabilitation for over 20 years with excellent

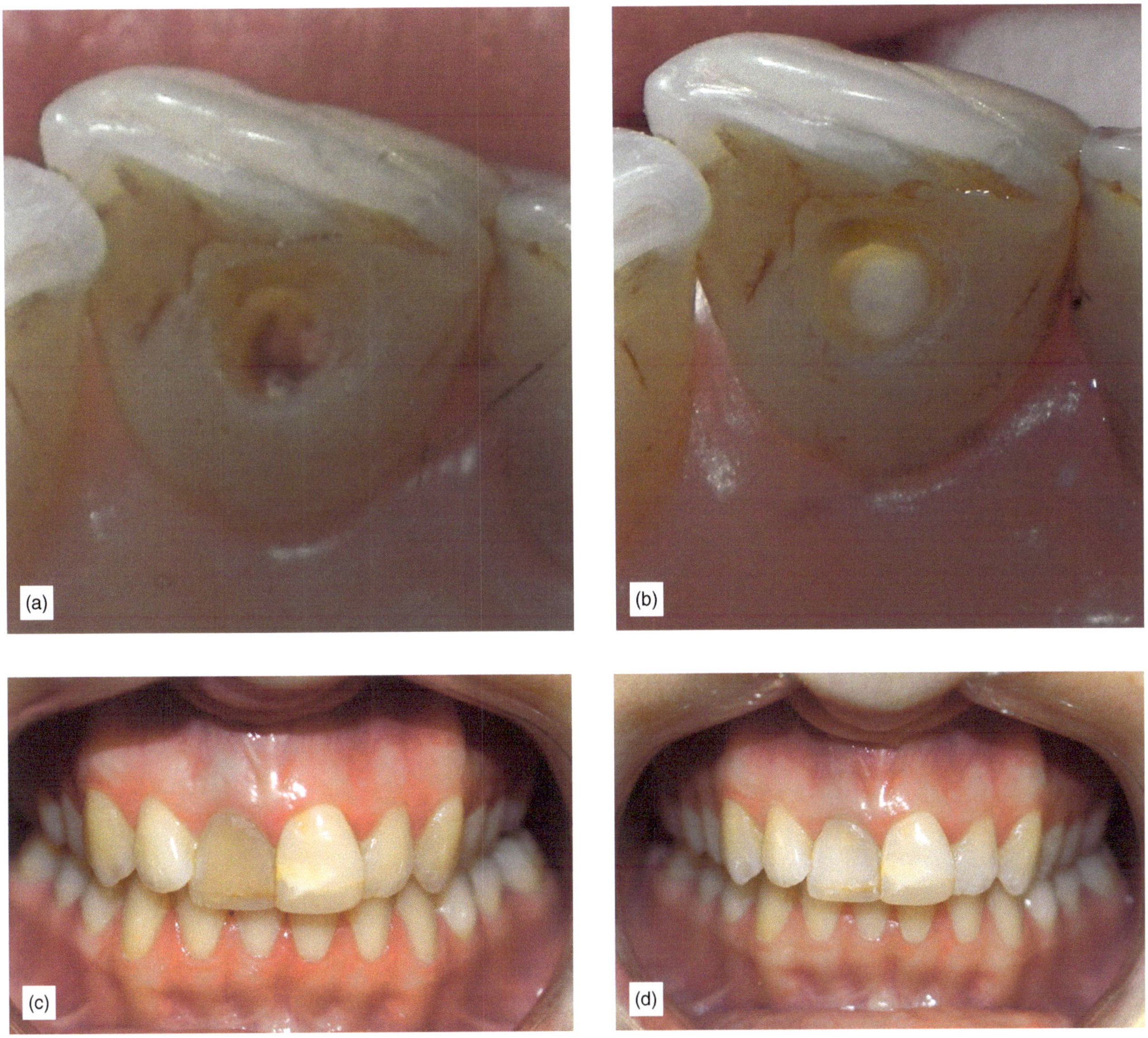

Figure 7.27 (a) Remove filling. (b) Seal gutta percha with Ionosel (VOCO). (c) Before internal bleaching (courtesy of Dr Nuria Fernandez Marmolejo). (d) After one application of internal bleaching (courtesy of Dr Fernandez Marmolejo).

results. When correct occlusal principles are used, porcelain veneers are an ideal means of restoring the worn dentition [50]. Traditionally, when the lingual surface of the tooth must be covered, as in cases where the anterior guidance must be altered, full-coverage crowns will be used. An alternative is a V-shaped veneer, which allows for partial lingual coverage, without having to break contact, create a taper and ending up cutting about 75% of the tooth away. An alternative would be a lingual wrap veneer that extends slightly beyond the desired occlusal contact. This lingual wrap design has been called a V-shaped or "taco-shell" veneer. This is commonly used to regain canine or anterior contact or guidance (Figure 7.28a–d). There are very small variations in the preparation when a lingual wrap is desired:

- The incisal edge will be prepared at 90 degrees from the gingival plane.
- The path of insertion of the V-shaped veneers will change to a facial–apical direction (Figure 7.29), which means that it is important to check the path of the insertion, and absence of undercuts.
- Make a small to moderate lingual bevel on the incisal edge, within the enamel, to modify path of insertion.
- Ensure that enough space is available in the lingual surface for the desired thickness of restorative material. When bonded to enamel, less than 1 mm is necessary for strength with either feldspathic porcelain or lithium disilicate.
- Mark with the veneer preparation, and bur the extent of the wrap desired into the lingual surface.

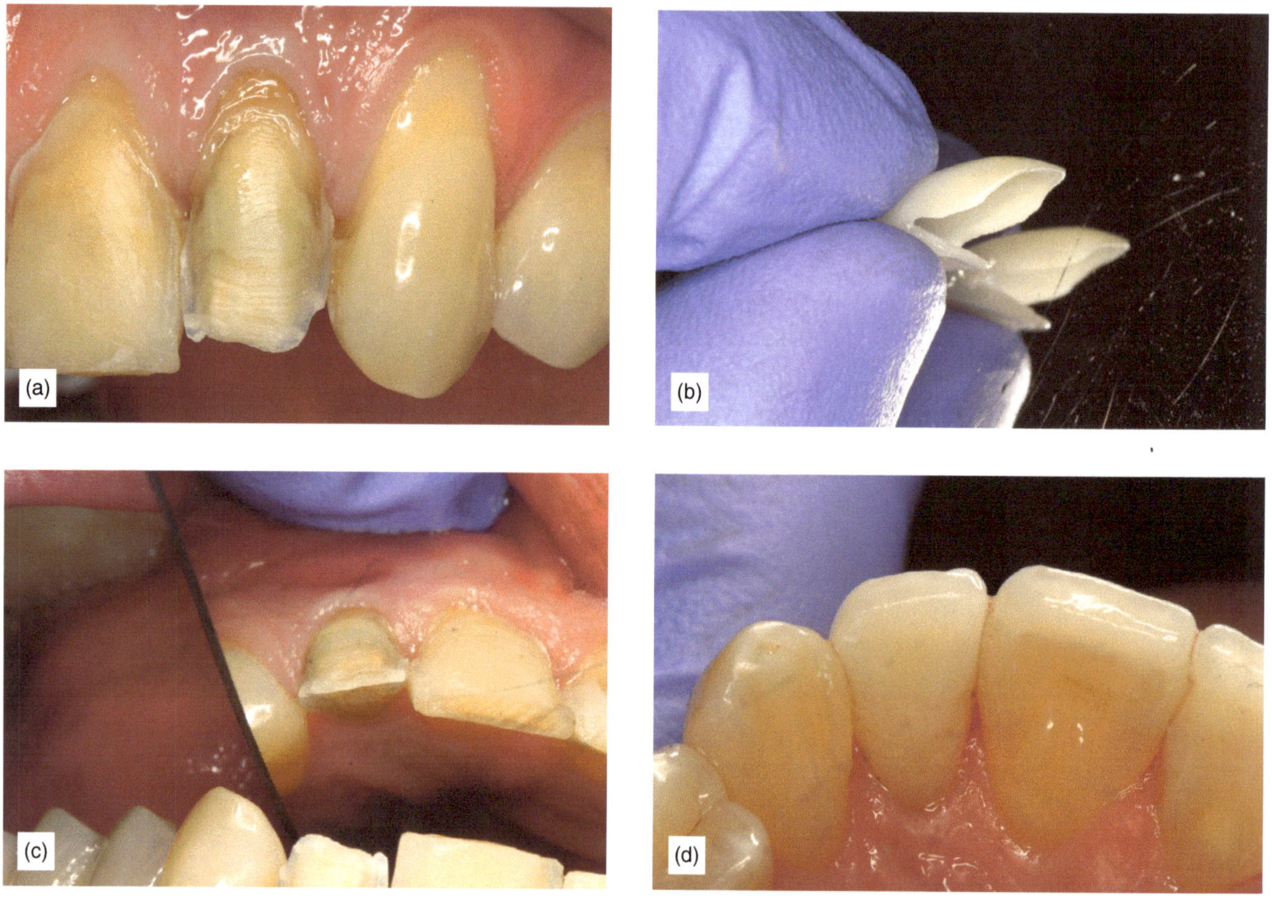

Figure 7.28 (a) V-shaped veneer preparation, facial aspect. (b) V-shaped porcelain veneer. (c) Lateral incisor needing lingual coverage to achieve centric contact. (d) Lingual appearance of a cemented V-shaped veneer.

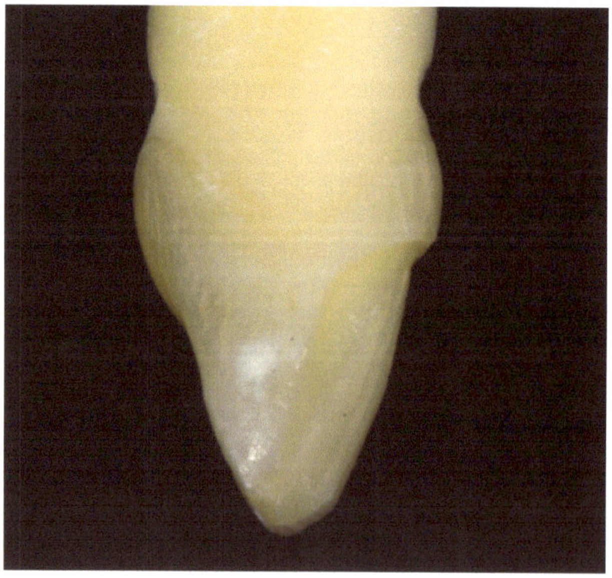

Figure 7.29 Lingual bevel for path of insertion, with no lingual reduction.

After preparation for a single porcelain veneer to repair a damaged tooth, the final impression and provisional restoration will be very similar to an onlay provisionalization, from a preoperative impression, although in some cases a wax-up may be required. Follow this with a final impression, usually using a polyvinyl siloxane material. For details of simple provisionalization and final impression techniques, see Chapter 8. When several porcelain veneers are being made as part of an esthetic rehabilitation, provisional veneers need to be made for a wax-up. Chapter 8 discusses how the wax-up is made, using smile design principles and provisionalization of more complex cases.

References

1 Castelnuovo J, Tjan AH, Phillips K, Nicholls JI, Kois JC. Fracture load and mode of failure of ceramic veneers with different preparations. *J Prosthet Dent*, 2000; 83(2): 171–180.

2 Schmidt KK, Chiayabutr Y, Phillips KM, Kois JC. Influence of preparation design and existing condition of tooth structure on load to failure of ceramic

laminate veneers. *J Prosthet Dent*, 2011; 105(6): 374–382.

3 Batalocco G, Lee H, Ercoli C, Feng C, Malmstrom H. Fracture resistance of composite resin restorations and porcelain veneers in relation to residual tooth structure in fractured incisors. *Dent Traumatol*, 2012; 28(1): 75–80.

4 Magne P, Perroud R, Hodges JS, Belser UC. Clinical performance of novel-design porcelain veneers for the recovery of coronal volume and length. *Int J Periodontics Restorative Dent*, 2000; 20(5): 440–457.

5 Peumans M, Van Meerbeek B, Yoshida Y, Lambrechts P, Vanherle G. Five-year clinical performance of porcelain veneers. *Quintessence Int*, 1998; 29: 211–221.

6 Walls AWG. The use of adhesively retained all-porcelain veneers during the management of fractured and worn anterior teeth: Part 2. Clinical results after 5 years of follow-up. *Br Dent J*, 1995; 178: 337–340.

7 Wilson C. Multidisciplinary treatment of anterior worn dentition: a staged approach. *Compend Contin Educ Dent*, 2015; 36(3): 202–207.

8 Castelnuovo J, Tjan AH, Phillips K, Nicholls JI, Kois JC. Fracture load and mode of failure of ceramic veneers with different preparations. *J Prosthet Dent*, 2000; 83(2): 171–180.

9 Fradeani M, Redemagni M, Corrado M. Porcelain laminate veneers: 6- to 12-year clinical evaluation: A retrospective study. *Int J Periodontics Restorative Dent*, 2005; 25(1): 9–17.

10 Geminiani A, Lee H, Feng C, Ercoli C. The influence of incisal veneering porcelain thickness of two metal ceramic crown systems on failure resistance after cyclic loading. *J Prosthet Dent*, 2010; 103(5): 275–282.

11 Chun YH, Raffelt C, Pfeiffer H, Bizhang M, Saul G, Blunck U, Roulet JF. Restoring strength of incisors with veneers and full ceramic crowns. *J Adhes Dent*, 2010; 12(1): 45–54.

12 Gurel G, Sesma N, Calamita MA, Coachman C, Morimoto S. Influence of enamel preservation on failure rates of porcelain laminate veneers. *Int J Periodontics Restorative Dent*, 2013; 33(1): 31–39.

13 Edelhoff D, Sorensen JA. Tooth structure removal associated with various preparation designs for anterior teeth. *J Prosthet Dent*, 2002; 87(5): 503–509.

14 Magne P, Douglas WH. Porcelain veneers: Dentin bonding optimization and biomimetic recovery of the crown. *Int J Prosthodont*, 1999; 12: 111–121.

15 Bertolotti R. Indirect veneers. *CDA J*, 1988; 16(3): 37–42.

16 Jones B. Changing lives with porcelain veneers. *J Cosmet Dent*, 2005; 21(3): 132–134.

17 Prevedello GC, Vieira M, Furuse AY, Correr GM, Gonzaga CC. Esthetic rehabilitation of anterior discolored teeth with lithium disilicate all-ceramic restorations. *Gen Dent*, 2012; 60(4): e274–e278.

18 Stappert CF, Stathopoulou N, Gerds T, Strub JR. Survival rate and fracture strength of maxillary incisors, restored with different kinds of full veneers. *J Oral Rehabil*, 2005; 32(4): 266–272.

19 Hui KK, Williams B, Davis EH, Holt RD. A comparative assessment of the strengths of porcelain veneers for incisor teeth dependent on their design characteristics. *Br Dent J*, 1991; 171(2): 51–55.

20 Burke FJ. Survival rates for porcelain laminate veneers with special reference to the effect of preparation in dentin: a literature review. *J Esthet Restor Dent*, 2012; 24(4): 257–265.

21 Peumans M, De Munck J, Van Landuyt K, Van Meerbeek B. Thirteen-year randomized controlled clinical trial of a two-step self-etch adhesive in non-carious cervical lesions. *Dent Mater*, 2015; 31(3): 308–314.

22 Donmez N, Bell S, Pashley DH, Tay FR. Ultrastructural correlates of in vivo/in vitro bond degradation in self-etch adhesives. *J Dent Res*, 2005; 84(4): 355–359.

23 Gurel G, Morimoto S, Calamita MA, Coachman C, Sesma N. Clinical performance of porcelain laminate veneers: outcomes of the aesthetic preevaluative temporary (APT) technique. *Int J Periodontics Restorative Dent*, 2012; 32(6): 625–635.

24 Crispin BJ. Margin placement of esthetic veneer crowns. Part III: Anterior tooth visibility. *J Prosthet Dent*, 1981;45(3): 499–501.

25 Shetty A, Kaiwar A, Shubhashini N, Ashwini P, Naveen D, Adarsha M, Shetty M, Meena N. Survival rates of porcelain laminate restoration based on different incisal preparation designs: An analysis. *J Conserv Dent*, 2011; 14(1): 10–15.

26 Magne P. Immediate dentin sealing; a fundamental procedure for indirect bonded restorations. *J Esthetic Restorative Dent*, 2005; 17(3): 144–155.

27 Sadighpour L, Geramipanah F, Allahyari S, Fallahi Sichani B, Kharazi Fard MJ. In vitro evaluation of the fracture resistance and microleakage of porcelain laminate veneers bonded to teeth with composite fillings after cyclic loading. *J Adv Prosthodont*, 2014; 6(4): 278–284.

28 Gresnigt MM, Ozcan M, Kalk W, Galhano G. Effect of static and cyclic loading on ceramic laminate veneers adhered to teeth with and without aged composite restorations. *J Adhes Dent*, 2011; 13(6): 569–577.

29 Chaiyabutr Y, Kois JC, Lebeau D, Nunokawa G. Effect of abutment tooth color, cement color, and ceramic thickness on the resulting optical color of a CAD/CAM glass ceramic lithium disilicate reinforced crown. *J Prosthet Dent*, 2011; 105(2): 83–90.

30 Barizon KT, Bergeron C, Vargas MA, Qian F, Cobb DS, Gratton DG, Geraldeli S. Ceramic materials for porcelain veneers: part II. Effect of material, shade, and thickness on translucency. *J Prosthet Dent*, 2014; 112(4): 864–870.

31 Guess PC, Schultheis S, Wolkewitz M, Zhang Y, Strub JR. Influence of preparation design and ceramic thicknesses on fracture resistance and failure modes of premolar partial coverage restorations. *J Prosthet Dent*, 2013; 110(4): 264–273.

32 Schmidt KK, Chiayabutr Y, Phillips KM, Kois JC. Influence of preparation design and existing condition of tooth structure on load to failure of ceramic laminate veneers. *J Prosthet Dent*, 2011; 105(6): 374–382.

33 Magne P, Douglas WH. Design optimization and evolution of bonded ceramics for the anterior dentition: a finite-element analysis. *Quintessence Int*, 1999; 30(10): 661–672.

34 Guess PC, Selz CF, Voulgarakis A, Stampf S, Stappert CF. Prospective clinical study of press-ceramic overlap and full veneer restorations: 7-year results. *Int J Prosthodont*, 2014; 27(4): 355–358.

35 Cheung W. A review of the management of endodontically treated teeth. Post, core and the final restoration. *J Am Dent Assoc*, 2005; 136(5): 611–619.

36 Sorensen JA, Martinoff JT. Intracoronal reinforcement and coronal coverage: a study of endodontically treated teeth. *J Prosthet Dent*, 1984; 51(6): 780–784.

37 Pereira JR, de Ornelas F, Conti PC, do Valle AL. Effect of a crown ferrule on the fracture resistance of endodontically treated teeth restored with prefabricated posts. *J Prosthet Dent*, 2006; 95(1): 50–54.

38 Magne P, Douglas WH. Cumulative effects of successive restorative procedures on anterior crown flexure: intact versus veneered incisors. *Quintessence Int*, 2000; 31(1): 5–18.

39 Stokes AN, Hood JA. Impact fracture characteristics of intact and crowned human central incisors. *J Oral Rehabil*, 1993; 20(1): 89–95.

40 Salameh Z, Sorrentino R, Ounsi HF, Sadig W, Atiyeh F, Ferrari M. The effect of different full-coverage crown systems on fracture resistance and failure pattern of endodontically treated maxillary incisors restored with and without glass fiber posts. *J Endod*, 2008; 34(7): 842–846.

41 Christensen GJ. Posts vs. no posts in endodontically treated teeth. *Clin Rep*, 2013; 6(11): 1–2.

42 Meijering AC, Creugers NH, Roeters FJ, Mulder J. Survival of three types of veneer restorations in a clinical trial: a 2.5-year interim evaluation. *J Dent*, 1998; 26(7): 563–568.

43 Amato M, Scaravilli MS, Farella M, Riccitiello F. Bleaching teeth treated endodontically: long-term evaluation of a case series. *J Endod*, 2006; 32(4): 376–378.

44 Rotstein I, Mor C, Friedman S. Prognosis of intracoronal bleaching with sodium perborate preparation in vitro: 1-year study. *J Endod*, 1993; 19(1): 10–12.

45 Rotstein I, Zalkind M, Mor C, Tarabeah A, Friedman S. In vitro efficacy of sodium perborate preparations used for intracoronal bleaching of discolored non-vital teeth. *Endod Dent Traumatol*, 1991; 7(4): 177–180.

46 Palo RM, Valera MC, Camargo SE, Camargo CH, Cardoso PE, Mancini MN, Pameijer CH. Peroxide penetration from the pulp chamber to the external root surface after internal bleaching. *Am J Dent*, 2010; 23(3): 171–174.

47 Plotino G, Buono L, Grande NM, Pameijer CH, Somma F. Nonvital tooth bleaching: a review of the literature and clinical procedures. *J Endod*, 2008; 34(4): 394–407.

48 Fradeani M, Barducci G, Bacherini L, Brennan M. Esthetic rehabilitation of a severely worn dentition with minimally invasive prosthetic procedures (MIPP). *Int J Periodontics Restorative Dent*, 2012; 32(2): 135–147.

49 Magne P, Magne M, Belser UC. Adhesive restorations, centric relation, and the Dahl principle: minimally invasive approaches to localized anterior tooth erosion. *Eur J Esthet Dent*, 2007; 2(3): 260–273.

50 Ruiz JL, Coleman TA. Occlusal disease management system: The diagnosis process. *Compend Contin Educ Dent*, 2008; 29(3): 148–158.

8

Esthetic Co-Diagnosis Using the Dentofacial Esthetic Diagnosis System

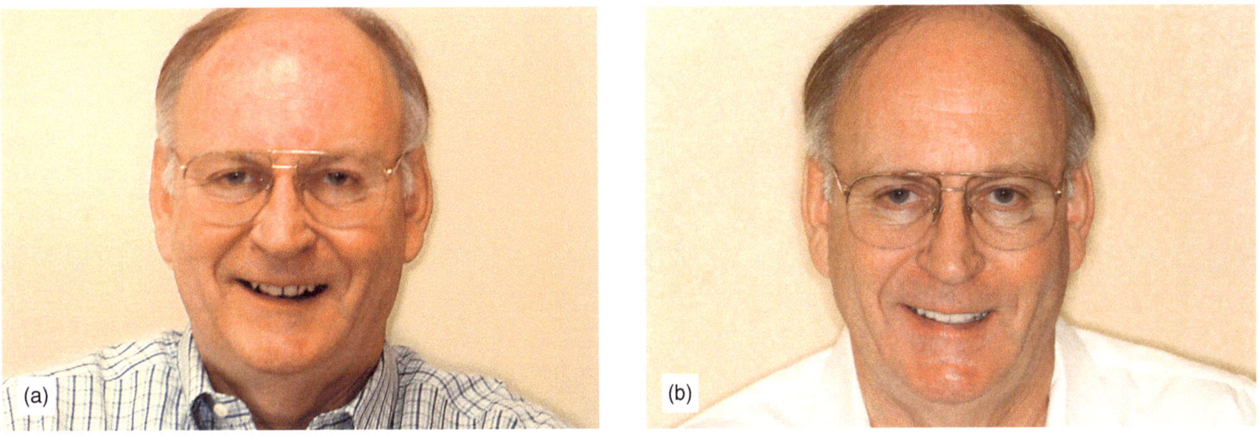

Proper dentofacial smile design allows enhancement not just of the teeth but of the entire facial appearance.

Introduction

Diagnosis and treatment planning is indispensable for treatment success. Detailed plans are always prepared and approved before any beautiful building is ever constructed (Figure 8.1a,b). Similarly, knowing the final restoration outline based on known dentofacial principles, the patient's esthetic goals and the occlusal requirements leads to predictable results, patient satisfaction and minimally invasive preparation, as described in Chapter 7. Smile design is not just a luxury; it is indispensable, and combined with occlusal analysis is an integral part of a thorough diagnosis. As clinicians, it can be easy to focus on the principles we know and overlook a patient's goals when they come in for esthetic improvement. Diagnosing on only retracted photographic views or a cast of the patient's teeth can lead to focusing on the tooth shape and gingival condition, while the overall appearance of

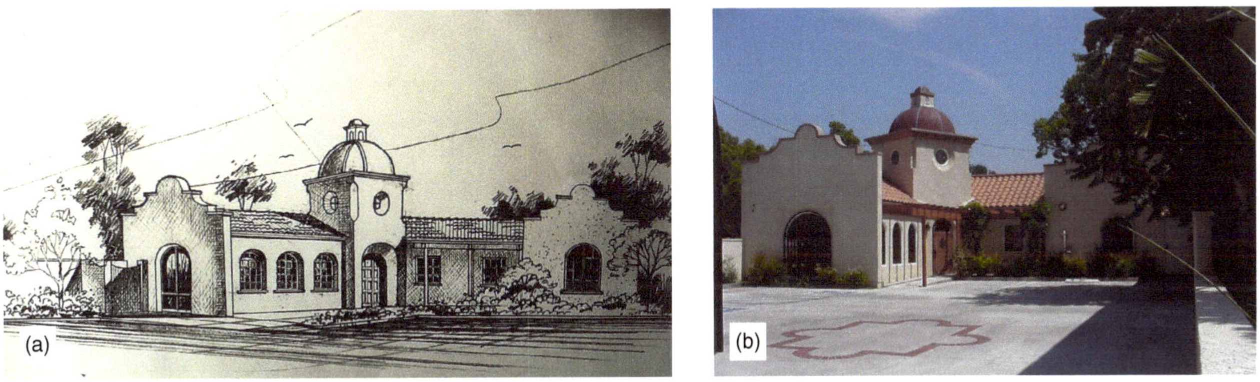

Figure 8.1 (a) Drawing of a building 2 years before construction. (b) After construction.

Supra-Gingival Minimally Invasive Dentistry: A Healthier Approach to Esthetic Restorations, First Edition. By Jose-Luis Ruiz.

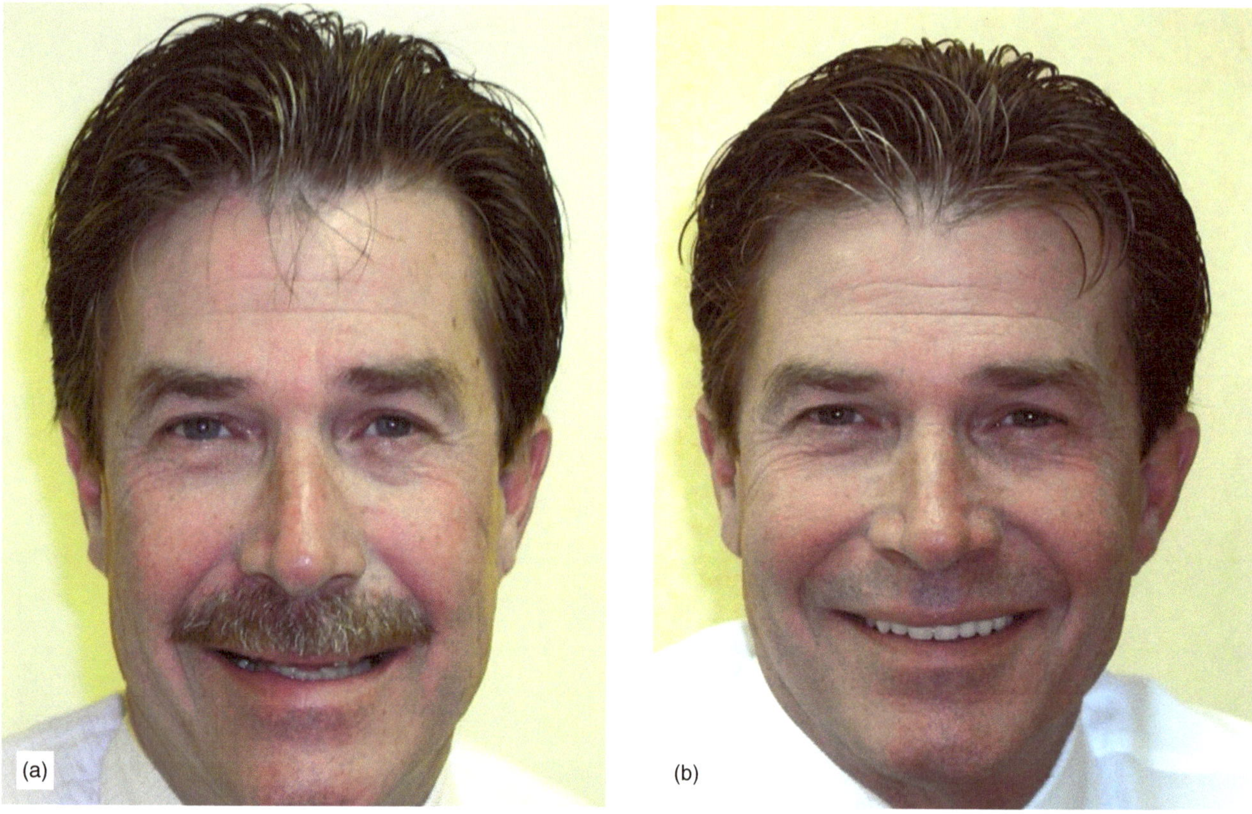

Figure 8.2 (a) Face before veneers. (b) Face enhancement after veneers.

how the smile should enhance the entire face can be lost. Similarly, sending a set of casts to a laboratory, and asking for wax-ups without detailed instructions is basically a Las Vegas style gamble.

The Psychology of the Smile

When patients come in for esthetic dental treatment, they are looking at the "big picture" – they want to look better, not just the teeth but the smile and thus the entire face, and so should clinicians, or unhappy patients will be the results (Figure 8.2a,b) [1]. Understanding the importance that the smile has in human social interaction and overall emotional wellbeing should increase awareness of the great importance that smile design has when treating the anterior dentition (Figure 8.3) [2,3]. Dentofacial esthetics is the evaluation of teeth as they relate to other facial structures and facial symmetry that is influenced by the teeth. As with anything related to esthetics, it is subjective, but has some basic rules [4,5,6].

Any time that multiple anterior teeth are being planned for treatment, a dentofacial evaluation and design should be the first step to ensure a harmonious dentofacial outcome. The evaluation and design should also take into consideration the entire occlusal scheme, which will lend to stability and longevity of the dentition (see Chapter 13). This process mirrors that of building construction or extensive remodeling. It always begins with an architectural design with the goal of beauty, and then ensuring proper engineering and function. X-rays and periodontal charting, caries assessment and periodontal therapy should be integrated with the overall diagnosis.

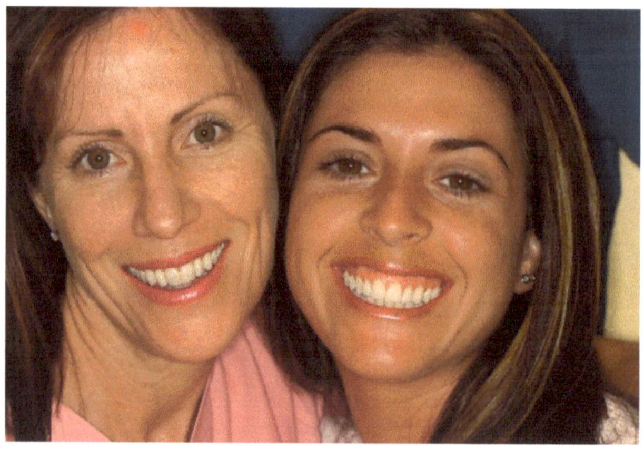

Figure 8.3 Beautiful smiles are contagious.

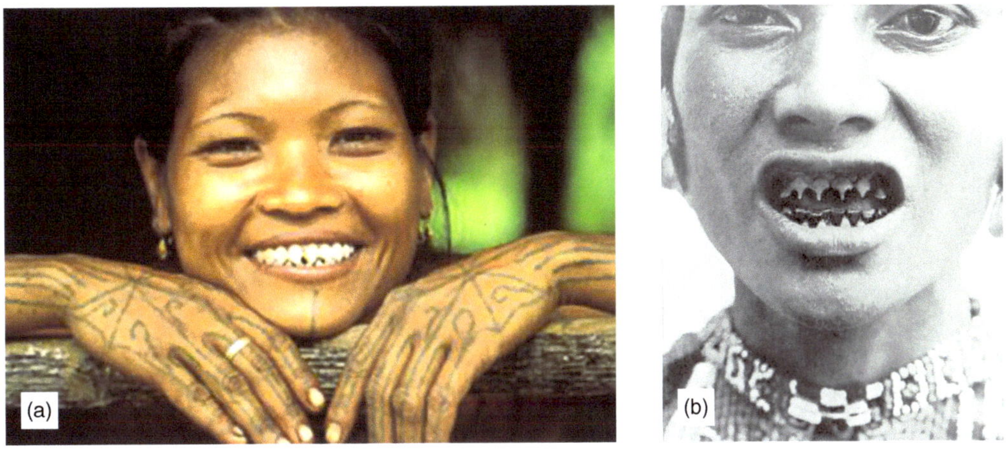

Figure 8.4 (a and b) Unusual dental beauty (tribal).

Parameters, Not Rules

Predictable results and patient satisfaction can be easily obtained by systematically recording the patient's goals and preferences and blending them with known esthetic parameters. Through a series of forms and two-way communication, the dentofacial esthetic diagnosis system takes a clinician step by step, guiding with principles, but not giving absolute rules, so as to allow for individual preference.

Some important parameters apply in this process. Again, the subjective nature of beauty requires latitude for choices and opinions (Figure 8.4a,b). There are, on the other hand, clinical parameters for ensuring a healthy occlusion, as well as esthetic parameters that are universal in the definition of beauty [7,8].

Record Gathering

Before the smile diagnosis can be completed with the patient, information must be gathered that can be used for diagnosis and presented to the patient. This information can also be used to communicate with members of the esthetic team, such as the restorative dentist (working as team leader), any specialists involved (orthodontist, periodontist, oral surgeon) and the laboratory technician. Photographs allow for the assessment of tooth position in relation to face and lips. Photography is an excellent way to show patients multiple views of their face, smile and teeth, in order to come to a mutual agreement on treatment. The following records can and should be completed by a well-trained dental assistant (local laws may limit auxiliaries' duties): A full set of periapical x-rays, panoramic x-ray (not required but highly recommended), six-point periodontal charting, and articulated casts mounted using a face bow and a semi-adjustable articulator. Finally, a high-quality 11-photograph series, which can be acquired with a simple point-and-shoot digital camera (Box 8.1).

Smile Design Step By Step

The 11 simple photographs (Box 8.1) [9] taken by the assistant are displayed on the computer screen or printed, allowing the patient to observe their own smile from different views. All findings are recorded on the dentofacial esthetic diagnosis form (Figure 8.6) [10]. The 25 parameters of dentofacial esthetics are best illustrated photographically, and it is a simple way to organize them. Each view and parameters therein will be assessed, and only those parameters with problems will be discussed by the clinician with the patient:

- Is the parameter within acceptable limits? If so, it is not necessary to discuss this with the patient.
- Can the problem be corrected with restorative dentistry? If yes, explain specific treatment to the patient, including options, and estimated cost to correct. If not correctable, explain limitations; or
- Suggest specialist referral option (orthodontist, periodontist, oral surgeon).

It is important to bear in mind that only a few parameters will need to be discussed. Usually only five or six problematic parameters will be addressed, and the entire smile design procedure should take approximately 10–15 minutes in most cases.

The 25 Parameters

The following are general guidelines for each of the 25 dentofacial parameters and should not be considered as rules. Each parameter discussed will be tempered by the patient's own preferences, their willingness to

Box 8.1 Dentofacial esthetic photographic series

2 x face – front smiling view and profile view (Figure 8.5a,b).

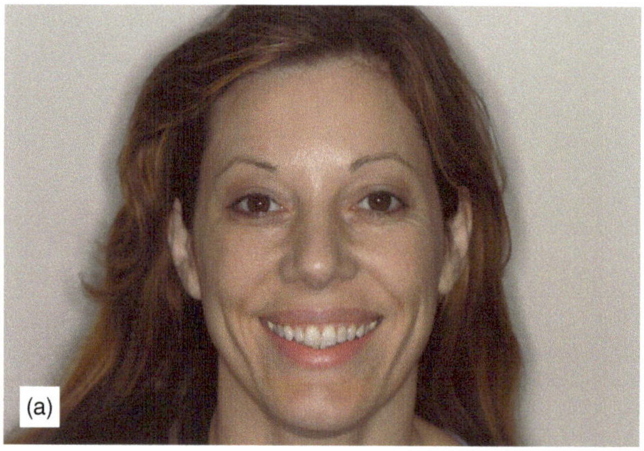

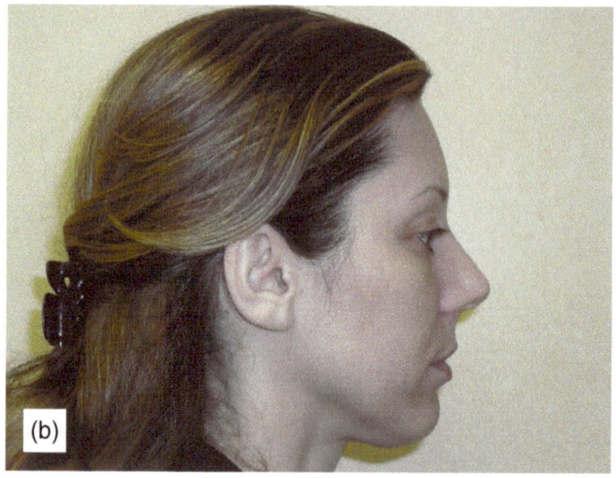

3 x non-retracted close-up shots – front, left and right smiling views (Figure 8.5c–e).

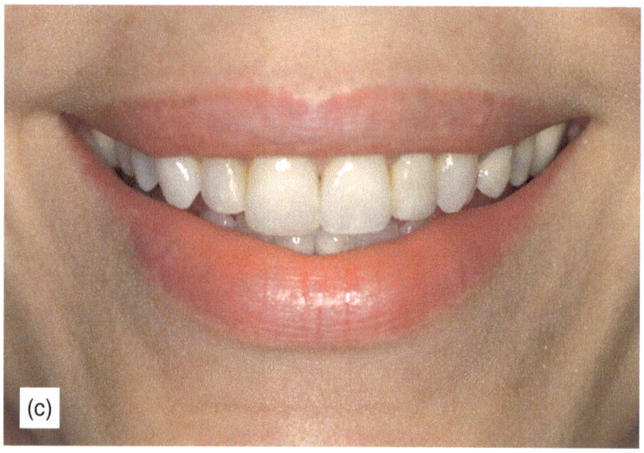

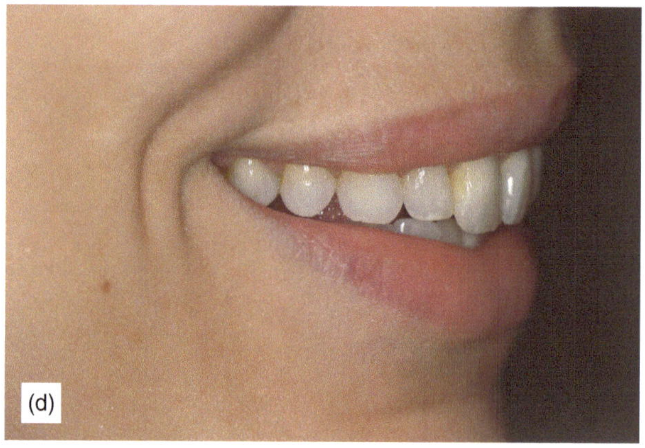

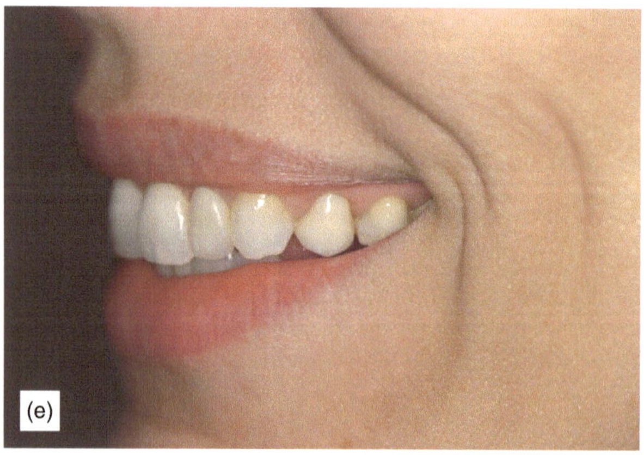

1 x conversational tooth show (Figure 8.5f).

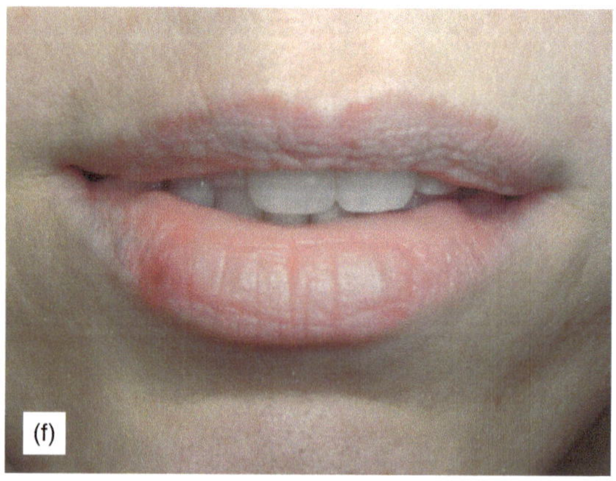

Figure 8.5 (a) Front full-face, smiling. (b) Profile. (c) Close-up smile, front. (d) Close-up right side. (e) Close-up left side. (f) Close-up, conversational view, repeating the number "66". (*Continued*)

3 x retracted close-up shots – front, left and right views (Figure 8.5g–i).

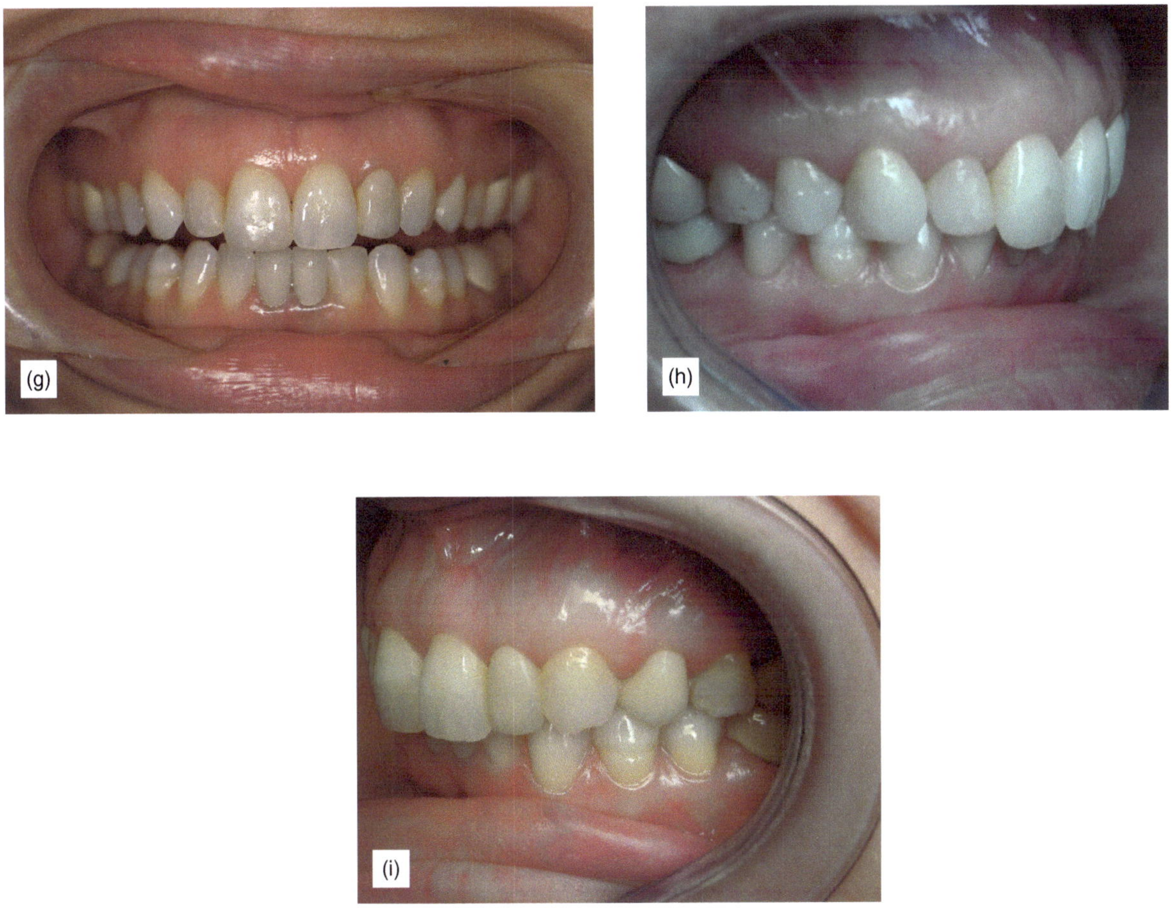

2 x occlusal – maxillary and mandibular, using a mirror (Figure 8.5j,k).

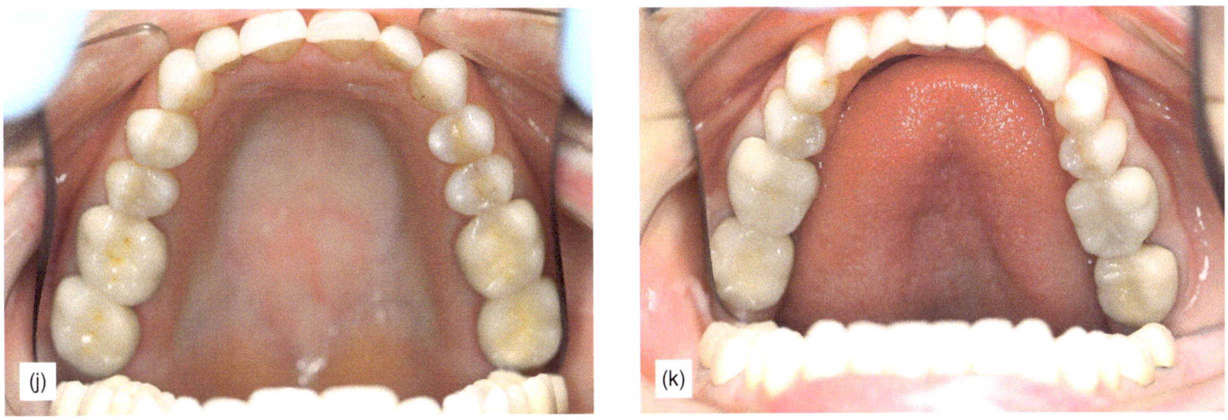

Figure 8.5 *(Continued)*
(g) Retracted front with teeth slightly separated. (h) Retracted right, biting. (i) Retracted left, biting. (j) Maxillary occlusal view. (k) Mandibular occlusal view.

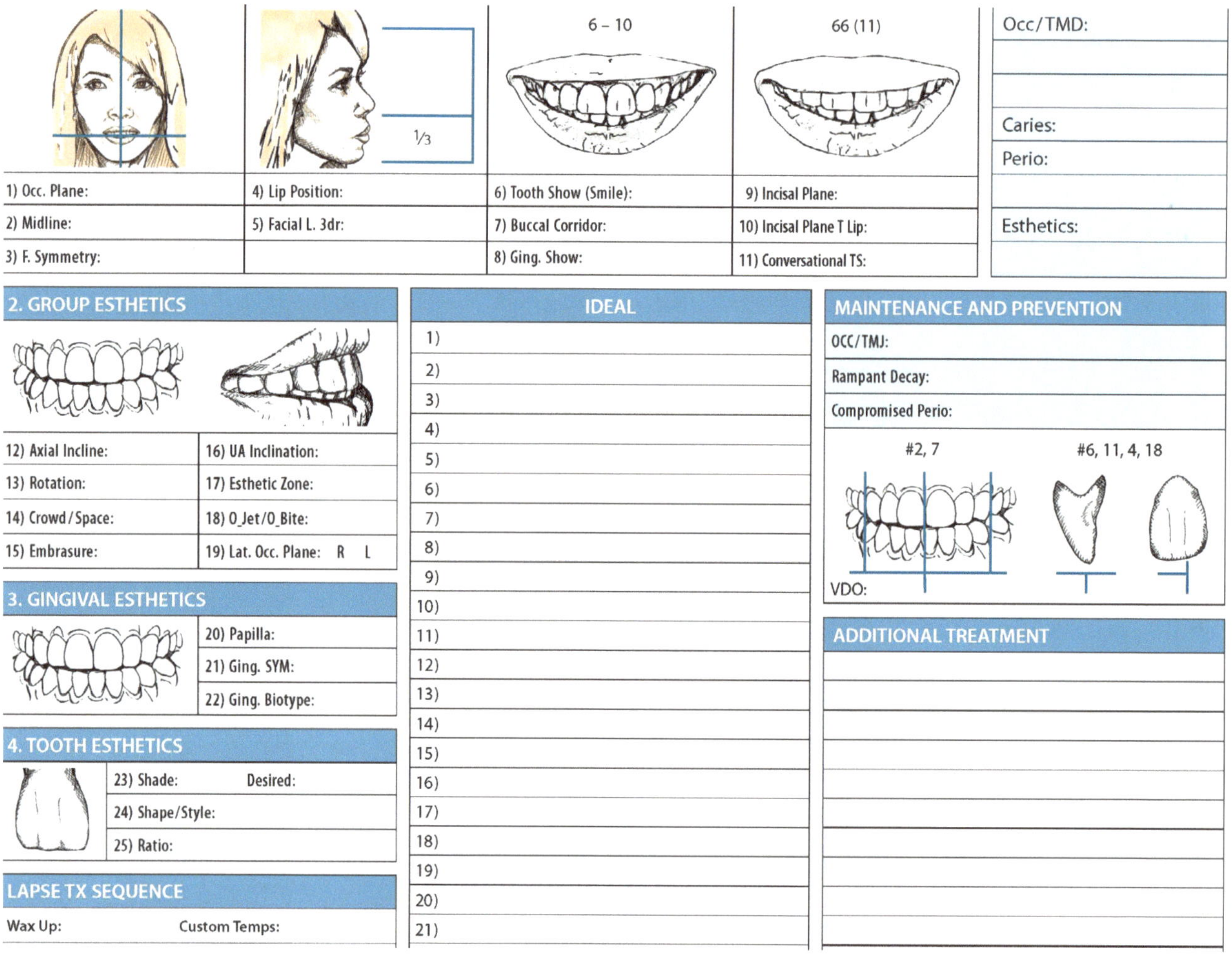

Figure 8.6 Close-up of the form with all the images.

proceed with any corrective treatment, balanced by the patient's budget. Using the dentofacial esthetic diagnosis form easily walks the clinician through the esthetic and clinical parameters, while allowing notes to be taken for review and diagnosis later on (Figure 8.7).

1 Occlusal Plane, Front Full-Face Smiling (Figure 8.8) [11]

Take an imaginary line parallel to the horizon and touching the incisal edges of both centrals, and either the incisal edge of the canines or equidistant to both canines, laterals and the rest of the dentition. (Figures 8.9, 8.10a–c). The use of a facebow-mounted cast can greatly help in evaluation and laboratory communication and correction (Figure 8.11a,b).

2 Midline (Front Full-Face Smiling) [12]

This is a vertical line which dissects the face vertically and can use glabella (the point where the nose and forehead connect) and filtrum or cupid's bow, as a facial reference. Ideally, the facial midline and the dental midline should coincide, but often they do not. As long as the midline is perpendicular to the occlusal plane, the dental midline can be up to 2 mm off-center and the human eye can barely detect the disparity (Figures 8.12a–c,

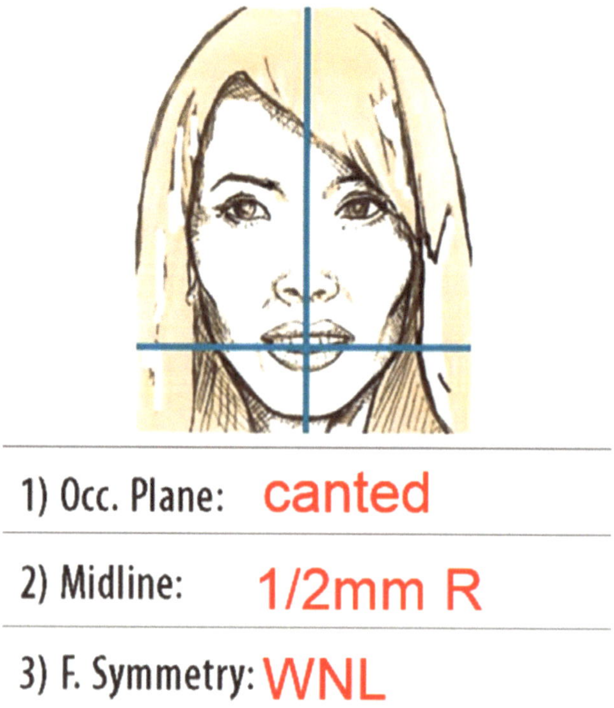

Figure 8.7 Close-up of section for notes on the form.

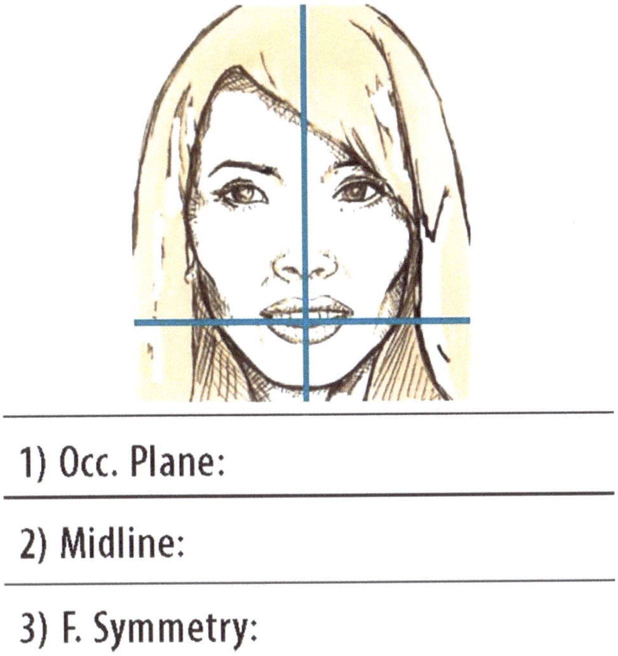

Figure 8.8 Front full face smiling form.

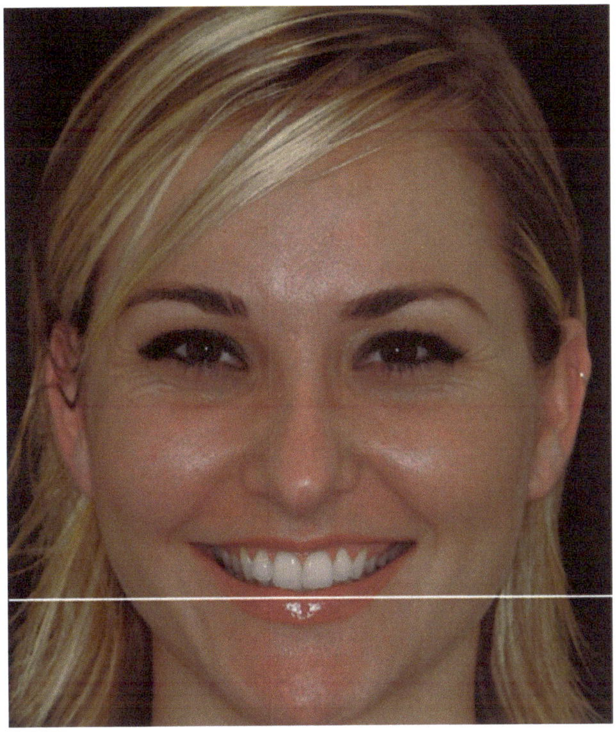

Figure 8.9 Full face ideal occlusal plane.

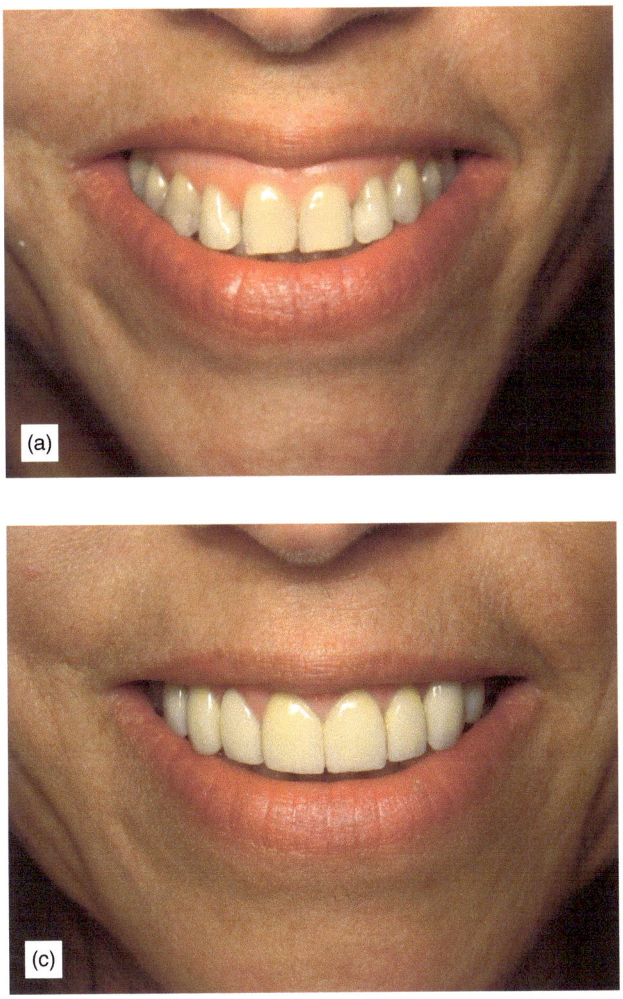

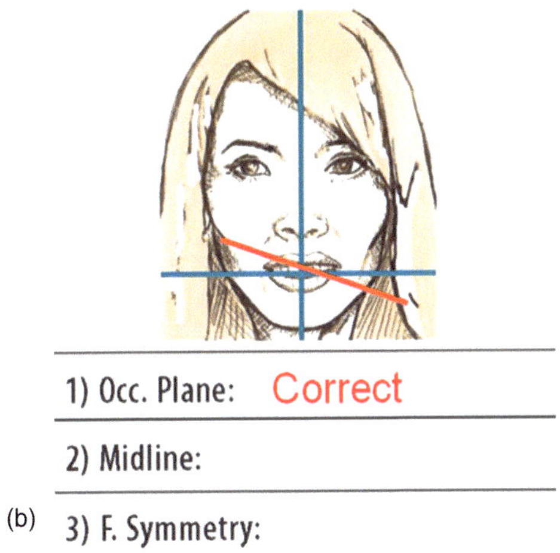

Figure 8.10 (a) Canted occlusal plane. (b) Form with correction notes. (c) After occlusal cant correction with veneers.

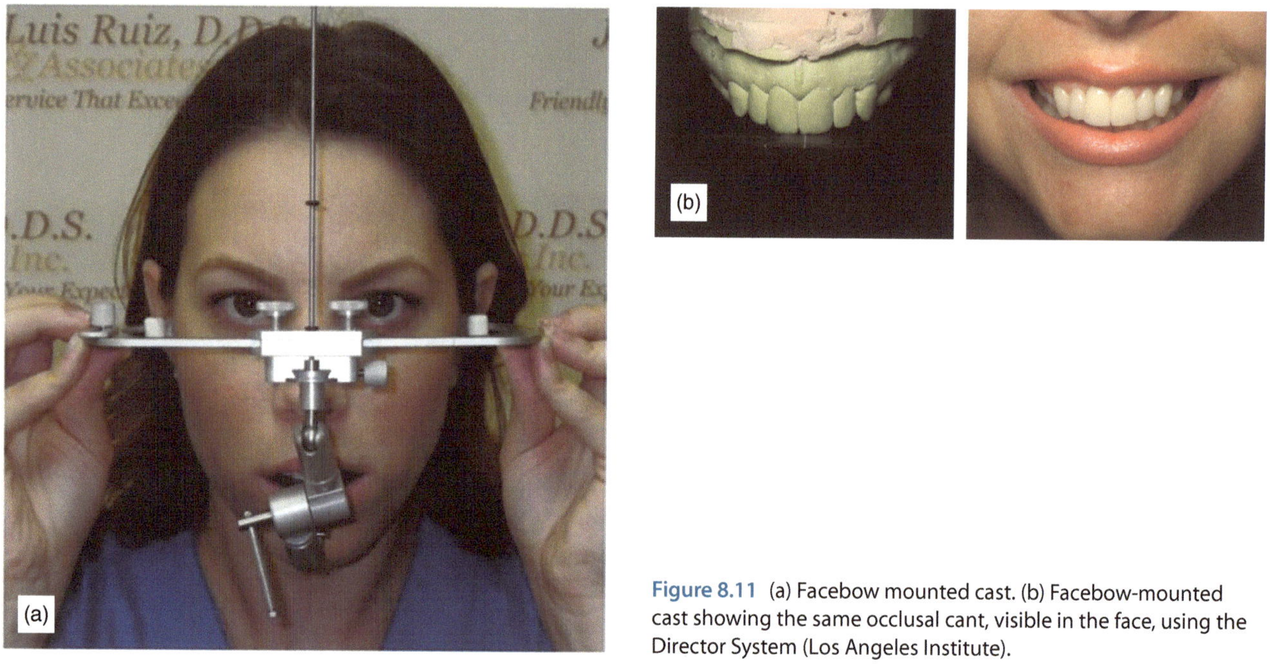

Figure 8.11 (a) Facebow mounted cast. (b) Facebow-mounted cast showing the same occlusal cant, visible in the face, using the Director System (Los Angeles Institute).

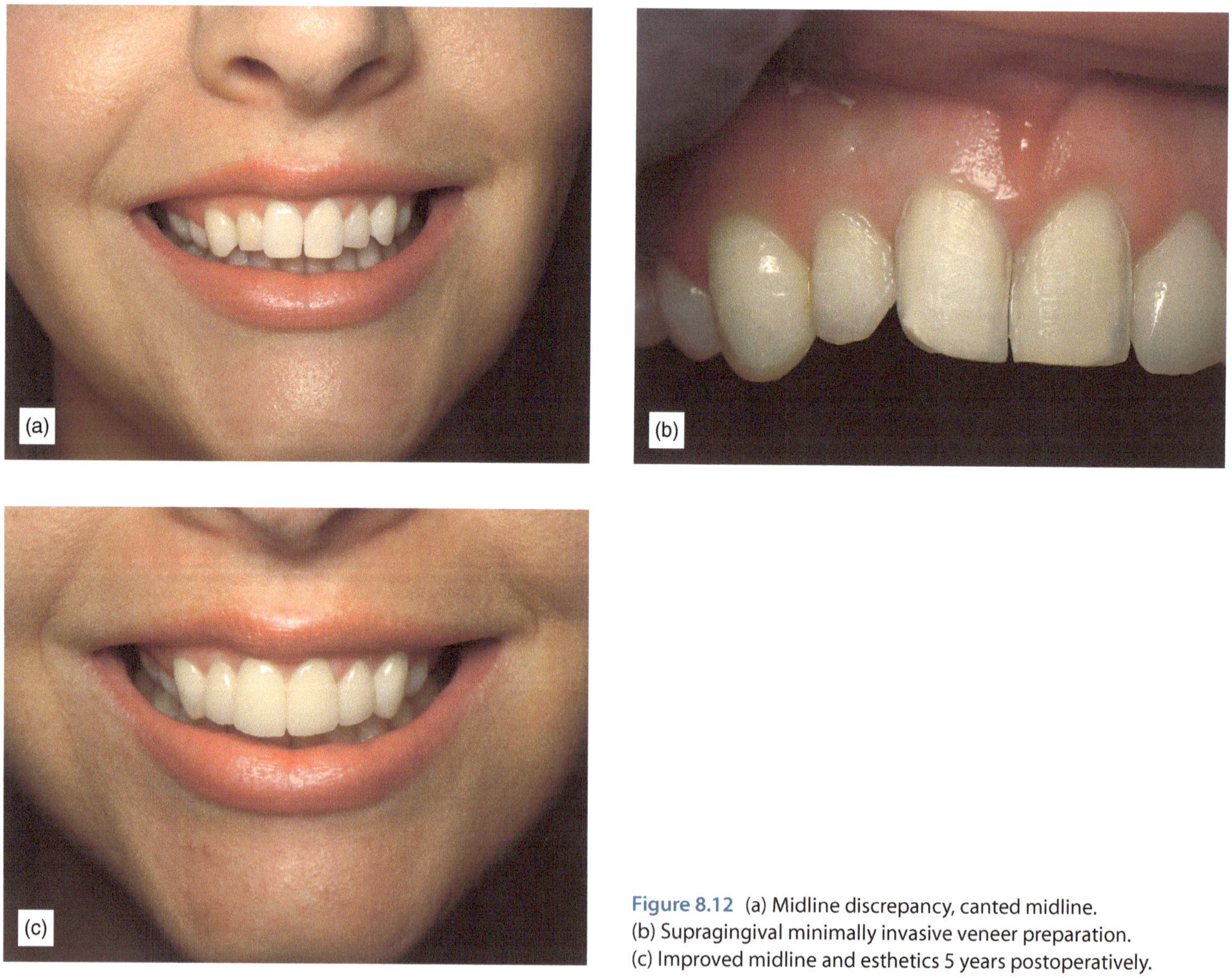

Figure 8.12 (a) Midline discrepancy, canted midline. (b) Supragingival minimally invasive veneer preparation. (c) Improved midline and esthetics 5 years postoperatively.

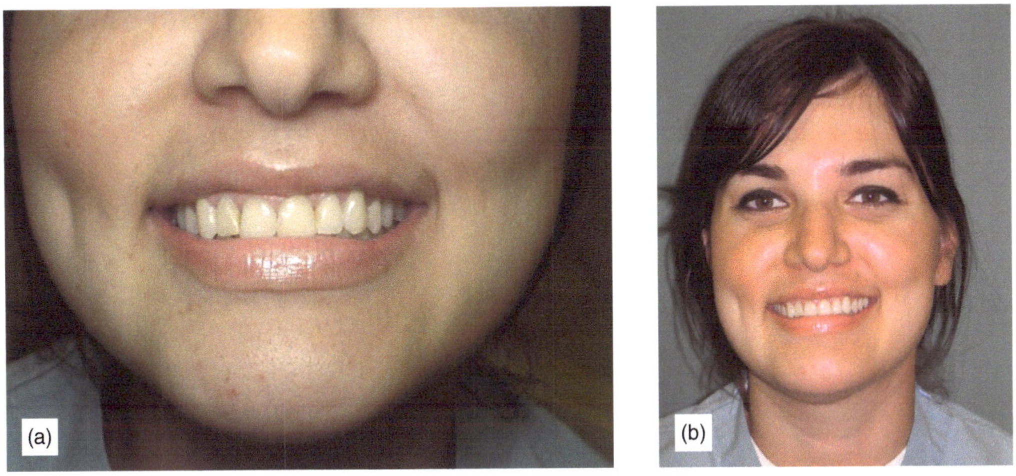

Figure 8.13 (a) Midline 2 mm to the right; close-up view. (b) Midline 2 mm to the right; full face view.

8.13a,b). The use of a facebow-mounted cast can greatly help in the evaluation, in communication with the laboratory and in correction (Figure 8.14a,b).

3 Facial Symmetry (Front Full-Face Smiling)

Any obvious facial asymmetry should be noted, as it can throw off the occlusal plane and midline. Facial asymmetries can greatly complicate the evaluation and communication with the laboratory, and may lead to compromised results. Only by the correct use of a calibrated facebow-mounted cast will good communication with the laboratory and acceptable corrections be possible (Figure 8.15a–d).

4 Lip Position (Profile)

It is important to consider the lip position and lip support when large changes in dental protrusion are being consider with orthodontics or restorative dentistry (Figure 8.16), as the lips are supported by the teeth [13], and changes will have a positive or negative effect on the look of the lips. Ricketts E-line [14] is an imaginary line drawn between the tip of nose and tip of chin, where the upper lip should be 1 mm from the line and the lower lip should touch it (Figure 8.17). This parameter is, however, subjective and dependent on ethnicity, and for these reasons the patient's opinion should be the primary guideline (Figure 8.18a–e).

5 Facial Lower Third (Profile view)

A collapsed lower third has an aging effect. The lower facial third collapses primarily due to a lack of posterior teeth to support the vertical dimension of occlusion and severe occlusal wear. This parameter should be considered when orthodontic or extensive restorative treatment is being planned, as improvements can be very rejuvenating (Figure 8.19) [15,16,17,18].

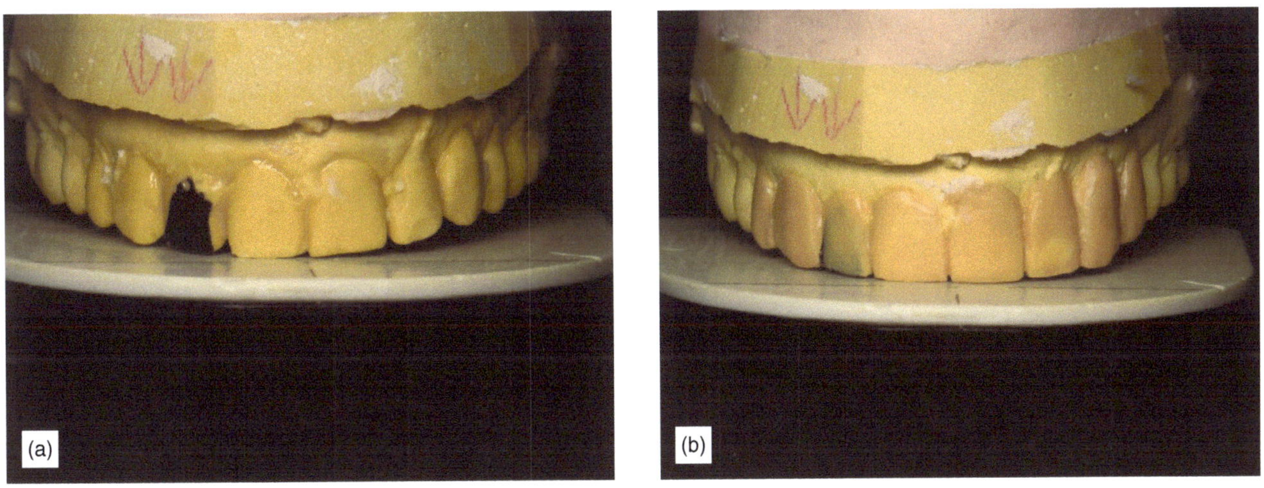

Figure 8.14 (a) Midline visibly incorrect on facebow. (b) Corrected with wax-up.

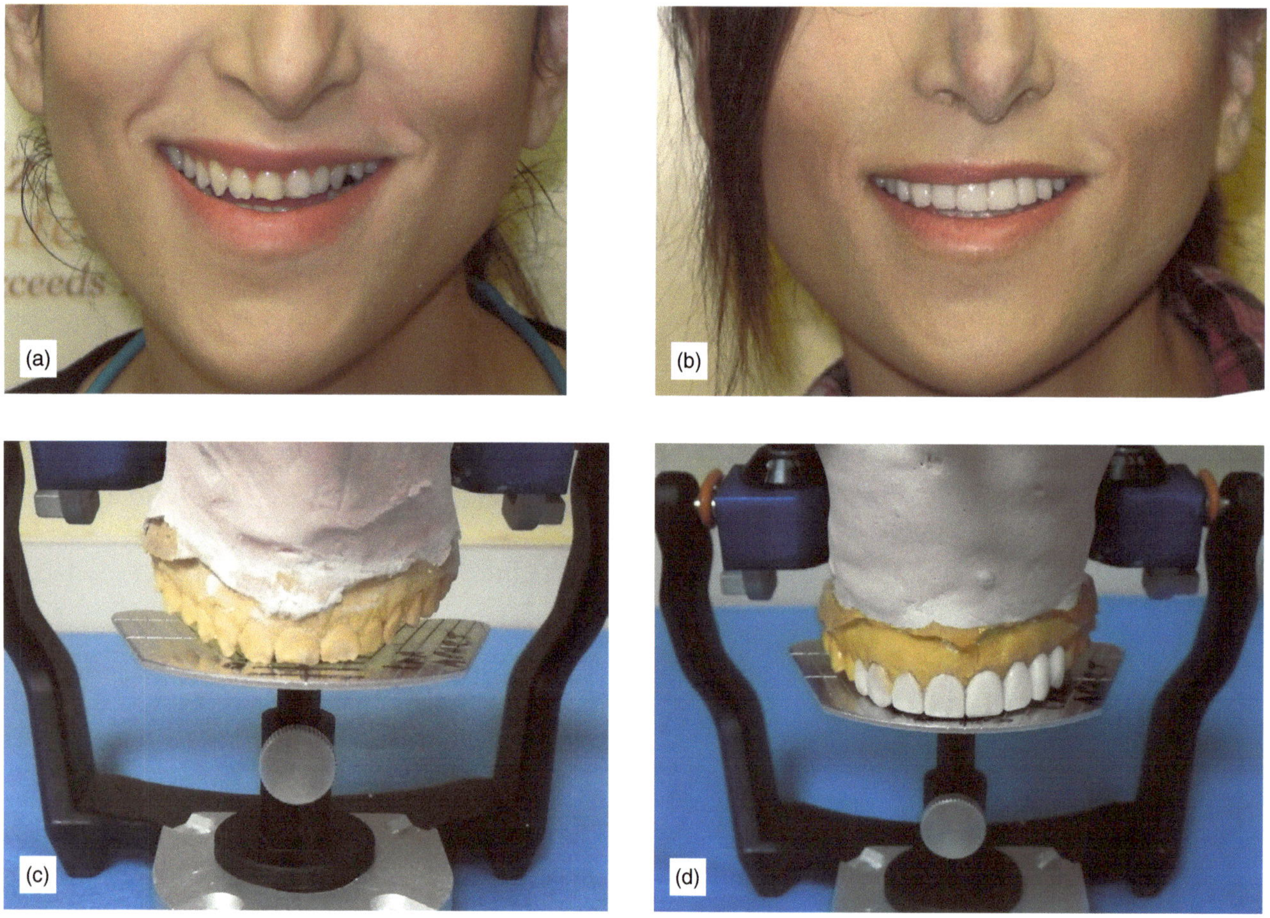

Figure 8.15 (a) Facial asymmetries will compromise diagnosis and final results, and must be assessed and discussed in advance to avoid unreasonable expectations. (b) Excellent results, still showing the complexity of correcting asymmetrical faces and smiles. (c) Facebow-mounted cast, using a diagnostic plate calibrated with the facebow and articulator (the Director, Los Angeles Institute). (d) Wax-up showing corrected midline and occlusal plane (the Director, at the prototype stage).

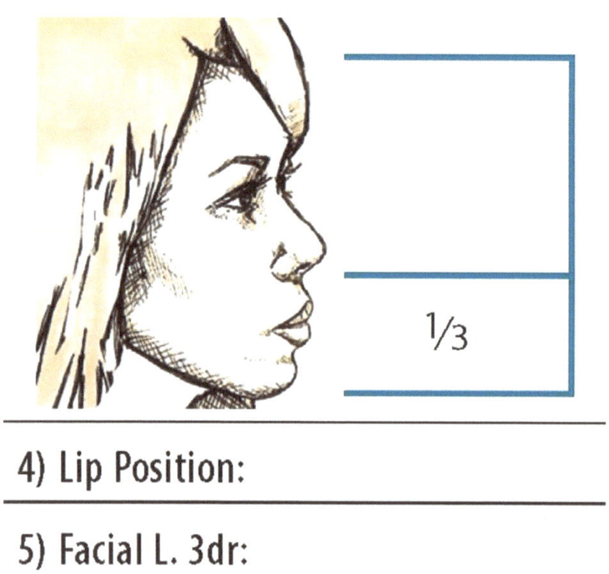

Figure 8.16 Parameters 4 and 5 are evaluated on this section of the form.

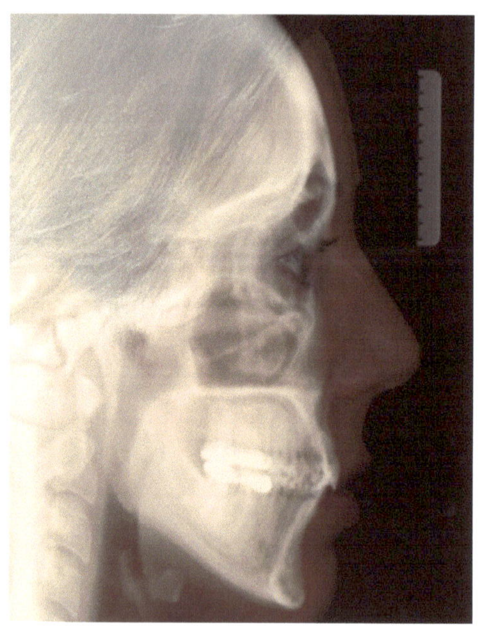

Figure 8.17 Cephalometry shows the lip being supported by the teeth.

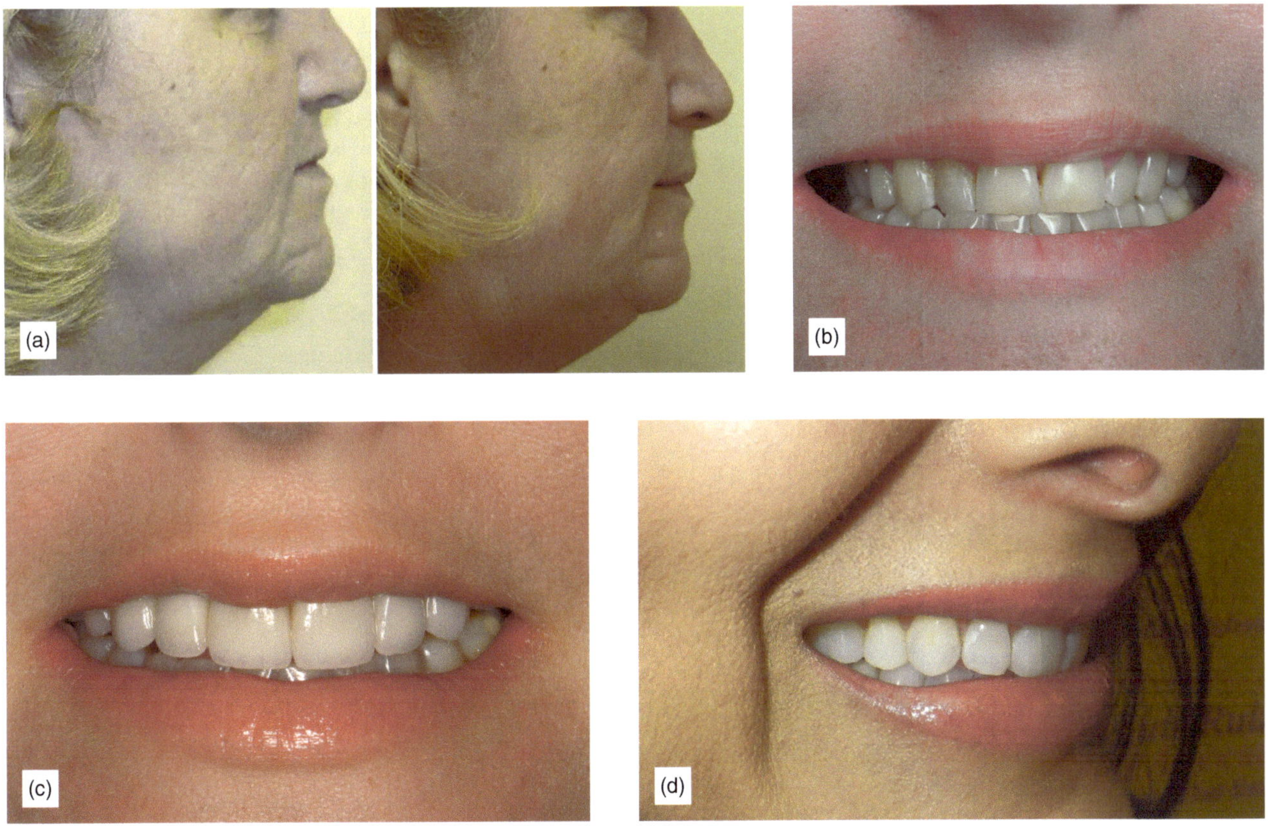

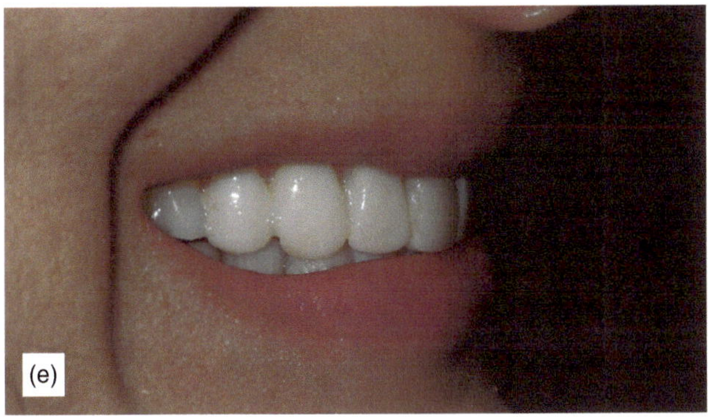

Figure 8.18 (a) Rejuvenating improvement by adding lip support. (b) Preoperative view of patient with unsupported lip. (c) Postoperative view of the patient, with improved lip support using minimally invasive veneers. (d) Side view of lip support. (e) Improved lip support at the provisional stage.

Figure 8.19 Collapsed lower third, compared after bite opening with a full upper arch rehabilitation.

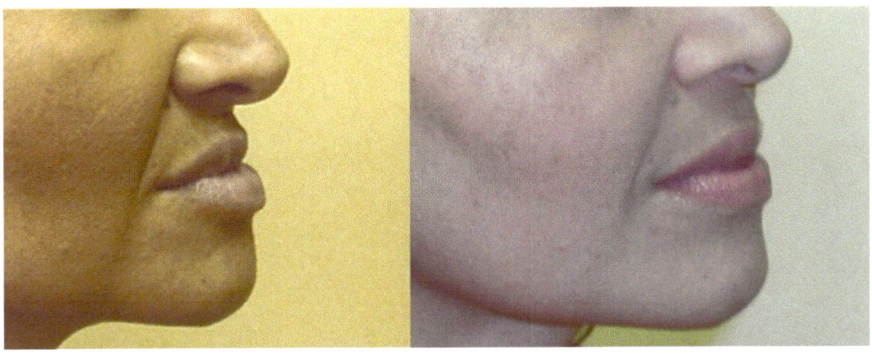

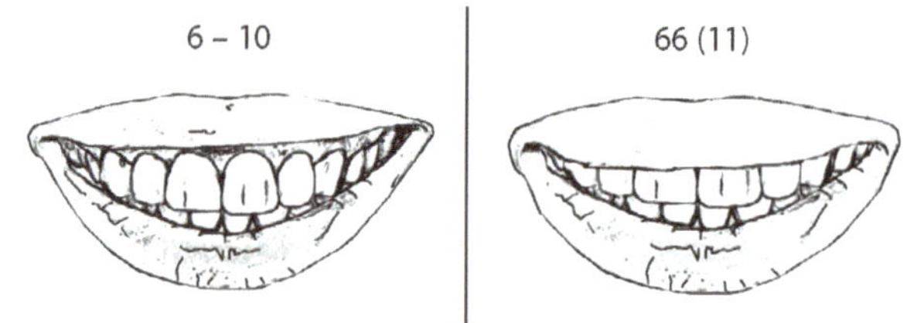

6) Tooth Show (Smile):	9) Incisal Plane:
7) Buccal Corridor:	10) Incisal Plane T Lip:
8) Ging. Show:	11) Conversational TS:

Figure 8.20 Parameters 6–11 are evaluated with smile close-up and conversational views.

6 Tooth Show (Front Smile View)

Tooth show is an age-defining parameter, and is one of the most often considered with the patient (Figure 8.20) [19,20]. Usually when teeth have severe wear, some incisal edge lengthening will have a rejuvenating effect on the smile. Ideally, the incisal edge of the maxillary teeth should be close to touching the lower lip. The further away the upper teeth are from the lip and the more lower tooth is visible during the smile, the older the smile will look. The patient's goals and preferences are crucial during the evaluative process (Figures 8.21a,b, 8.22a,b).

7 Buccal Corridor (Front Smile View)

The buccal corridor parameter is currently guided by a desire to have wide arches and very little buccal corridor shadow or space. Orthodontics with extracted bicuspids usually lead to a collapsed or narrow maxillary arch, although sometimes narrow arches are a natural occurrence. If during the evaluation the patient wishes to have a fuller smile, restorative or orthodontic options can be discussed (Figure 8.23a,b).

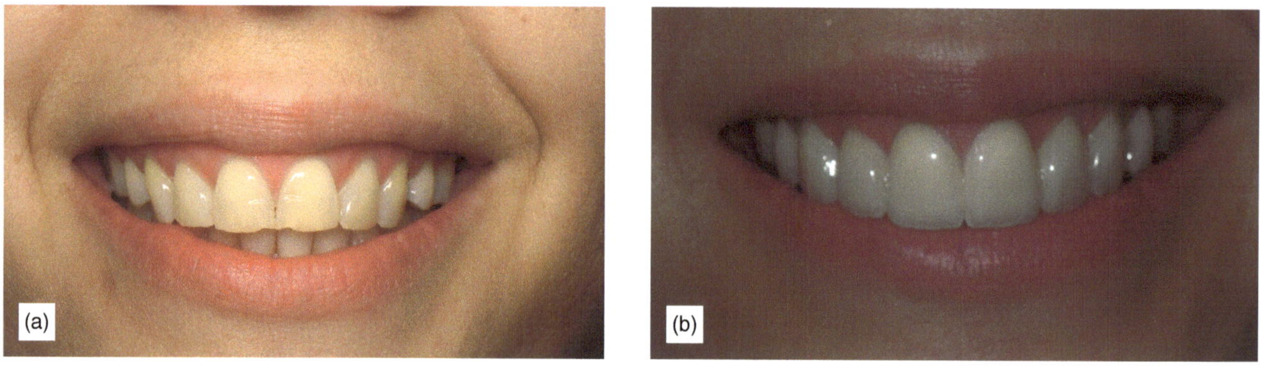

Figure 8.21 (a) Short anterior teeth due to incisal wear caused by occlusal disease. (b) Porcelain veneers with increased length, creating a more youthful appearance.

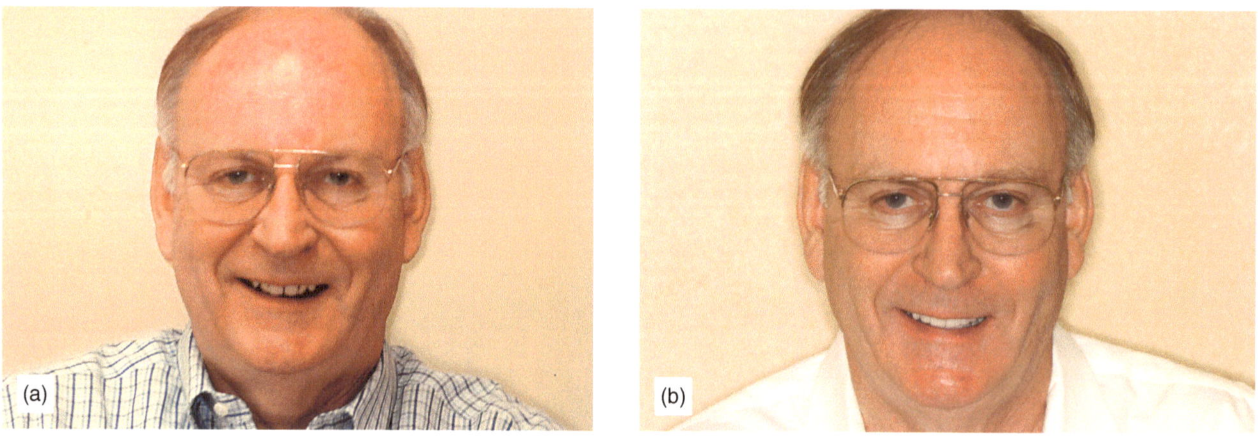

Figure 8.22 (a) Insufficient tooth show forces patient to smile very hard to show any teeth. (b) After increased tooth show, a more relaxed smile shows enough tooth and is highly esthetic.

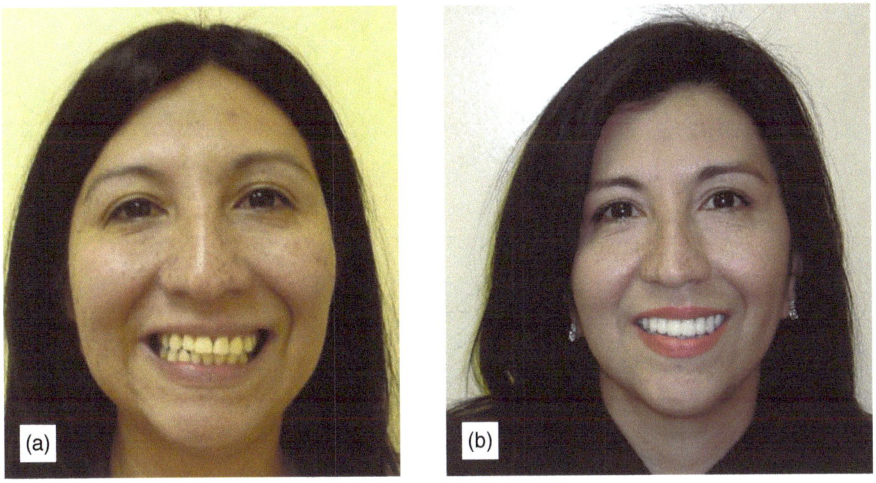

Figure 8.23 (a) Asymmetrical buccal corridor problem. (b) Corrected buccal corridor.

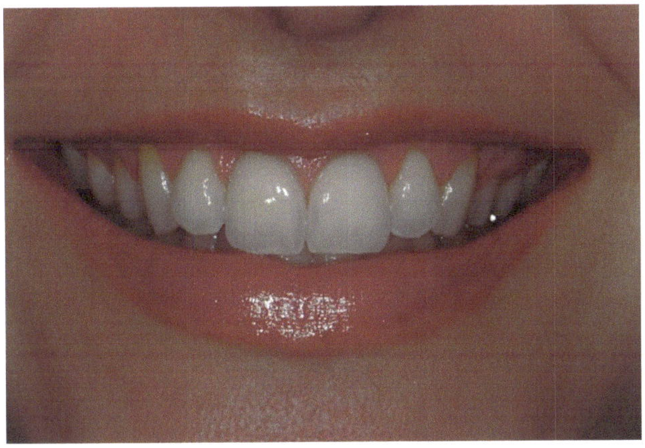

Figure 8.24 Acceptable gingival display.

8 Gingival Show (Front Smile View)

A gingival display is any gingiva that shows above the crown zenith of the teeth. The amount of gingiva displayed should be bilaterally symmetrical. Generally, up to 2 mm of display is acceptable for most women (Figure 8.24). Because men generally have longer lips, any amount of gingival display is not esthetically pleasing. Crown lengthening surgery can usually correct a "gummy" smile (Figures 8.25a,b, 8.26a,b).

9 Incisal Plane (Front Smile View)

The incisal plane, a line which touches the incisal edges of all visible teeth, should be continuous, not resembling a rollercoaster (Figure 8.27), and should have a positive curvature, like a happy face. Reverse curves are undesirable and should not be irregular or wavy (Figure 8.28a,b).

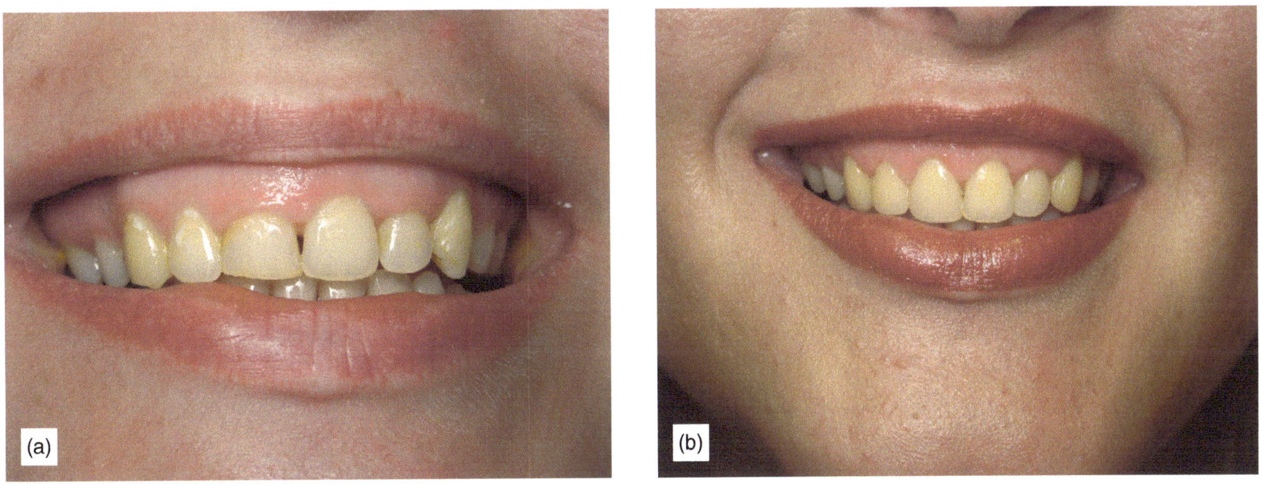

Figure 8.25 (a) Excessive and asymmetrical gingival display. (b) Corrected gingival display with crown lengthening surgery.

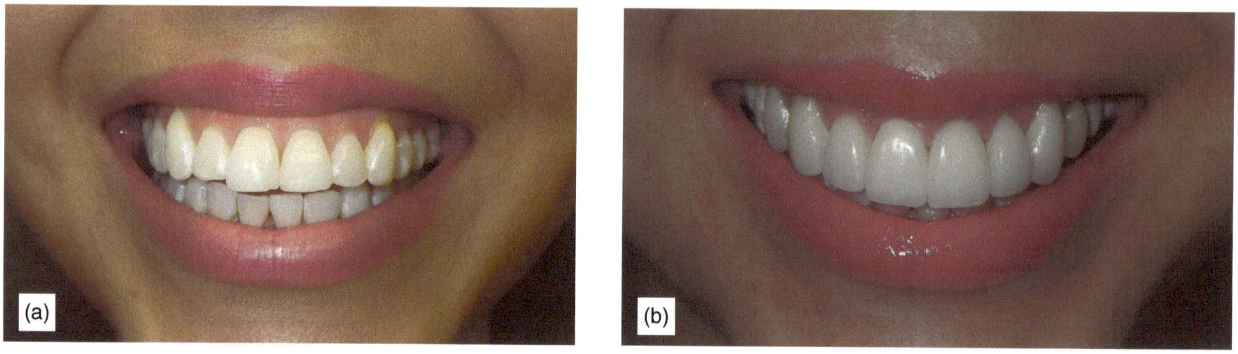

Figure 8.26 (a) Excessive and asymmetrical gingival display. (b) After crown lengthening surgery and porcelain veneers.

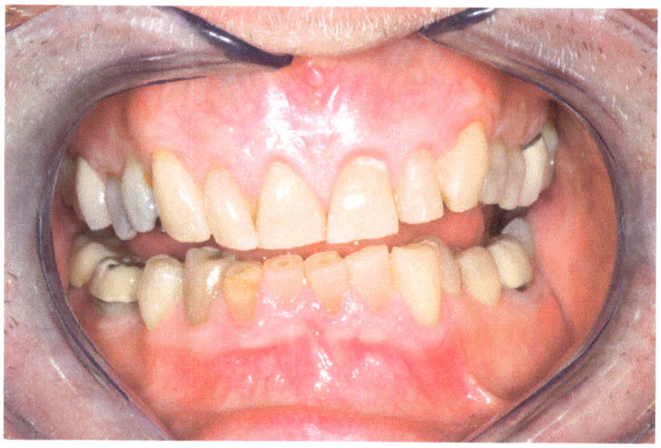

Figure 8.27 Wavy incisal plane caused by occlusal disease (courtesy of Dr Patricia Ryan).

10 Incisal Plane to Lip (Front Smile View)

It is desirable for the incisal edge to follow the curvature of the lower lip (Figure 8.29). Lips have different curvatures and ignoring the type of lip curvature can lead to unesthetic results (Figure 8.30).

11 Conversational Tooth Show [9] (Conversational View "66")

Some systems suggest taking a view with the lip in repose, to help to determine the appropriate amount of tooth show. It is, however, more important to know how much tooth shows when the patient is speaking, as this is the time when the teeth are being observed by others (Figures 8.31a,b, 8.32a,b). A conversational display can

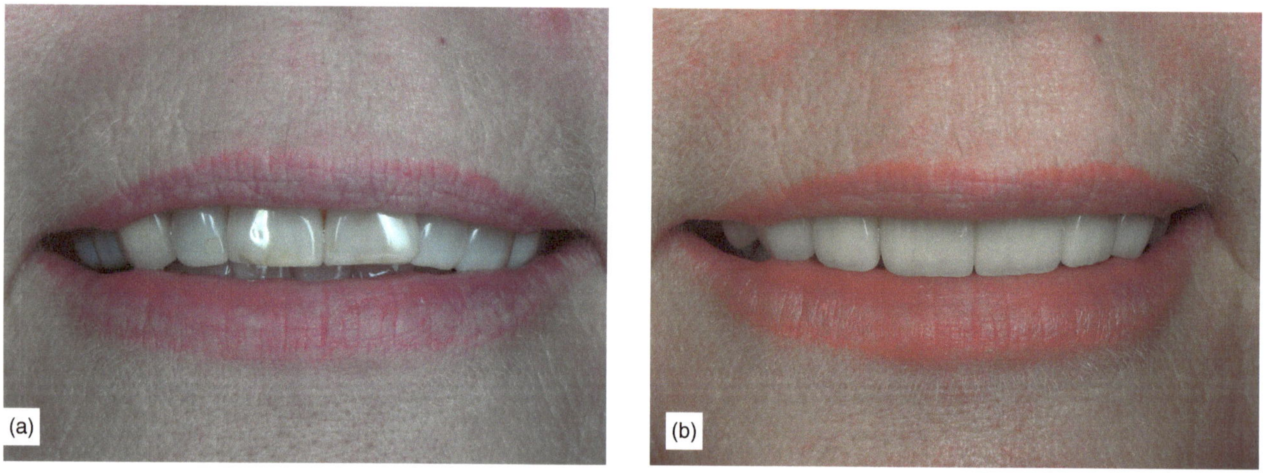

Figure 8.28 (a) Reverse curve. (b) After correction with veneers.

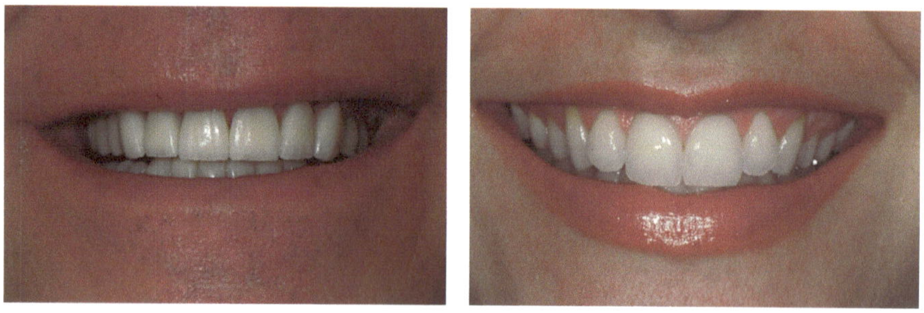

Figure 8.29 Incisal plane following lip curvature.

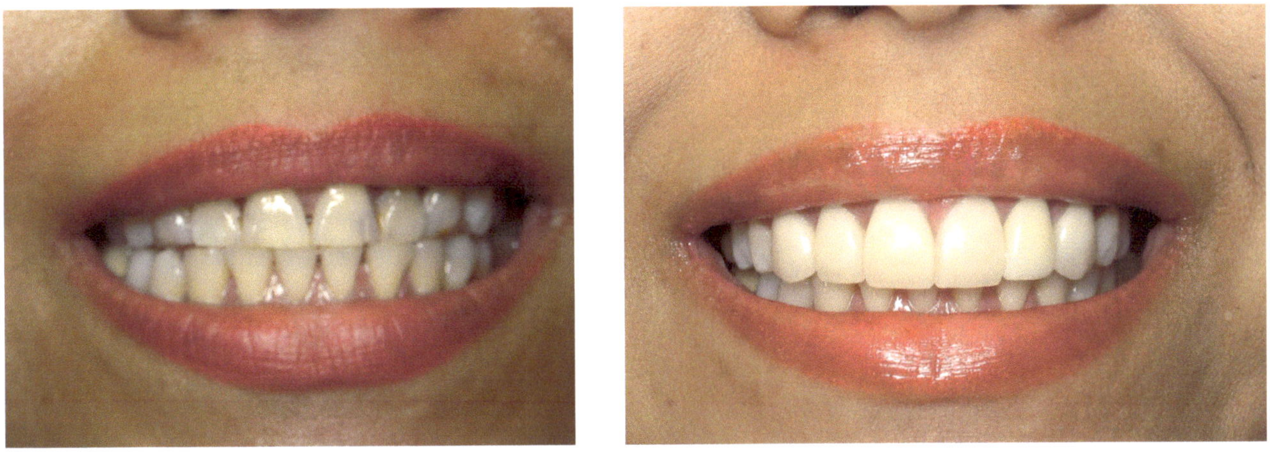

Figure 8.30 Incisal plane not following lip curvature.

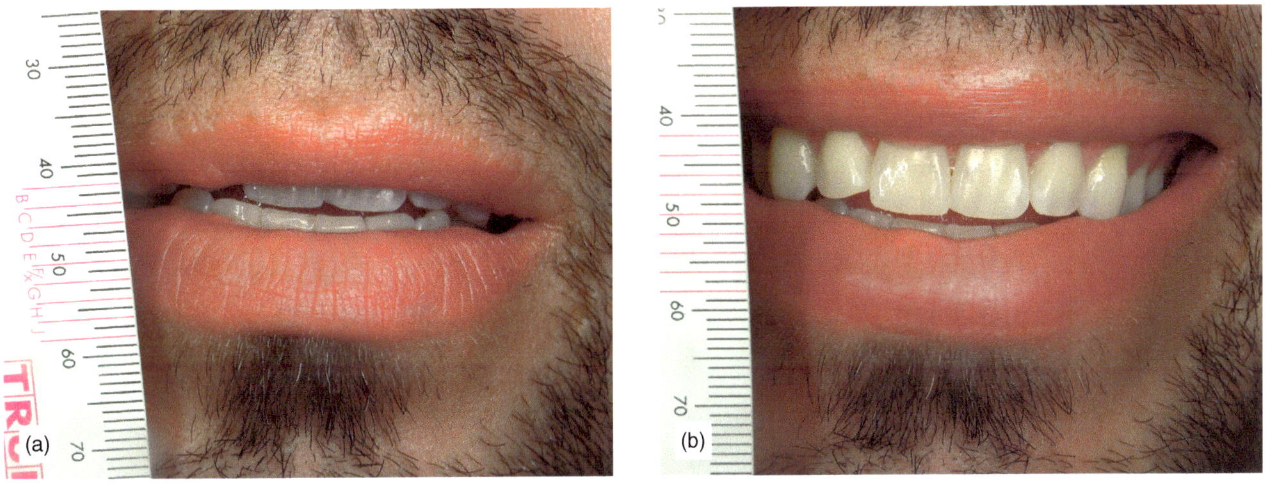

Figure 8.31 (a) Male repeating the number "66", a conversational tooth view. (b) Same male smiling.

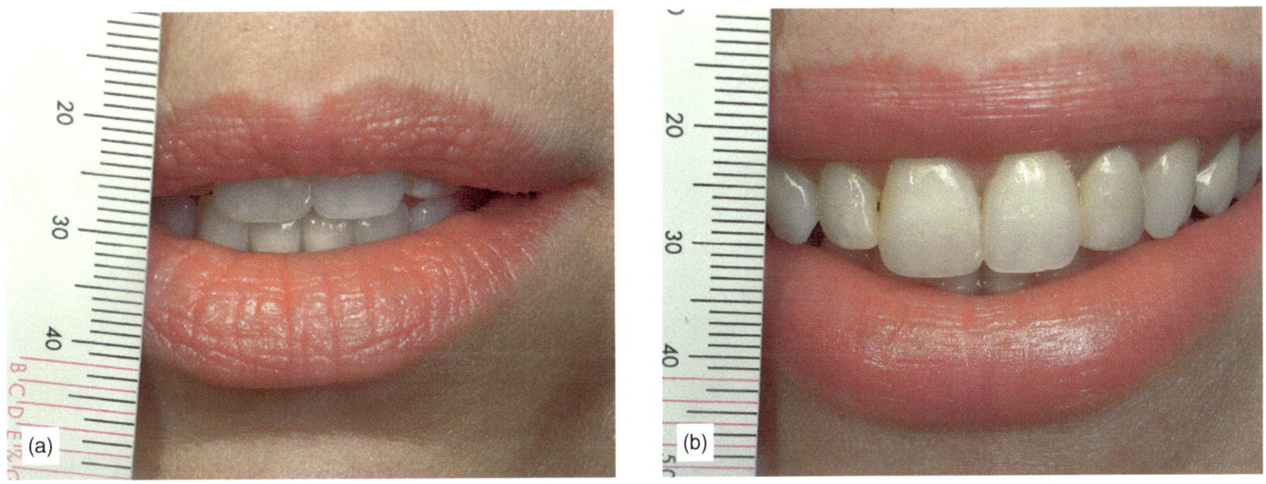

Figure 8.32 (a) Female repeating the number "66" for the conversational view. (b) Compare the amount of tooth shown when smiling.

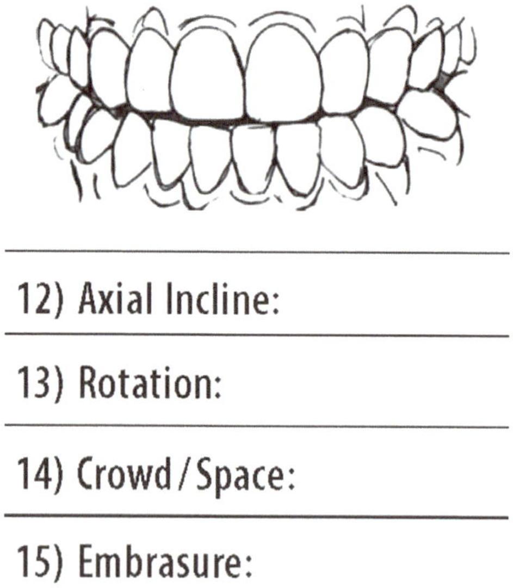

Figure 8.33 Close up of form with close retracted view.

be recorded by taking pictures while the patient repeats the number "66". In a similar way to the amount of tooth visible when smiling, the amount of conversational tooth show decreases with age.

12 Axial Inclination and Rotation (Front Retracted View)

The axial inclination (Figure 8.33) and rotation [21] are important parameters. They can easily make a smile look less attractive, and the patient should be involved in deciding whether restorative dentistry, preprosthetic orthodontic or orthodontic treatment may be the correct option to correct these discrepancies (Figure 8.34a–c).

13 Rotation of teeth

Rotation of the teeth is easy to spot, and a decision to correct with orthodontic procedures or by using restorative dentistry with all their benefits and consequences must be discussed with the patient.

14 Spacing/Crowding (Front Retracted View)

Often, spacing and crowding can be corrected with orthodontic therapy alone, while sometimes restorative correction can give fast results, and in some cases a combination of treatments may be required. Understanding the patient's goals, the timeline desired for results and their budget can help to make a final decision (Figures 8.35a,b, 8.36a–d).

15 Incisal Embrasures (Front Retracted View)

Incisal embrasures are the silhouette of the teeth and key to esthetic results. Evaluating what type of embrasures

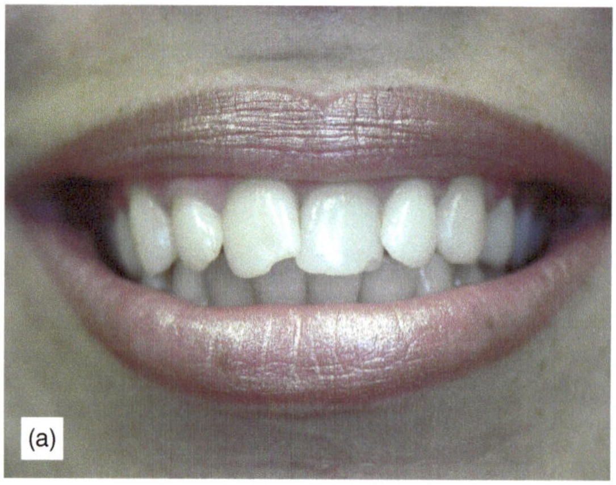

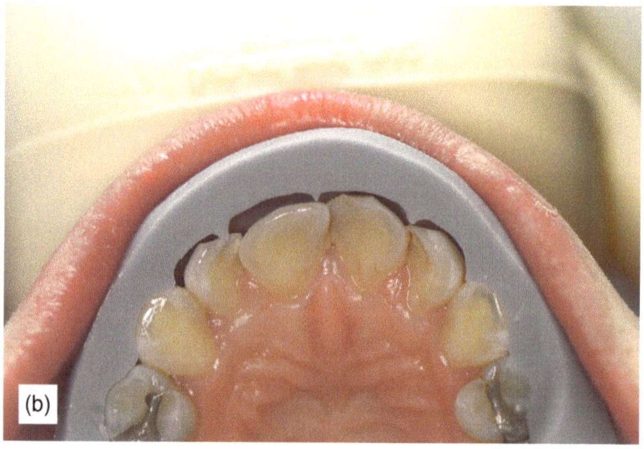

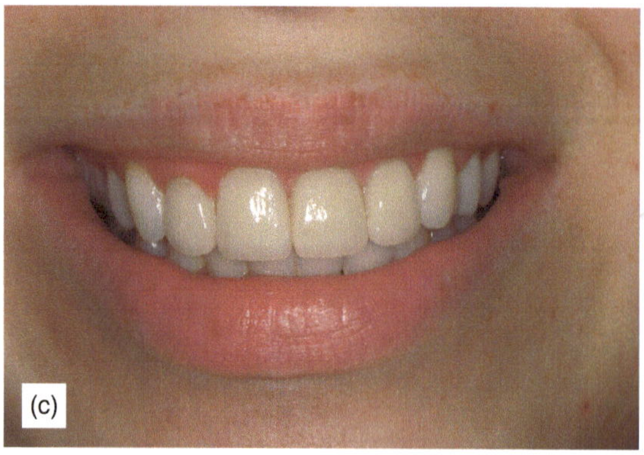

Figure 8.34 (a) Female patient with rotation and axial inclination problems who was unwilling to undergo orthodontics. (b) Using the silicon matrix to ensure separation in the correct area, to achieve correct tooth size. (c) Final result with four veneers.

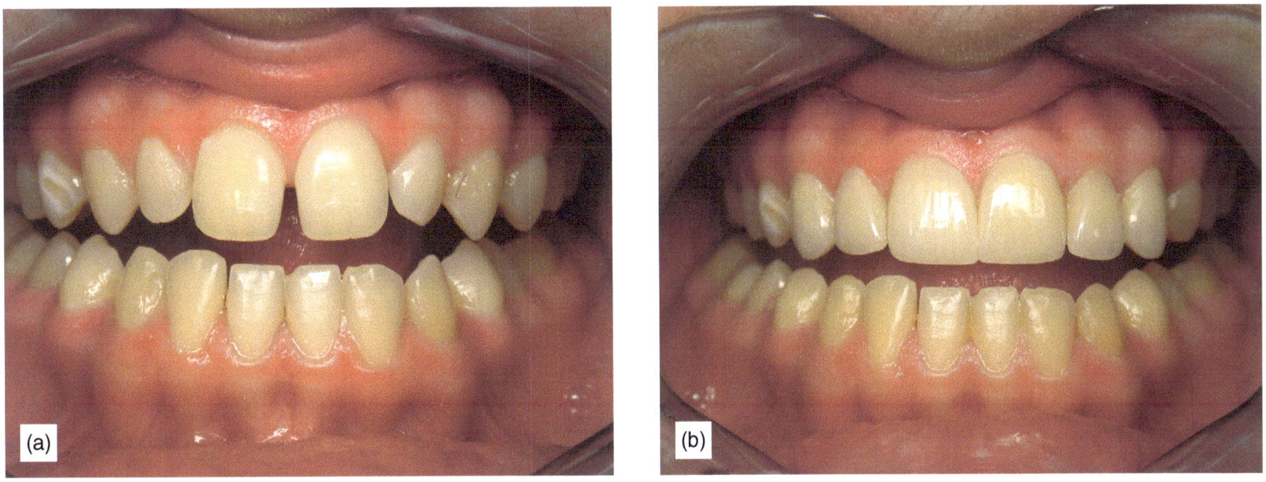

Figure 8.35 (a) Spacing was deemed to be possible without orthodontics. (b) Good results achieved with veneers only.

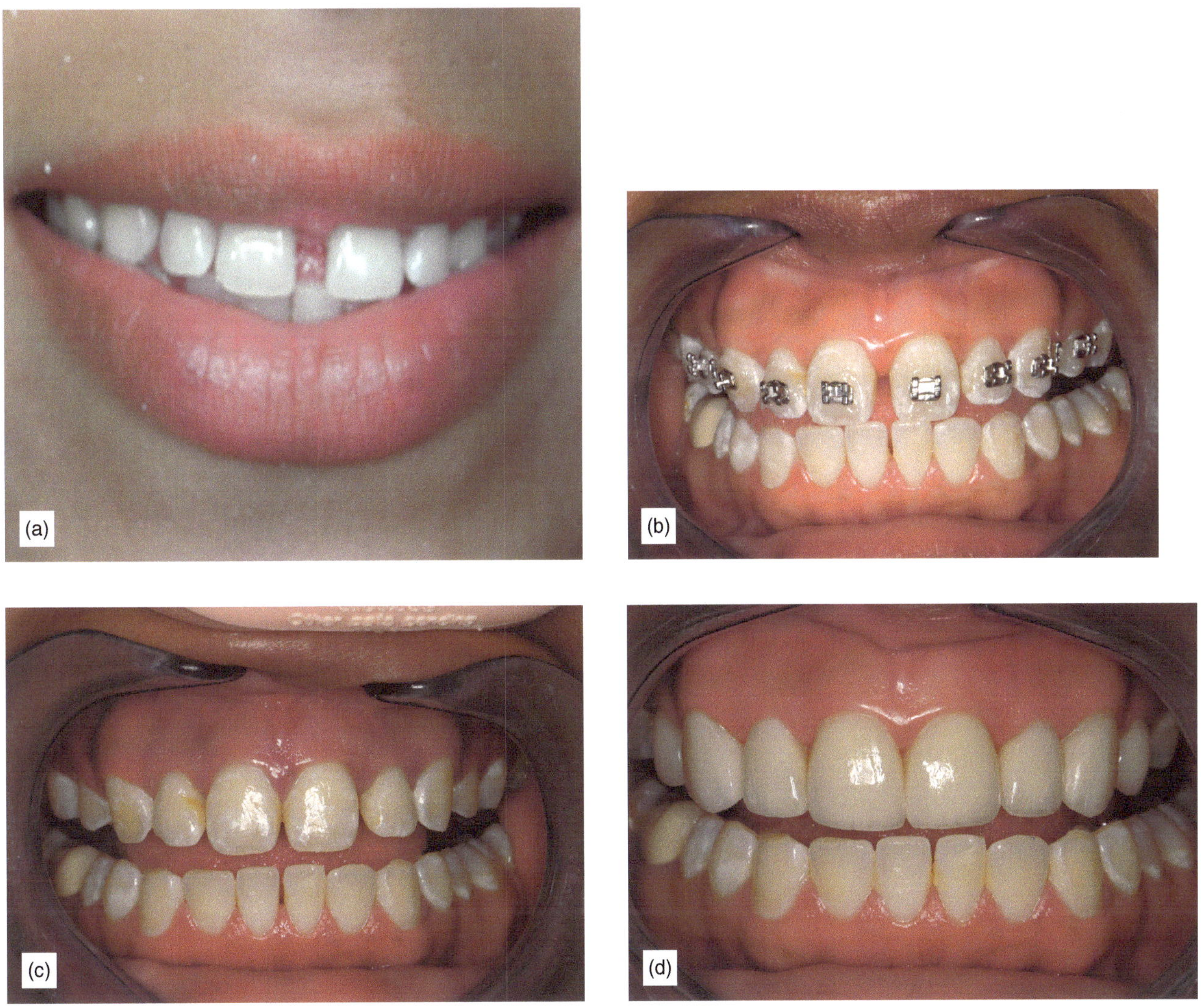

Figure 8.36 (a) Some cases should be treated with preprosthetic orthodontics to avoid ending up with asymmetries or excessively large centrals. (b) Preprosthetic orthodontics to improve spacing. (c) After bracket removal. (d) Postoperative view.

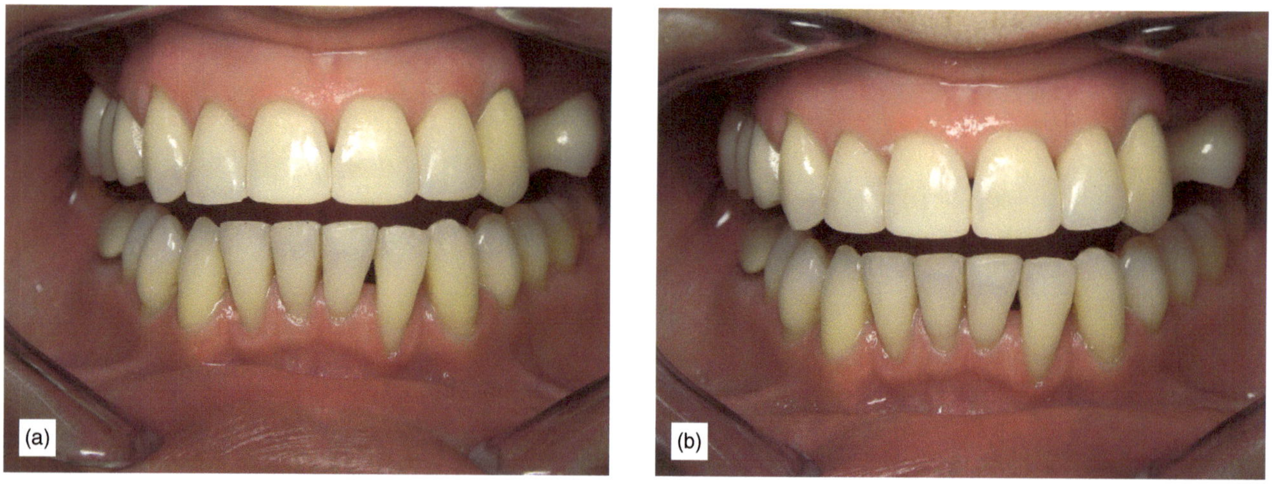

Figure 8.37 (a) Uneven incisal embrasures can create an undesirable esthetic appearance. (b) Minor enamel recontouring of the incisal edges and embrasures can have a very positive esthetic improvement.

currently exist and what type of final embrasures or shape of teeth the patient wishes to have will help to clarify the ultimate results. Using a smile book can be helpful to simplify the patient's selection (Figure 8.37a,b).

16 Maxillary Anterior Incisor Inclination (Smile Side View)

Maxillary incisors should have a slight forward inclination or proclination to the occlusal plane (Figure 8.38). Excessive proclination or retroclination is unesthetic, and if the patient finds it undesirable, treatment options including orthodontics must be discussed. Changes on inclination will alter the overjet and must be taken into consideration (Figures 8.39a–d, 8.40a,b).

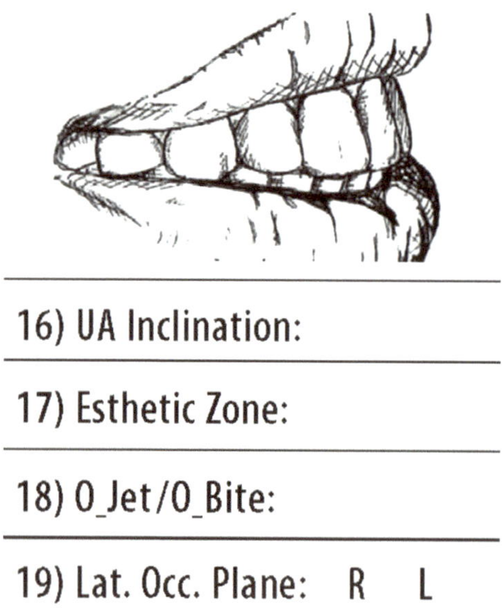

Figure 8.38 In both retracted and non-retracted lateral views, parameters 16–19 can be evaluated.

17 Esthetic Zone (Smile Side View)

Because patients usually only view themselves head on, the side photographic views are very revealing and valuable for diagnosis, often making the patient aware of unseen problems and sometimes requiring that restorations extend more distally (Figure 8.41).

18 Overjet and Overbite (Smile Side View and Retracted)

Overjet and overbite are important functional parameters (Figure 8.42a,b), which sometimes need to be altered to provide the necessary clearance for the envelope of function. It is interesting to realize that many patients think that the ideal position for the teeth is to be border to border, or with a minor overjet; they generally see overjet as undesirable. Education at this time is a must to avoid patient dissatisfaction (Figures 8.43, 8.44).

19 Occlusal Plane from the Lateral View (Smile Side View and Retracted)

It is important to evaluate the occlusal plane from the lateral view. Back teeth should be shorter than front; a reverse plane will have an unesthetic appearance and also has undesirable occlusal consequences (Figure 8.45a,b).

20 Papilla (Front Retracted View)

Papilla (Figure 8.46a,b), or lack of papilla, can lead to open gingival embrasures, which is a common patient complaint. Acknowledging and developing a treatment plan to correct missing papilla is important. Multiple options with variable results are available, and guided bone regeneration, orthodontic extrusion and

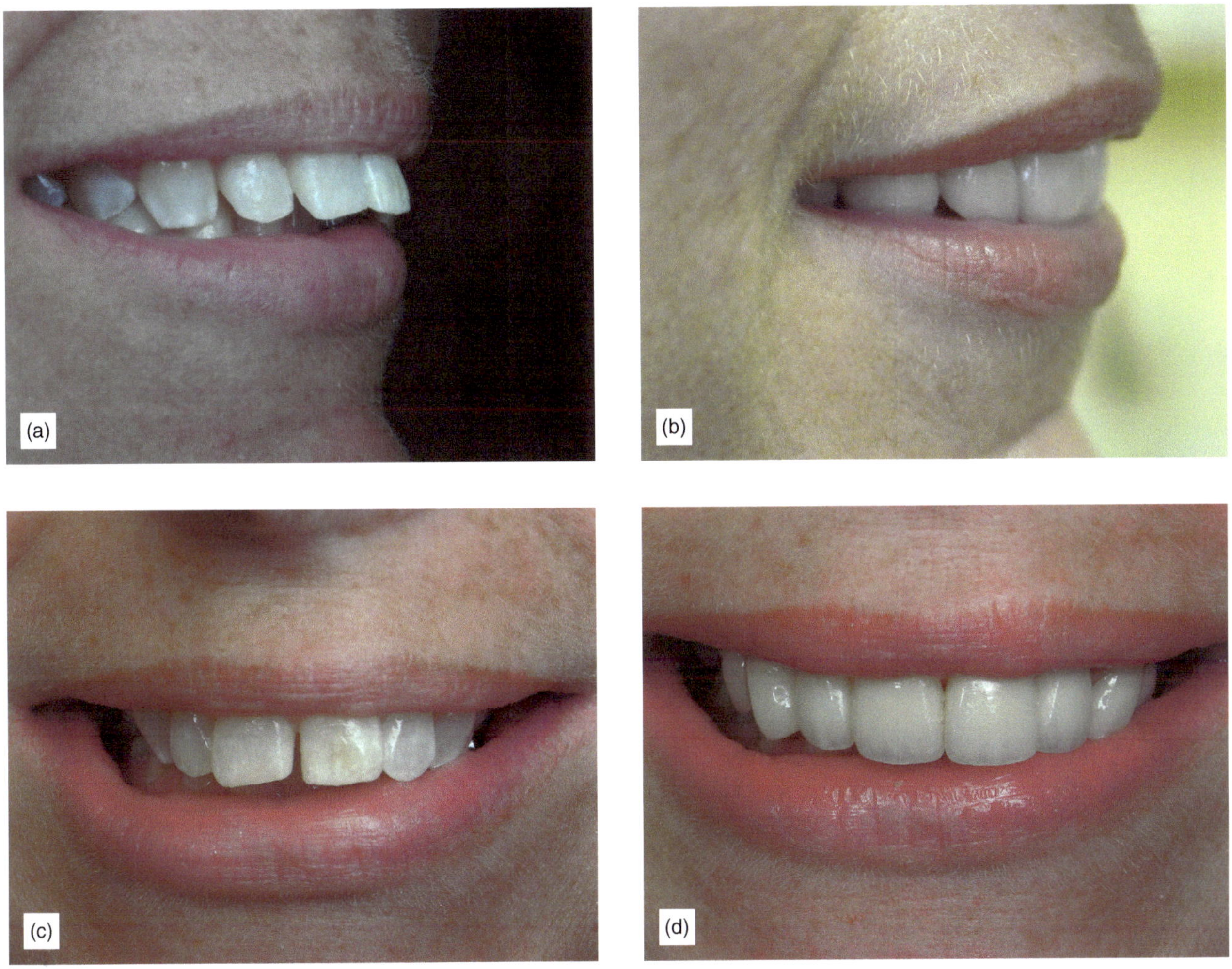

Figure 8.39 (a) Older case of female not wanting wires and brackets orthodontics, which was treated with aggressive tooth preparation for veneers to correct excessive proclination. (b) Final result, lateral view. (c) Front view. (d) Front view of finish veneers, with Invisalign® (Align Technology) or MTM® Clear Aligner (Dentsply) orthodontics. Aggressive preparation is less desirable and now less common.

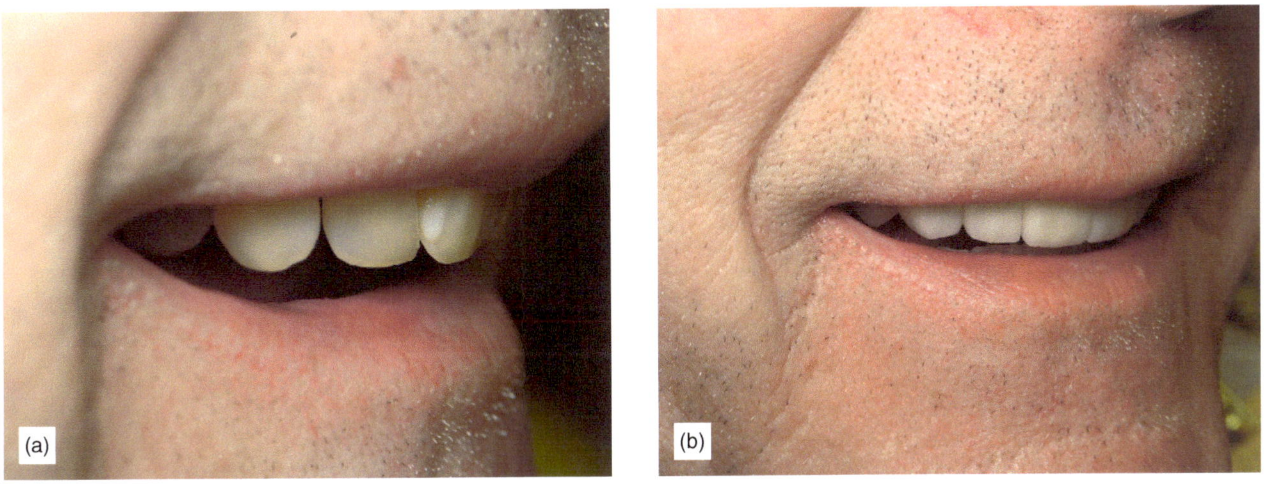

Figure 8.40 (a) Excessive retroclination of anterior teeth. (b) Improved retroclination and effect on lips.

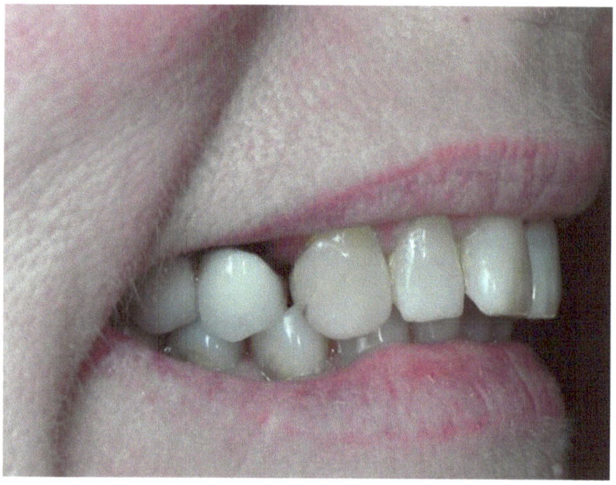

Figure 8.41 When the patient sees the side-view photographs, they usually see problems they do not see in the usual front mirror view.

restorative options should be discussed. If restorative closure of gingival embrasure is planned, the patient should be aware of the change in the shape of the tooth from a bell shape to a more square shape. Limitations and incomplete closure of the embrasure should also be discussed (Figure 8.47).

21 Gingival Symmetry (Front Retracted View)

Symmetry of the gingiva is of great esthetic importance when the entire tooth is visible. When the gingiva are visible and there are asymmetries, the patient should be made aware of it and asked if they would like improvement. Based on the severity and the patient's goals, periodontal correction can be included in the treatment plan.

22 Gingival Biotype (Front Retracted View)

Biotype is important when the esthetic plan includes extractions, implants or fixed partial dentures, or where gingival

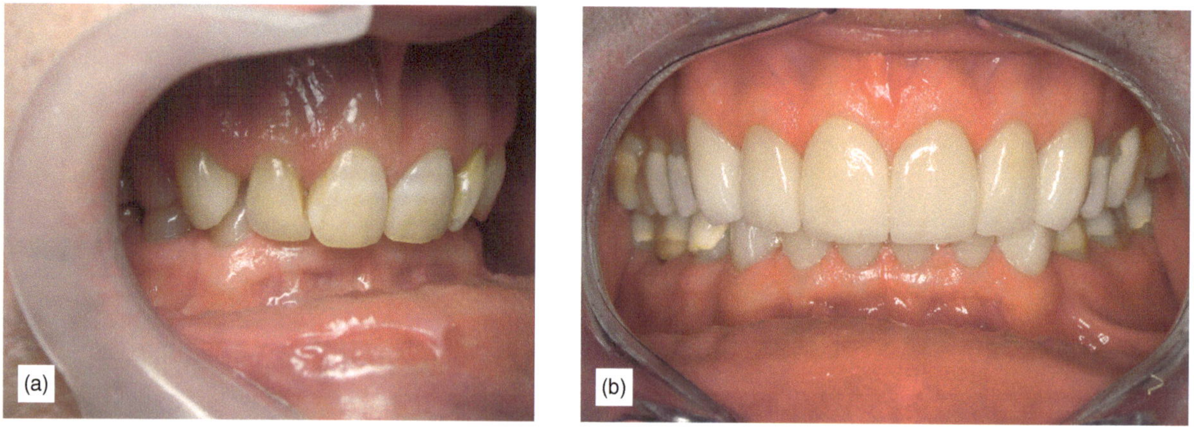

Figure 8.42 (a) 110% overbite and patient biting his palate. (b) After bite opening with bonded veneers and long-term onlay temporaries.

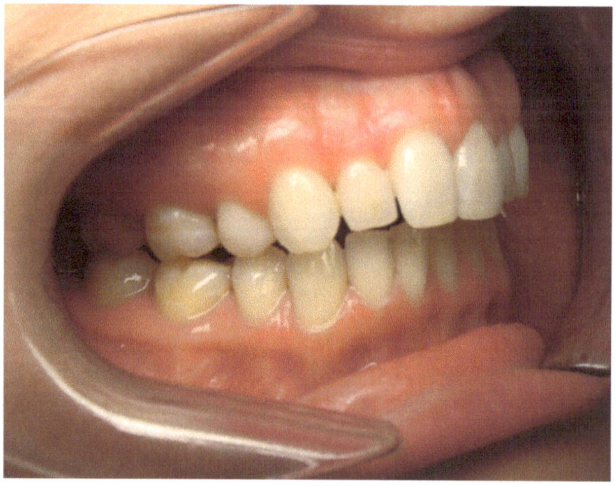

Figure 8.43 Excessive overjet.

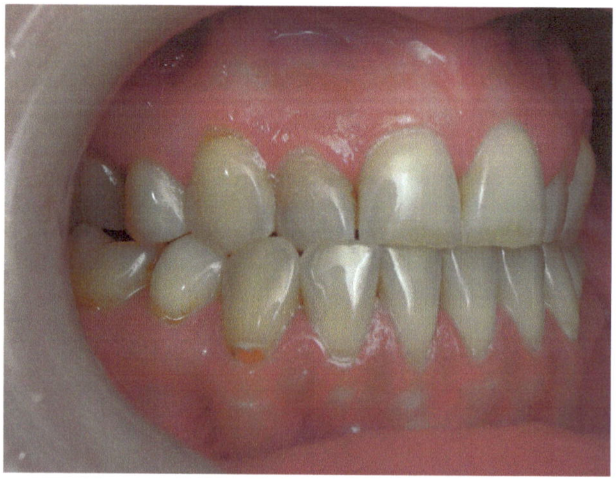

Figure 8.44 Insufficient overjet.

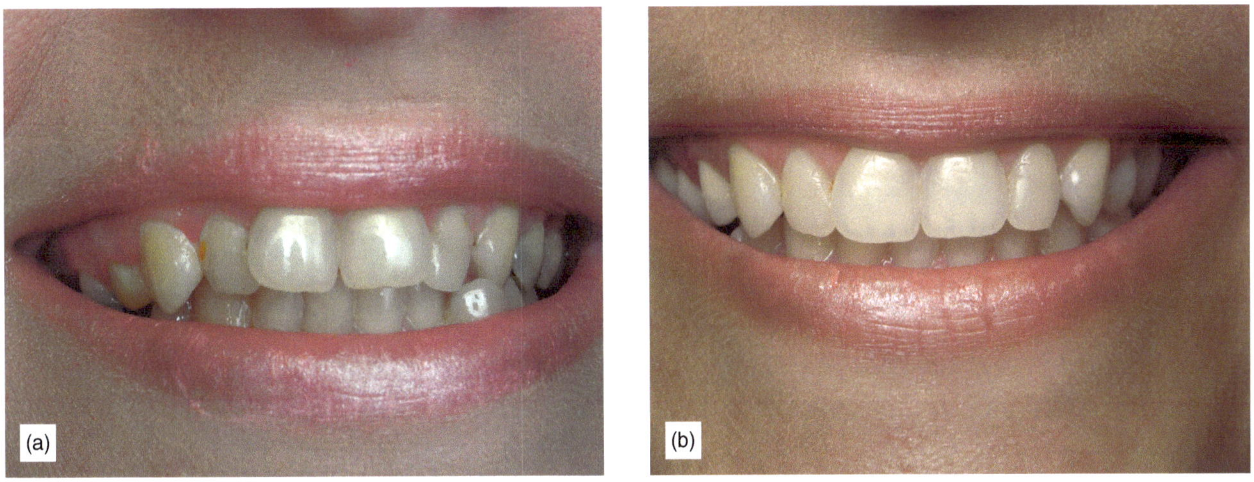

Figure 8.45 (a) Reversed plane, where the posterior teeth are longer than the anterior with a very unesthetic appearance. (b) Improved reverse plane with a combination of traditional orthodontics and some restorations.

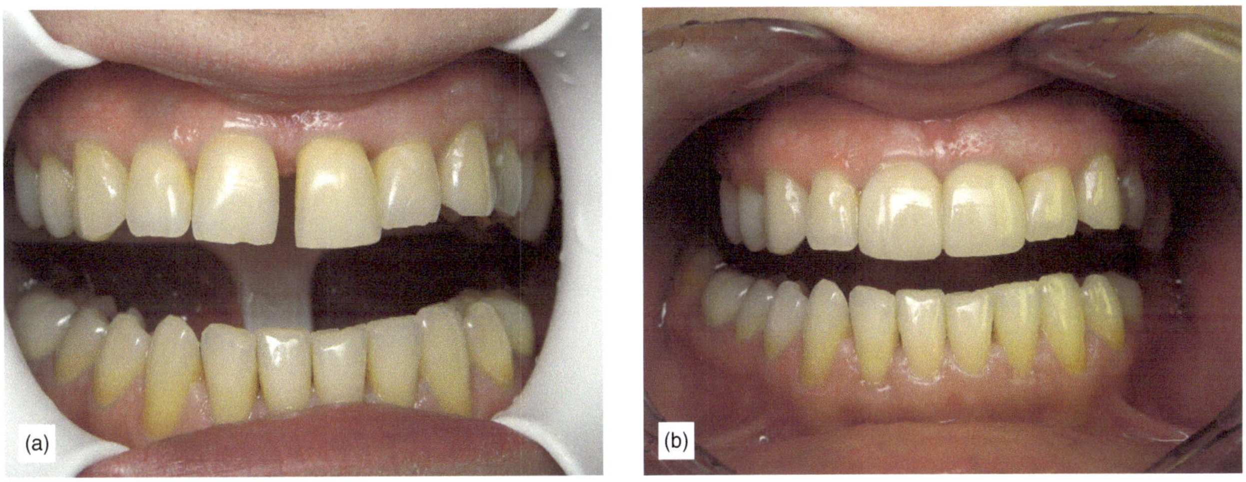

Figure 8.46 (a and b) Open gingival embrasures and large diastemas can be very challenging.

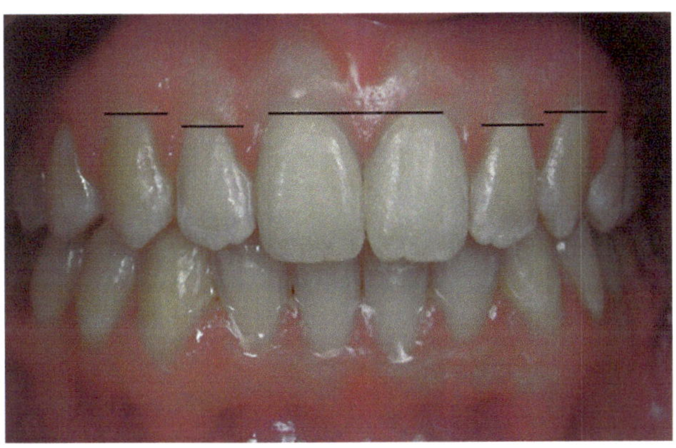

Figure 8.47 Gingival zenith of teeth has a great influence in esthetics.

line stability is important, as it is an important determinant of gingival recession and stability (Figure 8.48a,b).

23 Shade (Front Retracted View)

Many years in practice has shown me that the number one reason why patients end up unhappy after esthetic treatment is dissatisfaction with the shade of their teeth, and usually they wanted them to be whiter. A extremely effective and simple approach is to give the patient two primary options, with a third in special cases: "Natural White" or A1; "Hollywood White" or B1, with a third alternative for younger patients who may already have B1 and are looking for extra white results, "Extra White" or 1M1 – any whiter than this is usually artificial looking (Figures 8.49a,b, 8.50a,b).

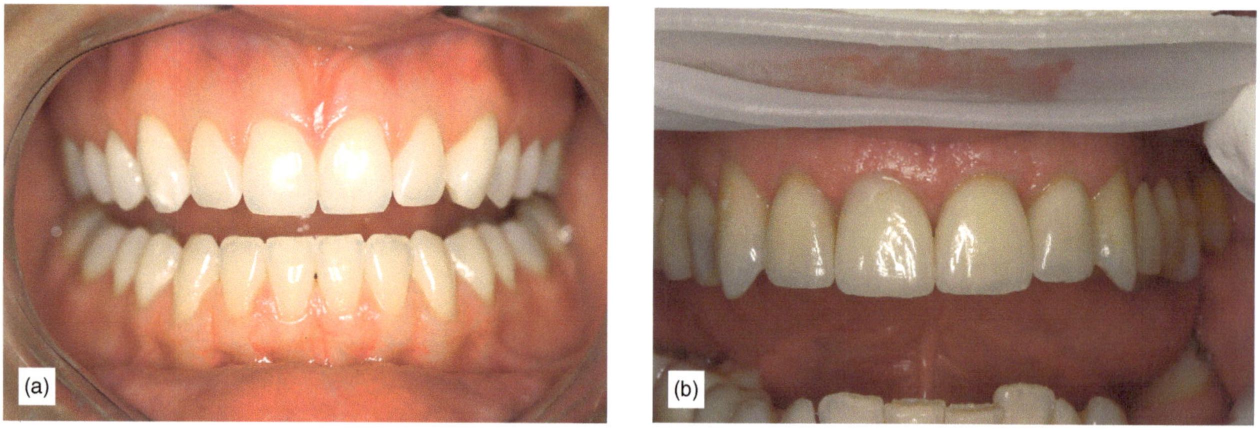

Figure 8.48 Biotype (a) Thin. (b) Thick.

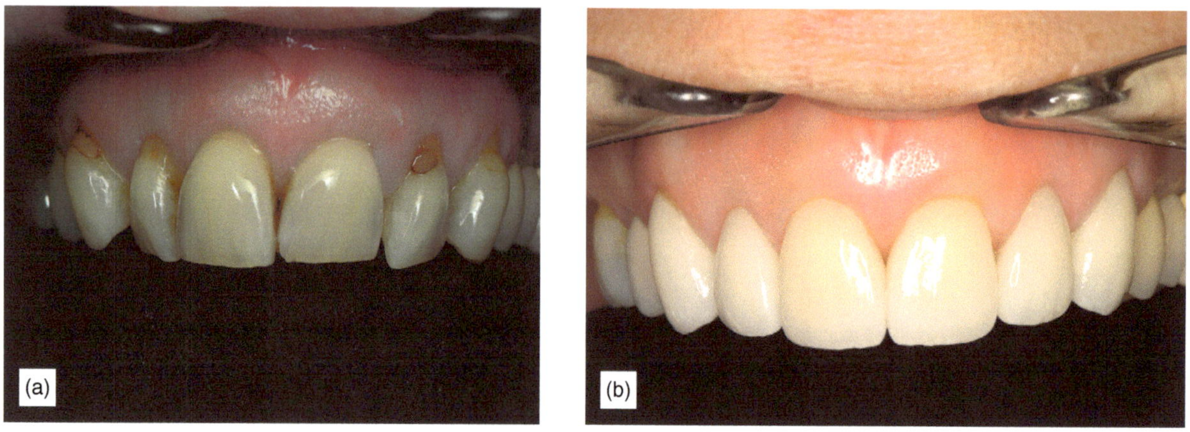

Figure 8.49 (a) Teeth dark and stained. (b) After bleaching and veneers.

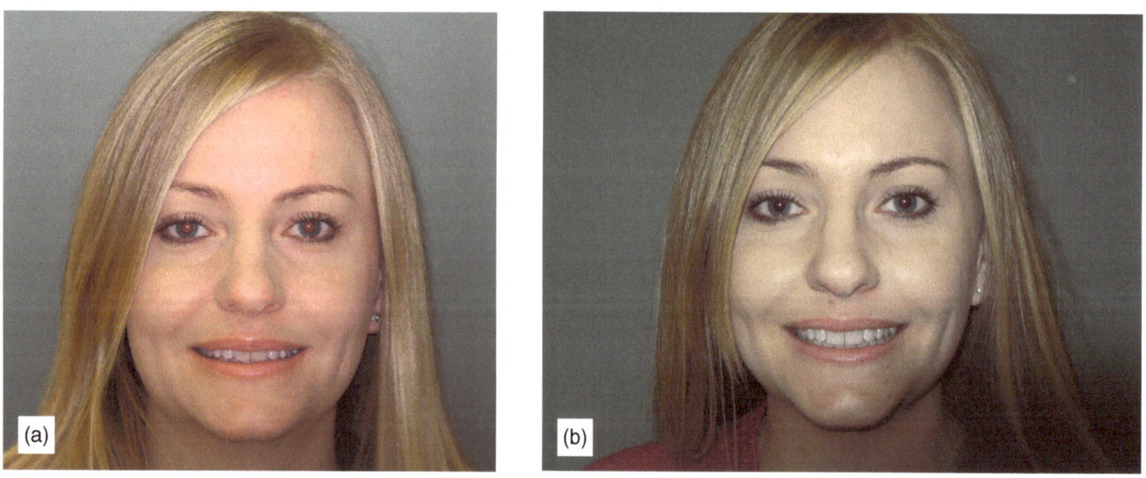

Figure 8.50 (a) Centrals are inset, which makes them appear darker. (b) After whitening and two central veneers.

24 Shape (Front Retracted View)

Tooth shape is not related to the shape of the face [22], but more related to patient's preference, gender and age. A simple way to determine the patient's preference is to use a smile design book, such as the LVI Smile Catalog or the Los Angeles Institute Smile Books.

25 Ratio (Front Retracted View)

Teeth look more symmetrical, and thus more beautiful if the correct ratio of height compared with width is present. This is important mostly when patients show the entire tooth and gum when smiling. Although this is subjective, the approximate

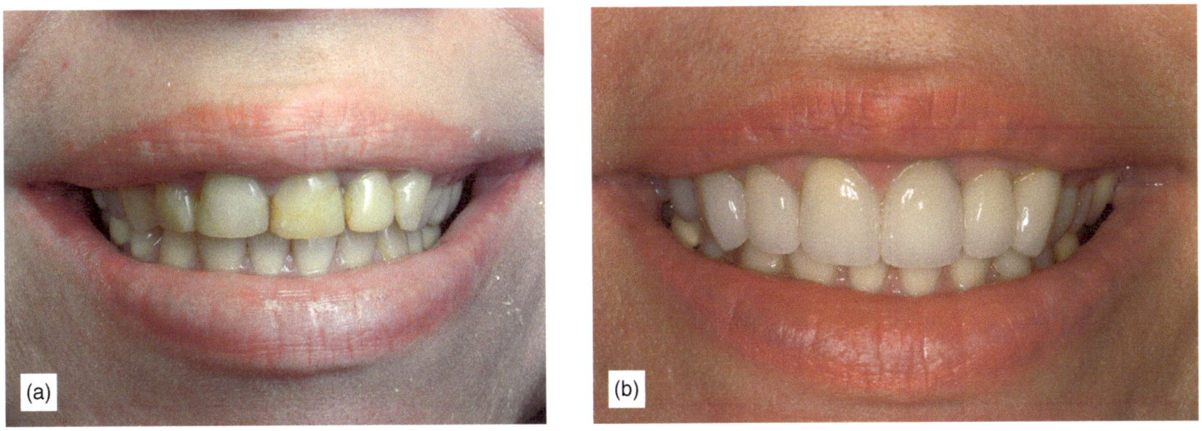

Figure 8.51 (a) The ratio of the teeth make them look square and anesthetic. (b) After some crown lengthening and veneers.

ratio is 100% height to approximately 80% width (Figure 8.51a,b).

Communication

Dentist and Patient

Much will be learned by both dentist and patient about the nature of their esthetic goals, available corrections, priorities for the patient, financial limitations and treatment limitations, during the few minutes that it takes to decide on a smile design with the patient. This will lead to a true esthetic co-diagnosis, and better patient satisfaction with the esthetic results. While it is important to involve the patient, it is also important to control this process, and not to over promise, especially with patients who are particular or may appear to have emotionally oriented goals. It is important to remind them that perfection is never the goal, to avoid creating unreasonable expectations, otherwise even beautiful results will be shadowed because there is always something that could be better.

Notes should be made on the form of the desired corrections and concerns of both patient and clinician (Figure 8.52). There is room at the top of the form for the patient's top priorities. The patient's main priorities must be addressed and every effort must be made to fulfill such priorities to the best of the clinician's ability. It is very important to talk about possible limitations to reaching such priorities, before the treatment starts.

Dentist And Laboratory Technician

Once the smile has been analyzed and the patient's preferences have been recorded, then the case can be sent to the laboratory for a "blue print" wax up. The cast sent to the laboratory should ideally be mounted using a facebow capable of providing information on the occlusal plane and midline. In addition, the cast provided should already be equilibrated (see Chapter 13) so when the wax-up is used to fabricate provisional veneers after equilibration, the fit will be more accurate. Communication between dentist and laboratory is as important as the communication between dentist and patient. The laboratory should be made aware of the decisions reached by the clinician based on the patient's desires related to length, shape, occlusal plane corrections, overjet changes, and so on. Good instructions on the laboratory slip will yield a good wax-up (Figure 8.53). It is always important to check the wax-up a few days before the preparation appointment to confirm that the laboratory has followed the instructions as desired. Sometimes misunderstanding may lead to a wax-up that is not a correct reproduction of what the clinician and patient wanted, and this will have an important influence

Figure 8.52 It is important to list the patient's primary esthetic goals on the form.

Patient Name: Date:

PATIENT'S MAIN CONCERNS

1.

2.

3.

4.

Pt. Esthetic Expectations:

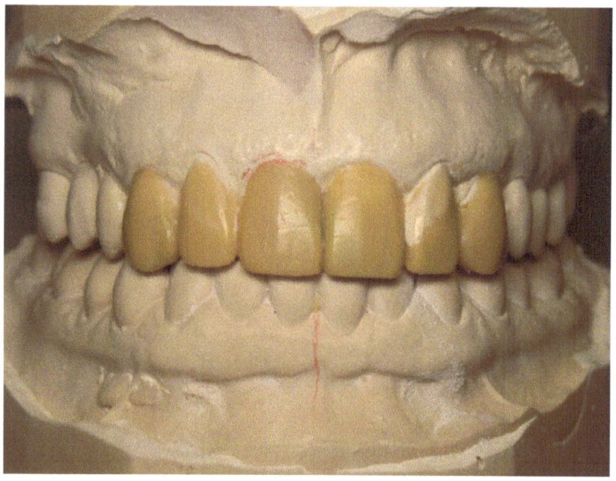

Figure 8.53 Nice wax-up.

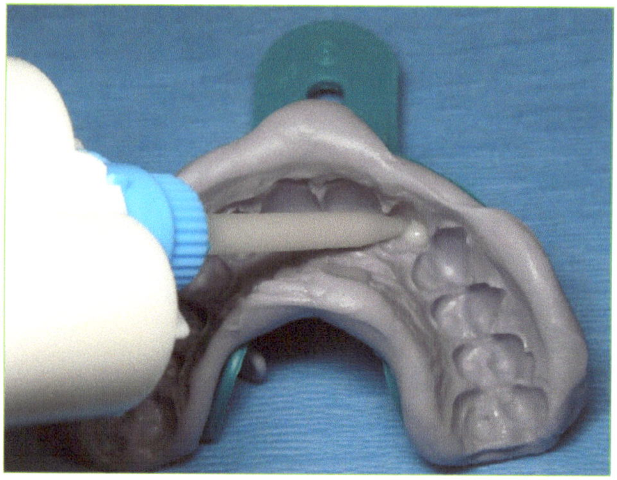

Figure 8.54 Matrix with midline marked and filled with bis-acryl composite material.

on the future of the rehabilitation, so a few minutes of checking is time well spent. If the wax-up is not ideal, it should be sent back for correction.

Making Provisional Restorations (Prototypes)

A silicone putty material such as Panasil (Kettenbach), should be used to fabricate two silicon matrices from the final wax-up. One should be used as a preparation guide and the other to fabricate prototype provisional restorations. The provisional should be made of a good quality bis-acryl composite material of the correct shade, such as Vysalis® (Kettenbach) or Structure 3 (VOCO). There are two ways to fabricate such provisionals using the putty matrix. One is to allow them to fully set in the mouth, polymerization shrinkage will help to retain the provisional. A second and more desirable way is to remove the provisional before full polymerization and trim outside the mouth, then clean and cement. This allows for better cleaning of the provisional material around the gums and usually yields better tissue health for cementation.

Steps for a Chairside Cemented Provisional

Step 1: Make sure the matrix extends at least three or four teeth past the ones being worked on, this will allow for enhanced indexing. Also check for a correct fit in the mouth.

Step 2: Mark the midline on the matrix with a pen, to allow for easy indexing (Figure 8.54).

Step 3: Fill matrix with bis-acryl composite material, making sure that no air bubbles are trapped. Always extrude a pea-sized amount, as the first material coming from an automix tip is usually not correctly mixed.

Step 4: Seat the matrix on the teeth using the midline as a guide. Avoid pressing the matrix on the prepared tooth area, as this could cause air bubbles. Gently hold it in place.

Step 5: Timing is important. When the material starts to get hard but still has some flexibility, after about 1 minute, this is the time to remove matrix from the mouth.

Step 6: Quickly remove any lingual excess to avoid having this interfere in the removal. Gently tease the provisionals off the teeth, using a sickle. It is desirable to take all the provisionals together, but if they break, it is easy to repair.

Step 7: Once the provisional is removed from the mouth, clean the teeth of the excess using gauze and re-seat the provisional, to avoid shrinkage occurring outside the mouth.

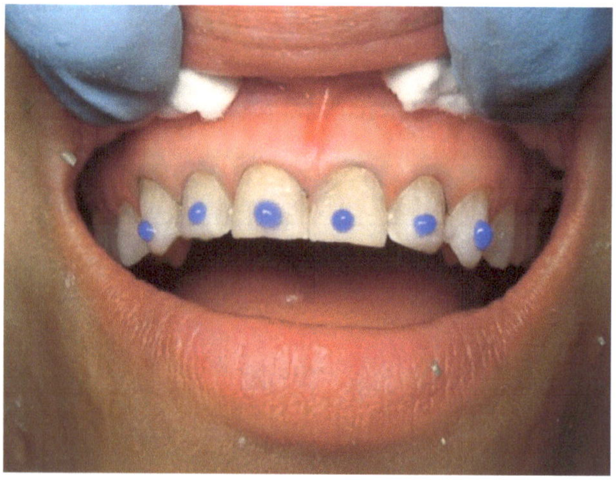

Figure 8.55 Spot etch and bond.

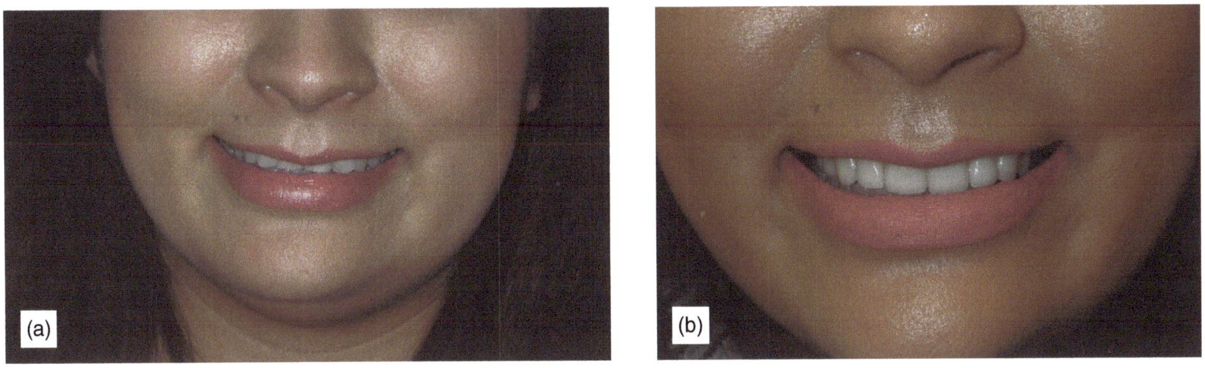

Figure 8.56 (a,b) Side by side photographs at the esthetic check visit.

Step 8: Wait 4 minutes for final polymerization and shrinkage. This is the perfect time to do all the repairs necessary with flowable composite. There is no need to apply a bonding system; these materials are compatible and will bond automatically.

Step 9: When it is evident that there is no retention or embrasures where the cement can lock in, it is desirable to spot etch and bond. Always place the spot etch and bond on the same location, so it is easy to identify and remove with the bur (Figure 8.55).

Step 10: Trim and cement with any resin temporary cement.

Step 11: Clean the cement, and adjust the bite. Make any corrections necessary to length, bulk, and so on.

Step 12: Educate the patient and the family that it is normal to feel that they look strange at first, and perhaps too long, because it is different than usual. Speech will be affected and it will take a few days to regain the full ability to pronounce certain words. All this will pass and the patient will adapt [19].

Esthetic and Bite Check

The provisional restoration will give the patient a chance to "test-drive" their new smile and changes to their bite. The one-week esthetic check appointment has the purpose of allowing the patient and dentist to go over what is liked, disliked, and desired to be changed before final restorations are fabricated. In this appointment, the assistant will take new photographs of the full face, smiling and close up, front, and sides. The photographs should be put side by side with the preoperative photos to have a real assessment of goals achieved (Figure 8.56a,b). Usually the patient will be satisfied with the improved smile. If there is a need to make corrections (shortening, lengthening, trimming, bulking, etc.), these should be made on the provisionals. If many corrections need to be made, it would be desirable to make a new esthetic check appointment for a week's time. The same corrections should be made relating to the bite. Once the provisional restoration is approved by the patient, an alginate impression of the provisional can be sent to the laboratory and they can be instructed to use the approved provisional cast as a guide to fabricate the final restoration (Figure 8.57).

Dentists who communicate their commitment to their patients, their esthetic goals, and overall oral health will undoubtedly increase treatment acceptance and patient satisfaction. When a systematic process such as the dentofacial esthetic diagnosis system is implemented, dentists obtain predictable results that make for happy, good-looking patients.

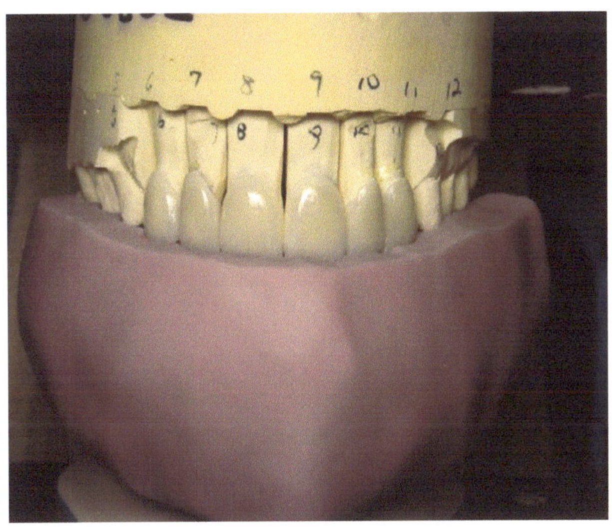

Figure 8.57 Silicon matrix used by a laboratory to replicate approved provisional restorations.

References

1 Ruiz JL. Achieving optimal esthetics on a patient with severe trauma: using a multidisciplinary approach and an all-ceramic fixed partial denture. *J Esthet Restor Dent*, 2005; 17: 285–292.
2 Ruiz JL. The psychology of a smile. *J Cosmetic Dent*, 2003; 19: 58–59.
3 Coffield KD, Phillips C, Brady M, Roberts MW, Strauss RP, Wright JT. The psychosocial impact of developmental dental defects in people with hereditary amelogenesis imperfecta. *J Am Dent Assoc*, 2005; 136(5): 620–630.
4 Morley J, Eubank J. Macroesthetic elements of smile design. *J Am Dent Assoc*, 2001; 132: 39–45.
5 Morr T. Understanding the esthetic evaluation for success. *J Calif Dent Assoc*, 2004; 32: 153–160.
6 Frese C, Staehle HJ, Wolff D. The assessment of dentofacial esthetics in restorative dentistry: A review of the literature. *J Am Dent Assoc*, 2012; 143(5): 461–466.
7 Atiyeh BS, Hayek SN. Numeric expression of aesthetics and beauty. *Aesthetic Plast Surg*, 2008; 32(2): 209–219.
8 Ricketts RM. The biologic significance of the divine proportion and Fibonacci series. *Am J Orthod*, 1982; 81: 351–370.
9 Ruiz JL. A systematic approach to dento-facial smile evaluation using digital photography and a new photographic view. *Dent Today*, 2006; 25: 82–86.
10 Ruiz JL. Achieving predictable, beautiful smiles using a dento-facial esthetic diagnosis system. *Compend Contin Educ Dent*, 2007; 28(1): 50–55.
11 Lee RL. Standardized head position and reference planes for dento-facial aesthetics. *Dent Today*, 2000; 19(2): 82–87.
12 Spear FM, Kokich VG, Matthews DP. Interdisciplinary management of anterior dental esthetics. *J Am Dent Assoc*, 2006; 137(2): 160–169.
13 Jacobsen A. *Radiographic Cephalometry: From Basics to 3-D Imaging*, 2nd ed. Hanover Park, IL: Quintessence Publishing, 1995, p. 239.
14 Ricketts RM. A foundation for cephalometric communication. *Am J Orthodont*, 1960; 46: 330–357.
15 Mack MR. Facially generated occlusal vertical dimension. *Compend Contin Educ Dent*, 1997; 18(12): 1183–1190.
16 Kois JC. Occlusal vertical dimension: Alteration concerns. *Compend Contin Educ Dent*, 1997; 18(12): 1169–1177.
17 McLaren EA, Rifkin R. Macroesthetics: Facial and dentofacial analysis. *J Calif Dent Assoc*, 2002; 30(11): 839–846.
18 Ricketts RM. The golden divider. *J Clin Orthod*, 1981; 15(11); 152–159.
19 Rivera-Morales WC, Goldman BM. Are speech-based techniques for determining OVD reliable? *Compend Contin Educ Dent*, 1997; 18(12): 1214–1215, 1219–1223.
20 Vig RG, Brundo GC. Kinetics of anterior tooth display. *J Prosthet Dent*, 1978; 39(5): 502–504.
21 Spear FM. The esthetic correction of anterior dental mal-alignment conventional vs. instant (restorative) orthodontics. *J Calif Dent Assoc*, 2004; 32(2): 133–141.
22 Wolfart S, Menzel H, Kern M. Inability to relate tooth forms to face shape and gender. *Eur J Oral Sci*, 2004; 112(6): 471–476.

Part IV

Bonded Cementation of Indirect Restorations

9

Bonded Cementation of Veneers and Onlays

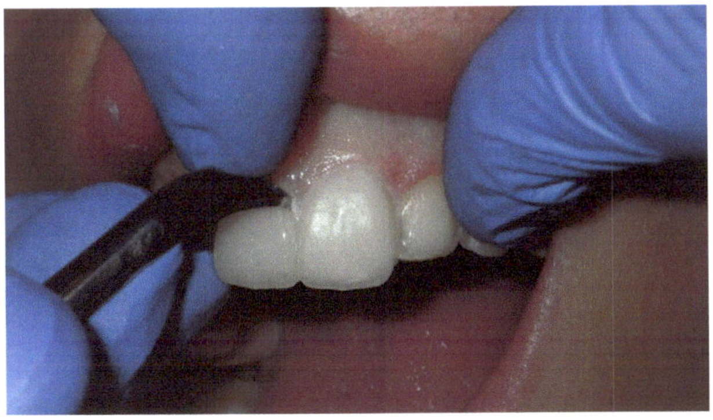

The proper technique during resin cement removal will ensure simplicity and safety, and improve margins.

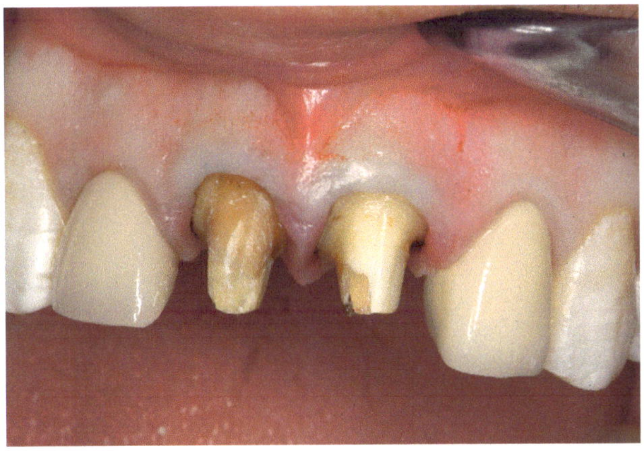

Figure 9.1 Crown being cemented with resin-modified glass ionomer cement (Meron Plus AC (VOCO)); note the amount of tooth removed and subgingival margins.

Cementing Bonded Restorations

Bonded cementation is a crucial step in ensuring correct retention and marginal seal of bonded restorations. It is the bonded cementation of indirect onlays or veneers that tends to greatly concern and sometimes dissuade clinicians from embracing this newer technique. The fact that traditional crowns and bridges can be cemented very successfully with traditional crown and bridge cements such as resin-reinforced glass ionomer cements, which are easy to use and rarely cause sensitivity [1,2,3], can be a reason why many people prefer a full crown procedure. They see those familiar procedures as easier. Nevertheless, the price paid by the tooth and the gingiva for this apparent simplicity at cementation may be too high (Figure 9.1).

It is easy to understand why some clinicians stay away from bonded restorations. First, postoperative sensitivity continues to irritate dentists and patients after the bonded cementation of indirect bonded restorations [4,5]. Second, the importance and complexity of isolation can be challenging. Some educators suggest, without good literature support, that unless a rubber dam is used, the adhesive procedure will not succeed or will be of inferior quality. Such statements can easily make many clinicians shy away from adhesive procedures. According to Christensen, less than 10% of restorative dentists use a rubber dam routinely [6]. Third, resin cementation is perceived to be a very sensitive and difficult technique, especially the removal of resin cement, because once it acquires its full hardness, removal of any excess can be very difficult. Additionally, previous failures may also be clear in some clinician's minds, which may prevent them from adopting these newer techniques. These concerns can easily be overcome with some additional training. It is important to remember that proper preparation will lead to a much easier cementation. Aggressive preparations with a great deal of dentin exposure and subgingival margin placement will make the cementation procedure very difficult. The implementation of a supragingival protocol can greatly simplify this process, as can choosing the appropriate materials correctly (Figure 9.2a–d).

Supra-Gingival Minimally Invasive Dentistry: A Healthier Approach to Esthetic Restorations, First Edition. By Jose-Luis Ruiz.

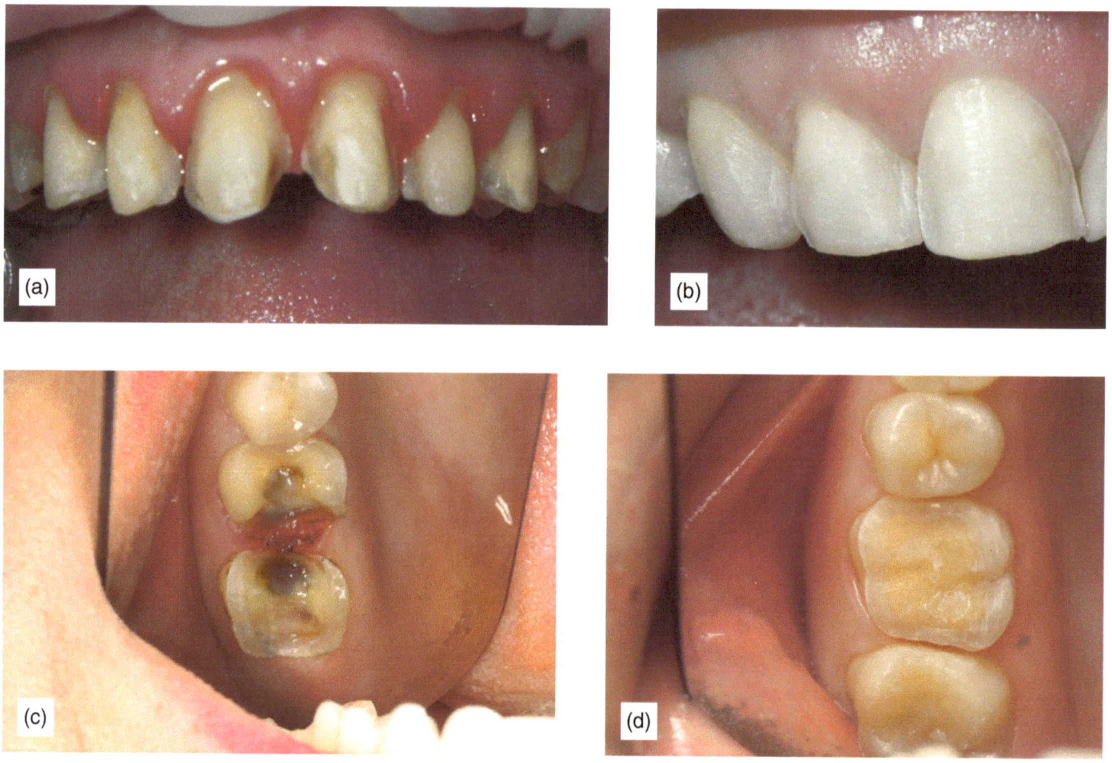

Figure 9.2 (a and b) These images depict how much easier and predictable the isolation is when margins are supragingival compared with bleeding subgingival margins for anterior porcelain veneers. (c and d) These images depict how much easier and predictable the isolation is when margins are supragingival compared with bleeding subgingival margins for bonded onlays.

Postoperative Sensitivity

Postoperative sensitivity after the cementation of bonded onlays and veneers is well documented [7,8]. One important reason for this sensitivity is the incorrect use of geometric preparation with mechanical retention, which can prevent full seating of the restoration, owing to the film thickness of the adhesive cement. Polymerization and contraction of the cement will continue after maximum seating and will form internal gaps, leading to bite pressure sensitivity if the dentinal tubules are not perfectly sealed (Figure 9.3). Nevertheless, supragingival minimally invasive preparation techniques, combined with correct bonded cementation techniques can virtually eliminate the problem of postoperative pain. Occlusal adjustment is also a contributory factor in postoperative sensitivity and is discussed in this chapter.

Isolation

Excellent isolation during bonded cementation is a must, as any contamination can lead to failure. This may lead some to suggest that unless a rubber dam is used, failures will occur. This is not supported by the literature or through clinical experience. Experience and the literature attest equal results with or without a rubber dam [9,10,11]. Correct preparation, choice of adhesive

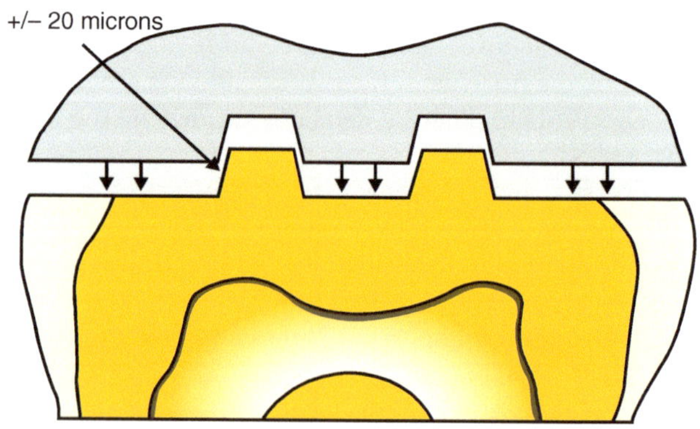

Figure 9.3 Resin cement film thickness plays an important role when the onlay preparation is geometric and has retention form, as it will prevent full seating and will increase the effects of polymerization shrinkage (courtesy of Dr Raymond L. Bertolotti).

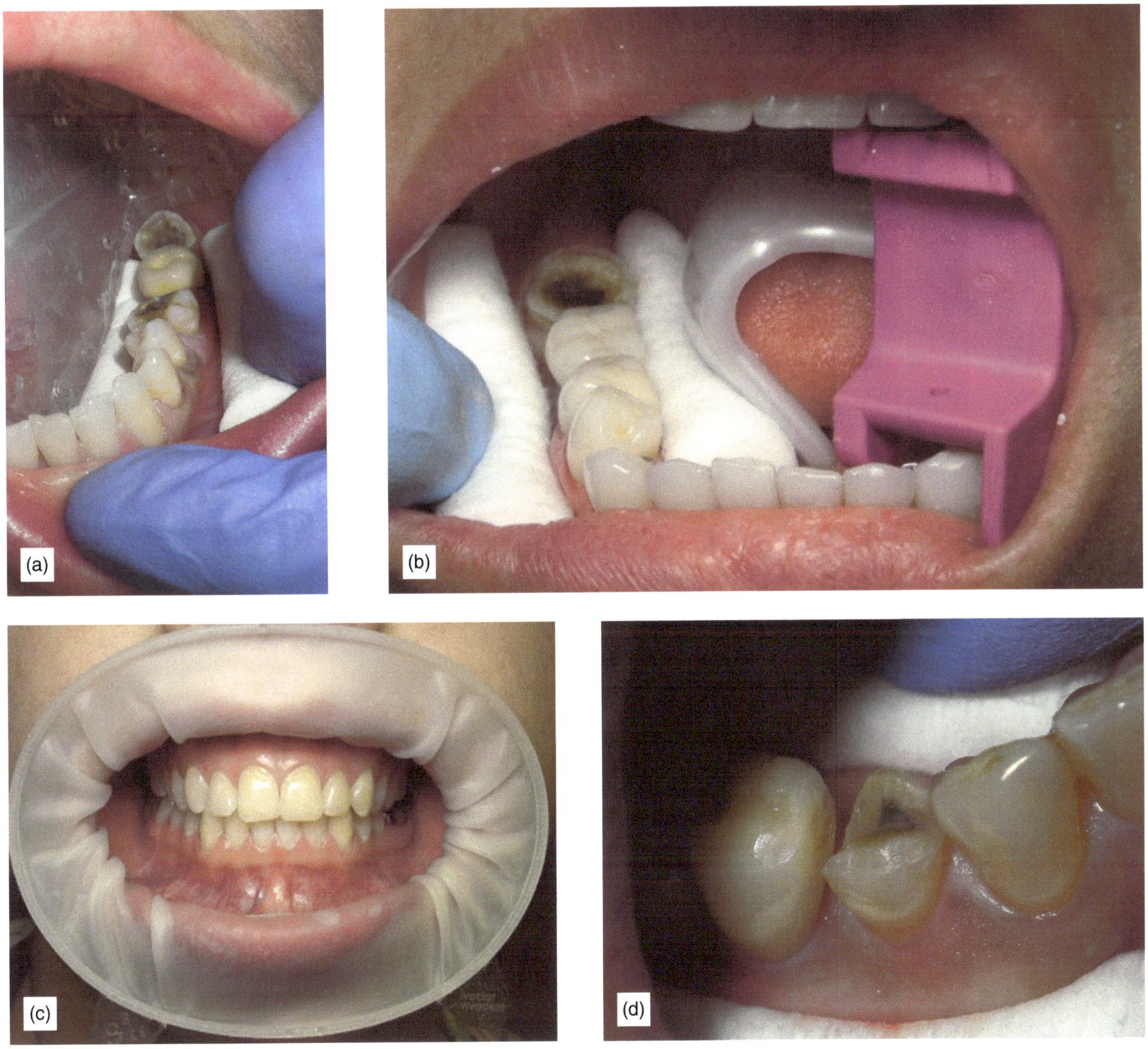

Figure 9.4 (a) DryShield® isolation system. (b) Mouth prop (Propgard®, Ultradent). (c) OptraGate® (Ivoclar). (d) Cotton roll isolation. (*Continued*)

[12,13] and technique can play a key role in simplifying isolation. The implementation of a supragingival protocol during preparation makes cementation easier. The choice of self-etch bonding systems is of great importance because the acidic monomer of this system is designed to work in multiple levels of moisture on the teeth, making the use of an oral humidity controller (rubber dam) unnecessary [14]. A number of simple devices for isolation are available and can be used during bonded cementation, including traditional cotton roll isolation (Figure 9.4a–e). Adhesive cementation requires excellent isolation.

Bonded Cementation has Multiple Layers

It must be remembered that when bonding an indirect restoration there will always be two substrates being bonded together by a resin cement and an adhesive, so there are multiple layers that require great attention (Figure 9.4a–e). The correct choice of adhesive and cement is of great importance. The two substrates or surfaces that are being joined together, the tooth surface (enamel and/or dentin) and the restoration surface or intaglio surface must be prepared prior to bonded cementation.

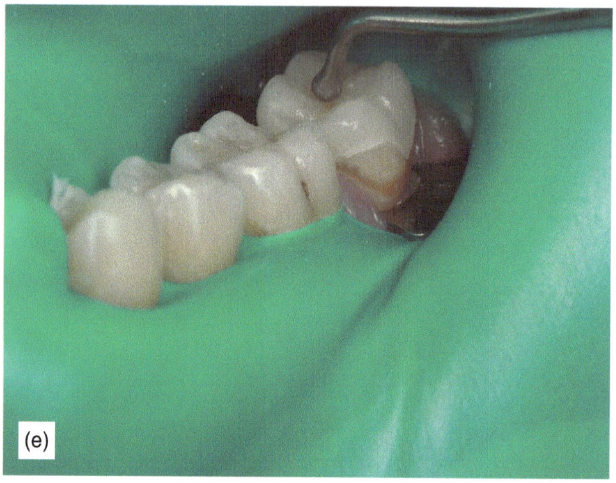

Figure 9.4 (*Continued*)
(e) Rubber dam isolation on a second molar, showing the imperfect nature of any system.

Choosing the Correct Resin Cement

Resin cements have characteristics which make them the ideal type of cement for bonded indirect restorations, like high tensile strength, high compressive strength, low modulus of elasticity and low solubility [15,16]. The use of these strong adhesive resin cements in fact enhances the strength of composite, feldspathic porcelain and lithium disilicate restorations [17], although they have minimal effect on zirconia and alumina. There are a number of different types of resin cements, each with their own advantages and disadvantages. Depending on the type of activator used for polymerization, the resin cements can be categorized as chemically (self) cured, light-cured and dual-cured. Most resin cements do not adhere to the tooth without the help of a dental adhesive or bonding system, with the exception of the self-adhesive type cements.

There are many other important differences between resin cements, including filler particle size (which affects the ability to polish the tooth), available colors, opacity, consistency, speed of curing [18]. A crucial characteristic of a resin cement required for the implementation of supragingival dentistry is optimal translucency, as rule 5 requires the proper use of translucency to achieve a good supragingival restorative margin blending, and the cement is one of the three components of this rule [19]. Attention must be paid to avoiding the use of opacious cements, which will decrease the translucency of the restorative material of choice, and will force the need to hide the margins subgingivally (Figure 9.5a–c). Finally, choosing a cement with excellent chameleon characteristics, the ability to blend with other colors and absorbing them is very desirable, as it simplifies the choice of cement shade.

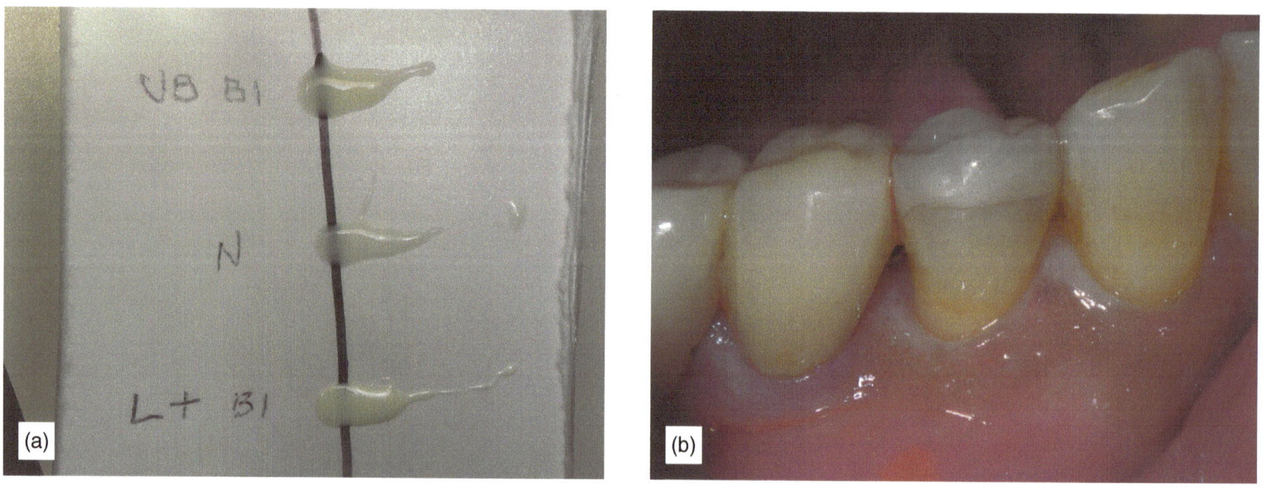

Figure 9.5 (a) Three drops of opacious, medium and translucent cements, showing different effects covering a line. (b) Without cement, the restoration lacks a visual connection with tooth. (*Continued*)

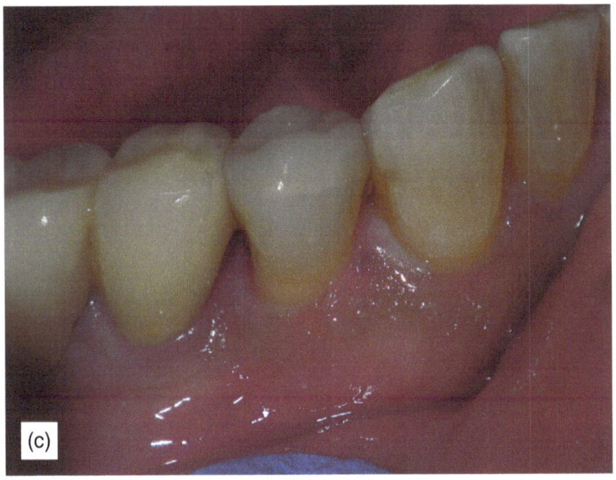

Figure 9.5 *(Continued)*
(c) Translucent cement (Clearfil™ Esthetic Cement, Kuraray) showing improved visual connection.

The Ideal Cement for Bonded Onlays

The first important consideration when choosing a resin cement is whether it will be light-curing, self-curing or dual-curing. Full self-curing cements are more hydrophilic, less color stable and harder to use because, after the restoration is fully seated, the clinician has to wait until the cement has set. This may compromise isolation, as the longer that isolation needs to be maintained the more difficult it is. The fact that onlays can vary in thickness anywhere from 2 mm to 5 mm (Figure 9.6) clearly makes light-cured cements unpredictable. Research has shown that an insufficient amount of light may reach the cement in thicker and darker restorations and may adversely affect the degree of conversion [20,21]. With light-cured cements it becomes worrisome, as there may be some parts of the cement under the onlay that will not cure correctly or fully. Some clinicians suggest warming the restorative composite regularly. This is impractical in a busy practice, as composite has to be warmed in advance to make it less thick. Additionally, the rigidity of a traditional resin cement may be undesirable for cementation, due to polymerization shrinkage.

For all of the above reasons, dual-cure resin cement is preferred (Figure 9.7). It sets on command, making isolation simpler and, in cases of thick porcelain areas where light may not fully penetrate, a chemical activator will polymerize the cement. The literature points to the fact that dual-cure cements that are not light activated will have less desirable mechanical properties [22,23].Attention must be paid to ensuring that the cement is compatible with self-etch bonding systems, as the acidity of self-etch can have a negative effect on some dual-cure cements [24,25]. I have used Clearfil™ Esthetic Cement (Kuraray) extensively with success. Simplicity in practice is a must and for posterior restorations only one shade is necessary: Universal. The great chameleon ability of this cement allows for an enhanced blending ability of the restoration, providing simple and predictable results. Other cements that

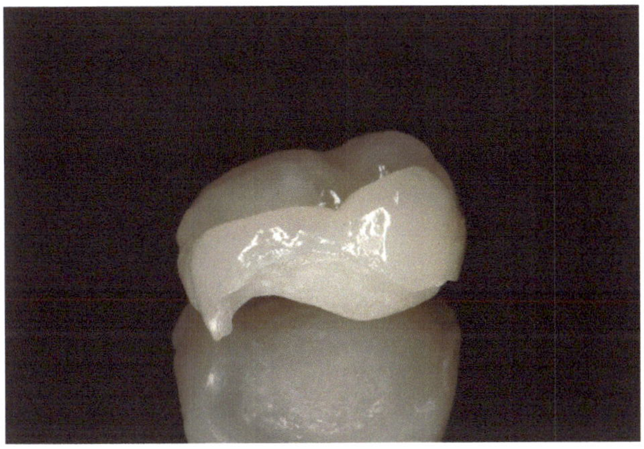

Figure 9.6 The curing light will have a difficult time passing through a 5-mm thick onlay.

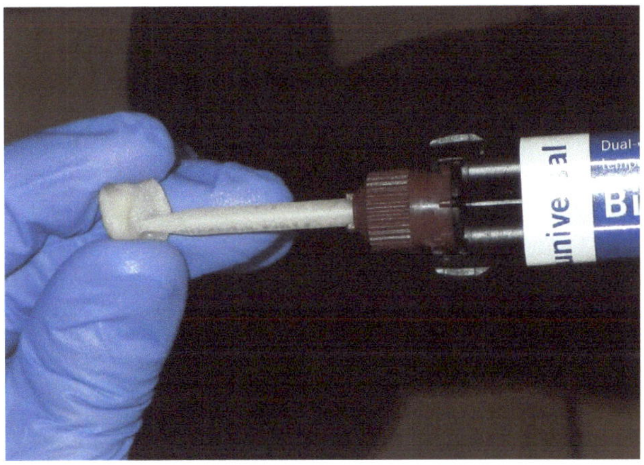

Figure 9.7 Dual-cure cement in an automix dispensing syringe, which makes it easy to dispense.

work well for onlays are Bifix QM (VOCO), Multi-Link (Ivoclar), Starfil 2B (Danville), NX3 Nexus™ Third Generation (Kerr) and Panavia V5 (Kuraray). Panavia F 2.0 also has the capability of direct adhesion. No primer is needed with metal oxides such as zirconia, alumina, and base metal ("non-precious") alloys. On these substrates (metal oxides), only sandblast conditioning is needed [26].

Self-adhesive resin cements also have a history of successful use, when used as indicated and in appropriate cases, such as mechanically retentive preparations with supragingival margins, where contamination and lower adhesion may not be a problem [27,28].A decrease in bond strength to enamel has been shown, so it may be risky to use self-adhesive resin cements with preparations with no mechanical retention [29]. With these materials, selective enamel etching is contraindicated because if any dentin is etched inadvertently, an important decrease in dentin bond strength will occur.

The Ideal Cements for Porcelain Veneers

Light-cured cements are considered to be more color stable because they do not include tertiary amine activators [30]. Combined with the fact that anterior porcelain veneers should be thin, light activation is predictable, which makes light-cured cement ideal for porcelain veneers. The most important characteristic of the cement becomes the proper translucency and the ability of the cement to enhance the blending of a thin, translucent restoration. Opacious cement would be contraindicated. The market is replete with veneer cement systems which offer different colors and levels of translucency. The most important determinants of the final shade and opacity of the finished restorations are the tooth (preparation) color and the type, and thickness of the ceramic veneer [31]. The veneer cement will influence the final color [32] to a lesser extent, unless opacious cements are used, but we already know that if supragingival margins are desired, opacious cement is contraindicated. Some techniques suggest using the cement to dramatically alter the color and value of the final restoration, or to mask the color under the restoration. This technique can be very complicated and can lead to some esthetic failures. Especially problematic are cases where there are variations of shade between the prepared teeth (Figure 9.8), and the different veneer and cement thickness, all which will make the perfect selection of different cements difficult and unpredictable. It is preferable to alter the color of the teeth prior to preparation by bleaching, internal bleaching or other means, and to allow a knowledgeable technician to undertake the necessary masking on the porcelain, as this will greatly simplify the results. Occasionally, a very difficult area such as a deep stain can be blocked out with a fully opaque flowable composite, (such as Accolade OP Mask™), which can be placed on the tooth before the impression is taken. The technician should always receive a photograph of the teeth next to a shade tab or tabs, if there is difference in shade between the teeth or parts of a tooth.

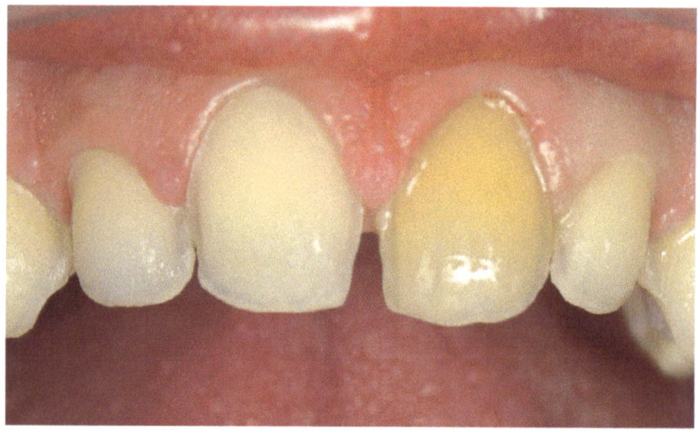

Figure 9.8 Difference in color on prepared teeth is very difficult and unpredictable to manage using different colored cements.

Trying-in the veneers before choosing a final cement is very important, as this will allow the clinician to have a preview of the approximate final shade. Most try-in pastes are not accurate. The clinician can perform the try-in procedure using a try-in paste with a good true-to-color characteristic, or with water. An accurate approach is to use Accolade™ PV Cementation System (Danville), which has a very accurate try-in "composite". This try-in composite has no light-cure initiators and the shades are adjusted to accurately duplicate the shade and translucency of the light-cured composite. By using composite and not a substitute such as glycerine-based pastes, a source of veneer bonding problems is eliminated. The try-in composite need not be fully removed and the residual is polymerized by "diffusion polymerization" when the composite is light-cured [33]. It is important to remember that if Accolade PV try-in paste is being used, the intaglio surface of the veneer must have been prepared with porcelain etch and silane.

My preferred choice is to assess the final shade with water as the medium to visually connect the veneer and the tooth. This will give the clinician a close idea as to how the final restoration will look with a fully clear cement, or without the influence of the cement, and from that point it is easier to select a cement option to either maintain the current value and brightness, or slightly increase or decrease them. Trying to change the shade with a cement is extremely complicated, as the

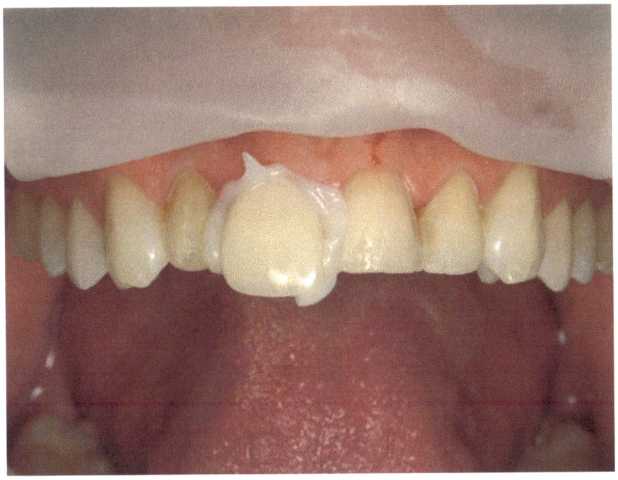

Figure 9.9 Try-in case with cement.

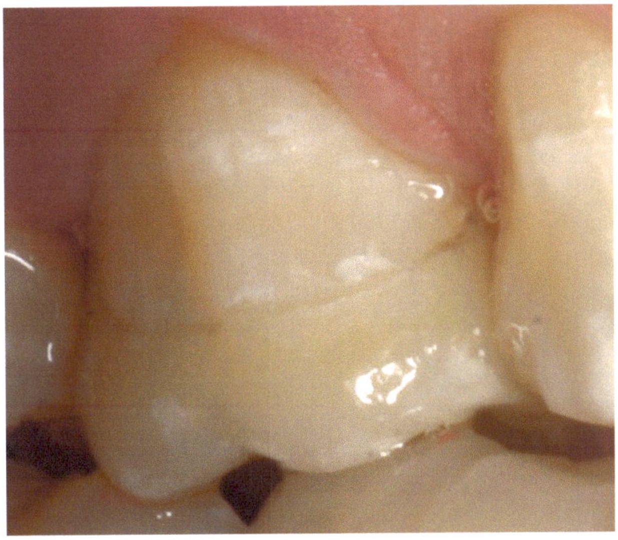

Figure 9.10 Observe, on the mesial margin of onlay cemented with clear cement, an apparent "gap". In reality, the margin is closed, but the clear cement appears to be missing.

possibilities are endless (Figure 9.9). For this reason, it is best to allow the experienced laboratory technician to have most of the control of the final shade and translucency, based on the existing tooth color. Small, final adjustments are done with the cement at the chairside, guided by the try-in procedure.

I use a simple and highly predictable approach of only three translucent veneer cements with slightly different values or brightness (degree of whiteness or blackness), which will be selected at the try-in. A light shade of cement, which is usually used for shade A1 or similar, will virtually maintain the same shade and level of translucency, with an insignificant increase in value achieved with the combined color of the tooth and the veneer. An extra-light cement used for shades B1 or 1M1 (the shades I most often use for porcelain veneers) will very lightly enhance the value and brightness of the final restoration with an insignificant decrease in translucency. A less frequently used yellow or universal shade used for shades A2 or darker will maintain the warm effect of darker shades without opacifying them. I also use the Accolade PV shades light, extra-light, and yellow, because of their high degree of translucency. Experience shows that a fully translucent or clear shade is undesirable because if there is an opening on the veneers, as often is the case, the clear cement will show grey and will adversely affect the esthetic results (Figure 9.10).

Bonding Systems

An absolutely crucial choice for success and longevity is the adhesive system (see Chapter 4). Postoperative sensitivity is not related to the resin cement, but to the adhesive being used, with the exception of self-adhesive cements. To avoid sensitivity, some suggest using an etch and rinse ("total etch") bonding system for veneers in mostly enamel situations and a self-etch for all other situations (Figure 9.11a,b). While this approach works, in clinical practice it can be very confusing for the dentist, and especially the clinical team, to change the protocol with veneers. In reality, there is no need to do this, as extremely predictable results can be achieved with self-etch systems on enamel using a selective etching protocol. Alternatively, a bonding system which allows either "etch and rinse" or self-etching may be used.

Figure 9.11 Veneer preparation: (a) Mostly in dentin. (b) Mostly in enamel.

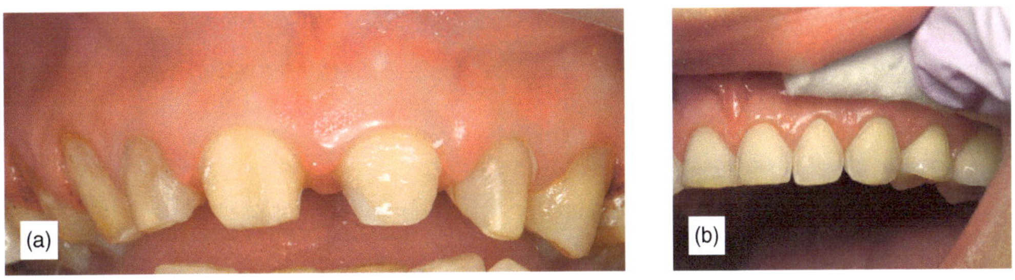

Preparing the Tooth for Adhesion

It is of great importance to have a properly cleaned and isolated tooth structure to bond to, as previously discussed. Any contamination from saliva or blood during cementation could result in deficient adhesion and could lead to eventual failure. Getting cement on the provisional can also be extremely deleterious to good adhesion. After the removal of the temporary restoration, any remnants of cement must be removed, as research clearly shows that any remaining cement will decrease the bond strength quite dramatically [34]. An ideal way of cleaning temporary cement from the tooth after the provisional is removed is the use of a simple sandblaster, such as the MicroEtcher IIA (Danville), with 27-micron or 50-micron alumina particles, or Consepsis® Scrub (Ultradent) chlorhexidine antibacterial slurry. The use of hemostatics can have a negative effect on veneers. Ferric sulfate should be avoided, because it has the potential to stain the resin cement over time when the residual ferrous sulfate oxidizes. Aluminum chloride is a better choice when hemostasis is needed. Research has shown that when hemostatics are used and not thoroughly cleaned, the bond strength can be seriously affected. Thorough cleaning of the tooth after the use of hemostatics is a must [35].

Preparing the Buildups for Bonded Cementation

During preparation, enamel margin preservation, margin elevation, immediate dentin sealing or any other type of composite, the buildup must be prepared to achieve ideal adhesion. There is a considerable amount of evidence to suggest that bonding to this composite is very predictable when performed correctly [36]. Proper preparation of the aged composite should include sandblasting with a microetcher and 27- or 50-micron alumina powder [37].

Preparation of the Porcelain Intaglio Surface

There is much research into the best protocol for the preparation of the intaglio (bondable) surface of the porcelain restoration. Most researchers agree that porcelain restoration is best treated with hydrofluoric acid, such as Ultradent® Porcelain Etch [38], followed by a good, fresh, silane coupling agent, such as Clearfil® Ceramic Primer (Kuraray) [39,40]. Attention must be paid to the etching protocol for each type of porcelain; incorrect etching time can decrease bond strength. Leucite-reinforced feldspathic porcelain, whether layered or pressed, should be etched for a full minute, whereas lithium disilicate need only be etched for 20 seconds. After etching, the intaglio surface must be washed very well with an air/water syringe, then dried completely. A ceramic primer should then be applied. Choose one that includes a solvent, silane, and MDP monomer, and does not need an additional coating of resin.

Zirconia is not a porcelain based on silicate. It is a metal oxide ceramic that will not etch with hydrofluoric acid, so the protocol for the intaglio surface is also different. The intaglio surface should be sandblasted and then a primer containing the MDP monomer should be applied, after which almost any resin cement (such as Clearfil™ Esthetic Cement) may be used. An alternative is to use a silica-coated aluminum oxide sand, which deposits an adhered silica layer onto the zirconia. The silica layer is then treated with silane to achieve a bond [41]. After sandblasting, a combination primer, containing both silane and MDP (the adhesive monomer in Panavia) [42], has been shown to further enhance adhesion to the silica layer [43]. When using an "adhesive built in" cement such as Panavia, the abrasive can be aluminum oxide, as Panavia bonds directly to metal oxides, and no primer is needed.

Step by Step Onlay Bonded Cementation

The Tooth

1) After dental anesthesia and the removal of the provisional, isolate using your method of choice (Figure 9.12a).
2) The tooth needs to be completely cleaned of remnant cement by using MicroEtcher (Danville). This is especially important if composite buildups were done. A scrub or pumice is a second option.
3) The onlay must be adjusted for proper proximal contacts and fit. Do not expect the fit of a porcelain onlay to match the fit of a gold onlay. Some slight opening in the margin is normal with porcelain, and resin cement will be used to seal those slight openings permanently (Figure 9.12b).
4) See Intaglio Onlay Preparation below.
5) Selectively etch the enamel for 10 seconds, carefully avoiding touching the dentin (Figure 9.12c).
6) Wash completely with water and dry. The tooth is dry when it is not shiny; desiccating the tooth is never desirable (Figure 9.12d).
7) Apply your bonding system of choice (such as Clearfil SE Protect primer) for 20–25 seconds over the

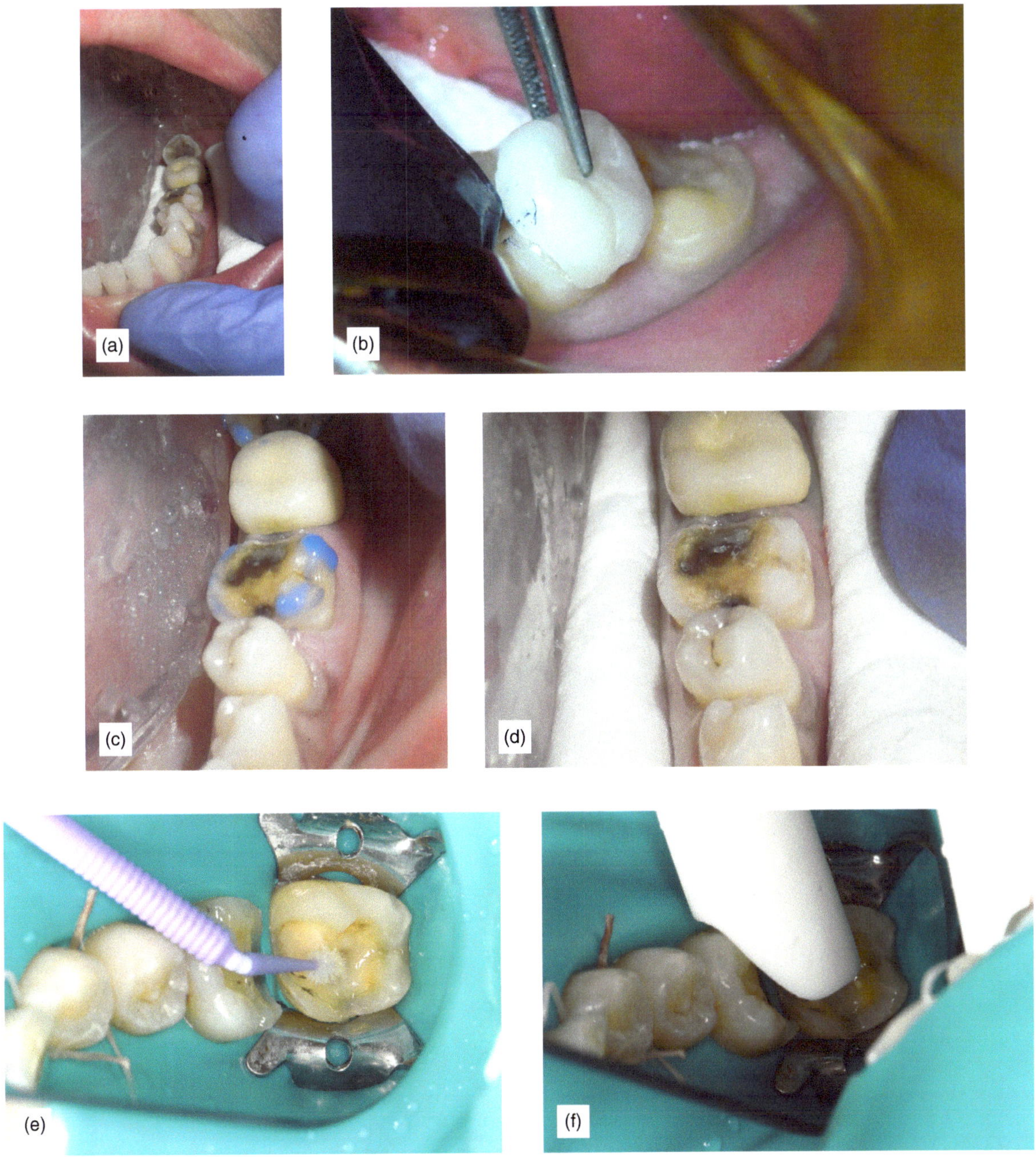

Figure 9.12 (a) Isolation. (b) Adjusting onlay. (c) Selective enamel etching. (d) After drying, frosted enamel. (e) Applying primer. (f) Removing solvent. (*Continued*)

dentin and the enamel, agitating it on the dentin (Figure 9.12e).

8) Remove the solvent with air until the liquid stops moving (Figure 9.12f).
9) Put one drop of the second bottle of Clearfil SE Protect in a well and mix with dual-cure activator, and apply thinly over enamel and dentin; do not cure.
10) Apply your cement of choice to either the tooth or the restoration and set the restoration (Figure 9.12g).
11) Clean gross excess cement with either a microbrush or plastic tip, avoiding removing it from the margin (Figure 9.12h).
12) Apply pressure to the onlay during cementation, as this increases the strength of the bond [44,45] and seats the restoration fully with less space taken by the cement.
13) Light cure for one cycle (time depends on light being used), leaving a cement that is hard, but not super hard. An alternative procedure is to spot cure facial and lingual margins to stabilize, then gel the remainder

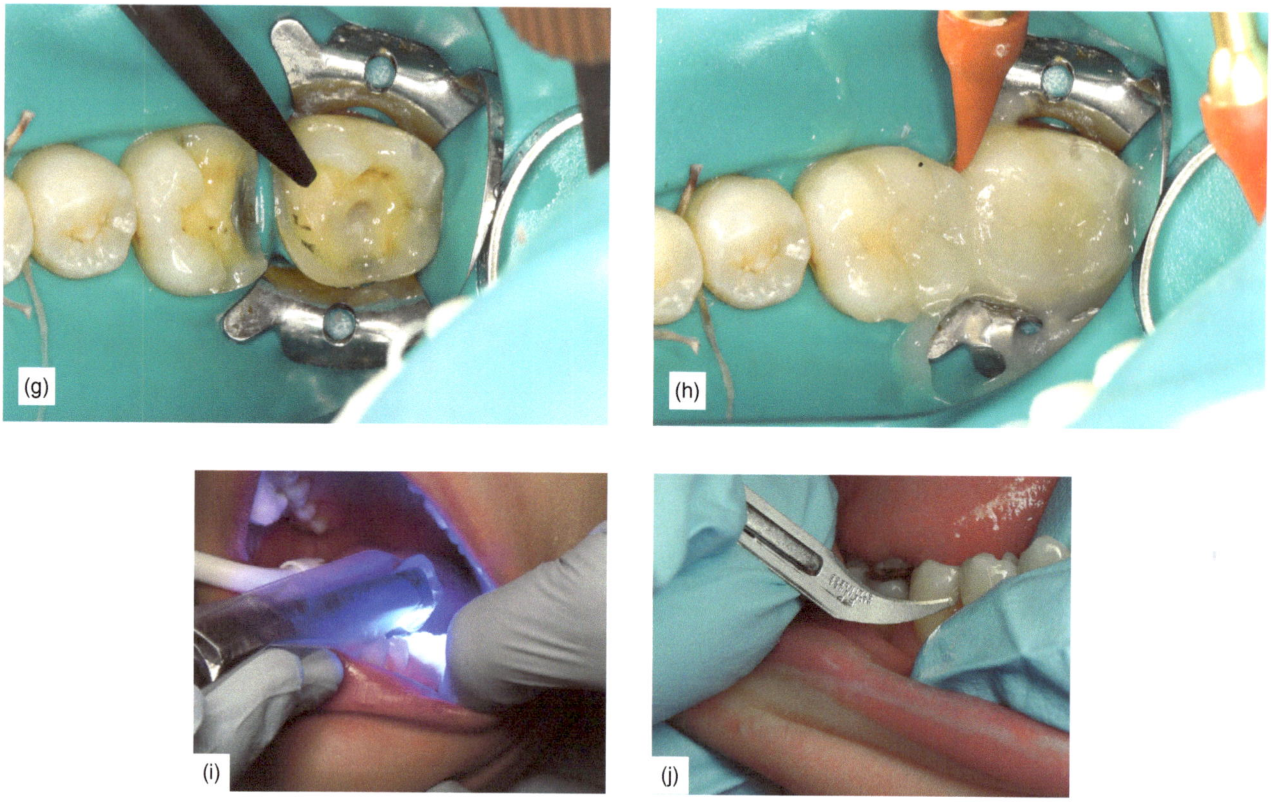

Figure 9.12 (*Continued*)
(g) Applying cement on onlay. (h) Removing excess using a gum massager. (i) Light-cure onlay for one cycle. (j) Using a no. 12 blade.

with brief light cure. Remove the gel. If desired, a metal matrix may be placed through the gel in the contact zones. Then fully light cure (Figure 9.12i).

14) After confirming that the cement is firm, use a no. 12 blade to remove excess cement (Figure 9.12j).
15) Attempt to pass some floss. If this is unsuccessful, use an interproximal finishing tool, such as a Cerisaw™ (DenMat).
16) After the cement is been removed, flood the tooth with an oxygen inhibitor (such as Liquid Lens™, Danville, glycerin-based gel), and do a final cure, one cycle facial, one cycle lingual, one cycle occlusal, using water to keep the tooth cool.
    a) Full polymerization of dual-cure cements is indispensable and increases success [46].
    b) Without this, a layer of resin will always be uncured, as resin cannot cure in the presence of oxygen. The oxygen-inhibited layer can be 0.25–0.5 mm of uncured resin. Incorrect curing of the cement will lead to the creation of a channel or ditch.
17) Make final bite adjustments:
    a) Isolate the area with cotton rolls, then use blue thin articulating paper (such as Artifol®, Bausch, metallic test film).
    b) Ask the patient to tap their teeth together hard, twice (it helps to say to the patient "tap, tap"). Marks will usually show on the working cusp and central groove (Figure 9.13a).
    c) As soon as there is equal contact throughout the area, use a differently colored paper (red) and ask the patient to grind their teeth ("grind, grind, grind, exaggerate the grind, forward, back, sideways") (Figure 9.13b).
    d) Whatever is marked in red outside the blue area is an interference and must be removed.
    e) Adjustments are complete when the centric contacts and the lateral movements are on top of each other.
    f) Having the patient sit up to do a final adjustment is an option, although the results will usually be the same. Sometimes you can find an additional adjustment that needs to be made, as there is a slight difference in the bite from laying back to sitting upright.
18) Polish the porcelain using the Sof-Lex™ (3M) or Dialite® (Brasseler) finishing and polishing system.

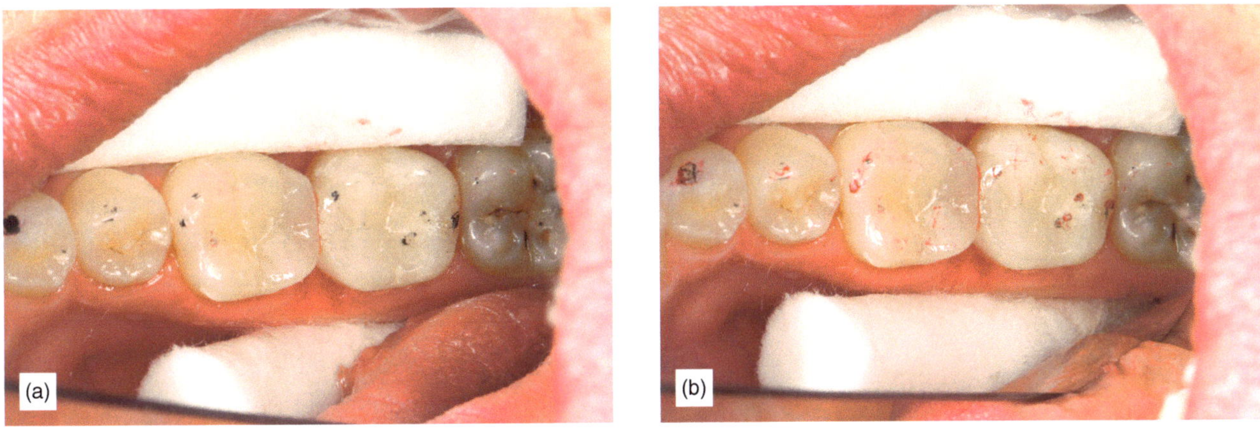

Figure 9.13 (a) After "tap tap," blue marks are visible. (b) Red marks outside the blue.

Intaglio Onlay Preparation

1) Prepare the porcelain for adhesion with hydrochloric acid, and Ultradent Porcelain Etch.
    a) Pressed feldspathic is etched for 1 minute, lithium disilicate for 20 seconds. Over-etching weakens the ceramic surface so it is undesirable.
    b) Note: Onlays may come pre-etched from the laboratory. If so, after making adjustments, only re-etch for 10 seconds or less, to remove contaminants. Alternatively, cleaning may be done with phosphoric acid.
2) Wash and dry the porcelain thoroughly. Porcelain needs to be bone-dry before applying the ceramic primer (silane).
3) Apply ceramic primer and leave for 1 minute, then air dry.
    a) Applying resin is not necessary.
    b) If using some brands of silane, apply for 1 minute, dry, then apply bond.
    c) The restoration is ready. When using a ceramic primer, there is no need to protect the onlay from ambient light.
4) If using zirconia, use these intaglio onlay preparation instructions.

Step By Step Veneer Bonded Cementation

The Tooth

1) After dental anesthesia, and the removal of the provisional, isolate using OptraGate® (Ivoclar) retractors, cotton rolls and good suction, or your isolation method of choice, including a rubber dam (Figure 9.14a).
2) The tooth needs to be completely cleaned of remnant cement by using a microetcher. This is especially important if composite buildups have been done. Consepsis scrub or pumice is a second option (Figure 9.14b).
3) Try-in all veneers with water. With teeth very wet, dip the veneer into water and set on the tooth. Repeat with the rest of the veneers. Alternatively, use the Accolade PV try-in system described above. Avoid desiccating adjacent teeth, which will then appear lighter.
4) When the water or try-in paste has created a visual connection with the tooth, check that the veneer has the look and color that the patient wishes (Figure 9.14c).
5) Choose an appropriate cement by try-in, as previously described.
6) I prefer to cement only two veneers at a time, to avoid the possibility of any restoration not seating fully, or moving during cementation. However, Dr R Bertolotti prefers to seat all six anterior veneers at once, and has many years of successful results. Readers should make the final decision based on their own skill and experience.
7) Carefully place triple-0 cord dipped in water to clearly uncover the margins for cementation. Should hemostasis be required, over the counter Visine works well to soak the cord (Figure 9.14d).
8) Adjust the contact and fit if necessary (Figure 9.14e).
9) It is common for some slight openings to be present on the margin with porcelain veneers. A resin cement should be used to permanently seal these slight openings.
10) See Intaglio Veneer Preparation below.
11) Selectively etch the enamel for 10 seconds, being careful to avoid touching the dentin. It is important to use a clear matrix, such as Blue View™ (Garrison), or plumber's tape to separate and isolate the adjacent prepared teeth from being etch or bonded (Figure 9.14f).
12) Wash thoroughly with water and dry. The tooth is dry when it is not shiny; desiccating the tooth is never desirable.
13) Apply your bonding system of choice (such as Clearfil SE Protect) for 20–25 seconds over the dentin and the enamel, agitating it on the dentin (Figure 9.14g).

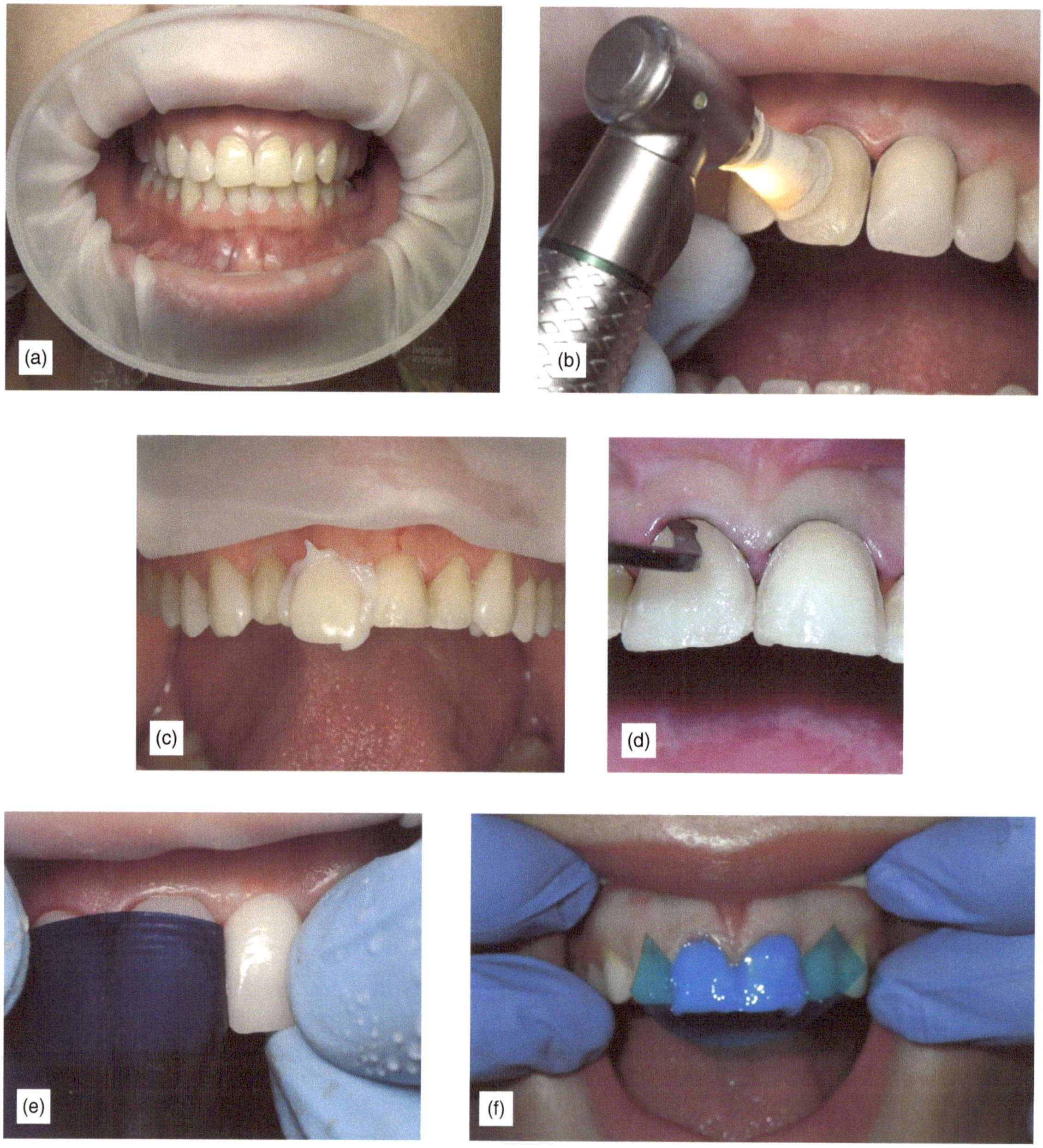

Figure 9.14 (a) Isolation veneers. (b) Cleaning teeth with Consepsis®. (c) Try-in with water or try-in paste. (d) Placing triple-0 cord. (e) Adjusting contacts. (f) Etching teeth, placing a matrix to isolate adjacent teeth from etch. (*Continued*)

14) Remove the solvent with air until the liquid stops moving.
15) Apply the second component of Clearfil SE Protect, the bond, thinly over the enamel and dentin, but do not cure.
16) Apply veneer cement to both veneer and seat.
17) Clean the gross excess cement with a plastic tipped massage gum (manufactured by GUM) (Figure 9.14h).
18) Light cure each veneer for one cycle, leaving a cement that is hard, but not super hard. Alternatively, Dr R. Bertolotti prefers to spot cure in the center, then gel the margins for easy removal of any excess (Figure 9.14i).
19) Cleanup can be done now, using a no. 12 blade (Figure 9.14j).
20) Try to pass floss through, but if unsuccessful, use a Cerisaw™ (DenMat; Figure 9.14k).
21) Repeat steps 7–20 for all the subsequent veneers, two at a time.
22) After all veneers are cemented, remove the cord and flood the tooth with an oxygen inhibitor liquid. Do the final cure, one cycle lingual, one cycle facial, on all restorations.

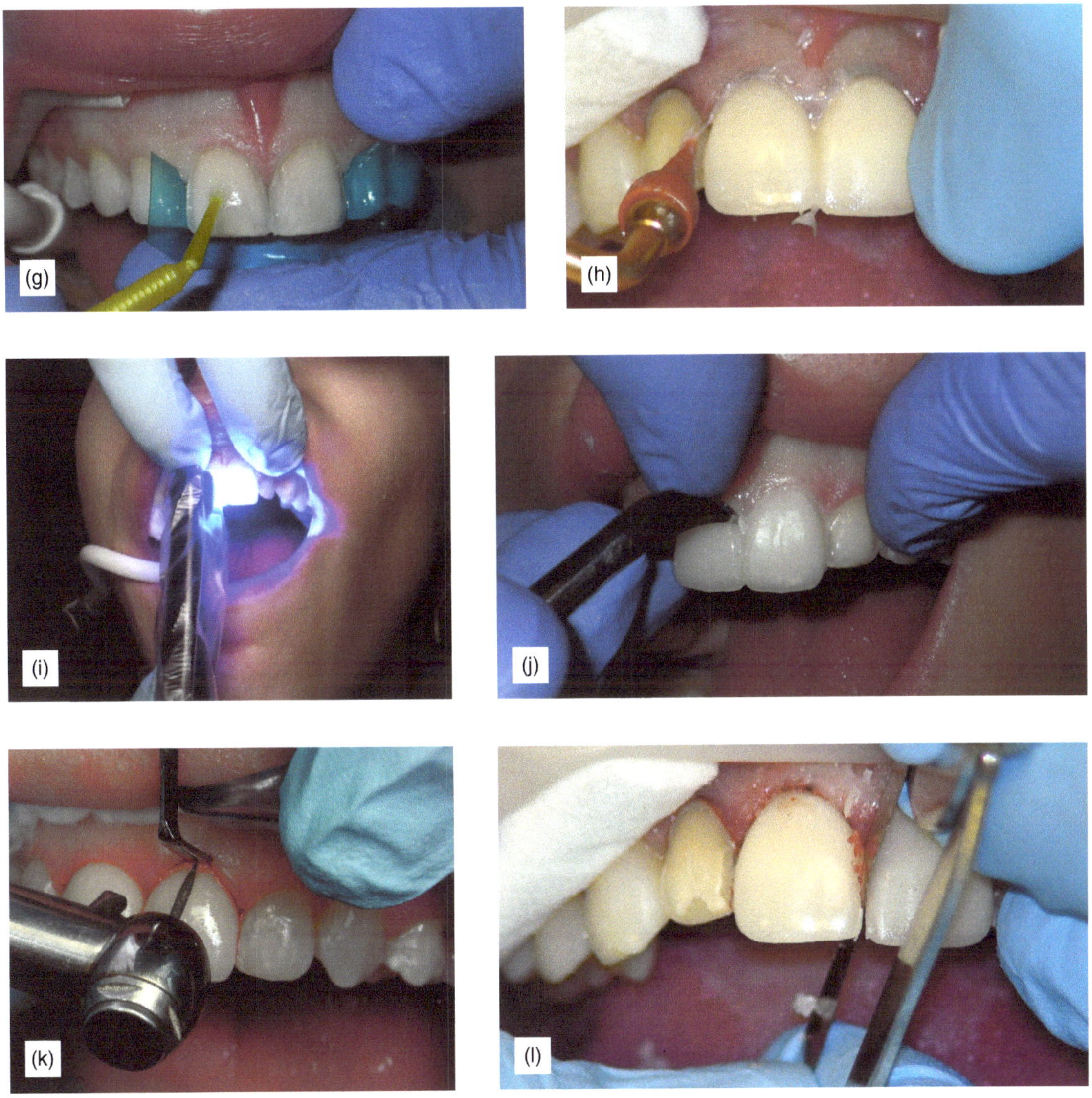

Figure 9.14 *(Continued)*
(g) Apply primer. (h) Removing cement with a gum stimulator (Buttler). (i) One cycle of curing. (j) Removing cement with no. 12 blade. (k) Using a Cerisaw™ (DenMat). (l) Using a Kincheloe (Hu-Friedy) gingival retractor to check margin integrity.

23) Use a gingival retractor to do a final check for margin quality. If necessary, use a flame diamond to smooth the margins (Figure 9.14l).
24) Polish with the Sof-Lex (3M) or Dialite (Brasseler) system.
25) Do a final bite adjustment (Chapter 12).

Intaglio Veneer Preparation

1) Prepare the porcelain for adhesion with a hydrochloric acid, Ultradent Porcelain Etch. Pressed feldspathic is etched for 1 minute, and lithium disilicate for 20 seconds. Over-etching weakens the ceramic surface, so it is undesirable.
   Note: Veneers may come pre-etched from the laboratory. If so, after making your adjustments, only re-etch for 10 seconds or less, to remove contaminants, or clean with phosphoric acid.
2) Wash and dry porcelain thoroughly. Porcelain needs to be bone-dry before applying the silane.
3) Apply ceramic primer and leave for 1 minute, then air dry.
   a) If using Kuraray ceramic primer, no additional step of applying resin is needed, since the silane itself contains resin.
   b) If using a silane without resin, wait 1 minute, dry, then apply the bond.
   c) The restoration is ready. When using Kuraray ceramic primer, there is no need to protect the onlay from ambient light.
4) Go back to step 11 in Step By Step Veneer Bonded Cementation above.

References

1 Ehlers V, Kampf G, Stender E, Willershausen B, Ernst CP. Effect of thermocycling with or without 1 year of water storage on retentive strengths of luting cements for zirconia crowns. *J Prosthet Dent*, 2015; 113(6): 609–615.
2 Lindquist TJ, Connolly J. In vitro microleakage of luting cements and crown foundation material. *J Prosthet Dent*, 2001; 85(3): 292–298.
3 Ruiz JL, Mitra S. Utilizing RMGI as a liner for direct composite restorations. *Compend Contin Educ Dent*, 2006; 27: 347–351.
4 Kramer N, Frankenberger R. Clinical performance of bonded leucite reinforced glass ceramic inlays and onlays after 8 years. *Dent Mater*, 2005; 21: 267–271.
5 Berkowitz G, Horowitz A, Curro FA, Craig RG, Ship JA, Vena D, Thompson VP. Postoperative hypersensitivity in class I resin-based composite restorations in general practice: Interim results. *Compend Contin Educ Dent*, 2009; 30(6): 356–363.
6 Christensen JG. Real-world moisture control: to dam or not to dam? *Clin Rep*, 2015; 8(5): 1–3.
7 Clinical Research Associates. Filled polymer crowns: 1- and 2-year status reports. *CRA Newsl*, 1998; 22(10): 1–3.
8 Christensen GJ. Resin cements and postoperative sensitivity. *J Am Dent Assoc*, 2000; 131(8): 1197–1199.
9 Thordrup M, Isidor F, Horsted-Bindslev P. A 5-year study of direct and indirect resin composite and ceramic inlays. *Quintessence Int*, 2001; 32(3): 199–205.
10 Reich S, Wichmann M, Rinne H, Shortall A. Clinical performance of large all ceramic CAD-CAM generated restorations. *J Am Dent Assoc*, 2004; 135: 605–612.
11 Van Dijken JWV, Horsted P. Effects of rubber dam versus cotton roll on marginal adaptation of composite resin fillings to acid-etch enamel. *Acta Odontol Scand*, 1987; 45: 303–308.
12 Feigal RJ, Hitt J, Splieth C. Retaining sealant on salivary contaminated enamel. *J Am Dent Assoc*, 1993; 124(3): 88–97.
13 Hebling J, Feigal RJ. Use of one bottle adhesive as an intermediate bonding layer to reduce sealant microleakage on saliva-contaminated enamel. *Am J Dent*, 2000; 13; 187–191.
14 Werner JF, Tani C. Effect of relative humidity on bond strength of self-etching adhesives to dentin. *J Adhes Dent*, 2002; 4(4): 277–282.
15 Stamatacos C, Simon JF. Cementation of indirect restorations: an overview of resin cements. *Compend Contin Educ Dent*, 2013; 34(1): 42–46.
16 Sakaguchi RL, Powers JM. Materials for adhesion and luting. *In Craig's Restorative Dental Materials*. 13th ed. Philadelphia, PA: Elsevier; 2012; pp. 327–348.
17 Christensen GJ. Are tooth colored onlays viable alternatives to crowns? *Clin Rep*, 2012; 5(1): 1, 3.
18 Christensen GJ. Best cement types for indirect restorations. *Clin Rep*, 2011; 4(10): 1–3.
19 Chaiyabutr, J. Effect of abutment tooth color, cement color, and ceramic thickness on the resulting optical color of a CAD/CAM glass-ceramic lithium disilicate-reinforced crown. *J Prosthet Dent*, 2011; 105(2): 83–90.
20 Simeone M, Lanza A, Rengo S, Aversa R, Apicella D, Apicella A. Inlay shading effect on the photopolymerization kinetic of a dental composite material used as bonding system in an indirect restoration technique. *Dent Mater*, 2005; 21(8): 689–694.
21 Runnacles P, Correr GM, Baratto Filho F, Gonzaga CC, Furuse AY. Degree of conversion of a resin cement light-cured through ceramic veneers of different thicknesses and types. *Braz Dent J*, 2014; 25(1): 38–42.
22 Aguiar TR, de Oliveira M, Arrais CA, Ambrosano GM, Rueggeberg F, Giannini M. The effect of photopolymerization on the degree of conversion, polymerization kinetic, biaxial flexure strength, and modulus of self-adhesive resin cements. *J Prosthet Dent*, 2015; 113(2): 128–134.
23 Foxton RM, Pereira PN, Nakajima M, Tagami J, Miura H. Durability of dual cure resin cement/ceramic bond with different curing strategies. *J Adhes Dent*, 2002; 4(1): 49–59.
24 Tay FR, Pashley DH, Yiu CK, Sanares AM, Wei SH. Factors contributing to the incompatibility between simplified-step adhesives and chemically-cured or dual-cured composites. Part I. Single-step self-etching adhesive. *J Adhes Dent*, 2003; 5(1): 27–40.
25 Pfeifer C, Shih D, Braga RR. Compatibility of dental adhesives and dual-cure cements. *Am J Dent*, 2003: 16(4): 235–238.
26 Kern M. Bonding to oxide ceramics: laboratory testing versus clinical outcome. *Dent Mater*, 2015; 31(1): 8–14.
27 Christensen GJ. Self-adhesive resin cements: are they working? *Clin Rep*, 2015; 8(5): 1–3.
28 Ruiz JL. Simplifying the cementation of porcelain onlays. *Dent Today*, 2004;. 23(3): 76–79.
29 Burgess JO, Ghuman T, Cakir D. Self-adhesive resin cements. *J Esthet Restor Dent*, 2010; 22(6): 412–419.
30 Peumans M, Van Meerbeek BV, Lambrechts P, Vanherle G. Porcelain veneers: a review of the literature. *J Dent*, 2000; 28(3):163177.
31 Barizon KT, Bergeron C, Vargas MA, Qian F, Cobb DS, Gratton DG, Geraldeli S. Ceramic materials for porcelain veneers: part II. Effect of material, shade, and thickness on translucency. *J Prosthet Dent*, 2014; 112(4): 864–870.
32 Chang J, Da Silva JD, Sakai M, Kristiansen J, Ishikawa-Nagai S. The optical effect of composite luting cement on all ceramic crowns. *J Dent*, 2009; 37(12): 937–943.
33 Dorsman GJ, Bertolotti RL. Shade accurate composite modified for long preview during veneer try-in.

International Association for Dental Research, General Session & Exhibition, June 28 – July 1, 2006, Brisbane, Australia. Abstract No. 1140.

34 Fonseca RB, Martins LR, Quagliatto PS, Soares CJ. Influence of provisional cements on ultimate bond strength of indirect composite restorations to dentin. *J Adhes Dent*, 2005; 7(3): 225–230.

35 O'Keefe KL, Pinzon LM, Rivera B, Powers JM. Bond strength of composites to astringent-contaminated dentin using self etch adhesives. *Am J Dent*, 2005; 18(3): 168–172.

36 Sadighpour L, Geramipanah F, Allahyari S, Fallahi Sichani B, Kharazi Fard MJ. In vitro evaluation of the fracture resistance and microleakage of porcelain laminate veneers bonded to teeth with composite fillings after cyclic loading. *J Adv Prosthodont*, 2014; 6(4): 278–284.

37 Gresnigt MM, Ozcan M, Kalk W, Galhano G. Effect of static and cyclic loading on ceramic laminate veneers adhered to teeth with and without aged composite restorations. *J Adhes Dent*, 2011; 13(6): 569–577.

38 Peumans M, Hikita K, De Munck J, Van Landuyt K, Poitevin A, Lambrechts P, Van Meerbeek B. Effects of ceramic surface treatments on the bond strength of an adhesive luting agent to CAD-CAM ceramic. *J Dent*, 2007; 35(4): 282–288.

39 Graiff L, Piovan C, Vigolo P, Mason PN. Shear bond strength between feldspathic CAD/CAM ceramic and human dentine for two adhesive cements. *J Prosthodont*, 2008; 17(4): 29–49.

40 Della Bona A, Anusavice KJ, Hood JA. Effect of ceramic surface treatment on tensile bond strength to a resin cement. *Int J Prosthodont*, 2002; 15(3): 248–253.

41 Wolfart M, Lehmann F, Wolfart S, Kern M. Durability of the resin bond strength to zirconia ceramic after using different surface conditioning methods. *Dent Mater*, 2006; 23: 45–50.

42 Bertolotti RL, Lacy AM, Watanabe LG. Adhesive monomers for porcelain repair. *Int J Prosthodont*, 1989; 2: 483–489.

43 Kern M. Bonding to oxide ceramics: Laboratory testing versus clinical outcome. *Dent Mater*, 2015; 31(1): 8–14.

44 Goracci C, Cury AH, Cantoro A, Papacchini F, Tay FR, Ferrari M. Microtensile bond strength and interfacial properties of self-etching and self-adhesive resin cements used to lute composite onlays under different seating forces. *J Adhes Dent*, 2006; 8(5): 327–335.

45 Chieffi N, Chersoni S, Papacchini F, Vano M, Goracci C, Davidson CL, Tay FR, Ferrari M. Effect of the seating pressure on the adhesive bonding of indirect restorations *Am J Dent*, 2006; 19(6): 333–336.

46 Foxton RM, Pereira PN, Nakajima M, Tagami J, Miura H. Durability of the dual-cure resin cement/ceramic bond with different curing strategies. *J Adhes Dent*, 2002; 4(1): 49–59.

Part V

Supragingival Dentistry and Direct Composite Restorations

10

Practical and Predictable Class II and III Direct Composite Restorations

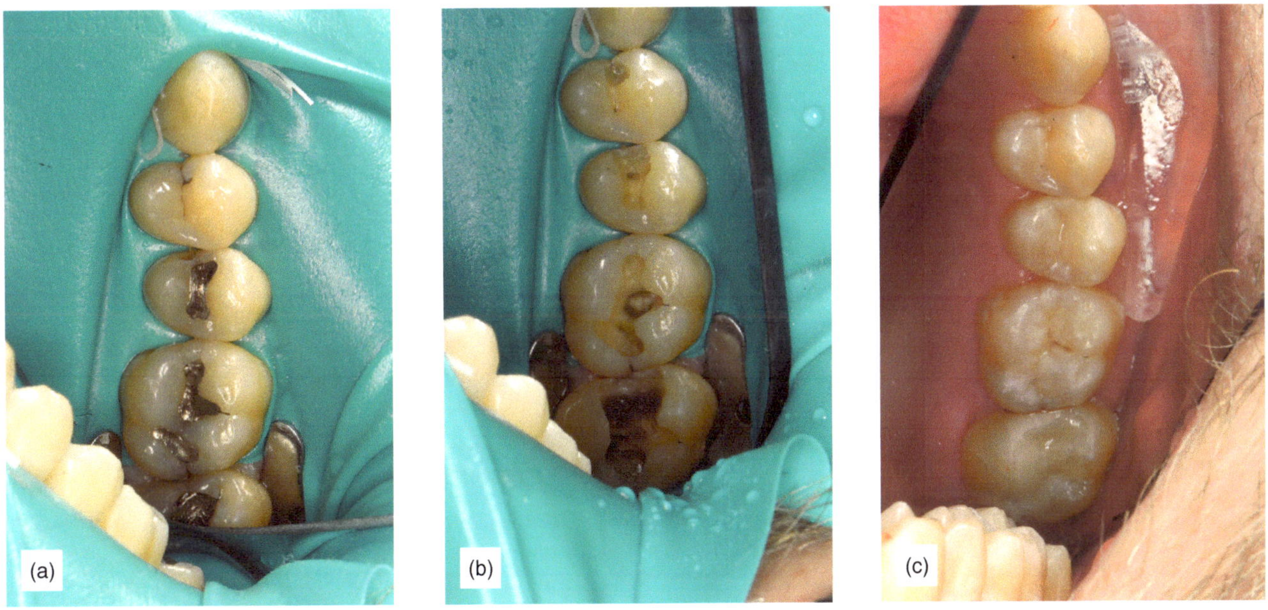

Direct composite restorations can be either predictable or a source of many problems.

Introduction

The most common procedures in restorative dentistry are direct composite restorations. Having a reliable, predictable, simple and efficient technique for direct composite restorations is paramount to a successful and happy professional life as a restorative dentist. If restorative dentists are not comfortable with these techniques or find them too time consuming and unprofitable, they will undoubtedly rely too much on indirect restorations. Many find direct composites to be complicated, unpredictable and sometimes unprofitable techniques. Since third-party compensation is in decline and clinicians contend with extreme fee competition, a time efficient, predictable and reproducible technique is a must. Supragingival minimally invasive adhesive techniques are the answer.

A Complicated and Unprofitable Technique

Most clinicians complain that direct composite restorations are considerably more time consuming and complicated than older techniques such as amalgam. This is often caused by a combination of incorrect techniques and some misunderstanding of the restorative material requirements. One major reason why the direct composite restoration procedure can be overcomplicated is the fact that traditional GV Black-based techniques of preparations are most often being used, followed by a resin-based composite filling. Clearly, the mechanically retentive, geometric GV Black-style preparation was designed for different materials and before adhesion became available (Figure 10.1). Bonded composite uses completely different materials with special characteristics, which require a completely different preparation

Supra-Gingival Minimally Invasive Dentistry: A Healthier Approach to Esthetic Restorations, First Edition. By Jose-Luis Ruiz.

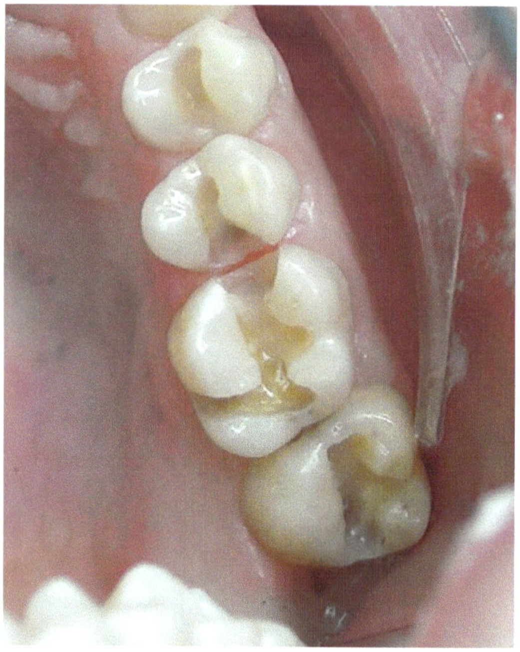

Figure 10.1 Geometric amalgam preparation.

(Figure 10.2). Supragingival minimally invasive adhesive preparations should be less complicated and time consuming than traditional preparations. The increase in time to perform an exacting traditional geometric preparation is not the only problem. In fact, a larger problem

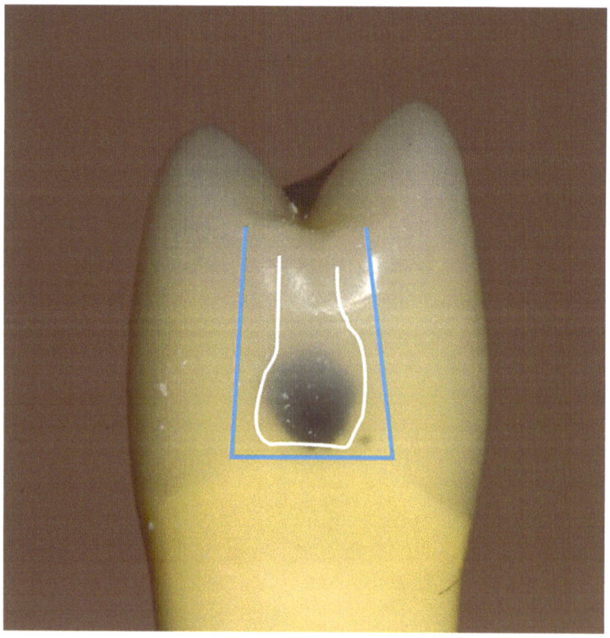

Figure 10.2 External outline of a traditional geometric preparation compared with the more tooth-preserving outline of a bonded composite preparation.

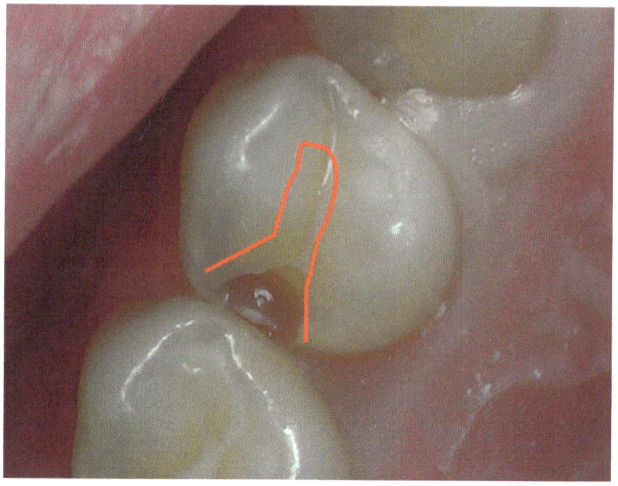

Figure 10.3 Tooth-conserving composite preparation compared with a traditional occlusal outline (dove tail) for amalgam preparation.

is that a traditional preparation makes the bonded restoration more complicated, time consuming and unpredictable. A proper preparation leads to an easier filling procedure.

The primary reason that direct composite preparations should be more widely used are:

- Composite does not require bulk for strength as does amalgam, so traditional preparations with external and internal outlines with minimum width and depth are unnecessary (Figure 10.3).
- Bonded composite reinforces tooth structure, including the enamel, so removal of a slightly undermined tooth is unnecessary [1,2].
- Bonded composites do not need mechanical retention, as they rely on adhesive.
- All of the abovementioned points lead to the all-encompassing fact that direct composites are and should be more minimally invasive than traditional restorations.
- Resin-based composite is intolerant of contamination, subgingival margins are undesirable and lead to higher chances for complications. A supragingival protocol is important. Supragingival protocols also simplify and shorten the preparation time. They simplify and make the filling procure time more predictable. Implementing the five principles of supragingival dentistry (Box 10.1) is equally important during direct restoration procedures as it is with indirect procedures (Figure 10.4).

Multicenter studies have reported excellent durability of direct composites [3]. One study looked at the 5-year durability of composites, and showed a 93% success rate,

Box 10.1 The five principles of supragingival dentistry

1) Careful removal of old restorations or caries close to the gingiva.
2) No boxes or unnecessary retention.
3) Enamel preservation and reinforcement.
4) Margin elevation.
5) Correct use of translucency.

which is almost equal to the 95.4% durability success of amalgam [4]. Although very durable, the literature shows that very large direct composite restorations fail faster and have shorter durability [5]. With improvements in techniques, the composite durability can be expected to increase.

Some clinicians who still desire the esthetic component for their patient but have difficulty in trusting direct composites default to diagnosing indirect inlays for durability's sake. Multiple studies fail to prove the superiority of indirect restorations. In fact, some studies suggest that direct composite outperforms indirect inlays (both composite and porcelain) [2,6,7]. Indirect restoration should be performed only when there is a large amount of damage to the tooth, which includes a missing or badly undermined cusp.

It is in the best interest of both clinician and patient that the clinician uses the proper techniques for direct composite. Every dentist should be able to perform this most common procedure with confidence, predictability and most importantly efficiency. In addition to the fact that indirect inlays are no more successful or durable than direct composites, they require less cutting of the tooth. As soon as an inlay is chosen, a taper is needed, requiring more aggressive tooth removal.

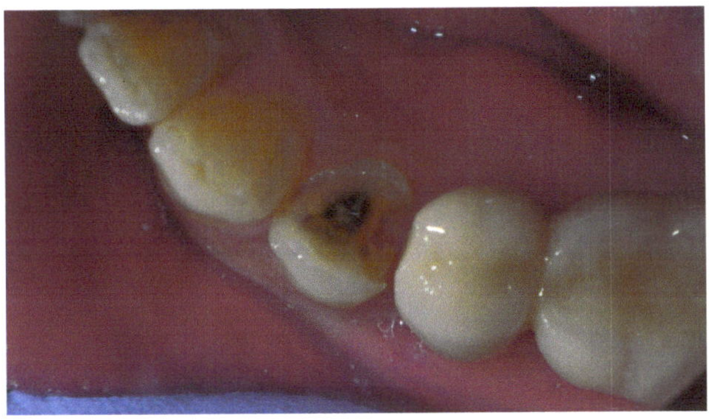

Figure 10.4 Deep subgingival caries deeply complicates the restorative procedure.

Universal Principles for Supragingival Minimally Invasive Preparation

Traditional GV Black-inspired preparation rules, such as extensions for prevention, no enamel without dentin support, geometric shape preparations and creating gingival clearance by dropping the box, do not apply to direct composite techniques. Understanding the specific requirements and characteristics of bonded composite allows for the development of more appropriate preparations for direct bonded composite restorations. The primary goals and universal rules for bonded composite preparations are as follows:

1) No specific outline, minimally invasive.
2) Caries removal should be performed using the most minimally invasive techniques available (supragingival principle 1).
3) No boxes or any unnecessary mechanical retention.
4) No need for unnecessary clearance.
5) Beveling.

No Specific Outline, Minimally Invasive

GV Black-inspired preparations, external or internal, serve to create geometric shapes which allow for the proper thickness of restorative material, sufficient access in to the cavity for instruments (condensers), or mechanical retentive features needed (e.g. preparation for amalgams). With direct composite, outlines are unnecessary, because composite does not require certain bulk for strength, condensation by instrument or mechanical retentive features. The primary goal of a direct composite preparation is the removal of caries and damaged old restoration, in the most minimally invasive form and to allow for the simple placement of the matrix band. It is acceptable for the access cavity in a proximal caries to be smaller than the internal cavity and to have an irregular shape (Figure 10.5). An internal outline can be irregular and only follow the shape created by the caries removal effort. The traditional need for bases to create a flat pulpal floor or forming geometric shapes is clearly unnecessary. Slightly undermined cusps can be preserved because bonded composite will reinforce the tooth structure (Figure 10.6).

Caries Removal Should be Performed Using the Most Minimally Invasive Techniques Available

Supragingival principle two indicates that when caries removal reaches close to the gingiva, extreme attention must be paid during caries and old restorative material removal. Clearly infected enamel and dentin must be eradicated from the tooth. Nevertheless, the traditional approach based on color and hardness and the effort to

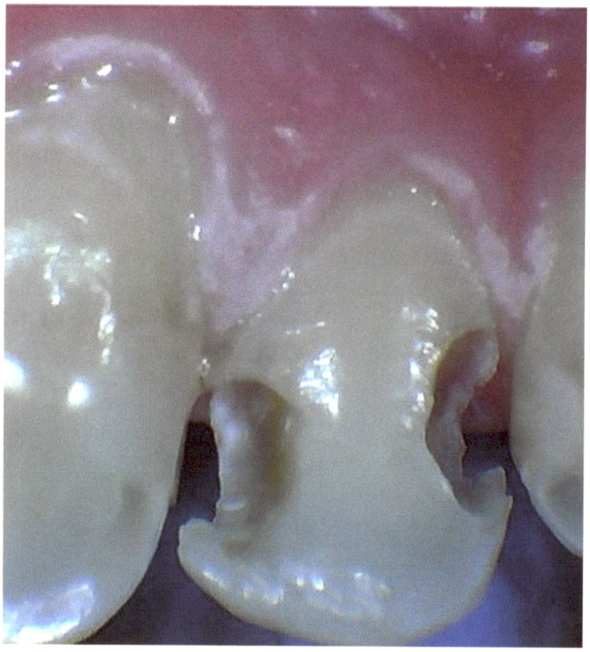

Figure 10.5 Class III preparation showing an internal outline larger than the external outline.

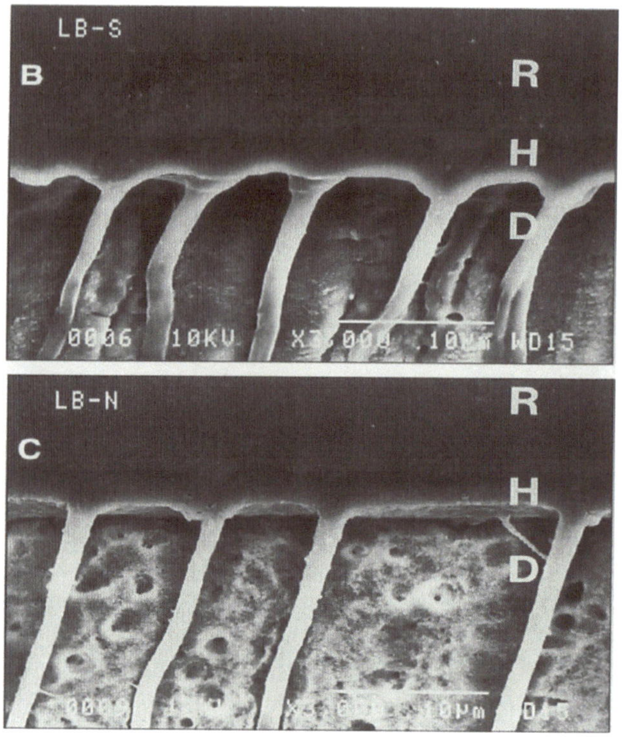

Figure 10.7 Scanning electron microscopy showing adhesive interfaces: slide B is an adhesive interface to normal dentin; slide C is an adhesive interface to caries-affected dentin (courtesy of Dr Masatoshi Nakajima).

remove all discolored dentin should be questioned, as it may be too destructive and may lead to a higher number of pulp exposures or subgingival margins [8]. Discolored dentin should not always be fully removed, as it has been well demonstrated that dentin caries has two layers [9], the superficial layer which is infected, not remineralizable and necrotic, and the deeper layer which is affected and stained but not infected, and is remineralizable and vital (Figure 10.7). With this understanding, preserving the stained but uninfected dentin can be a tooth- and pulp-saving procedure. Thorough and appropriate caries removal is indispensable, and the use of caries indicators has been demonstrated to be a great adjunct to catching hidden caries (Figure 10.8). At the same time, caries stains are also a method of detecting these two layers of carious dentin, as first described by Fusayama, followed by Nakajima [10].

Propylene glycol-based caries stains are often used. The outer infected carious dentin will be stained dark red. This dentin is removed. The inner affected dentin is stained very light pink, and is often referred to as a "pink haze" (Figure 10.9a–c). The concept of the peripheral seal is important, and special attention should be paid to ensuring healthy bondable enamel or dentin at the

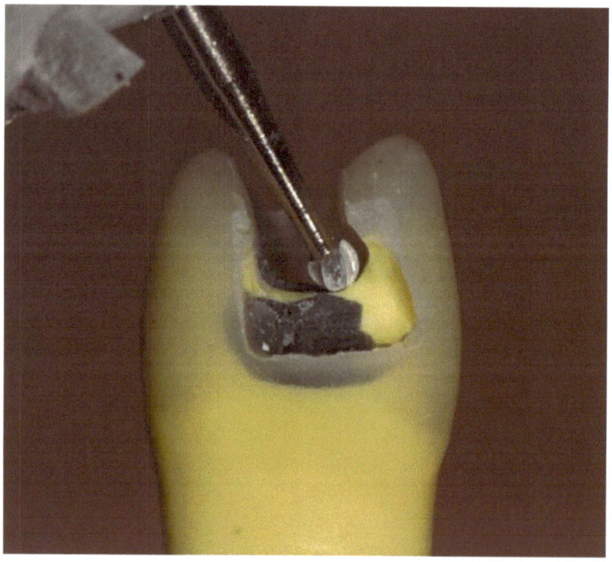

Figure 10.6 Cusps with an undercut and some unsupported enamel can be restored to close to their original strength, thanks to the reinforcement effect of adhesion.

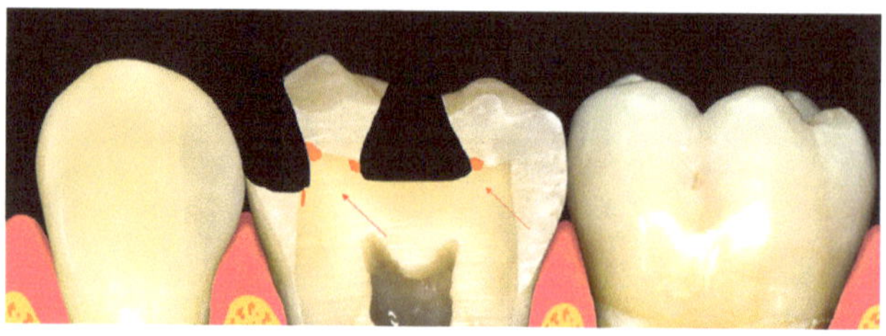

Figure 10.8 Areas where caries stain can uncover hidden caries.

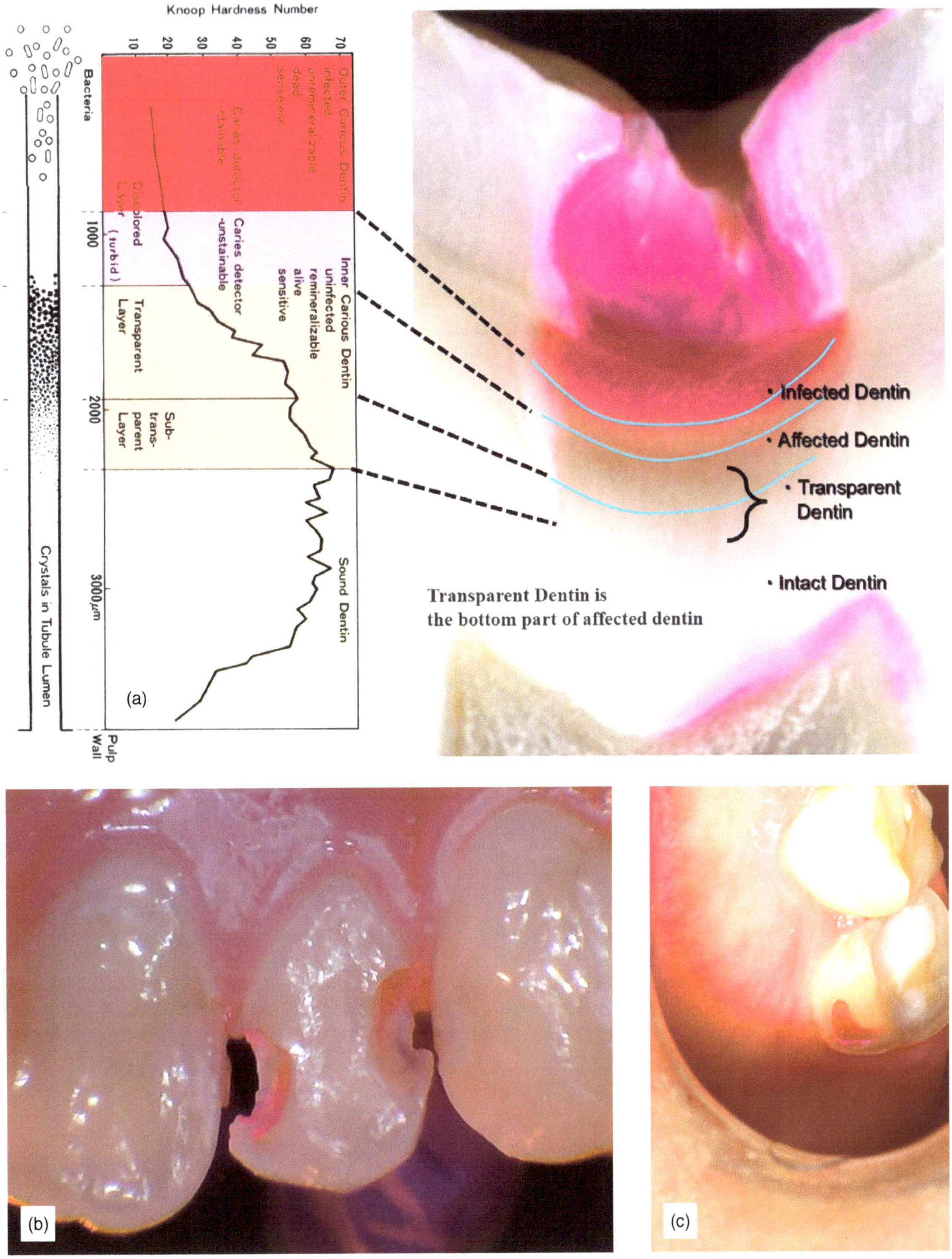

Figure 10.9 (a) Caries layers showing how they stain with red caries detector (courtesy of Dr Shigehisa Inokoshi). (b) Dentin stained red is carious and must be removed, pink staining shows non-infected tooth, which should be left, anterior. (c) Caries indicator used to uncover caries on a posterior tooth.

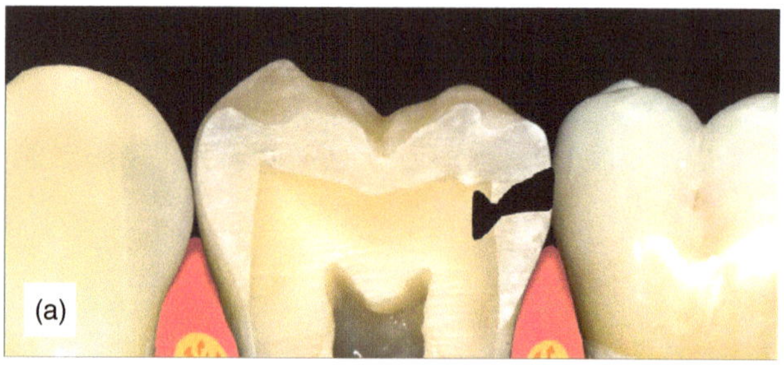

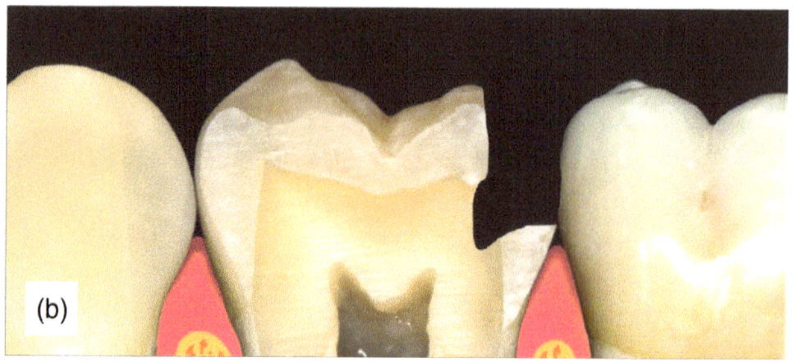

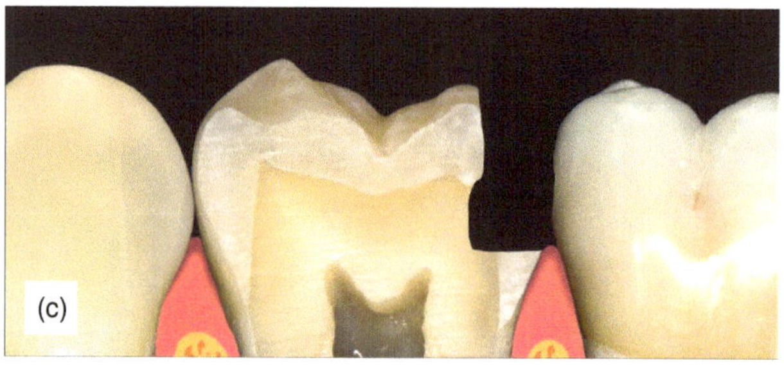

Figure 10.10 (a) Interproximal caries. (b) After careful caries removal, the margin is in contact and supragingival. (c) After traditional cervical contact breaking, the margin ends subgingivally.

restorative margins and around the pulp [11]. The inner affected dentin is not removed since it will remineralize. Affected dentin is bondable, although not as strongly as normal dentin, and research has shown that caries-affected dentin will remineralize [12,13].

The use of a base near the pulp is controversial. Currently, applying a self-etch bonding system directly onto deep or very deep dentin after cavity disinfection or, better still, using a self-etch bonding system with strong disinfectant characteristics, such as Clearfil™ SE Protect (Kuraray) is the treatment of choice and will provide excellent results [14].

The literature and clinical experience show that enamel margins are preferable and tend to be longer lasting [15]. Additionally, placing a matrix band and wedge when the margin goes considerably subgingival is more difficult. For this reason, the same care taken during caries removal should be taken during removal of caries on the cervical margin. To avoid subgingival margins, supragingival principles two and three must be considered, and enamel preservation techniques should be used [16] (the technique is discussed in detail in Chapter 3).

No Boxes or any Unnecessary Mechanical Retention

Intentionally cutting mechanical retentive features after caries is counterproductive and leads to unnecessary tooth removal, increased proximity to the pulp and subgingival margins. Traditional proximal boxes and dropping the gingival box for clearance are extremely undesirable. Interestingly enough, the difference between stopping after caries removal and continuing to drop the box is usually only a matter of one or two millimeters. However, that is all that prevents pulp exposure and subgingival margins or health and simplicity (Figure 10.10a–c).

No Need for Unnecessary Clearance

Mesial, distal and gingival clearances were mandatory with older less flowable materials like amalgam, which required strong packing to seal margins, and margin visibility was needed for margin seal confirmation (Figure 10.11a,b) Bonding systems and flowable composite can be used to seal margins reliably. Large clearances

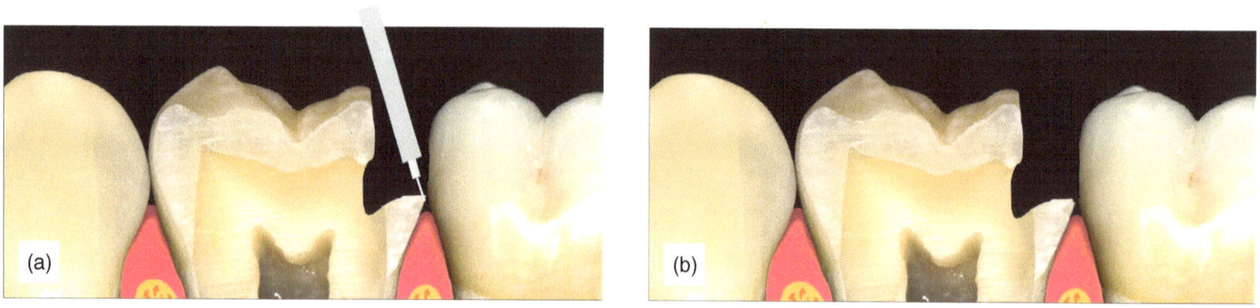

Figure 10.11 (a,b) The finished preparation with minor beveling.

are unnecessary. Supragingival principle two suggests creating clearance by using other more conservative means such as metal strips or a mosquito bur (Figure 10.11a,b). This is necessary for placing of the matrix band, but only minor separation is needed. Alternatively, wedging can allow for matrix placing. The use of a matrix retaining ring will cause tooth separation easily sufficient to compensate for the thickness of a matrix band.

Beveling

Research shows that when enamel is cut at an angle of 45 degrees, more rods are exposed, giving enhanced adhesion. Some studies suggest that this enhances the marginal seal [17] while others suggest minor benefits and that etching enamel can be sufficient preparation without beveling [18,19]. Some suggest convoluted beveling techniques that require special instrumentation. A meta-analysis has shown that a roughened surface seems to be sufficient to achieve excellent adhesion, while the adhesive system seems to have a large influence on lack of cervical leakage [20]. It is clinically impractical to create a perfectly even bevel. The few megapascals gained do not outweigh the additional time spent in creating such a bevel. Simply removing the sharp external cavosurface margin is sufficient and more practical. To complete this step, all that is necessary is to pass a diamond briefly along the cavosurface margin, just to purge any uneven enamel. No specific bevel or thickness of bevel is necessary. The exception, where longer bevels are needed, is when esthetic blending of the composite with the tooth is desirable, for example class III and VI with facial surface involvement. A 2–3 mm 45-degree bevel on the enamel will accomplish satisfactory blending when a composite with appropriate translucency is used.

Step by Step Preparation for Class II Caries

1) Enter the tooth through the occlusal surface using a small rotatory instrument to find the caries. A number 2 carbide round bur or number 1556 carbide will be suitable, depending on the size of the cavity. Maintain a small external outline while attempting to remove the occlusal and proximal caries. The size of the external outline needs to be appropriate to allow for visualization of the caries. No specific shape or outline is necessary, but the external outline needs to be on sound enamel or dentin. Decalcified enamel must be removed, as well as any old restorative material, which will expand the size of the external outline (Figure 10.12a).
2) Expand internally for initial removal of gross caries. Apply a caries finder for 10 seconds, and rinse. Remove caries until all infected dentin has been removed.
3) When breaking the proximal wall it is desirable to use a wedge guard or a metal matrix to protect the adjacent tooth. The external fluoride-rich layer should be protected to avoid the increased possibility of caries. Full interproximal clearance, which is needed for GV Black-influenced design of cavities, is not mandatory (Figure 10.12b).
4) A lack of proximal clearance may make it difficult to insert a matrix band. A margin separation technique using a "mosquito" bur through the contact can simplify matrix band insertion and will also work for minor interproximal beveling (Figure 10.12c). Using a wedge guard will protect the adjacent tooth. Placing a wedge to separate the tooth and a matrix band may be all that is necessary. Another possibility is to pre-separate the teeth by placing a ring in advance of the cavity preparation. The longer the ring is in place, the greater the separation. Danville's Mega-Ring is possibly the most powerful separator ring (Figure 10.12d).
5) When caries approaches the gingival margin, the supragingival protocol should be employed. Minimally invasive removal of caries and old restorations and enamel preservation techniques will make restoring easier, more predictable and healthier for the periodontium (see Chapter 3; Figure 10.12e).
6) Remove the sharp external cavosurface margin throughout, to remove loose enamel rods and enhance adhesion using a flame diamond (Figure 10.12f).

Step by Step Preparation for Class III Caries

1) Enter the tooth though the lingual surface using a small rotatory instrument to find the caries. A number 2 carbide round bur or number 1556 carbide will be suitable, depending on the size of the cavity. Maintain a small external outline while attempting to remove the proximal caries. The size of the external outline has to be appropriate to allow for visualization of the caries. No specific shape or outline is necessary, but the external outline needs to be on sound enamel or dentin. Decalcified enamel must be removed, as well as any old restorative material, which will expand the size of the external outline (Figure 10.13a).
2) Expand internally for the initial removal of gross caries. Apply a caries finder for 10 seconds and rinse. Remove dark red stained caries until all infected dentin has been removed, leaving a pink haze. Preservation of gingival dentin and enamel, even if unsupported, will simplify the restorative procedure.

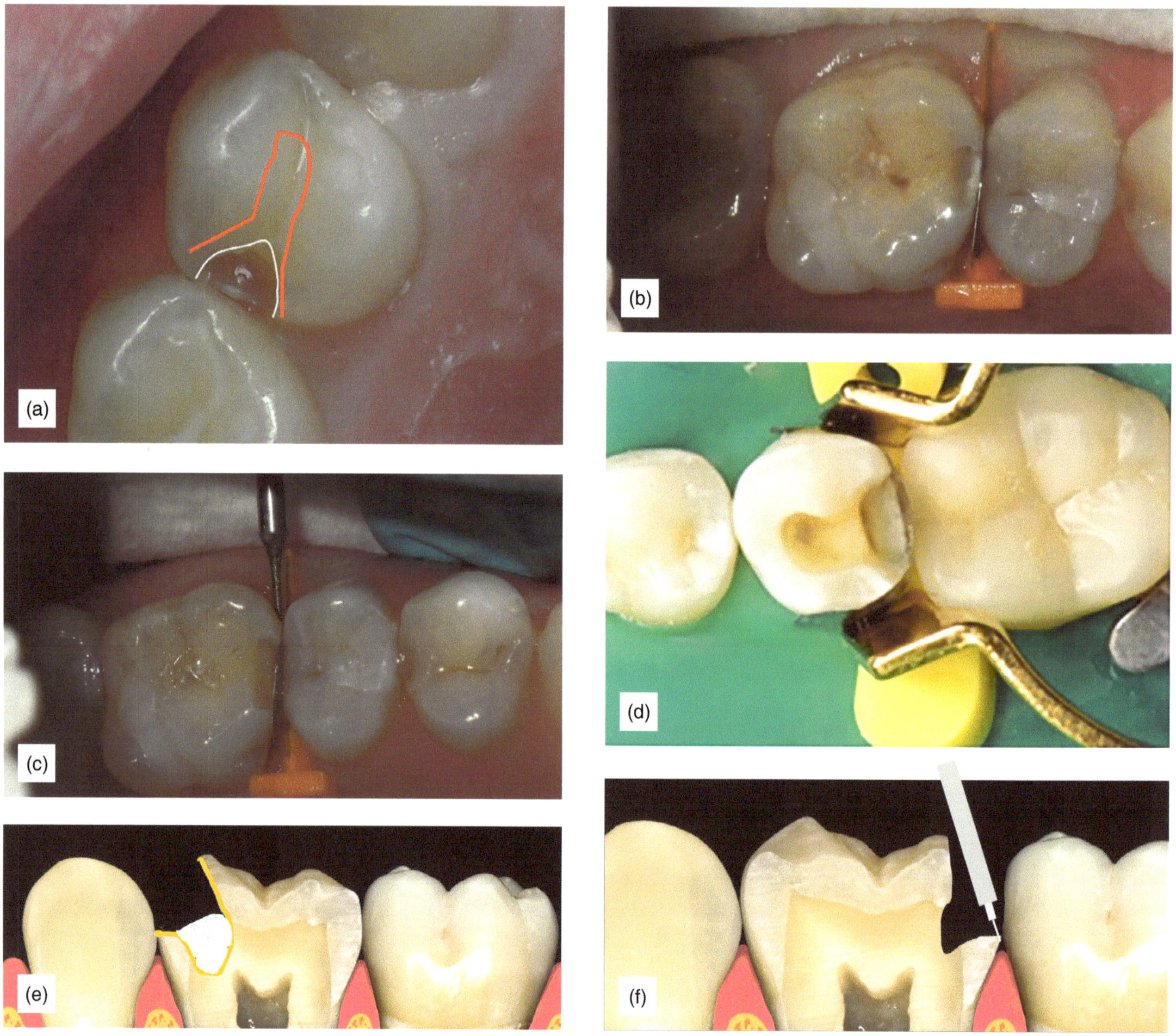

Figure 10.12 (a) External outline (preparation class II). (b) Wedge guard used to avoid nicking the adjacent tooth. (c) Using the mosquito bur is necessary to create clearance. (d) Mega Ring (Danville). (e) The enamel margin preservation procedure. (f) The finished preparation with minor bevels.

3) When breaking the proximal wall, it is desirable to use a wedge guard to protect the adjacent tooth, as the external fluoride-rich layer should be protected to avoid the increase possibility of caries. Full interproximal clearance, which is needed with the GV Black-influenced design of cavities, is not mandatory (Figure 10.13b).
4) Lack of proximal clearance may make it difficult to insert a matrix band. Placing a wedge or torqueing apart with a hand instrument to separate the tooth will usually allow a matrix band to be placed.
5) When caries approaches the gingival margin, use the supragingival protocol. Minimally invasive removal of caries and old restorations, and enamel preservation techniques will make restoring easier, more predictable and healthier for the periodontium (see Chapter 3; Figure 10.13c).
6) Remove the sharp external cavosurface margin throughout, to remove loose enamel rods and enhance adhesion, using a flame diamond.

Margins on Dentin and the Acid–Base Resistant Zone (or Super Dentin)

Knowing that enamel margins can improve marginal seal, concern may be raised when the margins end in dentin. Newer understanding and the use of some self-etch

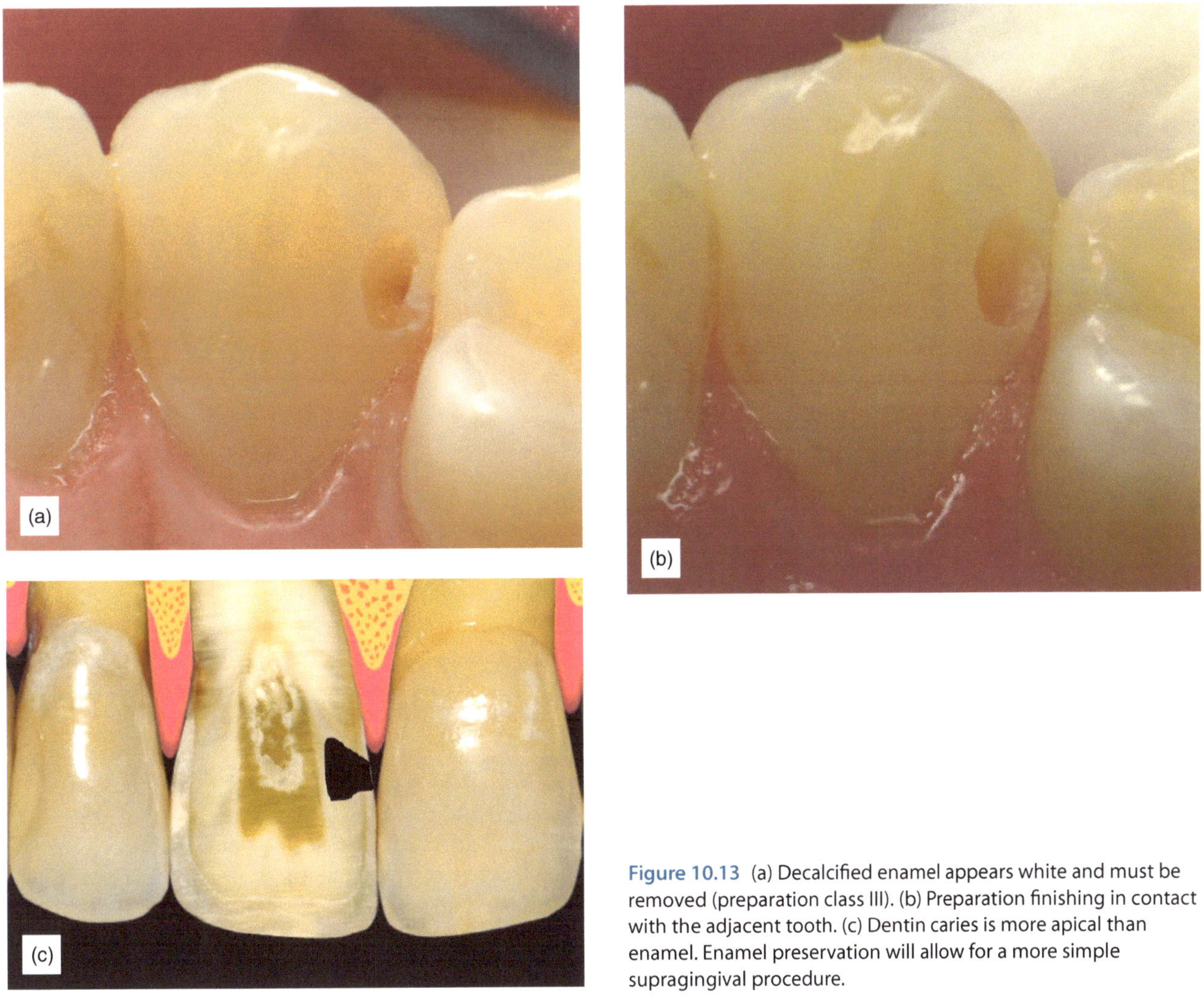

Figure 10.13 (a) Decalcified enamel appears white and must be removed (preparation class III). (b) Preparation finishing in contact with the adjacent tooth. (c) Dentin caries is more apical than enamel. Enamel preservation will allow for a more simple supragingival procedure.

bonding systems can help to mitigate such concerns. Current research is showing that, with proper conditioning and the use of some self-etch bonding systems with fluoride release abilities, such as Clearfil SE Protect, an acid–base resistant zone can form on the dentin (Figure 10.14) [21]. This zone may resist acid challenge, giving rise to the ability to resist demineralization and prevent secondary caries development. This layer is only encountered in self-etch adhesives [22]. The ultimate clinical effect of this layer remains to be understood and studied.

When the gingival margin is on the dentin, it is important to understand the concept of how composite will shrink toward the direction of the best bonded surface [15,23,24]. When shrinkage is correctly managed, this will in fact enhance the marginal seal. Incorrectly managed, it could lead to the exact opposite. After a bonding agent is cured, an effort should be made to build up the cervical

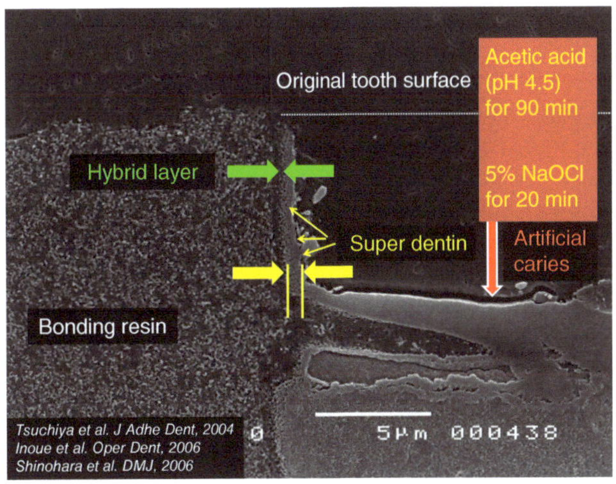

Figure 10.14 Super dentin (courtesy of Dr Jungi Tagami).

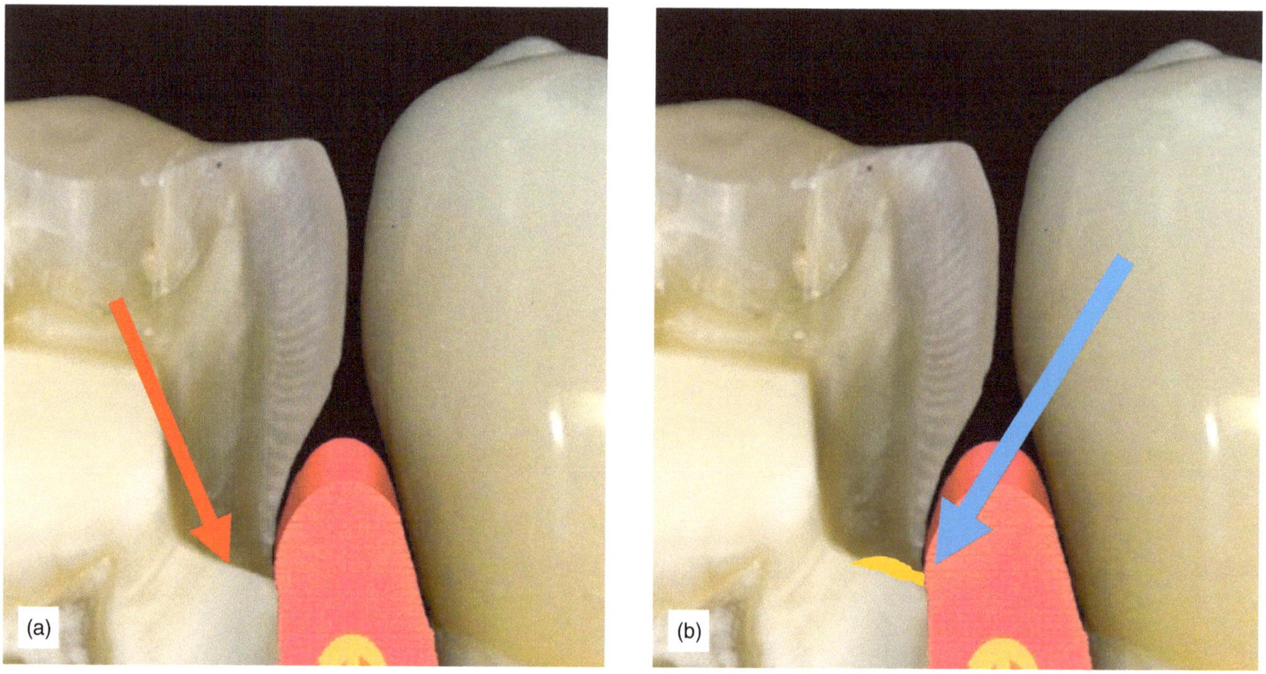

Figure 10.15 (a) The gingival floor is fully in the dentin and cementum, no enamel. (b) Placing the first increment only on the dentin gingival floor will enhance adaptation and avoid microgap.

margin with a thin layer of flowable composite, keeping it in contact with the dentin gingival floor alone (Figure 10.15a,b). Contact with the enamel walls could pull the composite in that direction and increase the chances of a gap forming at the gingival margin. The ideal flowable composite is one with excellent radiopacity.

Isolation

Correct isolation and uncontaminated surfaces when performing adhesive dentistry are essential. Contrary to many clinicians' vehement insistence, however, rubber dam isolation is not the only method for clinical success. Clinical studies have shown that rubber dam isolation or a correctly employed cotton roll isolation technique will give equal clinical success [25,26,27]. This is not to say that there is anything wrong with using the rubber dam method; it works perfectly well, if used correctly. It is known, however, that over 90% of dentists do not use rubber dam routinely, and making the use of a rubber dam mandatory for adhesive dentistry is not based on good evidence and is also clinically burdensome. Such dogmatic requirements can easily dissuade the quality clinician from using adhesive techniques. I have performed thousands of successful adhesive restorations for over 20 years, mostly without the use of a rubber dam.

Practice and efficient clinical techniques must be used to avoid compromising isolation. Lengthy and convoluted techniques require long periods of strict isolation and this may be one reason why it appears to be mandatory. The use of self-etch bonding systems, which are less technique and humidity sensitive is also desirable [28].

In addition to correctly performed cotton roll isolation, other options for isolation include an OptraGate® (Ivoclar), which is useful for anterior restorations (Figure 10.16), and PropGard® (Ultradent), which retracts the tongue as well, or DryShield® (Figure 10.17). Whichever method is used, it is imperative to remember

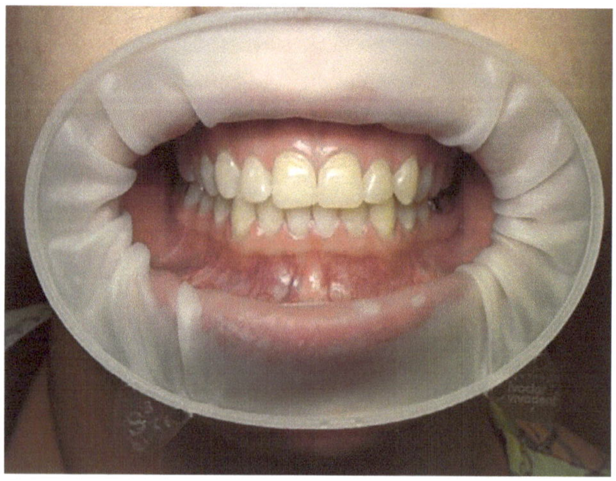

Figure 10.16 Isolation using OptraGate® (Ivoclar).

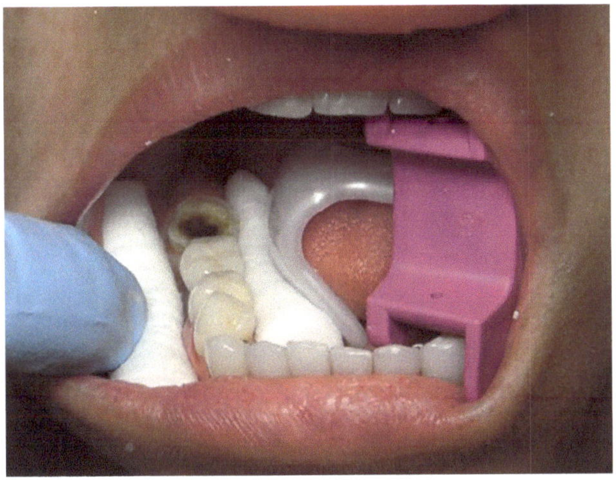

Figure 10.17 Isolation using PropGard® (Ultradent).

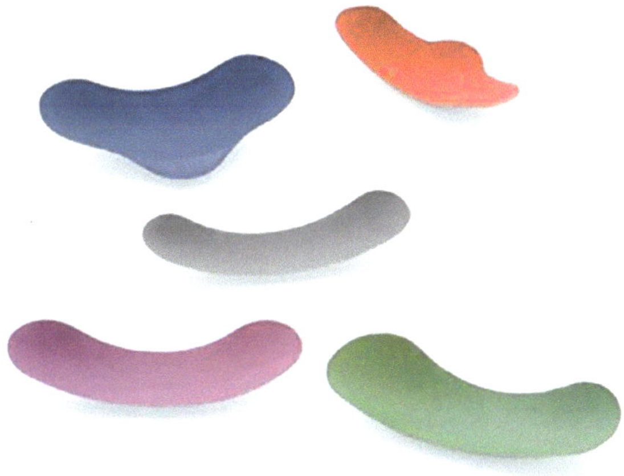

Figure 10.19 Teflon-coated matrix bands.

with adhesive dentistry that correct isolation is critical for clinical success. The slightest amount of blood, saliva, or crevicular fluid creates contamination, and a failed restoration.

Matrices and Wedges

The correct selection and use of matrix bands is of great importance. Traditional tofflemire (universal) retainers are not optimal, because they have flat surfaces, giving a restoration with flat proximal edges, with contact only at the very top of the tooth. The ideal matrix bands for class II bonded composites are rings and sectional matrices (Figure 10.18). The best type of matrix bands specifically for adhesive dentistry are Teflon-coated matrix bands (SlickBands™, Garrison), as most modern bonding systems can adhere to most surfaces including metal (Figure 10.19). Teflon-coated matrix bands prevent the bonding system from adhering to it, preventing small pieces of the proximal composite from being removed along with the matrix.

In reference to rings, the specific type used is up to the preference of the dentist. Any product with wider tines is highly recommended, similar to the Contact Matrix™ (Danville) sectional matrix system. The reason for this is that there is a wide separation between the cavosurface margin and the adjacent tooth. If smaller traditional tines (Figure 10.20) are used, they may invade the preparation, leading to a misshapen tooth. Wider tines also embrace the tooth and the adjacent tooth, which increases the adaptation of the matrix band. Increased

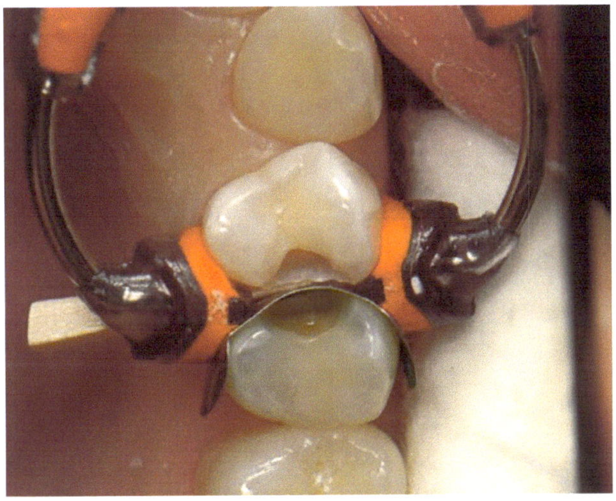

Figure 10.18 Garrison ring and matrix placed and ready to fill.

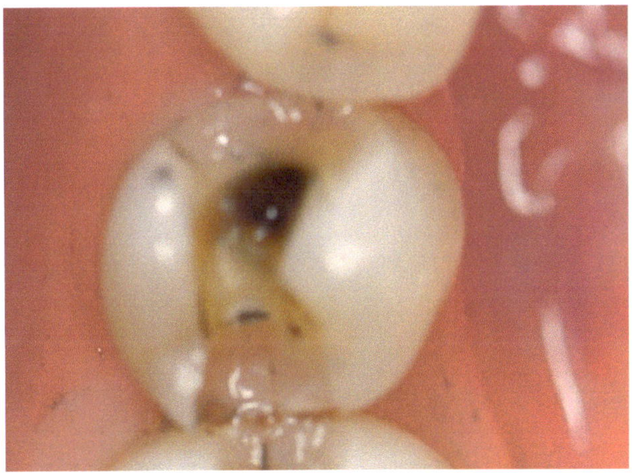

Figure 10.20 Large interproximal separation.

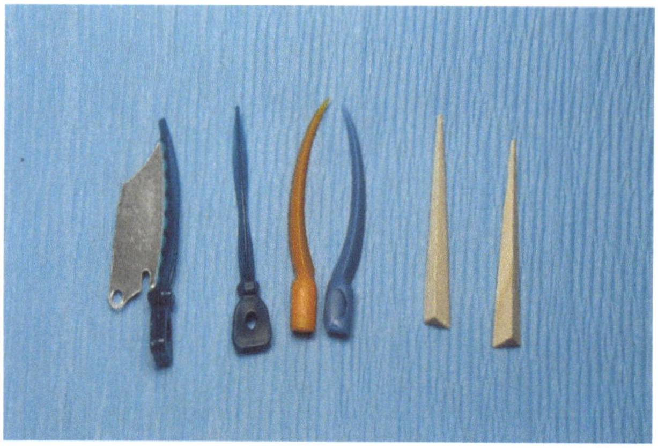

Figure 10.21 Many wedges are available, including Curvy wedges (VOCO).

adaptation to the adjacent tooth means less flash, and less cleanup afterwards, making the procedure much easier. While back-to back composite direct composite fillings cannot be done at the same time, it is possible, to do a mesial-occlusal-distal restoration on the same tooth using two rings.

There are a great variety of wedges on the market to choose from (Figure 10.21). Wooden wedges continue to work very well. Some more modern options offer curved wedges (such as those made by VOCO). These have the intention of better sealing the margin. The direction, either right or left, is important when using curved wedges, so care must be taken in choosing the correct one for each procedure.

Bonding

The bonding procedure is of great importance. Refer to Chapter 4 for full details of choice of materials and desirable techniques.

The Effects of Polymerization Shrinkage and Stress

Polymerization shrinkage of resin-based composite is unavoidable and the rate of shrinkage is between 1% and 3%. Research has shown that the force of this shrinkage is enough to break the adhesive bond between the composite and the tooth (microgap), and can even cause the thinner cusp to deflect [29,30]. Postoperative sensitivity, marginal leakage and recurring caries can be the consequences of shrinkage, which make this issue very clinically relevant (Figure 10.22). Some researchers have found the strategies used to minimize polymerization shrinkage and stress of restorative and flowable materials in relation to marginal microleakage to be less relevant than the bonding material used [31]. There are a number of available strategies to minimize polymerization shrinkage and stress. The incremental layering of composite, including specific layering protocols, while helpful, is of questionable efficacy [32]. Fibers and glass inserts have also been used [33]. Research has shown that after each composite increment is initially polymerized, the polymerization forces will stress the bonded surfaces, and the stress will continue for an extended period of time. Thus, cumulative polymerization stress to the bonded surface and the tooth is of concern. Other strategies used are liners or restorative materials with higher elasticity, as the elasticity or stiffness of the restorative material does play a large role in managing polymerization stress [34], in addition to stress-reducing curing protocols. A combination of such techniques is clinically reasonable.

Managing the Effects of Polymerization Shrinkage by the Use of Materials with Low Modulus of Elasticity

The desire to have the perfect liner or restorative composite which would minimize or eliminate the effects

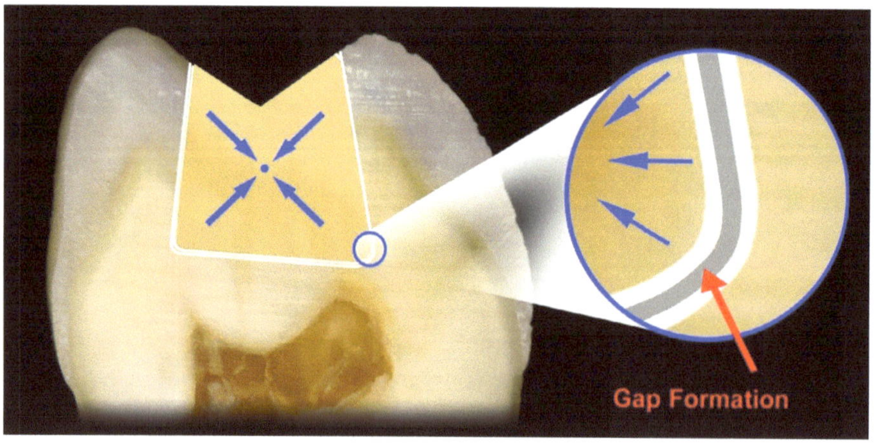

Figure 10.22 Microgap caused by polymerization shrinkage (reproduced with kind permission of *Compendium of Continuing Education in Dentistry*).

Table 10.1 Modulus of elasticity of resin-modified glass ionomer and resin-based composite.

	Source	Modulus of elasticity (GPa)	Volumetric shrinkage (%)
Low-viscosity resin (Revolution, Kerr)	Labella R, Lambrechts P, Van Meerbeek B, Vanherle G. Polymerization shrinkage and elasticity of flowable composites and filled adhesives. *Dental Materials*, 1999; 15(2): 128–137.	7.7	5.5
Resin-modified glass ionomer (Vitrebond™, 3M ESPE)	Tam LE, McComb D, Pulver F. Physical properties of proprietary light-cured lining materials. *Operative Dentistry*, 1991; 16(6): 210–217.	1.1	2.3

of polymerization shrinkage and stress is ever present in dentistry. While the perfect material has yet to be designed, some materials are available in dentistry which have been used as stress relievers to polymerization shrinkage.

Resin-modified glass ionomer (RMGI) has a low modulus of elasticity, and is considerably more elastic than resin-based composites, including flowable materials (Table 10.1) [35,36]. One study showed that the effect of polymerization shrinkage was decreased by close to 50% by the use of a 0.5 mm layer of RMGI liner (Vitrebond™, 3M) [37]. It is believed that when the composite shrinks, the high elasticity of freshly cured RMGI serves as a buffer, minimizing the effect of shrinkage and decreasing chances of a microgap. While many have reported excellent results with RMGI extended to the external part of the tooth [38,39,40], some have found it to increase failure [41].

RMGI internal liners are recommended for direct restorations deeper than 3 mm and with high configuration factors. An easy way of measuring the depth of a preparation is with a carbide bur, as the cutting blades of the bur are usually 4 mm in length. If the cavity is deeper than 4 mm, a liner could be considered (Figure 10.23). The liner should be thin – 0.5 mm. Some studies have shown superior results in dispersing stress using RMGI compared with flowable liners [42]. Controversy exists with this material, though, as some have found it to increase failure. Failures may relate to incorrect use, often the use of too thick a liner layer or placing the liner unnecessarily in cavities that are not sufficiently deep [41].

Bulk fill restorative composites are a newer and very promising approach to managing the effects of polymerization shrinkage and polymerization stress in particular. Bulk fill composites have a low modulus of elasticity and thus are intended to allow bulk filling of a cavity without the same amount of polymerization stress. The literature shows conflicting results. While some studies show a decrease in polymerization shrinkage and better marginal seal [43,44], others have found the amount of shrinkage and gap formation to be either the same or in some cases worse than traditional incremental filling [45,46]. As with most research, variations in results can be caused by technique, including over-bulking or using an inappropriate curing protocol [47].

Flowable composites have a slightly lower modulus of elasticity than a restorative composite, because of the lower fill content. While the use of flowable composite

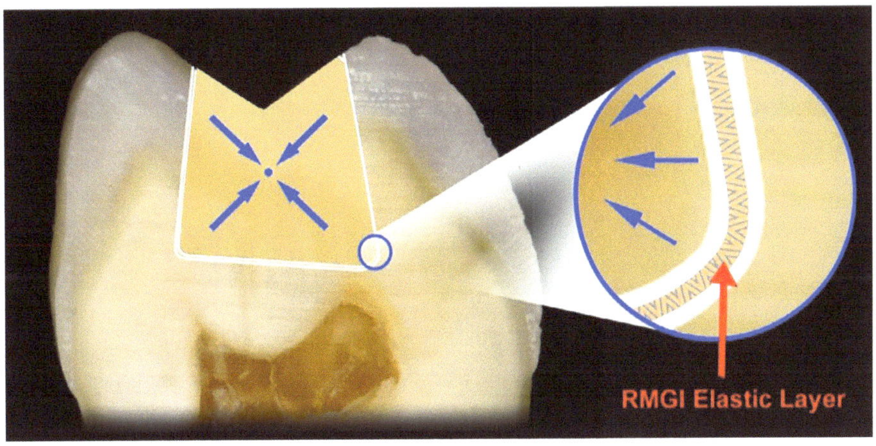

Figure 10.23 A liner can be used on very deep cavities (deeper than 4 mm), and placed thinly (reproduced with kind permission of *Compendium of Continuing Education in Dentistry*).

has been documented to improve margin adaptation and seal [48], the ability of flowable materials as liners to decrease the effects of polymerization shrinkage is questionable [49]. Incremental filling of the cavity is desirable for multiple reasons, a good protocol which includes understanding the effects of curing and layering is desirable to decrease polymerization shrinkage.

Managing the Effects of Polymerization Shrinkage by Layering and Curing: The Filling Procedure

A common approach to managing polymerization shrinkage and stress is to perform multiple increments (Figure 10.24). Multiple increments alone have been shown to have limited success and may not provide the complete answer [50]. The understanding that polymerization stress starts when composite is first cured and continues after curing, and that its effects are equally as important as polymerization shrinkages [51] has led to the use of a number of different filling and curing protocols, which combine low light intensity and periods of rest to allow for the stress in the composite to dissipate, such as soft start [52] and pulse cure [53], among others [54]. As for incremental filling of the cavity, there are benefits to managing stress, but the true extent of the clinical relevance has yet to be determined and studies are contradictory [54,55,56,57].

Curing speed, however, has been shown by some researchers not to be clinically relevant [55]. Ferracane has suggested that "while these results may be directly attributable to the generation of contraction stresses in dental composite restorations, and they provide a rationale for closely following a structured placement technique to minimize their effects, no direct clinical evidence currently exists to support a cause and effect relationship between contraction stress and clinical failure or longevity for these materials" [58]. Christensen showed no significant difference in composite properties when using either fast, slow or ramped curing speeds. A light with a 3-second cure has rendered much success for me over the years. It is also understood that the formulation of the restorative materials may have a greater influence in stress than the light-curing protocol [59].

In light of our knowledge, a realistic, practical and reasonable technique for minimizing the effects of polymerization shrinkage and stress, while understanding clinical reality, would include the reasonable use of each of the variables that can alter the effect of shrinkage and stress: the choice of materials, reasonable incremental filling, and a reasonable curing protocol. Always curing the bonding layer before filling provides a buffer layer, especially when using a thick bonding system such as Clearfil SE Protect. For practical reasons, a process with fewer increments is desirable, especially with the knowledge that increments alone do not decrease stress. Each increment should be no thicker than 2 mm and at no point should increments involve both dentin and enamel at the same time, as the stiffness and strength of adhesion are very different and will lead to increased stress, and possible microgaps. The first increment should be a thin layer of elastic liner, usually flowable composite. After each increment, a half-cycle of cure should be applied at a distance 10 mm from the composite to decrease light intensity, as research shows that distance decreases intensity [60]. After curing each increment, begin layering the next increment. It is desirable to allow 2 minutes to elapse before curing the next increment, to allow for the greatest amount of stress to dissipate from the previous increment. This will usually happen by default when the increment is layered carefully. Nevertheless, it is a good idea to keep track of time and not cure the next increment too quickly (Box 10.2).

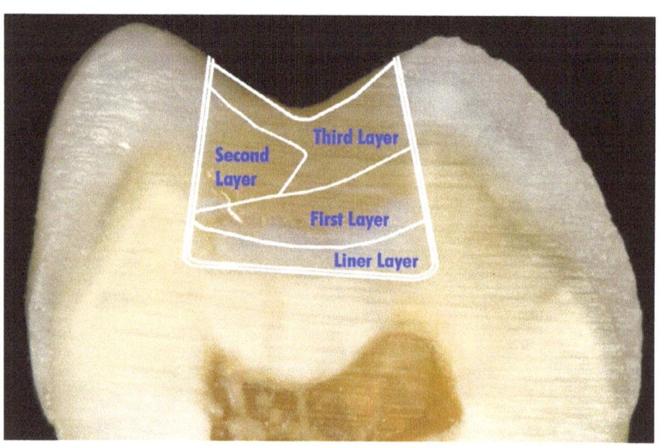

Figure 10.24 Multiple increments.

Box 10.2 The general rules for minimizing the effects of polymerization shrinkage and stress

- Use a thicker bond (e.g. Clearfil SE Bond).
- Always cure the bond.
- Avoid increments that include dentin and enamel together. These elements have different stiffness and initial bond and including them in the same increment is counterproductive.
- Increment cure should be at 10 mm from the composite and for half a cycle.
- Wait 2 minutes between cures (this generally happens without planning).
- After finishing, do a final cure before any bite adjustment.

The correct light curing of composite cannot be underestimated; the ultimate quality of the material can be dramatically affected if the composite is not correctly cured, and it can lead to weaker physical properties, color instability, and poor polish [61].

Developing Occlusal Morphology

The final stage of applying a composite is the enamel layer. This is where staining would be applied for characterization. However, this process is no longer popular with patients, so staining can easily be left out of the procedure. Developing a correct morphology of the enamel, conversely, is important and serves multiple purposes. It must be done before curing, because developing deep morphology allows for the segmentation of the occlusal composite surface, thus in theory decreasing stress during polymerization. Developing morphology with a drill after curing is also much more difficult and time consuming. A useful clinical technique to minimize excessive occlusal adjustment is to have the patient bite into the composite before the final cure. This will "mark" the bite and will allow for the development of morphology from that point, thus saving considerable time. It is important to remember that resin is hydrophobic, so water or saliva will not affect resin placed on the tooth. After applying the enamel composite, the uncured composite can be shaped using a deep acorn instrument, which will quickly form the grooves and marginal ridge (Figure 10.25). These instruments follow the morphology of the existing tooth.

First, place the acorn instrument in the center of the tooth, then drag the composite outwards to create each groove. Although rudimentary, a good comparison for this process is spreading butter on a flimsy piece of bread: To keep the bread from breaking apart, the best way is to place the butter in the center of the slice, and spread it outward, towards the crust. The excess composite should be wiped away after each drag of the acorn instrument, and the acorn should also be wiped every time.

The final step in shaping the occlusal surface is to create a triangular ridge. Place the acorn in the pit where the triangular ridge begins, then drag it outward twice diagonally toward the proximal side of the tooth in a "v" shape.

Finishing

After the final cure, there will always be flash remaining (Figure 10.26) on the facial and lingual cavosurface margins, but the most crucial area where flash will have the worst effect is in the gingival margin, because is hard to see and clean with traditional rotatory instrumentation. The risk of using a flame bur is that the tooth may be accidentally cut too much. The best way I have found to remove flash is with a sharp no. 12 blade (Figure 10.27). Using the blade to plane against the wall of the tooth, the flash is usually removed in seconds. Using this method leaves a beautiful, smooth tooth surface. There

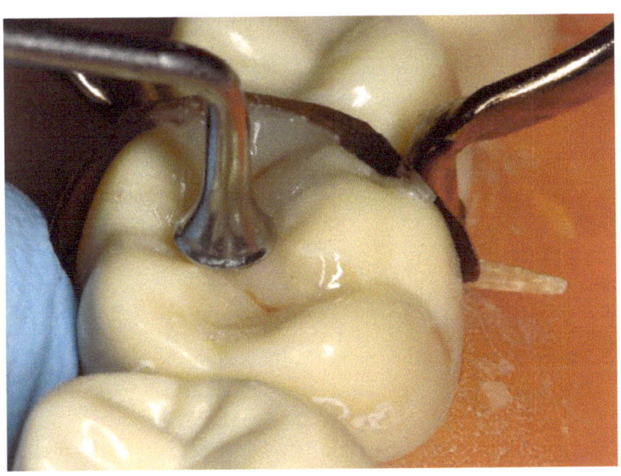

Figure 10.25 Using an acorn shape instrument (Ruiz 2 Instrument) to develop morphology.

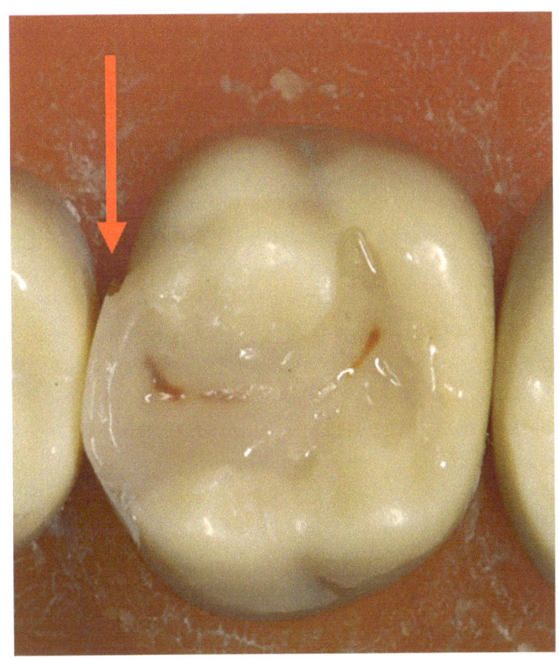

Figure 10.26 Flash is evident and it must be removed.

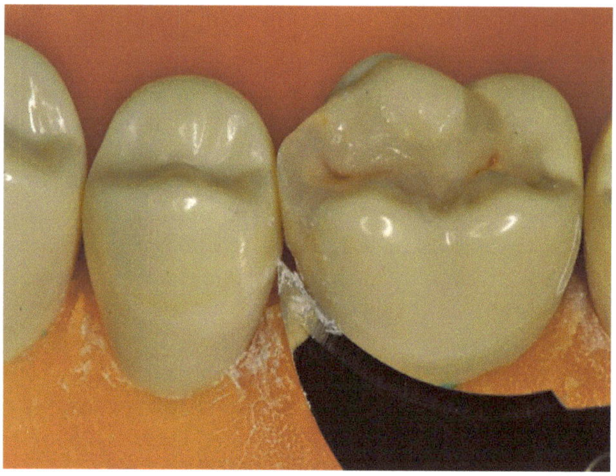

Figure 10.27 Using a no. 12 blade to remove the flash.

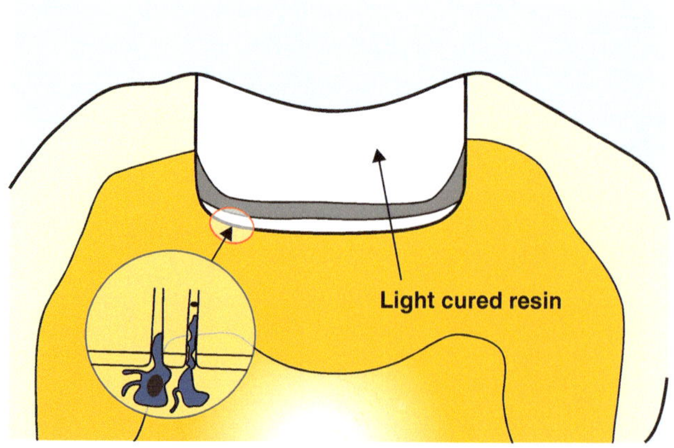

Figure 10.28 Gap formation on a shallow filling (courtesy of Dr Raymond L. Bertolotti).

are uncertainties about using a blade, as it may make the clinician nervous of cutting the patient or themselves. The following steps will assist in the safe use of this instrument:

1) Always use a round handle.
2) Always use two hands – one as a fulcrum, one to apply the force. This will minimize the risk of slipping.
3) Use a sharp blade.
4) Tactile sensation will guide and will inform when the surface is smooth.

A final cure is done next. The best way to ensure that the entire tooth is cured through is to place a 0.5 mm layer of oxygen inhibitor over the entire tooth prior to curing.

Postoperative Sensitivity

Postoperative sensitivity is still a major concern with direct composites. A common reason for this is a gap formation. If there is a gap (Figure 10.28), then biting down causes less pain than opening after the bite [62]. Fluid going out causes more pain then going in. This fact can separate the cause of sensitivity from occlusion issues. There is no good way of overcoming this problem after the fact. Following the protocol described in this chapter will minimize or eliminate postoperative sensitivity problems related to gap formation.

An additional and common cause of postoperative sensitivity is a restoration that does not take account of correct occlusion. There is a simple way to make sure the restoration will not cause sensitivity or pain due to occlusion. Place the patient in a supine position if not already. The tooth must be dry and isolated. The clinician must have two different colors of articulating paper on hand. Place the first color (blue) on the newly restored tooth or teeth and ask the patient to tap their teeth together twice firmly ("tap, tap"). If one area strikes more heavily than another, smooth it down and adjust accordingly. Everything must strike evenly (Figure 10.29). It is desirable to have contact along the central groove and the working cusp, but it may not be possible in every case, as the patient may have a malocclusion.

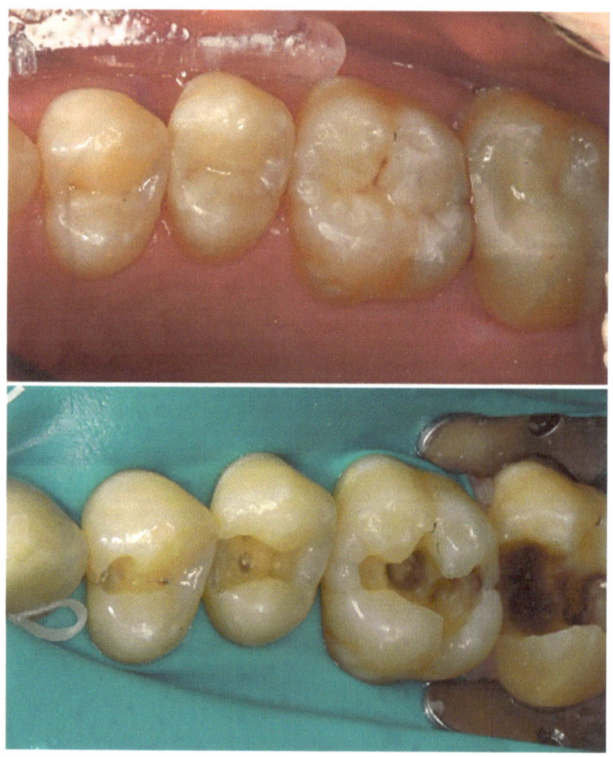

Figure 10.29 Before and after the finished restoration.

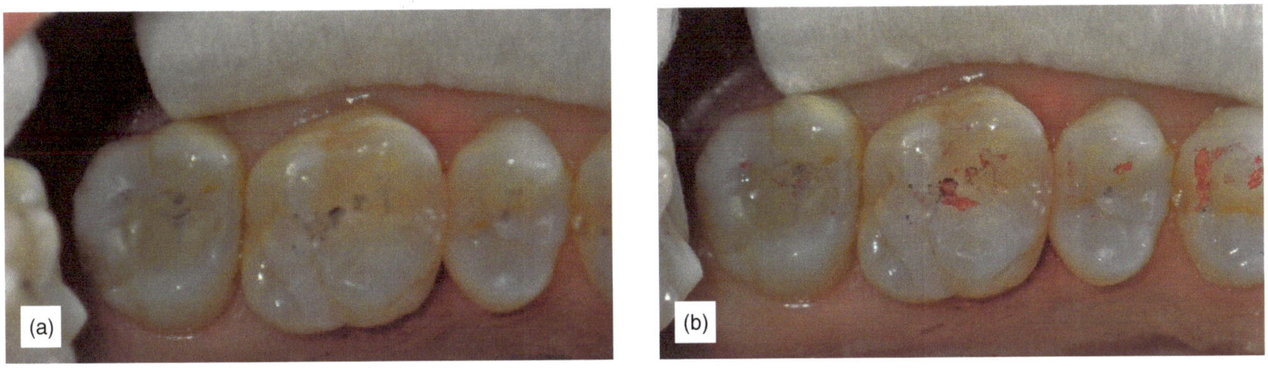

Figure 10.30 (a) Adjust maximum intercuspation contact. (b) Remove any red interferences; any red outside the blue must be removed.

After the initial adjustment, the second paper should be placed (red) and the patient should be asked to grind ("grind your teeth, slide your jaw front, back, sideways, and exaggerate the movements"). If there is any red apparent outside the blue on the patient's tooth, it must be removed (Figure 10.30). Red outside blue indicates a lateral interference, which can cause postoperative sensitivity.

If the clinician should notice that there is an interference in a part of the tooth that is unrestored, this should also be adjusted. Sometimes a patient may already have some minor or subclinical sensitivity on the tooth [63] to be restored due to hyperocclusion, and the restorative procedure may amplify the sensitivity. Any pain that the patient may feel after the restoration may be blamed on the procedure [64].

Step by Step Filling and Finishing Class II Direct Composite Restorations

Step 1: Isolate correctly and ensure that the adjacent tooth has correct morphology. Reshape if necessary (Figure 10.31a).

Step 2: Place a matrix band. If the band is too tight, a wedge can help to position the matrix, then remove wedge and replace the band, ensuring a tight gingival seal. Place the ring (Figure 10.31b).

Step 3: Selectively etch the enamel, especially uncut enamel, for 10 seconds, carefully avoiding dentin. Using a thick no-drip etch such as SureEtch® Gel (Danville) will make the process more predictable. Rinse well with water and air, then dry using air, until the dentin is not shiny and the etched enamel is frosty (Figure 10.31c).

Step 4: Apply primer for 20–25 seconds on enamel and dentin, followed by full removal of the solvent using visual confirmation (Figure 10.31d).

Step 5: Apply a thin layer of bond. If necessary, air thin and cure.

Step 6: Place a thin, (less than 1 mm) layer of flowable material along the proximal cavosurface margin and the occlusal floor. Perform an "incremental cure" (half of cycle at 10 mm from the composite; Figure 10.31e).

Step 7: Apply a 1.5 mm increment of restorative composite on the dentin, remaining within the dentin. Incrementally cure again (Figure 10.31f).

Step 8: Apply the final enamel increment of restorative composite. Develop morphology using an acorn instrument before curing. Deeper morphology and grooves will decrease stress. Incrementally cure (Figure 10.31g).

Step 9: Use a no. 12 scalpel blade to trim excess composite from the gingival margin and proximal flash (Figure 10.31h).

Step 10: Remove excess composite from the occlusal surface using a dry 12-bladed, carbide bullet-shaped bur (Figure 10.31i).

Step 11: Round the proximal marginal ridge with a Sof-Lex™ (3M) disc if necessary (Figure 10.31j).

Step 12: Apply the final cure using an oxygen inhibitor.

Step 13: Check occlusion (see Chapters 12 and 13).

Step 14: Give a final polish using a Jiffy brush (Figure 10.31k).

Step by Step Filling and Finishing Class III Direct Composite Restorations

Step 1: Do a shade test to make sure that the correct composite shade is being used. Place a small dot of composite on the facial surface of the healthy part of the tooth, cure and confirm the correct shade.

Step 2: Isolate correctly.

Step 3: Place a blue view matrix band. If the band is too tight, a wedge can help to position the matrix. Remove wedge and replace the band, ensuring a tight gingival seal.

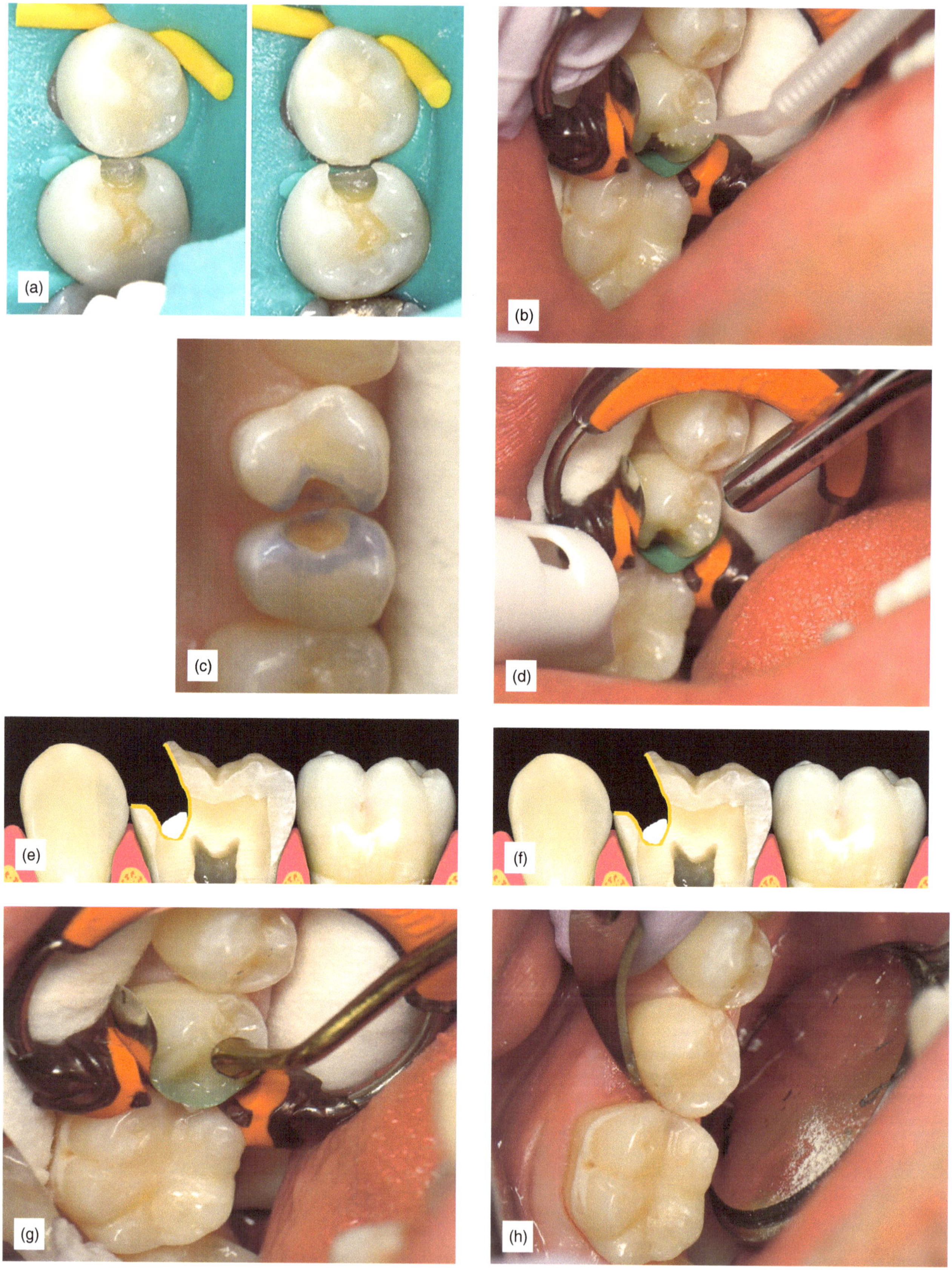

Figure 10.31 (a) Isolation. (b) Ring in place. (c) Selective etching for 10 seconds. (d) Drying of primer's solvent. (e) Placing the flowable material. (f) Two mm increments. (g) Developing deep morphology with an acorn instrument. (h) Number 12 Bard-Parker blade to remove excess. *(Continued)*

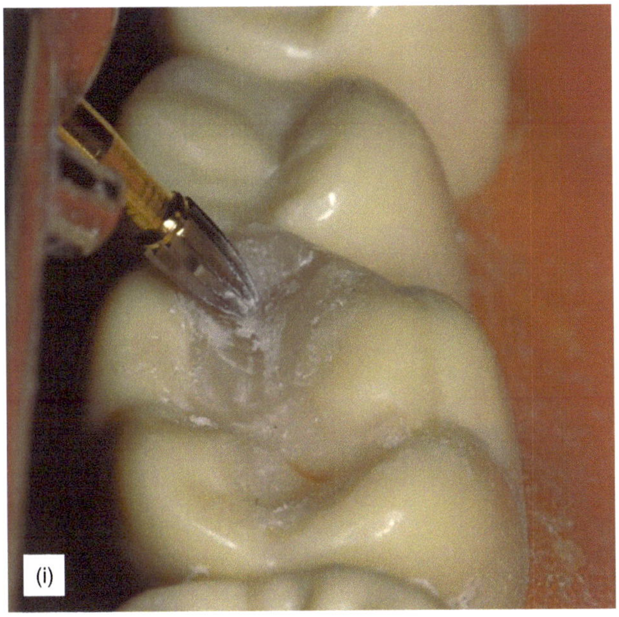

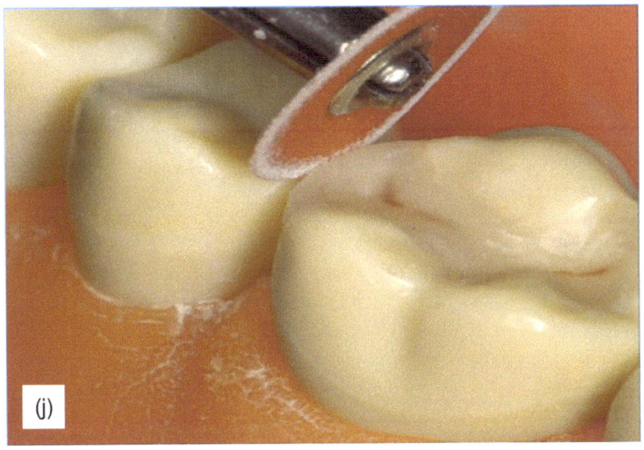

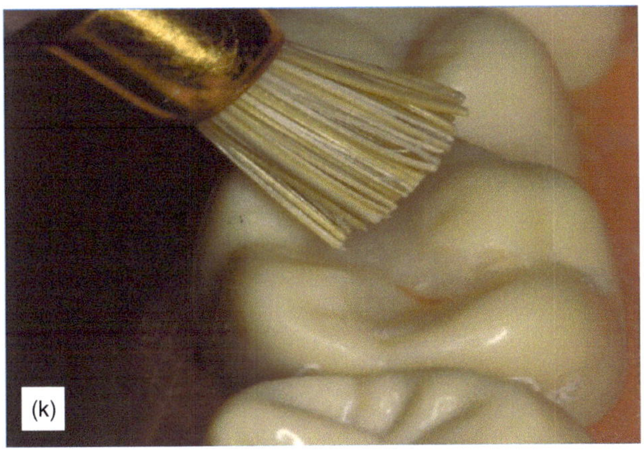

Figure 10.31 (*Continued*)
(i) Removing flash with 7406 (Brasseler) carbide. (j) Sof-Lex™ is used to finish and round marginal ridge. (k) Polishing with a Jiffy (Ultradent) brush.

Step 4: Selectively etch the enamel, especially the uncut enamel, for 10 seconds, carefully avoiding the dentin. Using a thick no-drip etch will make the process more predictable. Rinse very well with water and air, then dry using air, until the dentin is not shiny.

Step 5: Apply a primer for 20–25 seconds to enamel and dentin, then fully remove the solvent using visual confirmation.

Step 6: Apply a thin layer of bond. If necessary, air thin and cure.

Step 7: Place thin layer of flowable material which matches the restorative composite in the pulpal wall and the gingival floor. Cure for one cycle at 10 mm from tooth.

Step 8: Place a final increment of restorative composite, and shape. Cure for one cycle at 10 mm. Ideally, there should be 2 minutes between cures.

Step 9: Use a no. 12 scalpel blade to trim excess composite from the gingival margin and proximal flash.

Step 10: Remove excess composite from the occlusal surface using a dry 12-bladed, carbide bullet-shaped bur.

Step 11: Round the proximal marginal ridge with a Sof-Lex™ disc if necessary.

Step 12: Apply a final cure using an oxygen inhibitor.

Step 13: Check occlusion (see Chapters 12 and 13).

Step 14: Give a final polish using a Jiffy brush.

References

1 Santos MJMC, Bezerra RB. Fracture resistance of maxillary premolars restored with direct and indirect adhesive techniques. *J Can Dent Assoc*, 2005; 7(18): 585–590.
2 Shor A, Nicholls JI, Phillips KM, Libman WJ. Fatigue load of teeth restored with bonded direct composite and indirect ceramic inlays in MOD class II. *Int J Prosthodont*, 2003; 16(1): 64–69.
3 Gaengler P, Hoyer I, Hoyer I, Montag R, Gaebler P. Micromorphological evaluation of posterior composites: A 10-year report. *J Oral Rehab*, 2004; 31(10): 991–1000.
4 Anusavice KJ, Shen C, Rawls HR. *Phillips Science of Dental Materials*, 12th ed. St Louis, MI: Elsevier Saunders.
5 da Rosa Rodolpho PA, Cenci MS, Donassollo TA, Loguércio AD, Demarco FF. A clinical evaluation of posterior composite restorations: 17-year findings. *J Dent*, 2006; 34(7): 427–435.
6 St-George A, Sturdevant JR, Swift EJ Jr, Thompson JY. Fracture resistance of prepared teeth restored with bonded inlays. *J Prosthet Dent*, 2003; 89(6): 551–557.
7 Pallesen U, Qvist V. Composite resin fillings and inlays: An 11-year evaluation. *Clin Oral Invest*, 2003; 7: 71–79.
8 Heymann H, Swift E, Ritter A. Fundamentals of tooth preservation and pulp protection. In *Sturdevant's Art and Science of Operative Dentistry*, 6th ed. Mosby, 2013, pp. 141–163.
9 Fusayama T. Two layers of carious dentin; diagnosis and treatment. *Oper Dent*, 1979; 4(2): 63–70.
10 Hosoda H, Fusayama T. A tooth substance saving restorative technique. *Int Dent J*, 1984; 34(1): 1–12.
11 Alleman DS, Magne P. A systematic approach to deep caries removal end points: The peripheral seal concept in adhesive dentistry. *Quintessence Int*, 2012; 43(3): 197–208.
12 Akimoto N, Yokoyama G, Ohmori K, Suzuki S, Kohno A, Cox CF. Remineralization across the resin-dentin interface: In vivo evaluation with nanoindentation measurements, EDS, and SEM. *Quintessence Int*, 2001; 32(7): 561–570.
13 Nakajima M, Ogata M, Okuda M, Tagami J, Sano H, Pashley D. Bonding to caries-affected dentin using self-etching primers. *Am J Dent*, 1999; 12(6): 309–314.
14 Akimoto Momoi Y, Kohno A, Suzuki S, Otsuki M, Suzuki S, Cox CF. Biocompatibility of Clearfil Liner Bond 2 and Clearfil AP-X system on nonexposed and exposed primate teeth. *Quintessence Int*, 1998; 29(3): 177–188.
15 Van Meerbeek B, De Munck J, Yopshida Y, Inoue S, Vargas M, Vijay P, Van Landuyt K, Lambrechts P, Vanherle G. Buonocore Memorial Lecture. Adhesion to enamel and dentin: Current status and future challenges. *Oper Dent*, 2003; 28(3): 215–235.
16 Ruiz JL, Finger WJ. Enamel margin preservation and repair technique. *J Dent Res*, 2016; 95(Spec Iss 5): Abstract 2370749.
17 Swanson TK, Feigal RJ, Tantbirojn D, Hodges JS. Effect of adhesive systems and bevel on enamel margin integrity in primary and permanent teeth. *Pediatr Dent*, 2008; 30(2): 134–140.
18 Isenberg BP, Leinfelder KF. Efficacy of beveling posterior composite resin preparations. *J Esthet Dent*, 1990; 2(3): 70–73.
19 Perdigão J, Anauate-Netto C, Carmo AR, Lewgoy HR, Cordeiro HJ, Dutra-Corrêa M, Castilhos N, Amore R. Influence of acid etching and enamel beveling on the 6-month clinical performance of a self-etch dentin adhesive. *Compend Contin Educ Dent*, 2004; 25(1): 33–47.
20 Heintze SD, Ruffieux C, Rousson V. Clinical performance of cervical restorations: A meta-analysis. *Dent Mater*, 2010; 26(10): 993–1000.
21 Inoue G, Nikaido T, Sadr A, Tagami J. Morphological categorization of acid-base resistant zones with self-etching primer adhesive systems. *Dent Mater J*, 2012; 31(2): 232–238.
22 Nurrohman H, Nikaido T, Takagaki T, Sadr A, Waidyasekera K, Kitayama S, Ikeda M, Tagami J. Dentin bonding performance and ability of four MMA-based adhesive resins to prevent demineralization along the hybrid layer. *J Adhes Dent*, 2012; 14(4): 339–348.
23 Braga RR, Hilton TJ, Ferracane JL. Contraction stress of flowable composite materials and their efficacy as stress-relieving layers. *J Am Dent Assoc*, 2003; 134(6): 721–728.
24 Ferracane JL. Developing a more complete understanding of stresses produced in dental composites during polymerization. *Dent Mater*, 2005; 21(1): 36–42.
25 Swift, Edward Jr. Enamel bonding. *J Esthetic Restorative Dent*, 2003; (15)6: 325–326.
26 Thordrup M, Isidor F, Horsted-Bindslev P. A 5 year study of direct and indirect resin composite and ceramic inlays. *Quintessence Int*, 2001; 32(3): 199–205.
27 Reich S, Wichmann M, Rinne H, Shortall A. Clinical performance of large all ceramic CAD-CAM generated restorations after 3 years. *J Am Dent Assoc*, 2004; 135: 605–612.
28 Werner JF, Tani C. Effect of relative humidity on bond strength of self-etching adhesives to dentin. *J Adhes Dent*, 2002; 4(4): 277–282.
29 Alomari QD, Reinhart JW, Boyer DB. Effect of liners on cusp deflection and gap formation in composite restorations. *Oper Dent*, 2001; 26: 406–411.
30 McCullock AJ, Smith BG. In vitro studies of cuspal movement produced by adhesive restorative materials. *Br Dent J*, 1986; 161: 405–409.
31 Christensen JG. New resin-based composites: a shrinking problem? *Clin Rep*, 2010; 3(3): 1, 3.

32 Tjan AH, Bergh BH, Lidner C. Effect of various incremental techniques on the marginal adaptation of class II composite resin restorations. *J Prosthet Dent*, 1992; 67(1): 62–66.
33 Donly KJ, Wild TW, Bowen RL, Jensen ME. An in vitro investigation of the effects of glass inserts on the effective composite resin polymerization shrinkage. *J Dent Res*, 1989; 68(8): 1234–1237.
34 Yoshikawa T, Burrow MF, Tagami J. The effects of bonding system and light curing method on reducing stress of different C-factor cavities. *J Adhes Dent*, 2001; 3(2): 177–183.
35 Tolidis K, Nobecourt A, Randall RC. Effect of a resin-modified glass ionomer liner on volumetric polymerization shrinkage of various composites. *Dent Mater*, 1998; 14: 417–423.
36 Ruiz JL, Mitra S. Utilizing RMGI as a liner for direct composite restorations. *Compend Contin Educ Dent*, 2006; 27(6): 347–51.
37 Ruiz JL. Effect of new liner on polymerization shrinkage of resin cements. *J Dent Res*, 2007; 86(Spec Iss A): 2014.
38 Peumans M, Kanumilli P. Clinical effectiveness of contemporary adhesives: a systematic review of current clinical trials. *Dent Mater*, 2005; 21(9): 864–881.
39 Aboushala A, Kugel G, Hurley E. Class II composite resin restorations using glass-ionomer liners: microleakage studies. *J Clin Pediatr Dent*, 1996; 21(1) 67–70.
40 Miller MB, Castellanos IR, Vargas MA, Denehy GE. Effect of restorative material on microleakage of class II composites. *J Esth Dent*, 1996; 8: 107–113.
41 Opdam NJ, Bronkhorst EM, Roeters JM, Loomans BA. Longevity and reasons for failure of sandwich and total-etch posterior composite resin restorations. *J Adhes Dent*, 2007; 9(5): 469–475.
42 Alomari QD, Reinhart JW, Boyer DB. Effect of liners on cusp deflection and gap formation in composite restorations. *Oper Dent*, 2001; 26: 406–411.
43 Marovic D, Tauböck TT, Attin T, Panduric V, Tarle Z. Monomer conversion and shrinkage force kinetics of low-viscosity bulk-fill resin composites. *Acta Odontol Scand*, 2014; 29: 1–7.
44 Scotti N, Comba A, Gambino A, Paolino DS, Alovisi M, Pasqualini D, Berutti E. Microleakage at enamel and dentin margins with a bulk fill flowable resin. *Eur J Dent*, 2014; 8(1): 1–8.
45 Do T, Church B, Veríssimo C, Hackmyer SP, Tantbirojn D, Simon JF, Versluis A. Cuspal flexure, depth-of-cure, and bond integrity of bulk-fill composites. *Pediatr Dent*, 2014; 36(7): 468–473.
46 Benetti A, Havndrup-Pedersen C, Honoré D, Pedersen M, Pallesen U. Bulk-fill resin composites: polymerization contraction, depth of cure, and gap formation. *Oper Dent*, 2015; 40(2): 190–200.
47 Ilie N, Stark K. Effect of different curing protocols on the mechanical properties of low-viscosity bulk-fill composites. *Clin Oral Investig*, 2015; 19(2): 271–279.
48 Korkmaz Y, Ozel E, Attar N. Effect of flowable composite lining on microleakage and internal voids in Class II composite restorations. *J Adhes Dent*, 2007; 9(2): 189–194.
49 Kwon Y, Ferracane J, Lee IB. Effect of layering methods, composite type, and flowable liner on the polymerization shrinkage stress of light cured composites. *Dent Mater*, 2012; 28(7): 801–809.
50 Versluis A, Douglas WH, Cross M, Sakaguchi RL. Does an incremental filling technique reduce polymerization shrinkage stresses? *J Dent Res*, 1996; 75(3): 871–878.
51 Hardan LS, Amm EW, Ghayad A, Ghosn C, Khraisat A. Effect of different modes of light curing and resin composites on microleakage of Class II restorations. Part II. *Odontostomatol Trop*, 2009; 32(126): 29–37.
52 Kanca J III, Suh BI. Pulse activation: reducing resin-based composite contraction stresses at the cavosurface margins. *Am J Dent*, 1999; 12(3): 107–112.
53 Deliperi S, Bardwell DN. An alternative method to reduce polymerization shrinkage in direct posterior composite restorations. *J Am Dent Assoc*, 2002; 133(10): 1387–1398.
54 Muangmingsuk A, Senawongse P, Yudhasaraprasithi S. Influence of different softstart polymerization techniques on marginal adaptation of Class V restorations. *Am J Dent*, 2003; 16(2): 117–179.
55 Friedl KH, Schmalz G, Hiller KA, Märkl A. Marginal adaption of Class V restorations with and without "softstart-polymerization". *Oper Dent*, 2000; 25(1): 26–32.
56 Christensen GJ. Save time, effort, and money with fast, new LED curing lights. *Clin Rep*, 2010; 3(10): 1–3.
57 Bouschlicher MR, Rueggeberg FA, Boyer DB. Effect of stepped light intensity on polymerization force and conversion in a photoactivated composite. *J Esthet Dent*, 2000; 12(1): 23–32.
58 Ferracane JL. Buonocore Lecture. Placing dental composites: A stressful experience. *Oper Dent*, 2008; 33(3): 247–257.
59 Christensen JG. Save time, effort, and money with fast, new led curing lights. *Clin Rep*, 2010; 3(10): 1–3.
60 Felix CA, Price RBT. The effect of distance from light source on light intensity from curing lights. *Adhes Dent*, 2003; 5(4): 283–291.
61 Patel SB, Gordan VV, Barret AA, Shen C. The effect of surface finishing and storage media on bi-axial flexure strength and microhardness of resin-based composite. *J Am Dent Assoc*, 2003; 28(5): 560–567.
62 Fusayama T. Factors and prevention of pulp irritation by adhesive composite restorations. *Quintessence Int*, 1987; 18: 633–641.
63 Berkowitz G, Horowitz A Curro FA, Craig RG, Ship JA, Vena D, Thompson VP. Postoperative hypersensitivity in class I resin-based composite restorations in general practice: Interim results. *Compend Contin Educ Dent*, 2009; 30(6): 356–363.
64 Ruiz JL. Occlusal disease: Restorative consequences and patient education. *Dent Today*, 2007; 26(9): 90–95.

Part VI

Crown Replacement

11

Full Crowns: Are They Still Necessary?

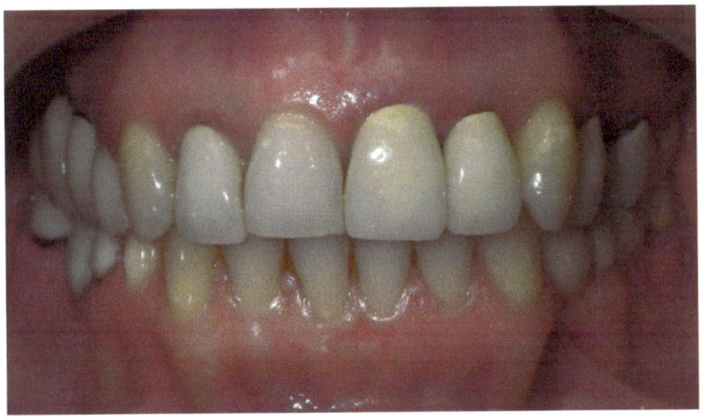

A mouth full of crowns.

Indications for Full Non-Metal Crowns

Most of the time, the indication for a full non-metal crown will be replacing an existing full crown (Figure 11.1a–e). On rare occasions, caries literally envelopes every surface of the tooth, and a full coverage crown is indicated. Even in such cases, however, the additional removal of healthy tooth to create the axial wall and any other form of mechanical retention is unnecessary. Crowns may also be used as abutments for a fix prosthesis, although adhesive techniques and improved materials offer new options, such as bonded bridges (Figures 11.2a–e, 11.3a–d). Full crowns are used as a final restoration covering the abutments of an implant, and even in these cases supragingival margins are desirable and make it easier to remove cement on cemented crowns (Figures 11.4a–d, 11.5a,b). Regardless of the indication, thanks to better restorative materials, full crowns today should be very different from those used in the past. More translucent restorative materials for crowns allow for a more supragingival margin placement whenever possible. The choice of restorative material for a full crown is very important. The correct choice of restorative material for the specific needs of full crowns will dictate the amount of tooth reduction required, margin placement and choice of cement to be used.

The Options in Non-Metal Restorative Materials for Full Crowns

There are several choices for restorative materials specifically for full crowns, each with different characteristics, and it would be a mistake to use one for all cases. The choice of the restorative material depends on the condition of the tooth after the removal of the old crown, the margin location, the cement to be used, and where the tooth is located in the mouth (anterior or posterior area). Understanding that anterior and posterior teeth have very different thresholds for esthetic requirements, as well as occlusal loads and forces, means that material choices will vary based on those requirements.

The indications and space requirements for each material differ, with specific consideration for full crowns. This chapter considers the current most popular restorative materials for crowns, discussed from the weakest and most translucent to the strongest and least translucent [1]. An important additional consideration is that the thickness of the material alters its level of translucency [2], so its blending ability will contribute to its strength as well as the thickness of the material [3].

Leucite-reinforced feldspathic porcelain

Leucite-reinforced feldspathic porcelain, layered or pressed, is an option in the anterior region when margins are supragingival and there is a good amount of remaining enamel for adhesive luting, the adjacent teeth are being treated with feldspathic veneers and the esthetic demands are great (Figure 11.6a–d). Using leucite-reinforced feldspathic porcelain for full crowns in the posterior area is questionable, although it has been popular with computer-aided designed and manufactured (CAD-CAM) crowns. Because of its intrinsic weakness, this material depend on adhesion for its strength and a strong enamel substrate is very desirable. Subgingival margins are undesirable because they complicate adhesion. Generally speaking, this material

Supra-Gingival Minimally Invasive Dentistry: A Healthier Approach to Esthetic Restorations, First Edition. By Jose-Luis Ruiz.

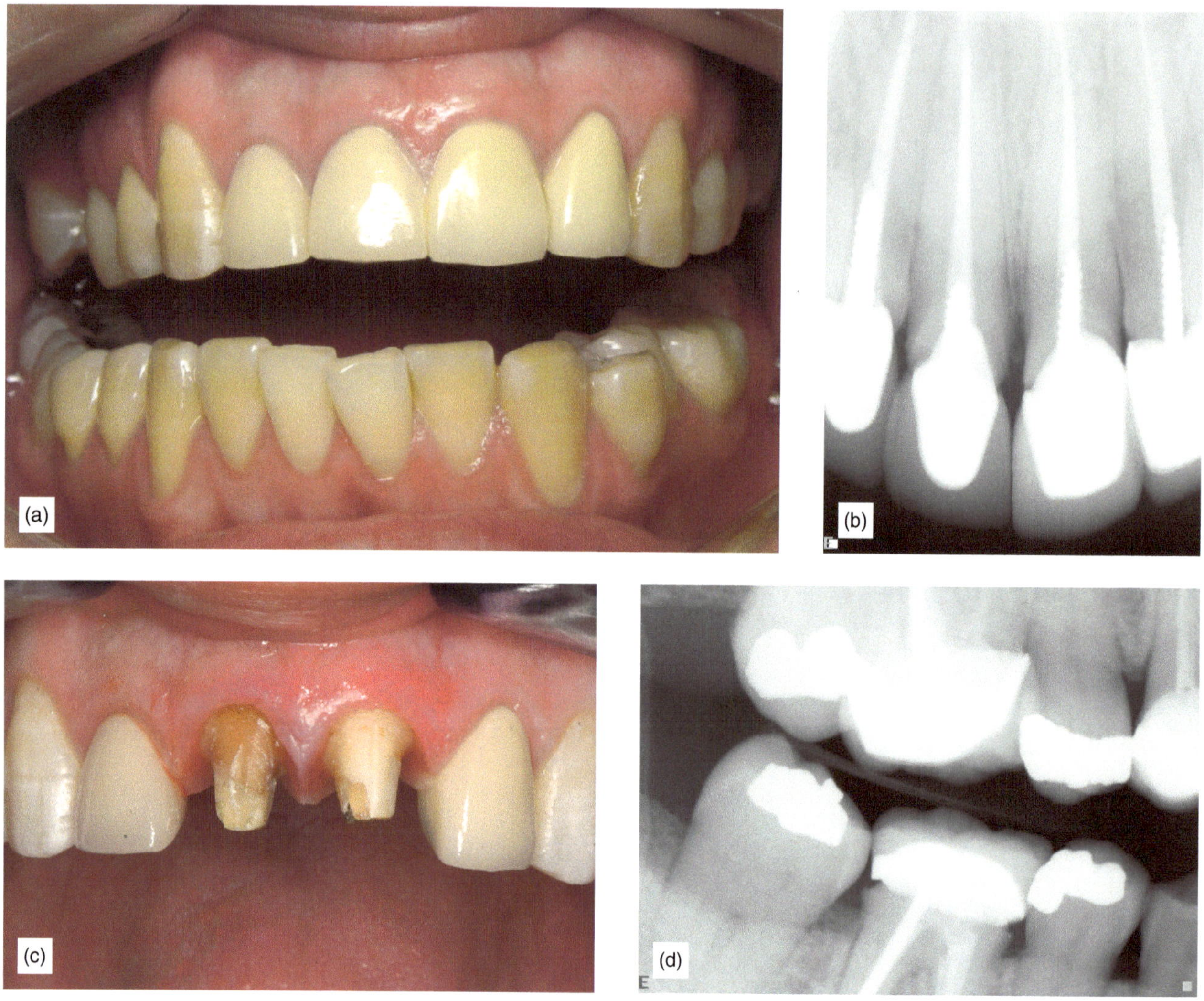

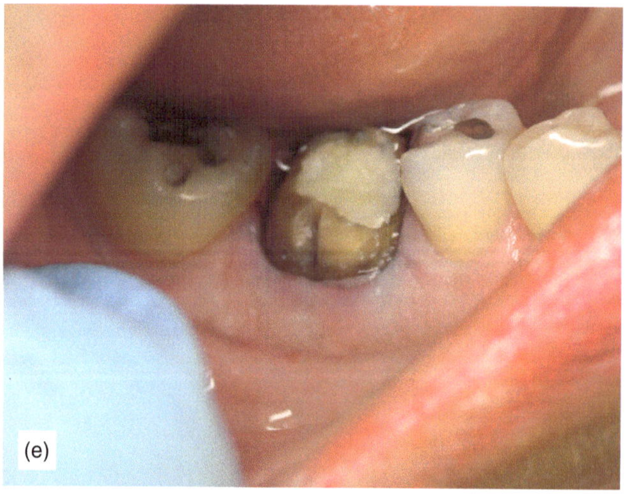

Figure 11.1 (a) While the clinical appearance is acceptable, the patient experienced bad odor and inflammation. (b) Radiographically, it is clear why subgingival margins can be so unhealthy. (c) After crowns were removed, it is evident that the proximal margins are very subgingival, which made good results difficult to achieve. (d) A separate posterior case, showing wide open subgingival margins. (e) It is clear how a short clinical crown was the reason that margins were placed so far subgingivally looking for mechanical retention, a facial groove was added for retention. Subgingival margins are usually very unpredictable.

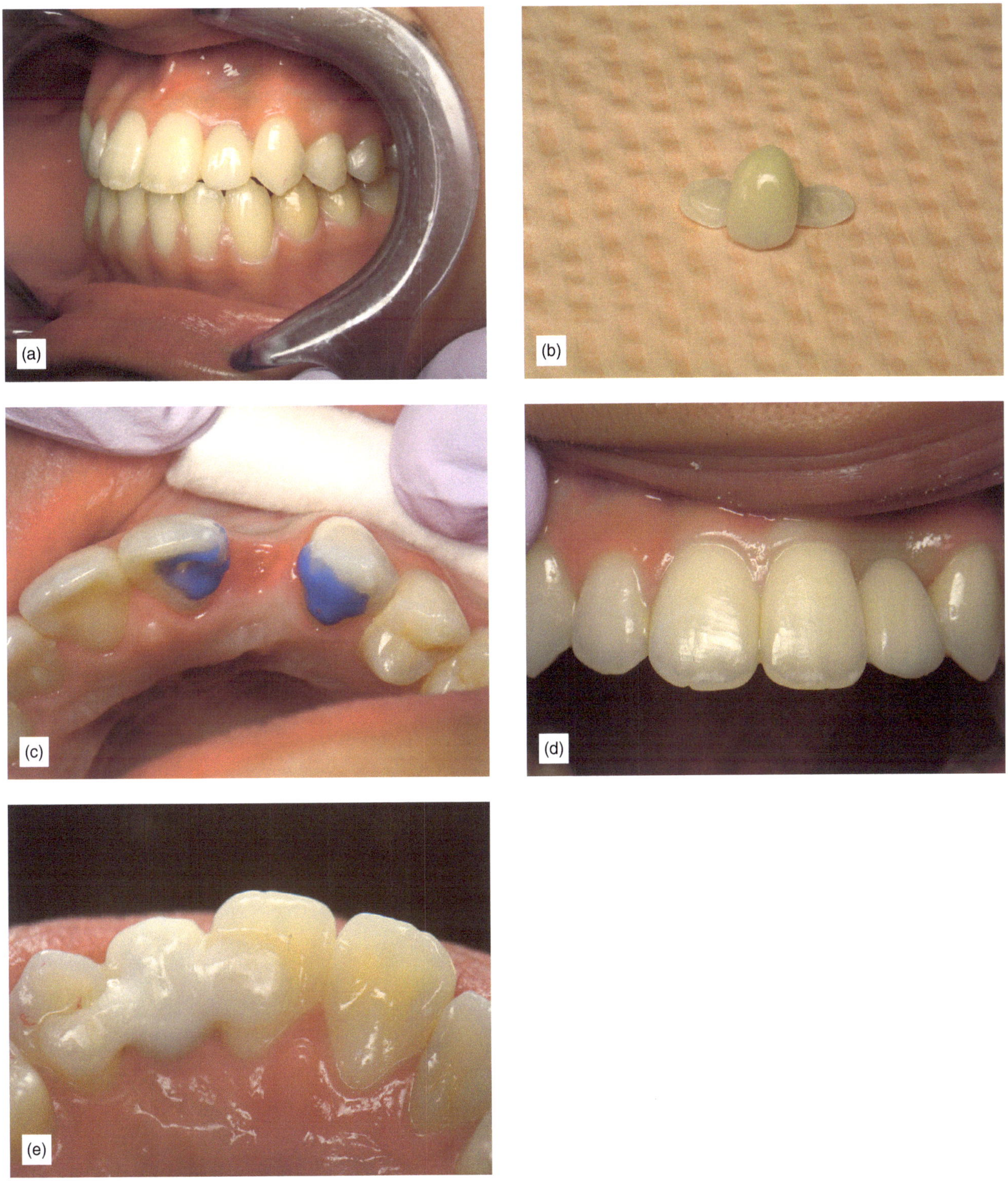

Figure 11.2 (a) Nice results on a bonded bridge case. The left lateral incisor is the pontic, and very little overbite gives the necessary space for lingual wings. (b) Zirconia Maryland bridge. (c) Bonding procedure, etching of enamel. (d) Facial view. (e) Large lingual wings are possible because, as (a) shows, there is minimal overbite and there is no occlusion on them.

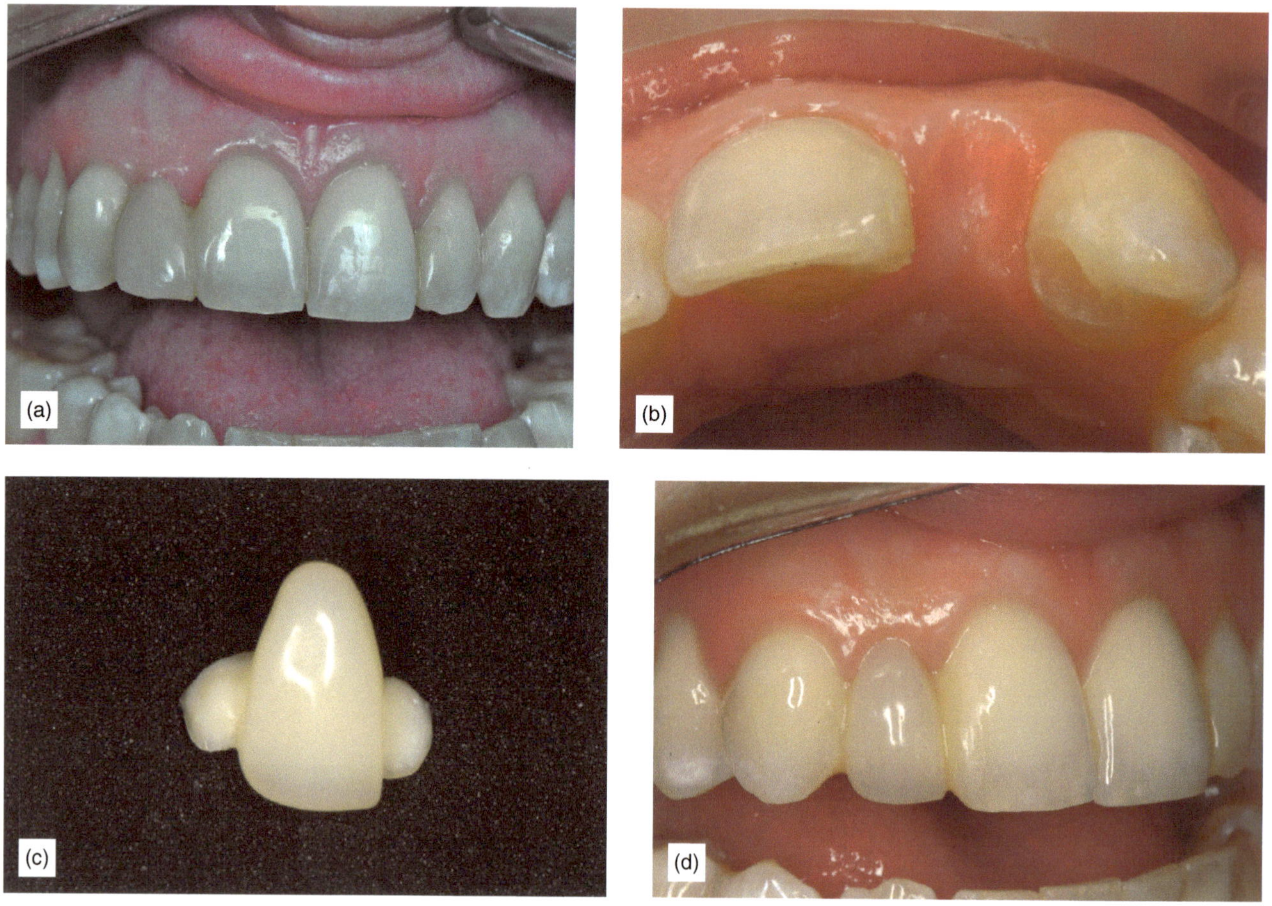

Figure 11.3 (a) A 3-year-old, chairside composite bonded bridge, with an unhygienic pontic and embrasures. (b) After an ovate pontic was developed. (c) Zirconia Maryland bridge. (d) A very esthetic and hygienic result.

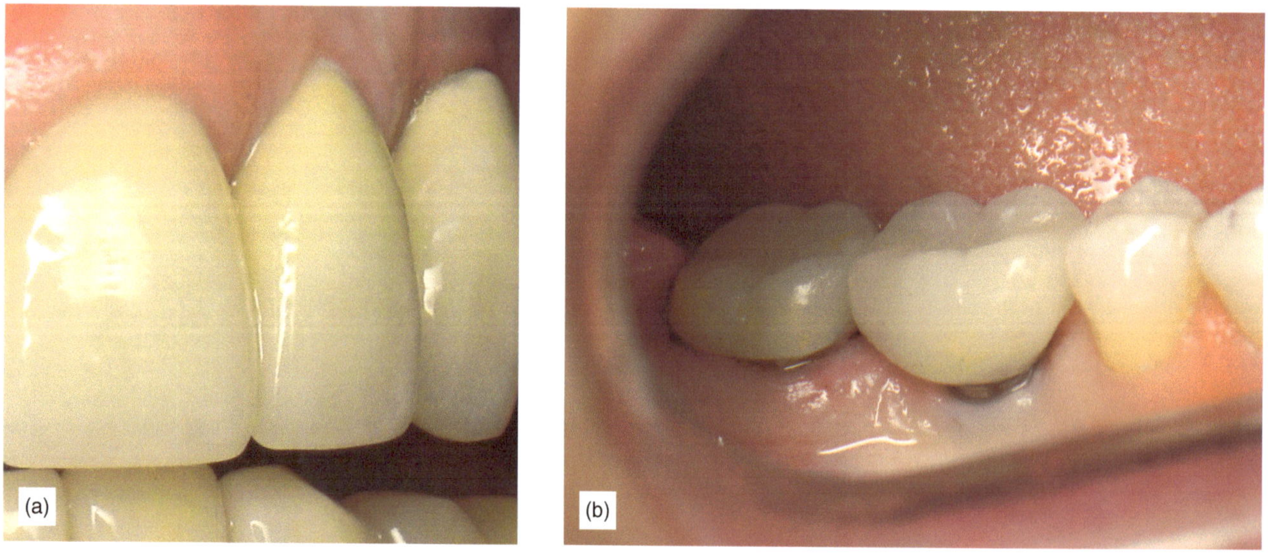

Figure 11.4 (a) Supragingival zirconia abutment, showing excellent esthetic results, with almost zero risk of subgingival leftover cement. (b) Supragingival crown on a titanium abutment. Some visible metal has no esthetic consequences in the lower posterior area. *(Continued)*

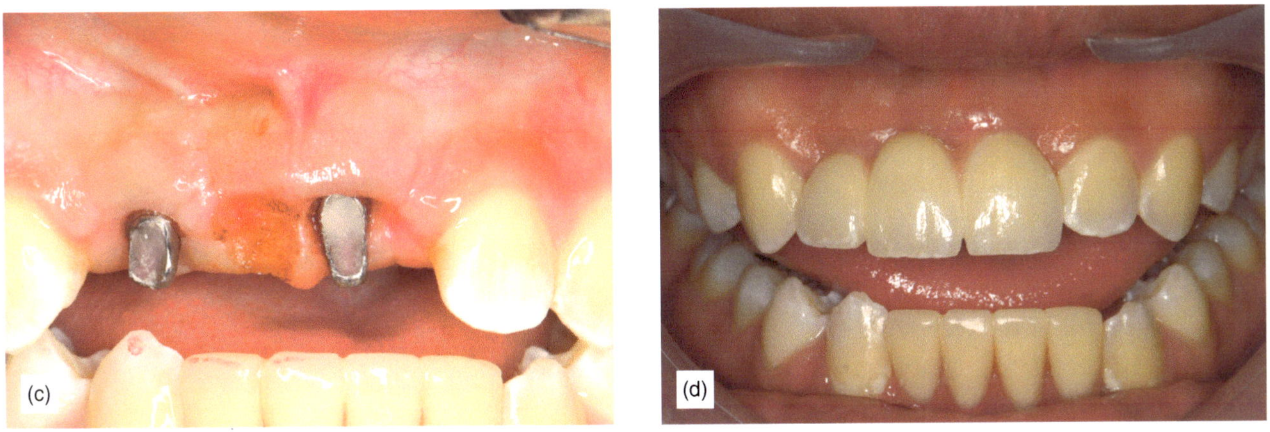

Figure 11.4 (*Continued*)
(c) Traditional deep subgingival pontic margins, which will compromise the cement cleanup. (d) An acceptable esthetic result.

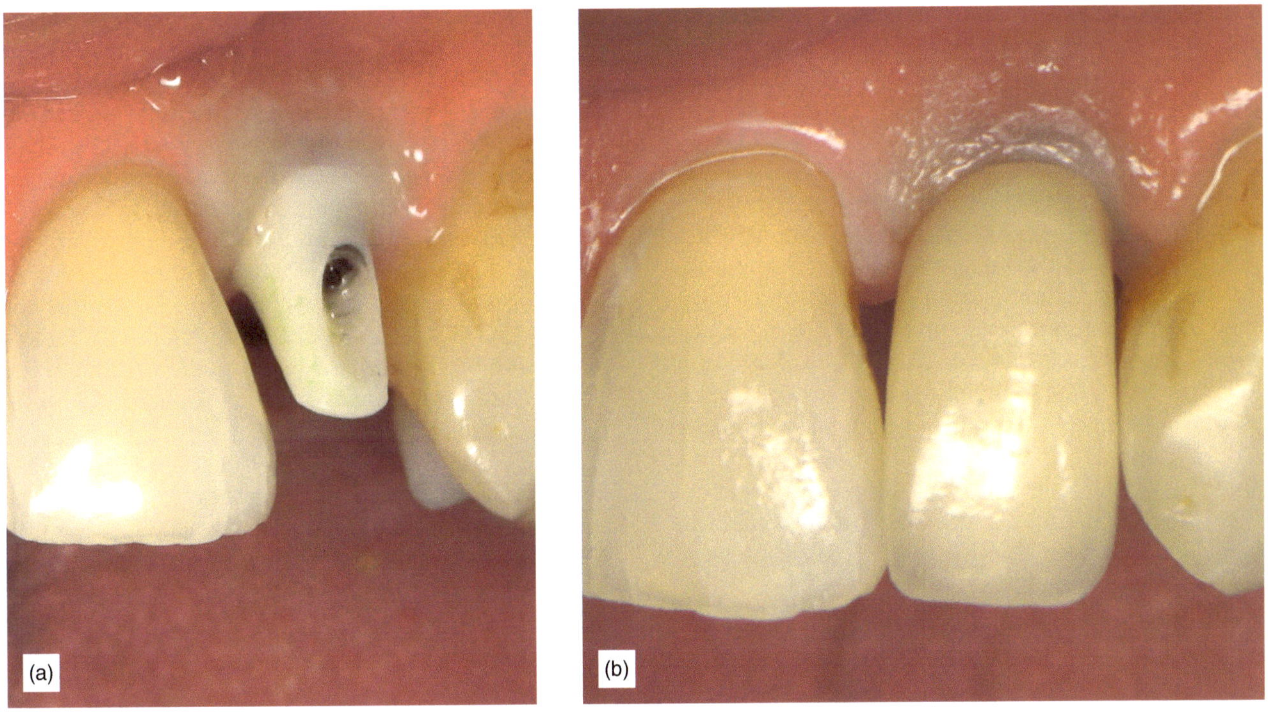

Figure 11.5 (a) Zirconia abutment in the esthetic zone with equigingival to supragingival margins. (b) Supragingival implant crown with excellent results.

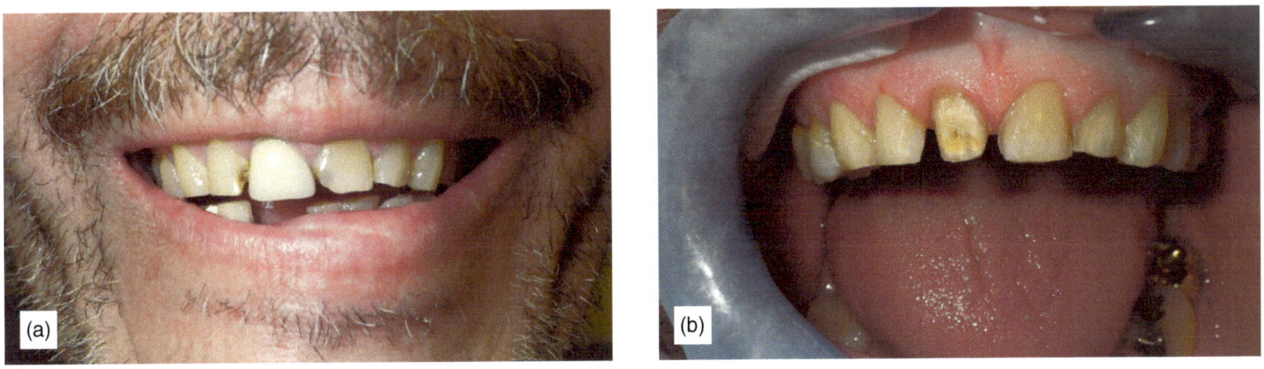

Figure 11.6 (a) Existing unesthetic porcelain-fused-to-metal crown on a right central incisor. (b) Leucite-reinforced feldspathic crown preparation (right central incisor) used along several feldspathic veneers. (*Continued*)

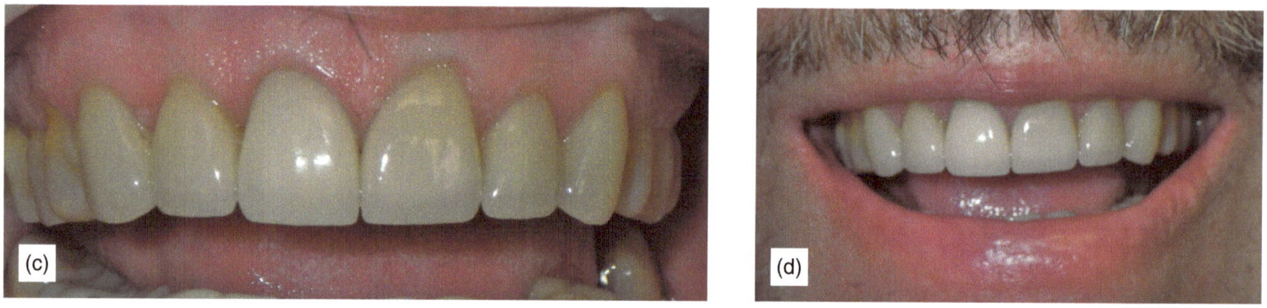

Figure 11.6 *(Continued)*
(c) Close-up of final feldspathic crown and veneers. (d) Improved smile; compare with (a).

is better used for bonded partial coverage veneers and, in rare situations, onlays [4,5]. The mode of failure of crowns made from this material is fracture of the restorative material, and for this reason they are not a primary choice (Figure 11.7a,b) [6,7].

Lithium disilicate

Lithium disilicate is unique because it can be used in two different modalities. First, bonded lithium disilicate may be used when margins are supragingival, to allow for predictable adhesive luting, because lithium disilicate is much stronger when bonded to the tooth, space requirements are less, 1 mm axial, 1.5–2 mm occlusal (Figures 11.8, 11.9). Lithium disilicate (e-Max, Ivoclar) is much stronger when bonded than when cemented. When it is bonded to mostly rigid tooth structures such as enamel, its strength can be close to that of zirconia, even when it is thinly applied, but when bonded to a less rigid structure like dentin, it is considerably less strong [3]. Lithium disilicate can be pressed or milled in a CAD-CAM machine. For many reasons, this material has quickly become the most ideal for bonded onlays [8,9]. The pressed version of e-Max appears to be a little stronger, with a better fit [10]. It comes in high-translucency and low-translucency versions. High translucency is preferable for most cases of partial coverage and supragingival margins where the cavosurface margin is considerably coronal to the gingival line and good blending is very important. Low translucency may be preferred if the color of the tooth needs to be hidden, but the disadvantage of opacious materials is that the margin line of the tooth and restoration will be very visible and will often need to be hidden, subgingivally. E-Max can also be layered, but its strength decreases considerably [11].

Second, cemented (not-bonded) lithium disilicate can be used when margins are subgingival and isolation will be difficult, requiring the use of more contamination resistant traditional crown and bridge cement, such as RMGI

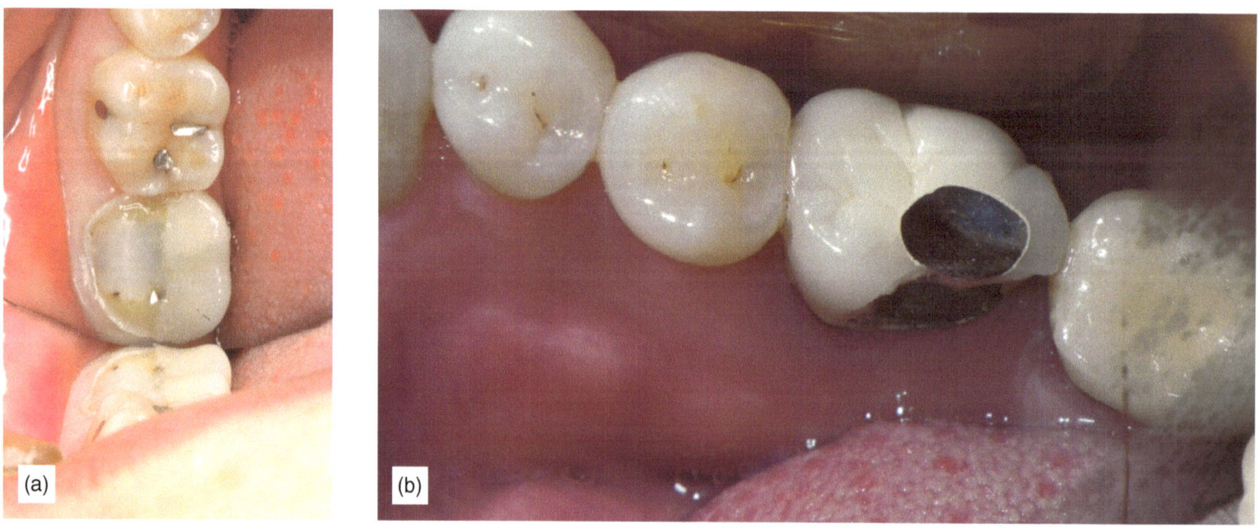

Figure 11.7 (a) Fractured feldspathic Empress crown. (b) Fractured feldspathic porcelain layered over a porcelain-fused-to-semi-precious metal.

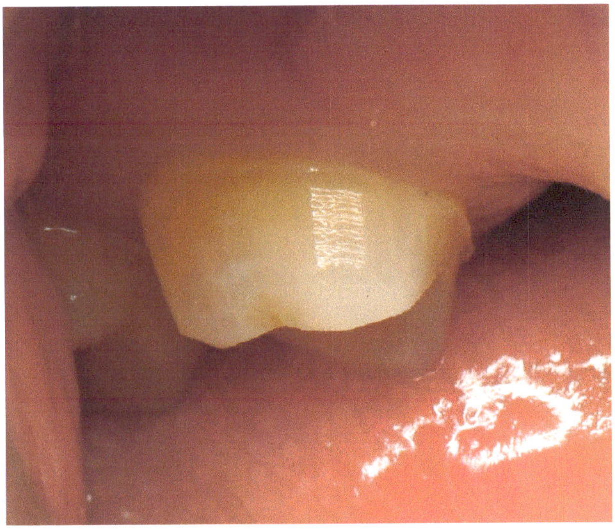

Figure 11.8 Preparation of posterior cemented e-Max.

Meron Plus AC (VOCO; Figures 11.10a,b, 11.11). Because e-Max is considerably weaker when it is cemented, the material must be thicker to increase strength, thus the space-reduction requirement will be 1.5 mm axial and 2 mm occlusal, requiring more aggressive tooth removal.

Laboratory-quality composite

Laboratory-quality composite such as Lava™ Ultimate may be used when margins are supragingival, to allow for

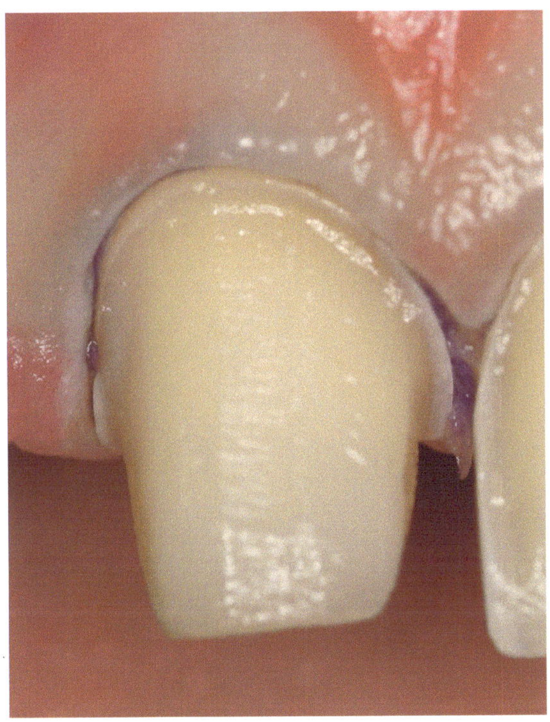

Figure 11.9 Preparation ideal for lithium disilicate-bonded anterior crown.

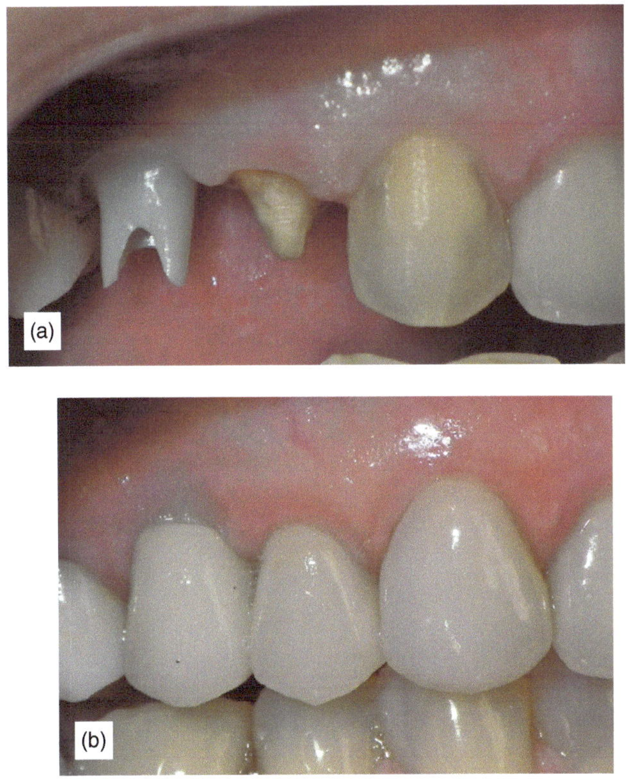

Figure 11.10 (a) The flexibility of lithium disilicate allows for use in cases with multiple substrates, the deep subgingival margins on the first premolar demand cementation versus bonding of the crowns. (b) Excellent esthetic result with two lithium disilicate-cemented crowns and one veneer.

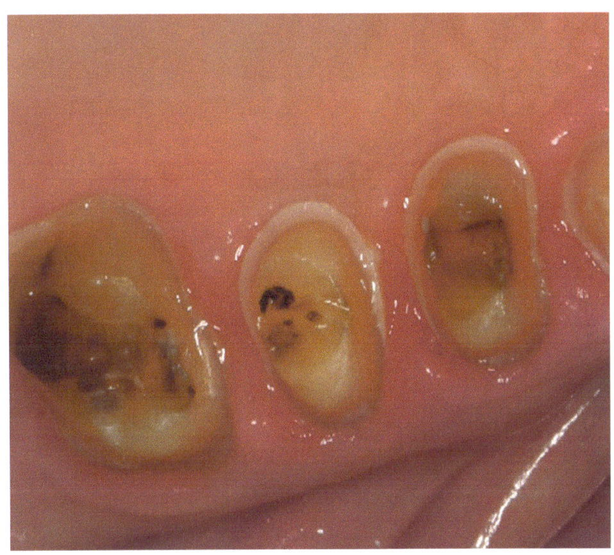

Figure 11.11 Situation in which isolation and bleeding control may be compromised, cemented lithium disilicate would be desirable choice.

adhesive luting. Because of its low flexural strength it requires more space-reduction even if bonded, 1.5 axial and 2 mm occlusal. Composite is also a popular material for CAD/CAM fabricated full crowns, and has shown good strength in this situation [12]. Composite crowns require aggressive preparation because they must be thick. Composite lacks rigidity and when the crown is thin, bending forces may lead to an increased chance of debonding, and possibly a shorter life [13,14]. Composite crowns also should be thick because of occlusal wear, and this can be considered a disadvantage in the durability of a full crown [15,16]. Finally, composite crowns should be cemented with adhesive and resin cement to increase strength, which means that subgingival margins would be contraindicated. 3M issued a statement in June 2015, indicating that Lava Ultimate should no longer be used for full crowns [17].

Zirconia

There are also two options for zirconia: monolithic and layered (PFZ). Layered zirconia can be used in the anterior and posterior area as it is esthetically pleasing and is the only non-metal material that can be used predictably for fixed partial dentures or bridges (Figure 11.12a–d). Zirconia can also be used when the margins are subgingival and adhesive cementation is very complicated. Because of its great strength, space and preparation requirements are low, at 1 mm axial and 1.5–2 mm occlusal, allowing for tooth preservation. Layered zirconia has a long history of success in dentistry [18,19,20]. Its intrinsic strength is remarkable, exceeding 1000 MPa. It can be milled into a thin coping, then a layered or pressed ceramics veneer can cover the coping, creating a layered restoration PFZ, similar to the porcelain-fused-to-metal (PFM) restorations of old.

Zirconia is very opacious unless it is used thinly. Thus, a correctly designed thin facial coping and translucent layer of porcelain allows PFZ to be far more translucent than a PFM or full zirconia crown (Figure 11.13a–e); this is not possible with full zirconia. In the anterior area, a very thin coping of 0.3 mm can be requested to allow for a restoration

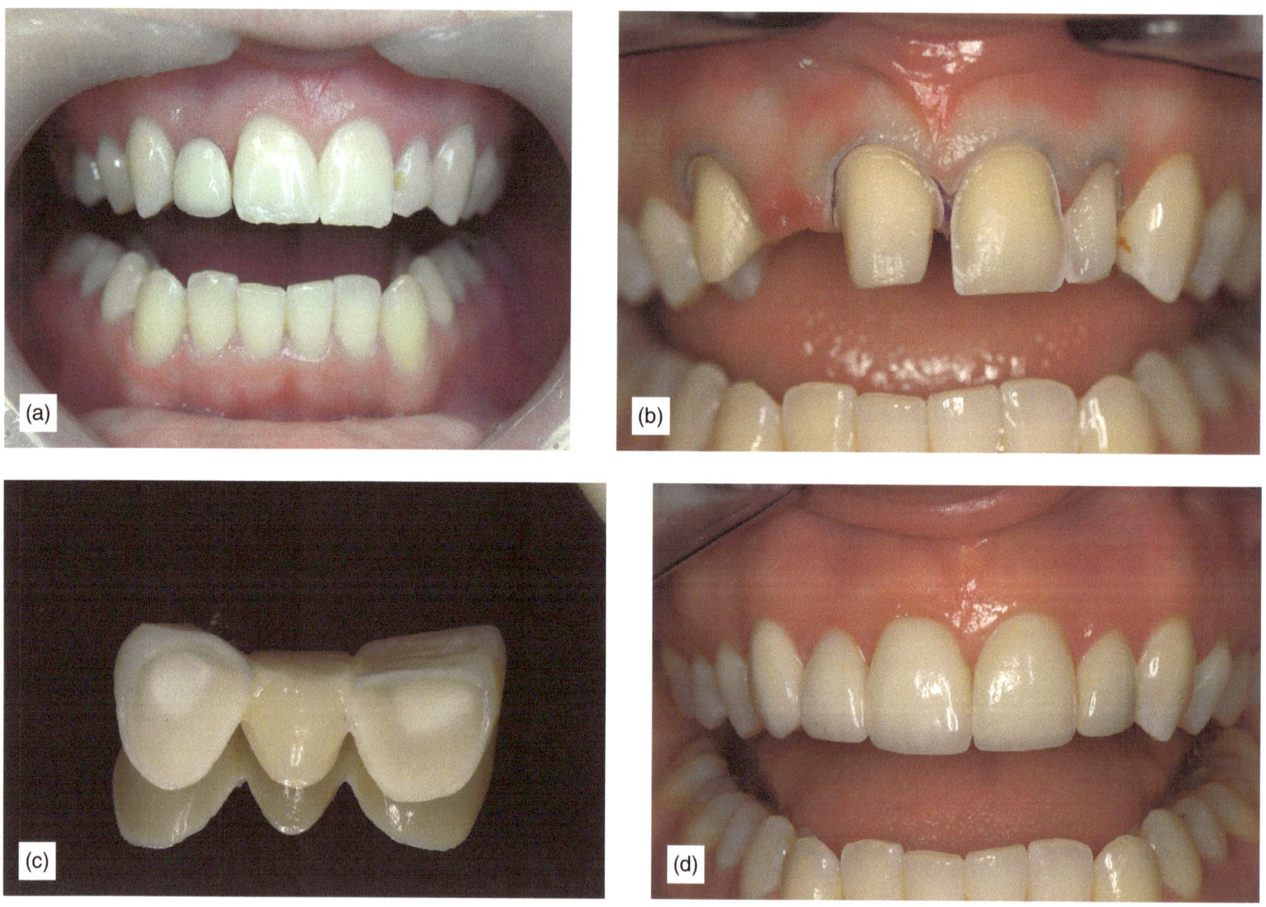

Figure 11.12 (a) Failing metal Maryland bridge. (b) Conservative supragingival preparation for layered zirconia bridge and two veneers. (c) Layered zirconia bridge with Noritake ZCR Press. (d) Excellent esthetic result combining layered zirconia bridge with Cerabien ZR Press (Kuraray) and layered Noritake veneers.

with some translucency and better marginal blending (Figure 11.13e). In the posterior, a default 0.5 mm coping is recommended, and the design of the coping is essential for success. In a long study conducted by Rella Christensen (the author is part of this study) the importance of a proper coping design was established, as well as the importance of correctly calibrated porcelain ovens and the use of the ideal veneering porcelain, such as Cerabien ZR Press (Kuraray) [18,21]. Too often, laboratories leave too much unsupported porcelain, as shown in Figure 11.14a,b, compromising the results. The coping must be designed using an anatomical design (Figure 11.15a–c). Figure 11.15b displays red wax, showing that there is 0.5 mm coping for maximum translucency on the facial and occlusal surfaces of the coping. The marginal ridges are reinforced with thicker zirconia, supporting the veneer porcelain that will be placed on top.

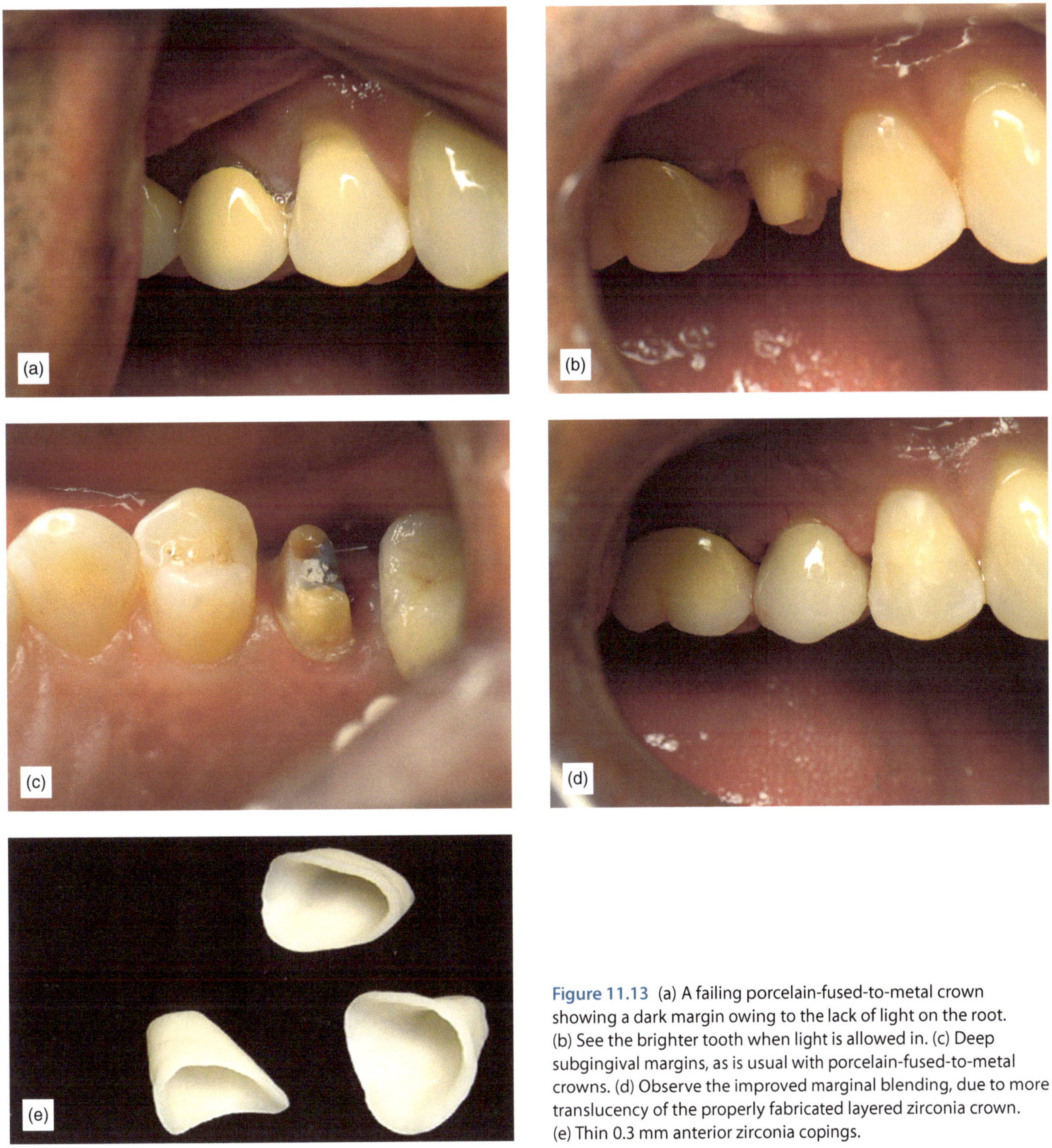

Figure 11.13 (a) A failing porcelain-fused-to-metal crown showing a dark margin owing to the lack of light on the root. (b) See the brighter tooth when light is allowed in. (c) Deep subgingival margins, as is usual with porcelain-fused-to-metal crowns. (d) Observe the improved marginal blending, due to more translucency of the properly fabricated layered zirconia crown. (e) Thin 0.3 mm anterior zirconia copings.

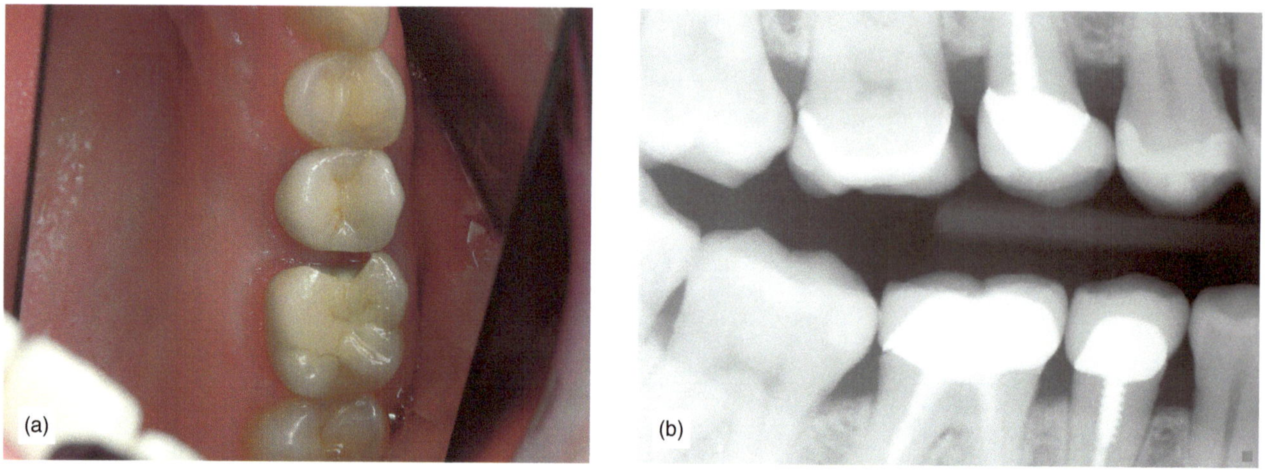

Figure 11.14 (a) Fractured veneer porcelain on marginal ridge of a layered zirconia crown. (b) X-ray shows the reason for the previous veneer porcelain fracture: an excessive amount of unsupported layering porcelain.

Monolithic zirconia may also be used when margins are subgingival, when esthetics are not important or a very thin restoration is desired, because of strength an axial reduction of 0.5 mm and 1–1.5 mm occlusal is all that is needed, allowing for tooth preservation (Figure 11.16). Monolithic or full zirconia with no external veneers has become extremely popular in recent years. Full zirconia is very opacious and unesthetic. Marginal blending is very poor and, for that reason, margins usually have to be placed subgingivally when

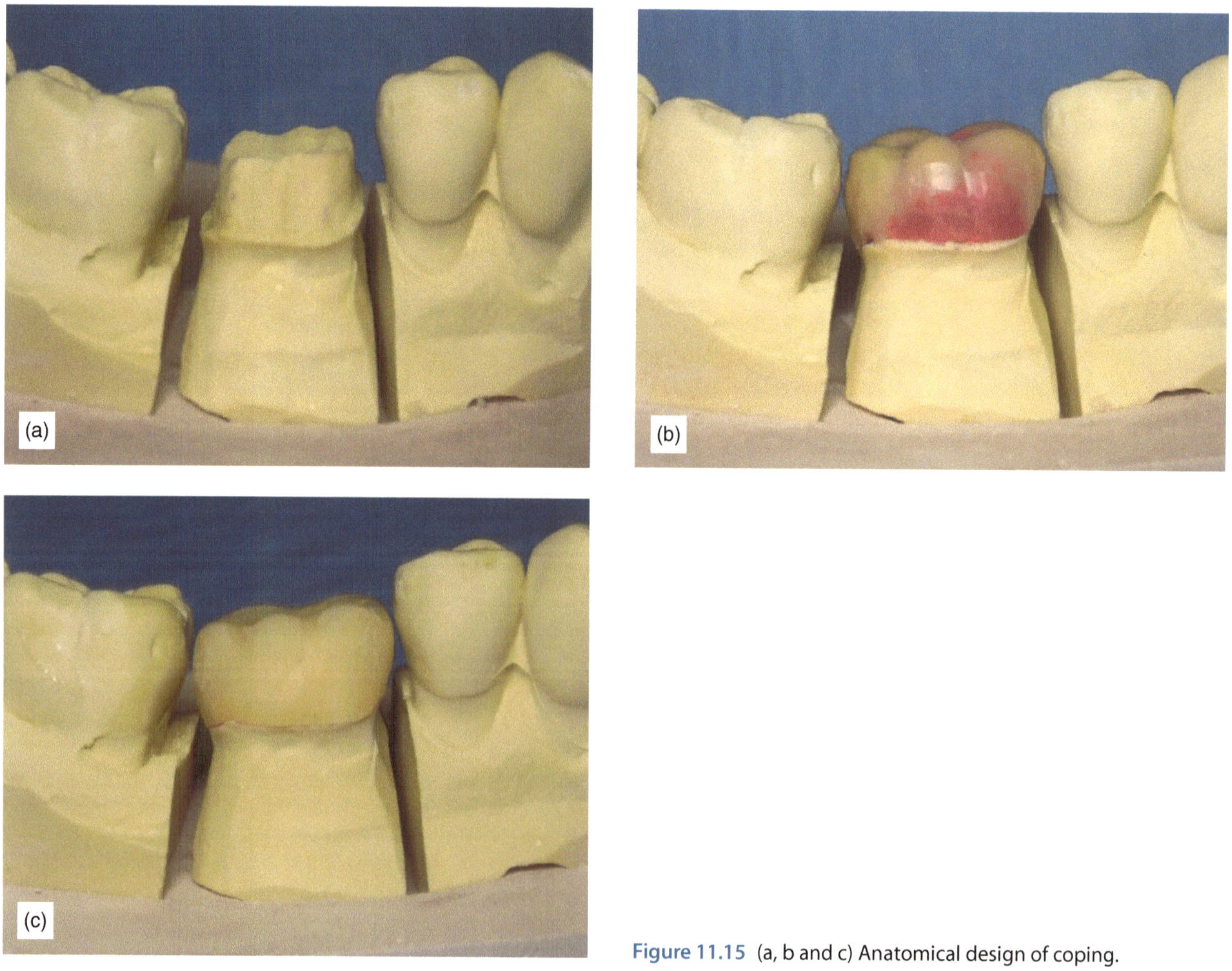

Figure 11.15 (a, b and c) Anatomical design of coping.

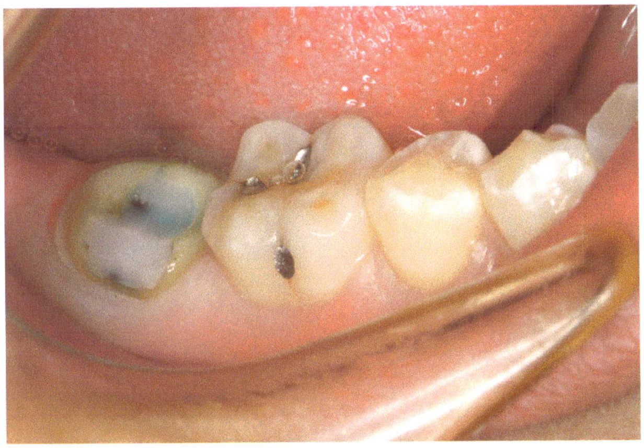

Figure 11.16 A full zirconia or monolithic crown may be desirable for a heavy bruxer with a short clinical crown on a second molar.

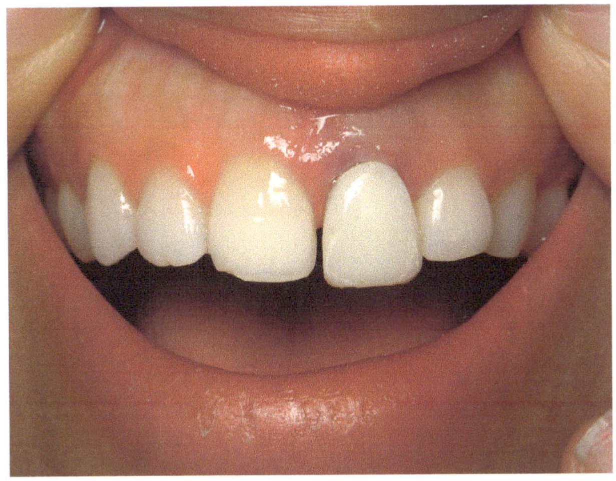

Figure 11.18 Unesthetic full zirconia margins.

used in areas that patients can see (Figures 11.17a,b, 11.18), usually forward from the molars. Outside the second and sometimes the first molars, full zirconia is usually contraindicated when supragingival minimally invasive dentistry is the goal. This material may be indicated for full crowns on second molars with limited occlusal space, where there is a high risk of fracture, and in teeth that have lost their rigidity, such as endodontically treated teeth with lower esthetic requirements. One serious disadvantage of full zirconia crowns is that removal can be an extremely time-consuming task, often requiring the use of several diamonds. This can be further compromised if the zirconia crown is bonded.

Layered Zirconia, Full Zirconia or Lithium Disilicate?

For most crown replacements, a layered zirconia crown (PFZ) is preferable to full zirconia (monolithic) or lithium because, when crowns are being replaced, the restorative margin will most often be subgingival. Layered and full zirconia crowns can be cemented with the less contamination-sensitive resin-modified glass ionomer (RMGI) without compromising on strength. The zirconia will not then require additional tooth reduction to create more space for the thickness and strengthening of the restoration that cemented lithium disilicate requires. When correctly fabricated, PFZs have marginally

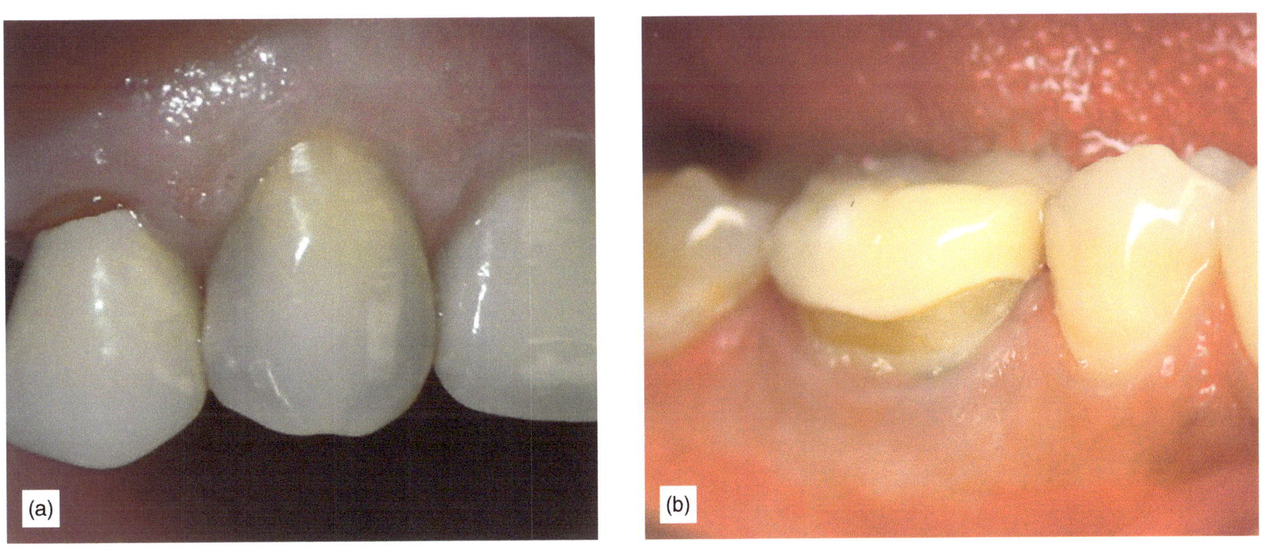

Figure 11.17 (a, b) Unesthetic full zirconia crowns.

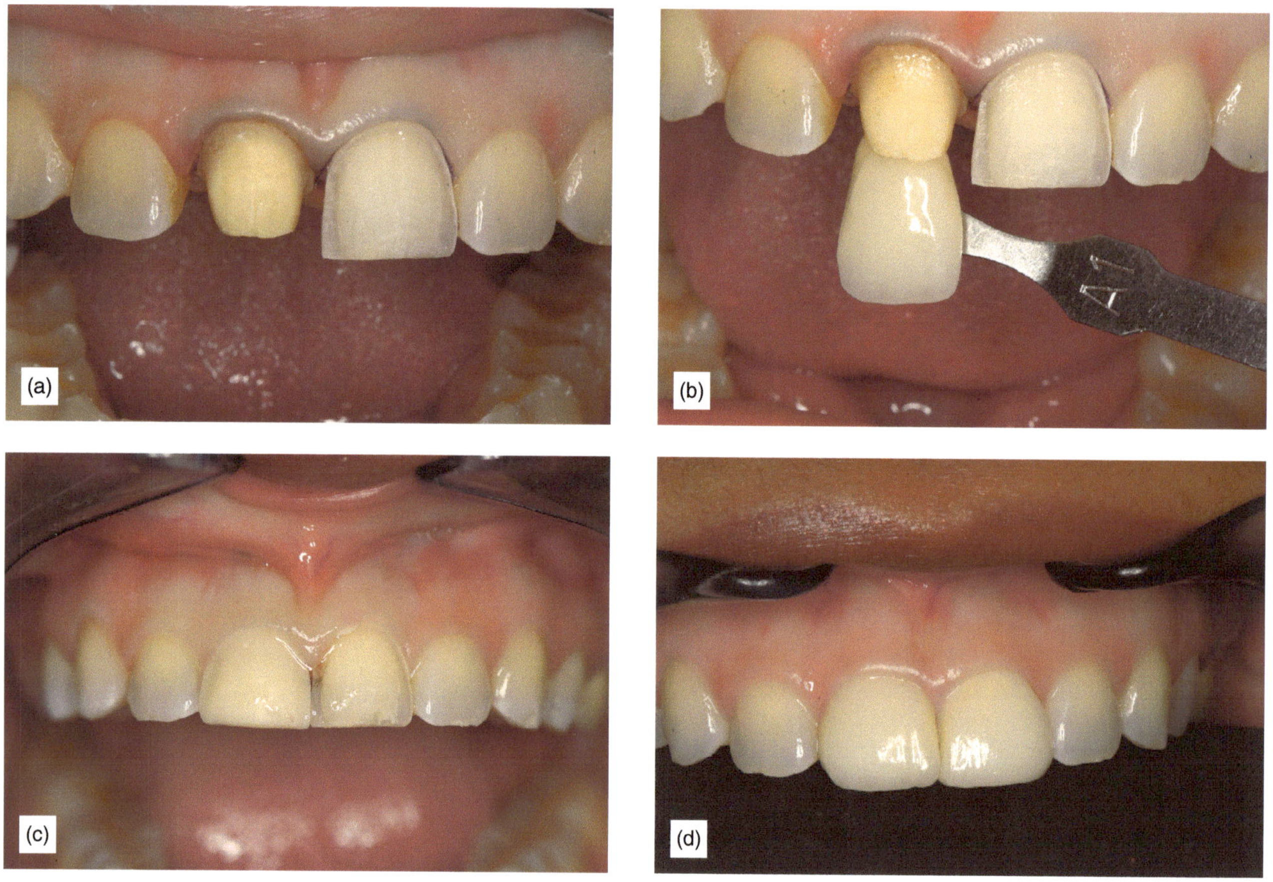

Figure 11.19 (a) A highly complicated situation, trying to match colors with two centrals, one a crown and one a veneer. (b) Communicate preparation (or stump) shade to the laboratory to fabricate a matching zirconia coping. (c) Zirconia coping attempting to match adjacent preparation; this will allow for an equal thickness of porcelain veneers over crown and tooth of the same material, Noritake Z porcelain. (d) A highly esthetic result.

acceptable translucency, allowing for a slightly supragingival margin placement in the non-esthetic zone, with acceptable esthetics. PFZs can be highly esthetic and when properly made very predictable (Figure 11.19a–d). Finally, when the restoration needs to be replaced, the removal is considerably simpler than full zirconia or lithium disilicate, especially when cemented with RMGI.

Preparation for a Full-Coverage All-Ceramic Crown

Supragingival minimally invasive crown preparation is highly encouraged. A tooth preparation is performed to create space for the restorative material, removal of caries and old failing restorations, and to facilitate laboratory fabrication, so the choice of material will dictate the amount of tooth to be removed and conversely, the amount of remaining tooth structure and gingival margin location will dictate the choice of material. In cases where an old crown is being replaced, the goal will be to limit further tooth reduction. Table 11.1 shows tooth conditions and the best choice of material based on the conditions. One material does not fit all situations.

The tooth preparation technique is similar to the familiar PFM crown preparation but different material

Table 11.1 Choice of material and tooth condition.

Tooth condition	Material
Crown option based on condition of existing preparation	Best restorative material option and cement
Subgingival margins	Zirconia layered or monolithic (RMGI)
Supragingival margins with medium esthetic	Layered zirconia (RMGI) or lithium disilicate (resin)
Supragingival margin and highly esthetic	Lithium disilicate (resin)
Second molar/esthetics do not matter	Full zirconia or gold (RMGI)

RMGI, resin-modified glass ionomer.

requires different amounts of space and reduction. Occlusal reduction will be completed first, followed by axial reduction with a chamfer diamond in three planes, as teeth have three different planes. Single-plane axial reduction is always more destructive. Because most ceramic crowns are milled and the impression laser scanned, clear butt margins avoiding a lip or 'J-margins' on the preparation are important (Figure 11.20).

Cementation of Full Crowns

The choice of cementation material for full crowns is of great importance. It is driven by the location of the margin and the condition of the tooth. Zirconia (or alumina) are highly sintered, which means that they cannot be etched and are not reinforced structurally with resin cement. Additionally, the strength of zirconia exceeds 1000 MPa, so resin cement reinforcement is unnecessary. This means that regular crown and bridge cement can be used without compromising strength. Lithium disilicate, conversely, contains glass, and can be etched and reinforced with resin cement. It is a weaker material than zirconia, and using a regular (non-resin) cement will weaken the restoration. If it is thinly applied, this will increase the chances of fracture or failure, which I have experienced multiple times with cemented e-Max.

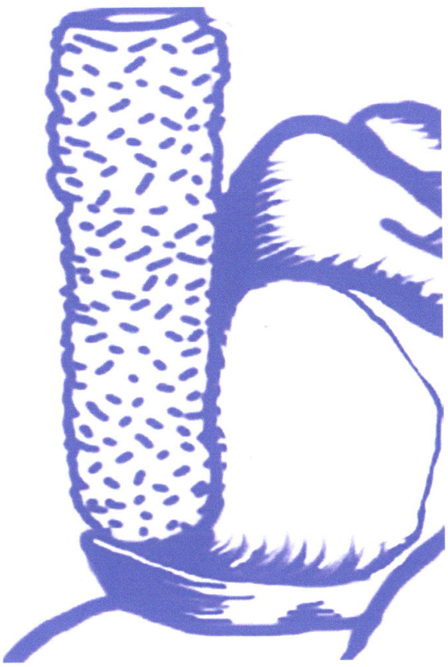

Figure 11.20 Avoid J-margins caused by chamfer burs.

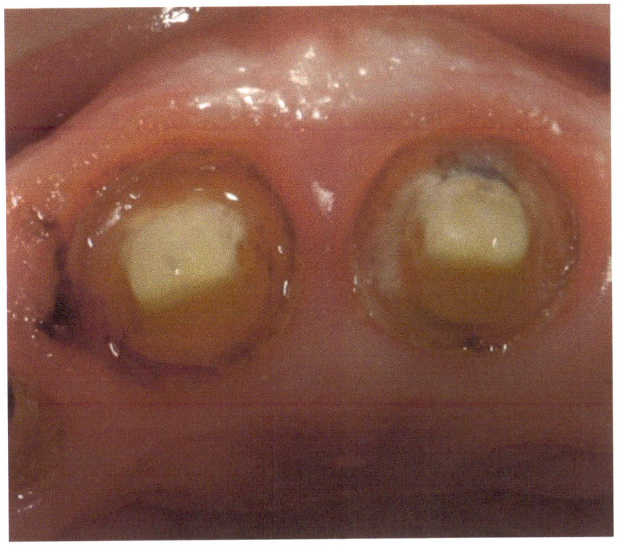

Figure 11.21 Subgingival margins are difficult to isolate.

Subgingival Margin Cementation

The ideal cement for a crown with existing subgingival margins is RMGI. The rationale for this preference is that RMGI such as Meron Plus AC (VOCO) [22] or RelyX™ Luting Cement (3M), is the most forgiving of all restorative cements where there is moisture or contamination [23]. Subgingival margins make it very difficult to have 100% predictable isolation (Figure 11.21) and, as previously discussed, ensuring that there is no contamination from saliva, blood or crevicular fluid is a must with bonded resin cements. Sandblasting the intaglio surface of the zirconia crowns with Siljet, followed by a coat of ceramic primer, and then cementing the crown onto a nicely clean and dry tooth (not desiccated) with RMGI cement will provide simple, sensitivity free, excellent results.

Cementing Crowns with Resin Cement

Without a doubt, a crown will have superior retention if it is bonded with resin cement [24]. However, bonded resin cement needs perfect isolation, which is extremely difficult to achieve with subgingival margins. Even if the isolation requirement can be met, the question should be asked whether resin cementation is in fact necessary for the super-strong ceramics such as zirconia. In general terms, zirconia does not need resin cement and, over the long term, bonding all zirconia crowns will end up being a nightmare for the future, as removing this restoration is extremely difficult. When bonded cementation is actually necessary because of a lack of retention (and isolation is achievable), resin cements are excellent (see Chapter 9 for step by step instructions).

References

1 Barizon KT, Bergeron C, Vargas MA, Qian F, Cobb DS, Gratton DG, Geraldeli S. Ceramic materials for porcelain veneers: Part II. Effect of material, shade, and thickness on translucency. *J Prosthet Dent*, 2014; 112(4): 864–870.
2 Dietchi D. Adhesive metal-free restorations: Current concepts for the esthetic treatment of posterior teeth. *Pract Periodont Aesthet Dent*, 1998; 10(1): 47–54.
3 Ma L. Load-bearing properties of minimal-invasive monolithic lithium disilicate and zirconia occlusal onlays: Finite element and theoretical analyses. *Dent Mater*, 2013; 29(7): 742–751.
4 Frankenberger R, Taschner M, Garcia-Godoy F, Petschelt A, Krämer N. Leucite-reinforced glass ceramic inlays and onlays after 12 years. *J Adhes Dent*, 2008; 10(5): 393–398.
5 Ruiz JL, Christensen GJ, Sameni A, Vargas L. Clinical performance of bonded ceramic and resin-based composite inlays and onlays using a self-etch bonding system; a 51-month report. *Inside Dent*, 2007; 3(5): 62–65.
6 El-Mowafy O, Brochu JF. Longevity and clinical performance of IPS-Empress ceramic restorations: A literature review. *J Can Dent Assoc*, 2002; 68: 233–237.
7 Lehner C, Studer S, Brodbeck U, Schärer P. Six-year clinical results of leucite-reinforced glass ceramic inlays and onlays. *Acta Med Dent Helv*, 1998; 3: 137–146.
8 Culp L, McLaren EA. Lithium disilicate: The restorative material of multiple options. *Compend Contin Educ Dent*, 2010; 31(9): 716–725.
9 Fasbinder DJ, Dennison JB, Heys D, Neiva G. A clinical evaluation of chairside lithium disilicate CAD/CAM crowns: A two year report. *J Am Dent Assoc*, 2010; 141(6 Suppl): 10s–14s.
10 Anadioti E, Aquilino SA, Gratton DG, Holloway JA, Denry IL, Thomas GW, Qian F. Internal fit of pressed and computer-aided design/computer-aided manufacturing ceramic crowns made from digital and conventional impressions. *J Prosthet Dent*, 2014; 113(4): 304–309.
11 Ereifej N, Rodrigues FP, Silikas N, Watts DC. Experimental and FE shear-bonding strength at core/veneer interfaces in bilayered ceramics. *Dent Mater*, 2011; 27(6): 590–597.
12 Belli, R. Mechanical fatigue degradation of ceramics versus resin composites for dental restorations. *Dent Mater*, 2014; 30(4): 424–432.
13 Magne P, Belser UC. Porcelain versus composite inlays/onlays: effects of mechanical loads on stress distribution, adhesion, and crown flexure. *Int J Periodontics Restorative Dent*, 2003; 23(6): 543–555.
14 Hopp C, Land MF. Considerations for ceramic inlays in posterior teeth: A review. *Clin Cosmet Investig Dent*, 2013; 5: 21–32.
15 Yesil ZD, Alapati S, Johnston W, Seghi RR. Evaluation of the wear resistance of new nanocomposite resin restorative materials. *J Prosthet Dent*, 2008; 99(6): 435–443.
16 Magne P, Stanley K, Schlichting LH. Modeling of ultrathin occlusal veneers. *Dent Mater*, 2012; 28(7): 777–782.
17 3M Science. Notice: Change in Indication – Lava™ Ultimate CAD/CAM Restorative. http://www.3m.com/3M/en_US/dental-us/products/lava-ultimate (accessed December 10, 2016).
18 Christensen RP, Ploeger BJ. A clinical comparison of zirconia, metal and alumina fixed-prosthesis frameworks veneered with layered or pressed ceramic: A 3 year report. *J Am Dent Assoc*, 2010; 141(11); 1317–1329.
19 Keough BE, Kay HB, Sage RD, Keen E. Clinical performance of scientifically designed, hot isostatic-pressed (HIP'd) zirconia cores in a bilayered all-ceramic system. *Compend Contin Educ Dent*, 2011; 32(6): 58–68.
20 Albashaireh ZS, Ghazal M, Kern M. Two body wear of different ceramic materials opposed to zirconia ceramics. *J Prosthet Dent*, 2010; 104(2): 105–113.
21 Christensen R. CZR Press by Noritake: Veneering ceramic for zirconia with least chipping and surface crumbling. *Clin Rep*, 2010; 3(8): 1.
22 Ehlers V, Kampf G, Stender E, Willershausen B, Ernst CP. Effect of thermocycling with or without 1 year of water storage on retentive strengths of luting cements for zirconia crowns. *J Prosthet Dent*, 2015; 113(6): 609–615.
23 Shimazu K, Karibe H, Ogata K. Effect of artificial saliva contamination on adhesion of dental restorative materials. *Dent Mater J*, 2014; 33(4): 545–550.
24 Piwowarczyk A, Lauer HC, Sorensen JA. In vitro shear bond strength of cementing agents to fixed prosthodontic restorative materials. *J Prosthet Dent*, 2004; 92(3): 265–273.

Part VII

The Occlusal Disease Management System: A Key to Success

12

The Importance of Occlusion and Occlusal Diagnosis in Restorative Dentistry

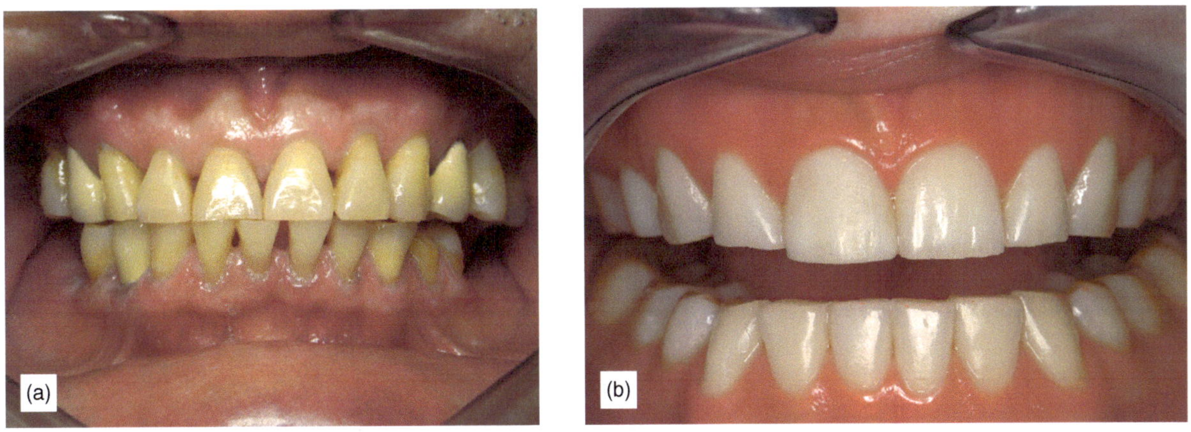

(a) Fifty-five-year-old with severe occlusal disease, who has severe wear, multiple fractures, missing multiple teeth, as well as many other signs and symptoms. (b) Eighteen-year old with severe occlusal disease, showing severe wear, as well as many other signs and symptoms.

The Occlusal Connection to Restorative Dentistry Success

Ceramic restorations are at an increased risk when a patient suffers from a traumatic occlusion combined with a parafunctional activity (occlusal disease). In fact, longevity studies point to the decrease in durability of ceramic restorations in patients with parafunctional habits (Figure 12.1a,b) [1]. The reality of the shorter durability of bonded ceramic restoration should be tempered with the reality that *all* restorations and the teeth restored, including porcelain-fused-to-metal and gold crowns, will have shorter durability and other problems when the patient has a severely traumatic occlusion and parafunctional activity (Figure 12.2a,b) [2]. Because of the fear of fractured restorations, many

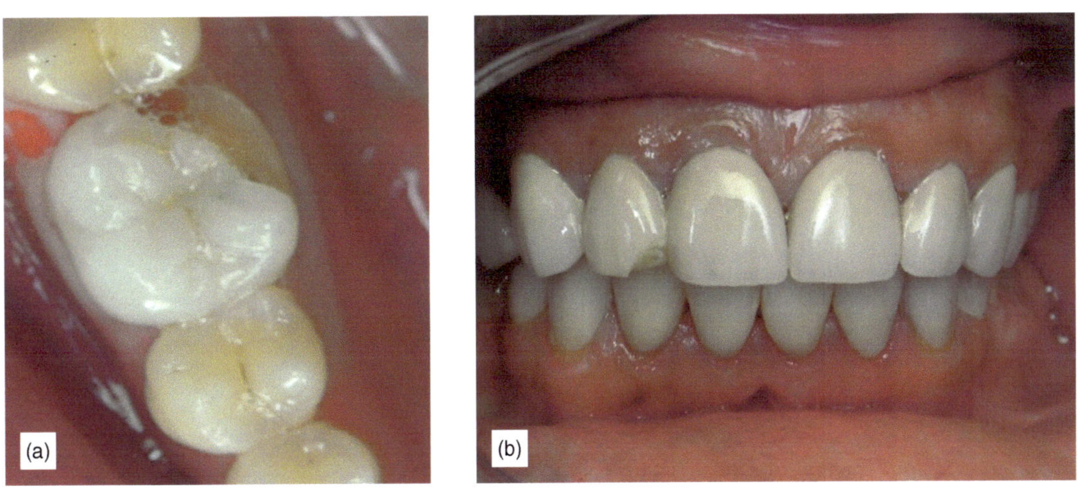

Figure 12.1 (a) Fractured onlay. (b) Fractured veneers.

Supra-Gingival Minimally Invasive Dentistry: A Healthier Approach to Esthetic Restorations, First Edition. By Jose-Luis Ruiz.

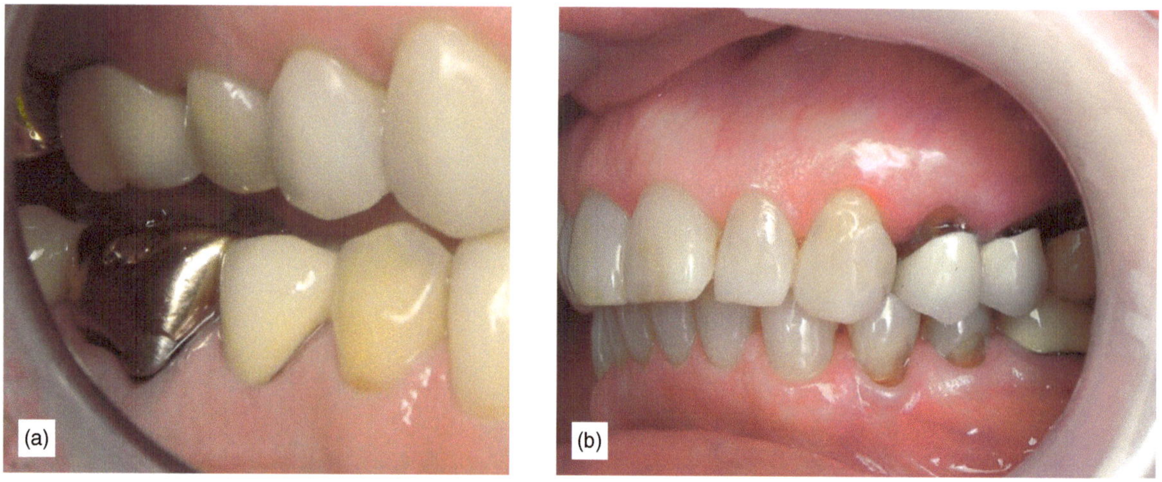

Figure 12.2 (a) Cervical abfraction compromising a gold crown. (b) Failing porcelain-fused-to-metal restoration caused by occlusal disease.

contraindicate partial coverage ceramic restoration, thus suggesting the use of more aggressive procedures such as full crowns of any type, including full zirconia crowns [3,4,5,6]. Ultimately, parafunctional activity combined with a traumatic bite (occlusal disease) is the reason for restoration failures [7], and good occlusal management can lead to success even in difficult cases (Figure 12.3a–h).

If unbreakable restorations are used without proper occlusal management, the unbreakable restoration will only transfer the forces and the damage into deeper tissues, or create other problems. The uncontrolled occlusal

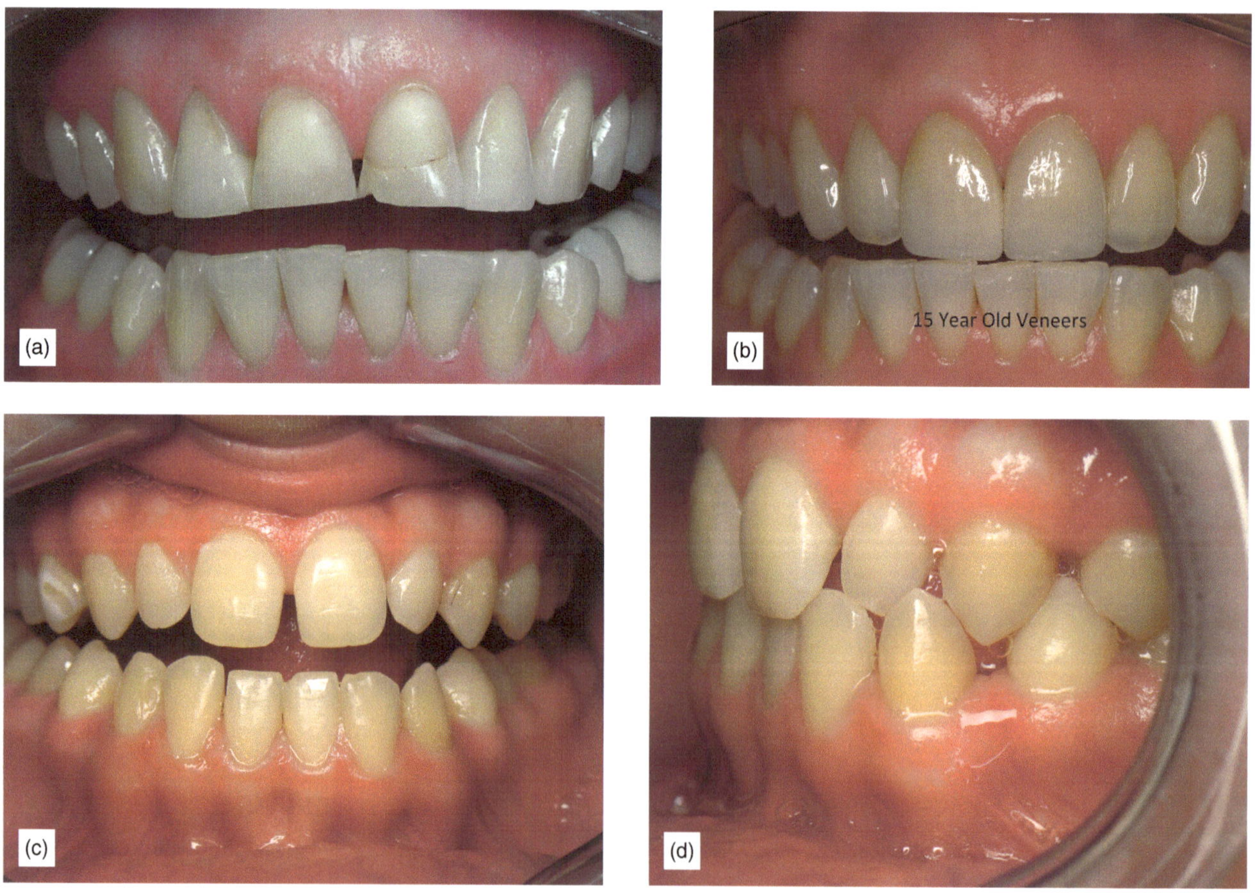

Figure 12.3 (a) Severely worn dentition. (b) A 15-year postoperative image of porcelain veneers with Noritake feldspathic porcelain. (c) Patient in need of esthetic treatment. (d) Traumatic occlusion, which can lead to failure of any restoration. (Continued)

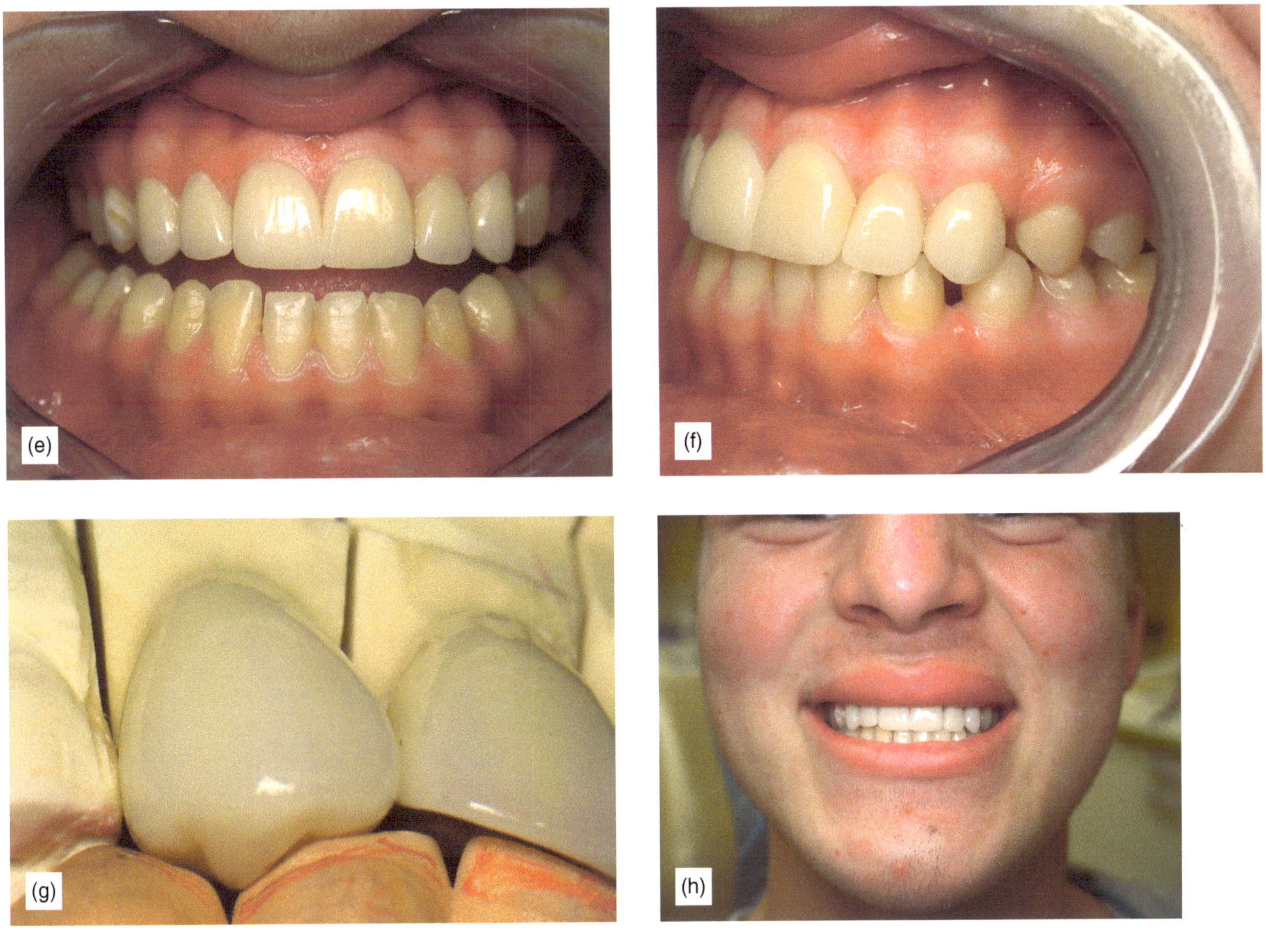

Figure 12.3 (*Continued*)
(e) Finished esthetic rehabilitation using Noritake feldspathic porcelain veneers. (f) Restorative correction of the cross-bite using porcelain veneers. (g) Canine guidance to manage forces. (h) 3-years postoperatively.

forces are great and will be expressed in many other ways, such as loose restoration, loose teeth, pain and sensitivity, tooth fractures at the neck or root level (Figure 12.4a,b), periodontal damage, headaches, migraines, and others. The following is a clinical example of how improper occlusal management can lead to restorative failure (Figure 12.5a–c). Figure 12.5a shows the gold onlay of a patient who suffered from postoperative pain and sensitivity for almost 2 years. She was scheduled for root canal treatment in the next few days. After differential diagnosis, occlusal trauma was considered to be a possible etiology for the pain, and within 2 days of a

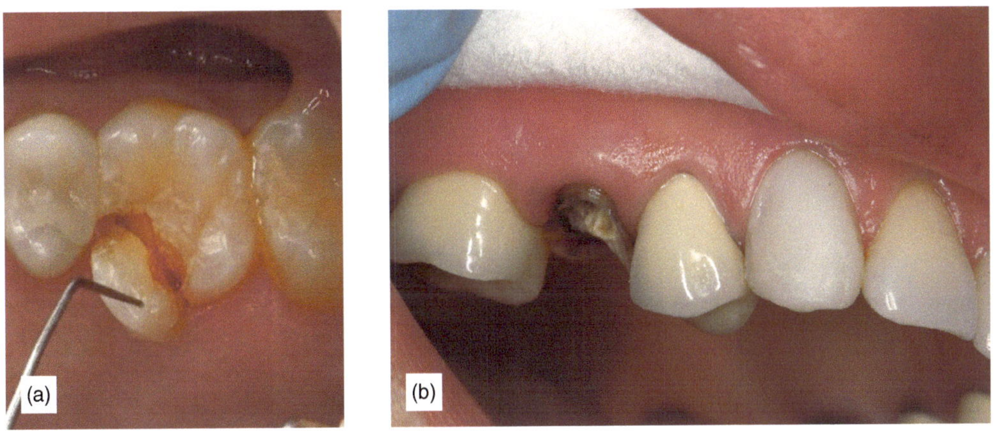

Figure 12.4 (a) Tooth fractures. (b) Tooth fractured to gum line.

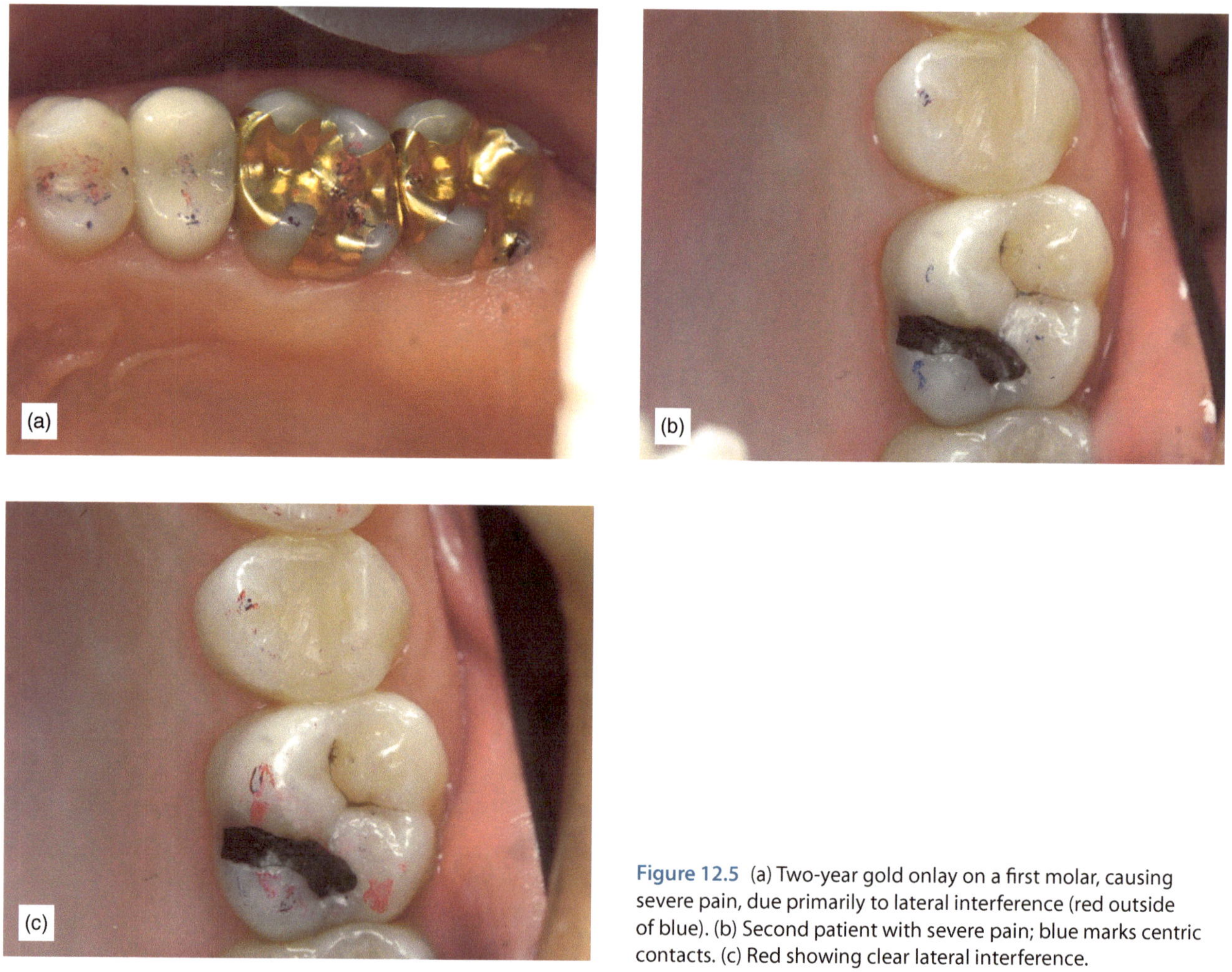

Figure 12.5 (a) Two-year gold onlay on a first molar, causing severe pain, due primarily to lateral interference (red outside of blue). (b) Second patient with severe pain; blue marks centric contacts. (c) Red showing clear lateral interference.

bite adjustment, the tooth stopped hurting permanently. Although the restoration did not break and it had great margins, the improper occlusal management led to patient dissatisfaction, long-term discomfort and almost an unnecessary endodontic procedure. Restorative success is far more than a restoration which does not break. Restorative success will encompass leaving the teeth needing repair or restoration in a healthy state, free of pulpal damage, and periodontal disease, and a patient who is satisfied with the esthetics of the restoration.

Understanding the great importance of occlusion and occlusal management improves the quality of dentistry, and the health of patients because:

- It allows better differential diagnosis in complicated cases, because undiagnosed occlusal problems are responsible for many catastrophic treatment decisions and results.
- It encourages healthier dentistry, more supragingival minimally invasive dentistry, because the fear of fractured restorations forces the dentist to cut crowns, rather than using partial coverage.
- It permits better, more comprehensive treatment for patients. Fear of fractures or failure prevents the dentist from undertaking single-tooth dentistry and encourages them to shy away from more comprehensive cases.
- Ultimately, it provides a healthier dental life for patients with occlusal disease. Early diagnosis and minimally invasive management permits patients to have a more satisfying, healthier dental life.

Attention to occlusion goes beyond restorative success, as occlusion is one of the leading causes of tooth loss and is also one of the three main enemies of human dentition, alongside caries and periodontal disease [8]. An excellent example is shown in the comparative photographs in Figures 12.6 and 12.7 of two patients, both in their early thirties, which show the devastating effect of occlusal disease. The patients are of similar age, both with good home care, free of caries and periodontal disease, but one has normal-looking dentition and the other has fractures, chips, abfractions and excessive incisal wear. There are similar examples in every practice. In this way, patients' dentition is compromised by occlusal disease, and it must be treated. Dentistry's goal is to help patients to keep their teeth for life, and occlusal disease can compromise this goal, inasmuch as caries and periodontal disease. Excessive incisal wear, fractures and other signs of occlusal disease are not an inevitable result of aging (Figure 12.8).

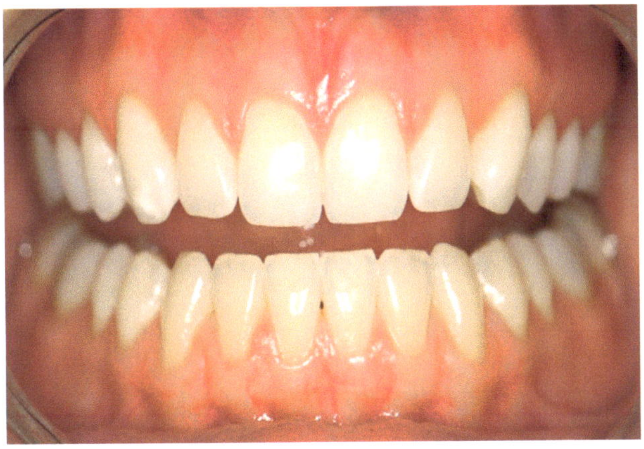

Figure 12.6 Healthy patient in her early 30s.

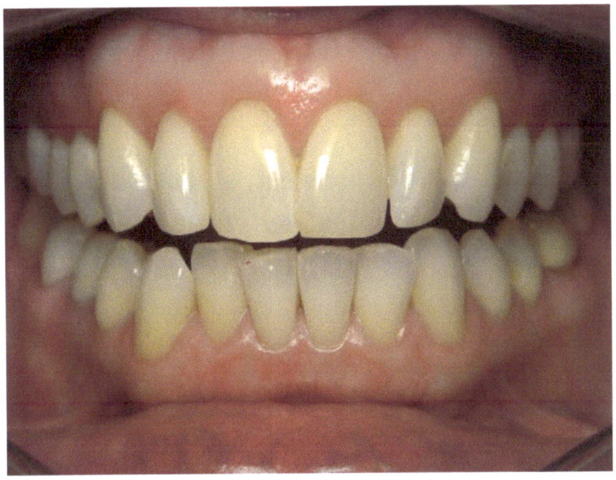

Figure 12.8 Fifty-seven-year-old patient with excellent barely worn dentition.

Occlusion: The Untreated Enemy

Occlusion and the treatment of occlusal disease is completely vital to dentistry. This is because everything that a dentist does affects the patient's occlusion, and in turn everything a dentist does is affected by the patient's occlusion (Figure 12.9). Even so, millions of patients with severe occlusal disease go untreated [9]. A primary obstacle for managing occlusal disease is the patient's absolute disinterest in their bite and refusal to accept grinding, clenching, or the importance of wearing a night guard. This leads to the question: whose fault is it that patients are so ignorant of the very negative effects of occlusal disease? Yes, the dental community. The problem is the failure to explain to the patient how occlusal disease is not just wear. There are, however, other deeper and more damaging signs and symptoms occurring beneath the visible wear. Another major obstacle in implementing occlusal diagnosis and management is the erroneous idea that extensive rehabilitation is the best way of managing worn dentition. The idea that function follows form instigates full rehabilitations. Occlusal management can and should be minimally invasive.

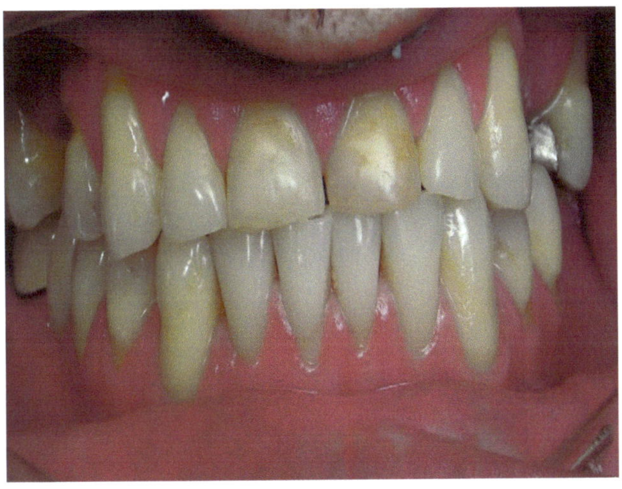

Figure 12.7 Male patient in his early 30s with severe occlusal disease.

Occlusal Disease Defined

The dictionary definition of disease is "an impairment of the normal state of the living animal or plant body or one of its parts that interrupts or modifies the performance of the vital functions, is typically manifested by distinguishing signs and symptoms, and is a response to environmental factors, to specific infective agents, to inherent defects of the organism (as genetic anomalies), or to combinations of these factors" [10]. Negative effects of occlusion have typically been referred to as "problems" or "conditions".

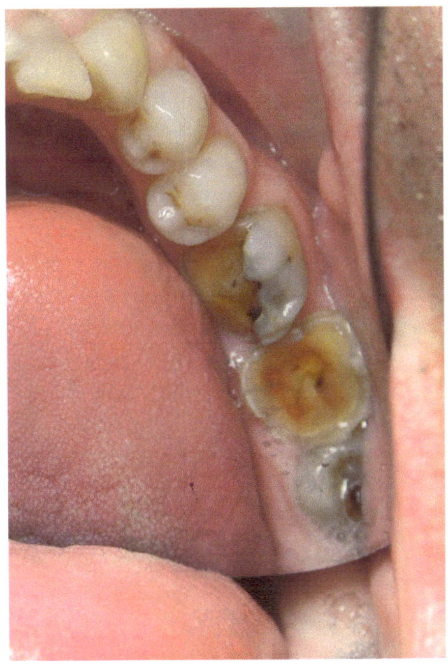

Figure 12.9 Badly worn dentition.

Based on the definition above, however, disease is the more appropriate term, giving the term "occlusal disease". The etiology of occlusal disease is a combination of inherent defects or malocclusion (traumatic bite), environmental factors or maladjusted restorations, and abnormal masticatory parafunctional activities, which will lead to degeneration and dysfunction of the masticatory system, expressed in signs and symptoms. For occlusal disease to exist, both conditions must coexist. Because a perfectly balanced, atraumatic bite does not usually exist in nature, and parafunctional activities are uncontrollable central nervous system activities that can be exacerbated by stress and certain drugs, it can be said that occlusal disease is extremely common, and it is also a chronic, incurable disease [11,12]. A more appropriate definition would be; "Occlusal disease is a chronic destructive process evident in any part of the masticatory apparatus (joint, muscles, periodontium or teeth), as a consequence of occlusal disharmony and parafunction. It has specific signs and symptoms and as any chronic disease it cannot be cured, but it can be managed" [7].

It is important to differentiate temporomandibular joint disease (TMD) from occlusal disease. Occlusal disease is the damage caused by the combination of parafunctional activity and a traumatic occlusion, while TMD is associated with internal damage of the joint. Occlusion and the management of occlusal disease is more mechanical, with the goal of harmonizing the occlusion based on well-known functional principles, as well as protecting the masticatory structures from the damage from parafunctional habits with appliances. Early diagnosis and management of occlusion is of great importance to any dentist, as occlusion affects every aspect of dental treatment. While all dentists need to be experts in occlusion, it is also important to be able to diagnose when there is true temporomandibular joint damage. The treatment of TMD is more complicated, because it is a joint condition and as such requires a more medical approach, as would any other joint. The restorative clinician can choose to train in the treatment of TMD or can choose to refer such cases to other experts or specialists.

A crucial step in implementing occlusal management is patient education. Once the patient accepts the importance of occlusal health, appropriate occlusal therapy will be a regular part of their oral health maintenance (Figure 12.10). Using the word "disease" instead of "condition," "wear," or "aging" is important in patient education. The latter terms lead the patient to perceive occlusal problems as a natural consequence of wear or aging. The first step in educating and managing occlusal disease is the implementation of a simple, yet effective system for accomplishing early diagnosis. It is also important to evaluate the severity of the disease (signs and symptoms) to present the most minimally invasive management possible, appropriate to the severity of the condition. Diagnosis using the seven signs and symptoms of occlusal disease makes this possible.

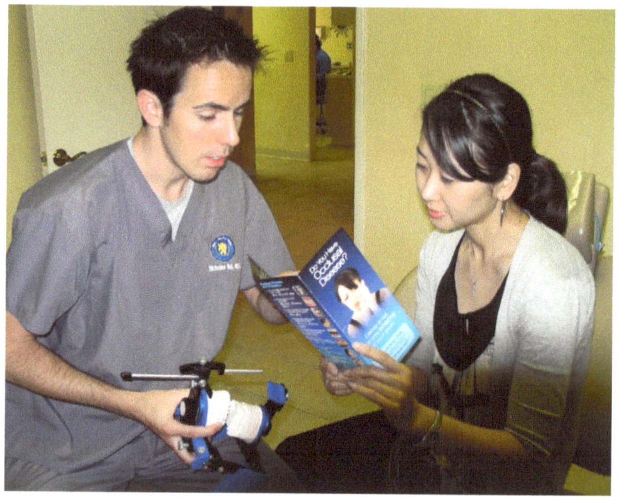

Figure 12.10 Patient being educated about occlusal disease.

Diagnosis Using the Seven Signs and Symptoms of Occlusal Disease

Regardless of what we choose to call occlusal problems, it is paramount to have a simple, methodical and fast way of diagnosing occlusal problems. Traditionally, diagnosing occlusal problems has been via a mounted cast and extensive interviews. It is virtually impossible and impractical for most dental practices to mount a cast on each patient, and it has been an obstacle in the implementation of routine occlusal diagnosis. Diagnosis of occlusal disease should not be limited to patients with severely damaged teeth, nor should the ability to diagnose be limited to certain dentists. Early diagnosis can prevent many problems from occurring (Figure 12.11) or worsening, so it is vital that dentists have a simple way of quickly and efficiently implementing occlusal examination and diagnosis into their routine examinations.

The Occlusal Disease Management System [7,13] is incremental, based on severity, and incorporates patients' willingness to accept diagnosis and treatment. It allows even the busiest of dentists to incorporate occlusal diagnosis and

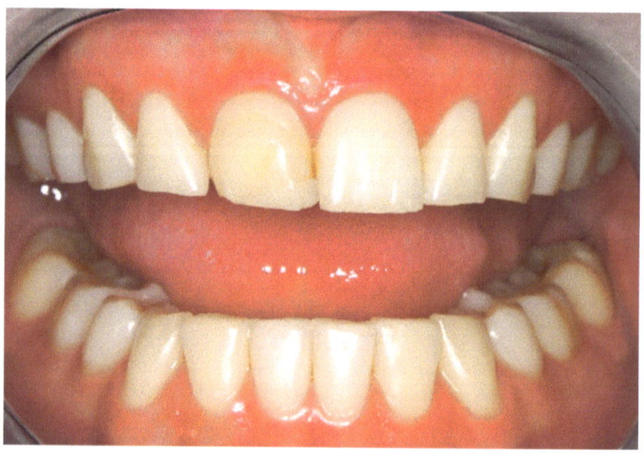

Figure 12.11 Eighteen-year-old patient with occlusal disease.

therapy for every patient, as it only takes 3 minutes to do a simple occlusal diagnosis. Knowing the seven signs and symptoms of occlusal disease (Box 12.1) is part of the first stage, aiding in diagnosis [14]. Every patient in the practice must have an occlusal examination as part of a comprehensive examination, as well as at periodic examinations; this is Stage 1. Stage 2 is reserved for patients with moderate to severe signs and symptoms or those who wish esthetic rehabilitations or are in need of extensive restorative dentistry and are motivated to pay for a complete occlusal analysis with mounted casts (see Chapter 13). Stage 3 is when the patient is diagnosed with true joint disease or TMD, which usually means referral to a specialist or treatment if the clinician is trained to treat those cases.

Initial Occlusal Examination

Every new patient who needs a comprehensive examination, and any existing patient who is due for a comprehensive examination, in addition to periodic examinations, should have an occlusal examination, which only takes 3 minutes. Occlusal examination should follow caries and periodontal examinations. A form listing the seven signs and symptoms should be used to record the findings (Figure 12.12). Each sign or symptom should be

Box 12.1 The seven signs and symptoms of occlusal disease

1) Pathological tooth wear, chipping or fractures.
2) Cervical dentin hypersensitivity.
3) Hypermobility.
4) Fremitus
5) Abfractions (non-carious cervical lesions).
6) Severe localised bone destruction, secondary to periodontal disease.
7) Muscle and temporomandibular disorder.

INITIAL EXAM FORM

Copyright©2004/2007 Ruiz Dental Seminars

PATIENT NAME: DATE:

Concerns	Solutions
1.	1.
2.	2.
3.	3.
4.	4.

Hygiene/Perio	Initial OD Examination	Medical & Dental Referral
Last Recall: Brush	Occ. Wear/FX:	Ref Endo: Ref OS:
Floss: Bleed w Flos:	CDH:	Ref Perio:
Tartar: Bone Loss:	Hypermobility:	Ref Ortho:
Inflam: Bleed U Prob:	Vert. Bone Loss:	Ref TMJ:
Esthetics	Abfractions:	Oral Cancer:
Smile Score:	Fremitus:	Medical Clearance:
Whitening:	Muscle or TMJ Pain:	
Diagnosis/Prevention	TX PLAN #1 - BASIC	Records
Periodontal:		MIP: CR:
OD:		OD:
Caries:		DFED:
EXISTING CONDITIONS		TX PLAN #2 - IDEAL

1		1		1	
2		2		2	
3		3		3	
4		4		4	
5		5		5	
6		6		6	
7		7		7	
8		8		8	
9		9		9	
10		10		10	
11		11		11	
12		12		12	
13		13		13	
14		14		14	
15		15		15	
16		16		16	

Figure 12.12 Form showing the seven signs and symptoms of occlusal disease.

evaluated as within normal limits, incipient, moderate, or severe. The patient should be listening to the findings to become aware of their own condition. When a patient presents with one or more of the seven signs and symptoms, it can be assumed the patient has occlusal disease, and, depending on the severity, a course of treatment will be suggested. If the patient does not display any signs or symptoms, it is safe to assume that they are well adapted to their occlusion, have no pathology, and are not in need of occlusal management.

Pathological Tooth Wear, Chipping, or Fractures

It only takes seconds to diagnose pathological tooth wear, chipping, and fractures. This is accomplished simply by a visual examination of the teeth. Occlusal wear is multifactorial, but acid may have an accelerating effect. Nonetheless, when excessive wear is present, the clinician should suspect occlusal disease. Multiple chips on the teeth (Figure 12.13), or small and large fractures of both teeth and restorations should be an indicator to the dentist of a pathological occlusion. It is important to identify the severity of the condition, within normal limits, incipient (Figure 12.14), moderate (Figure 12.15) or severe pathological tooth wear (Figure 12.16a,b), chipping or fractures, and record it. Severity is also dependent on the age of the patient. Restorative treatment should be attempted with caution when severe wear is present. Early diagnosis and management is much better than waiting until serious damage is already present [15].

Cervical Dentin Hypersensitivity

Cervical dentin hypersensitivity is one of the most common signs of occlusal disease. Patients come in daily

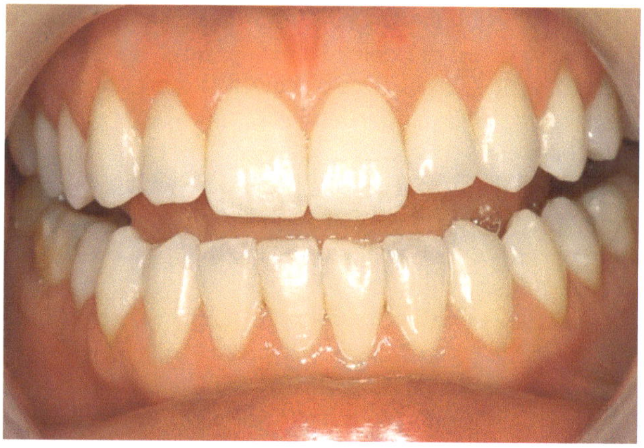

Figure 12.14 Incipient tooth wear.

with sensitivity issues, "I cannot eat ice cream," "I have to brush my teeth with warm water," "This tooth hurts tremendously when I drink cold water." Tooth hypersensitivity is multifactorial, and the etiology is often debated in the literature, ranging from gingival recession and root exposure to acidic foods and improper brushing as some of the factors. Hypersensitivity is still mostly treated with desensitizing toothpastes and topical agents, with very limited and temporary success [13,16], and with restorations, with equally short-term success (Figure 12.17) [17]. Much controversy exists about the role of occlusion in hypersensitivity [18]. Many studies which discredit the occlusal component lack a good method of diagnosing occlusal problems or a way of treating it, and thus are inconclusive [19]. All experienced clinicians know that occlusal trauma can cause sensitivity, even severe sensitivity. In a three-part clinical study, Coleman and colleagues ascertained that occlusal trauma was the primary source of cervical dentin hypersensitivity, and

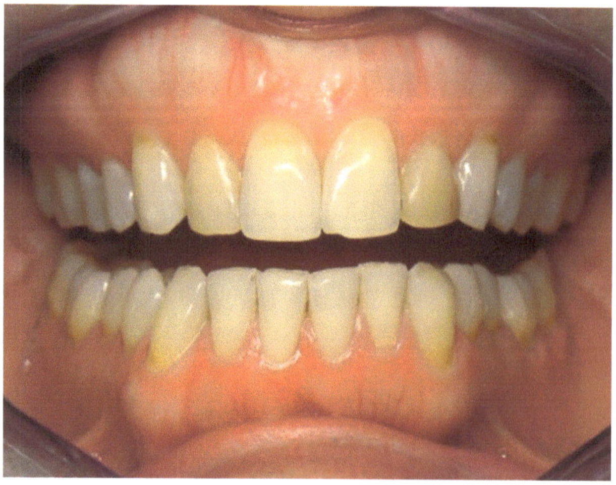

Figure 12.13 Multiple chips on posterior teeth.

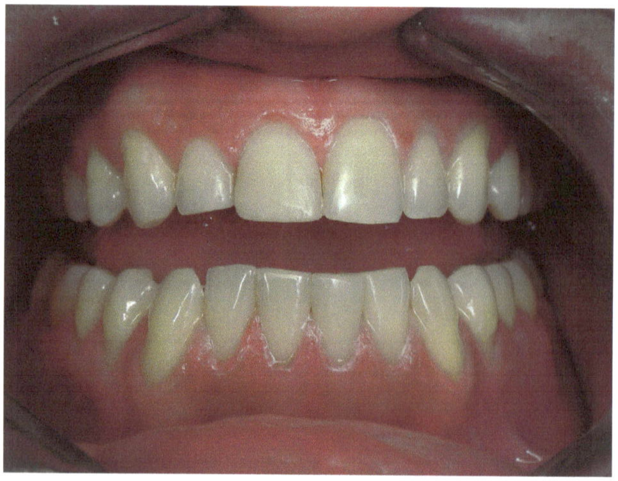

Figure 12.15 Moderate tooth wear.

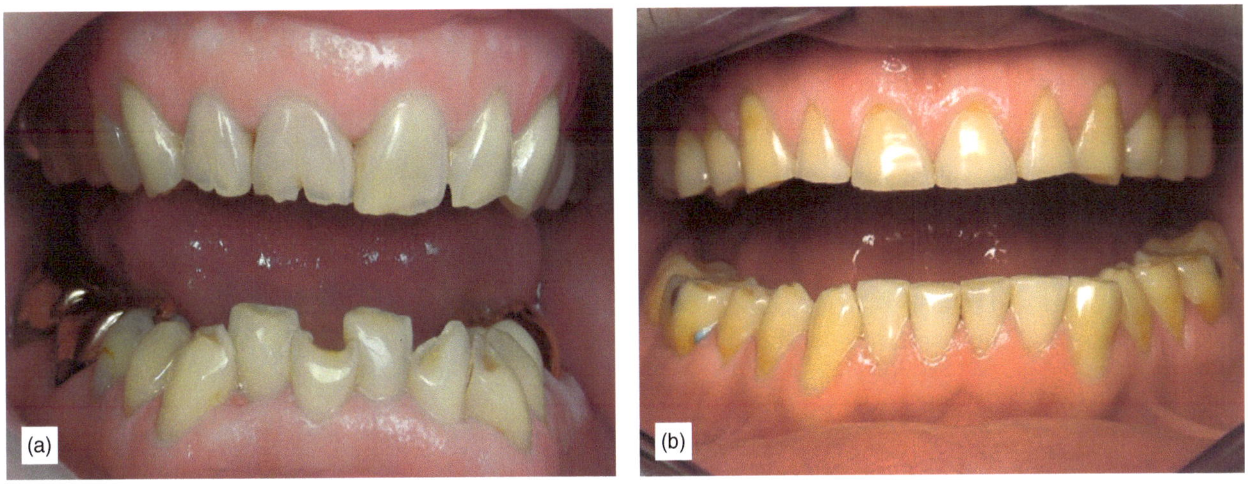

Figure 12.16 (a) Severe tooth wear in a 55-year-old patient. (b) Severe tooth wear in a 27-year-old adult.

the results showed that occlusal adjustment was the best modality of treatment that gave long-term resolution [20]. My extensive clinical experience in diagnosing tooth hypersensitivity and occlusal disease, and treating it with occlusal therapy, agrees with Coleman's findings.

Hypermobility

When the amount of tooth mobility present exceeds what would be expected with the level of attachment and bone present we can say that the tooth has hypermobility. Thus, when a patient presents with mobility of 2, 3 or even 4 on a tooth, but they show good or acceptable attachment level and good bone support (Figure 12.18a,b), this should serve as a clue to occlusal

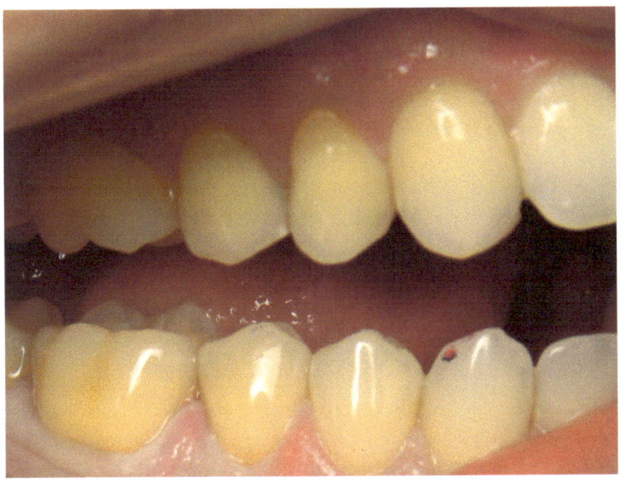

Figure 12.17 Three overhanging class V fillings to treat sensitivity; 1 year later, the patient still has severe sensitivity.

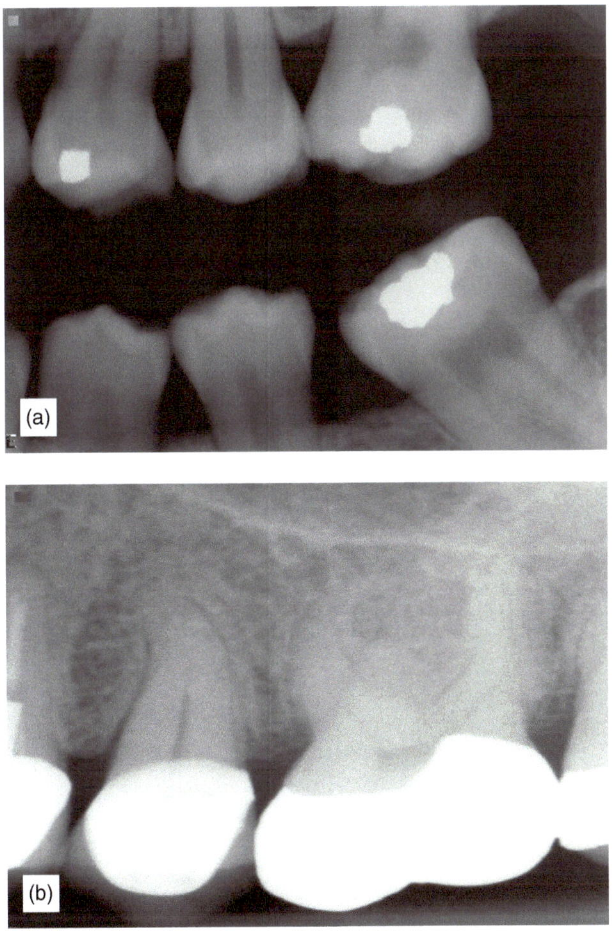

Figure 12.18 (a) A lower second molar having acceptable periodontal support, but severe mobility. (b) Tooth with acceptable periodontal support but severe mobility; sometimes the periodontal ligament is widened, but sometimes it is not.

interference and occlusal trauma [21,22]. Often, tooth mobility serves as an indicator for an eventual extraction, because there is usually no clinical technique to reverse the looseness of that tooth. Clinical experience shows that it is completely possible to take away the occlusal interference, by a proper limited or full occlusal equilibration, and have that tooth or teeth stabilize and mobility decrease or disappear. This should always be attempted prior to an extraction diagnosis; this will save many teeth. For a patient, the idea of their teeth becoming loose is very unappealing, so when they are informed that teeth are becoming loose as a consequence of their occlusal disease, they become far more interested in managing it.

Fremitus

Fremitus is mobility of the anterior teeth caused by occlusal interference, usually an envelope of function violation, and can be felt by the dentist placing their finger on the front teeth of the patient, and asking the patient to tap their teeth together (Figures 12.19, 12.20). Movement felt on any front tooth as the teeth hit together means that there is occlusal trauma causing mobility. The consequences of the untreated occlusal trauma which causes fremitus is proximal contact opening and teeth separating, broken incisal edges, broken incisal restorations and fractured teeth.

Abfractions

Abfractions are quite controversial in dentistry. A more popular term today is "non-carious cervical lesions" (NCCL), nevertheless the term "abfraction" denotes its occlusal origin. Many dentists believe that NCCL is caused by brushing, or abrasive toothpastes [23]. While NCCL have a multifactorial etiology [24], including toothpaste abrasion, acidic drinks, habits and other factors, the primary cause of their formation is lateral interference, as many studies have suggested (Figure 12.21a,b) [12,24,25,26,27,28].

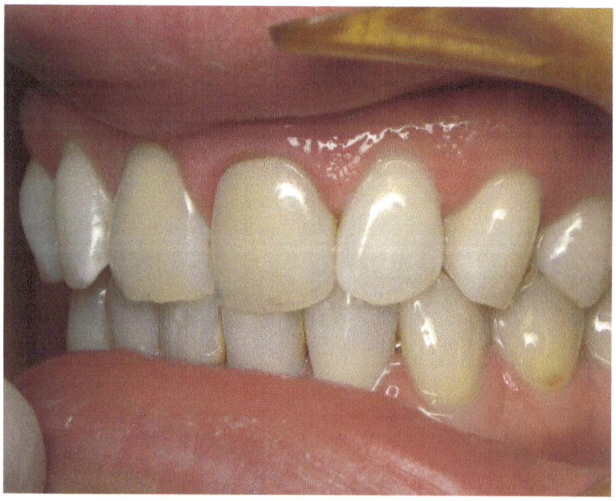

Figure 12.19 Tooth with fremitus.

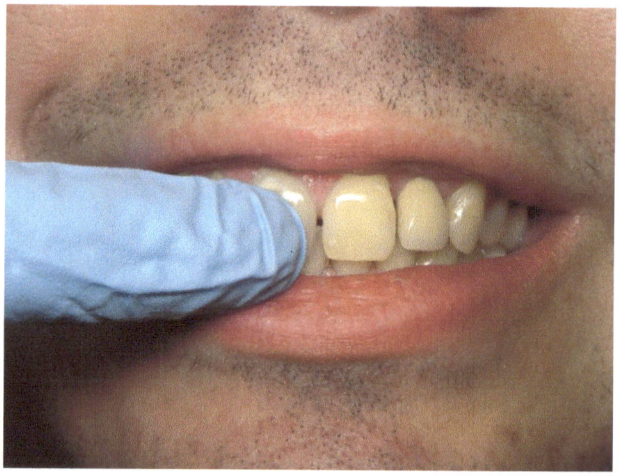

Figure 12.20 Finger testing for fremitus.

A clear example of the effects of flexion on the crown of a tooth is the large failure rate of class V restorations (Figure 12.22). When Class V restorations are placed without paying heed to the occlusal source, that tooth will continue to flex just as it did before the restoration [29], which will lead to the restoration being stressed, marginal deterioration, staining and eventual expulsion of the cavity. A simple way to increase class V durability is to remove the lateral interferences at the time of the restoration. Often, NCCL are restored because they are associated with hypersensitivity, but with proper occlusal equilibration, the sensitivity can be controlled and the tooth does not need to be restored.

Severe Localized Bone Destruction, Secondary to Periodontal Disease

An almost unknown consequence of occlusal disease is localized bone destruction, secondary to periodontal disease. For example, a full mouth x-ray will show that a patient has periodontal disease throughout their entire dentition, but it is common to see that only one or a few teeth have severe bone loss (Figure 12.23). An often forgotten source of accelerated bone loss, as the literature points out, is occlusal trauma secondary to periodontal disease [30,31]. Most periodontists are aware that there is an increase in success with periodontal procedures when occlusion is taken into consideration [32]. It is then important to acknowledge that occlusal disease leads to

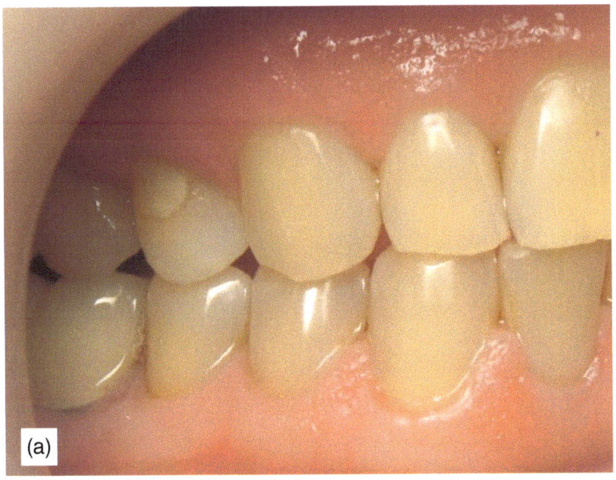

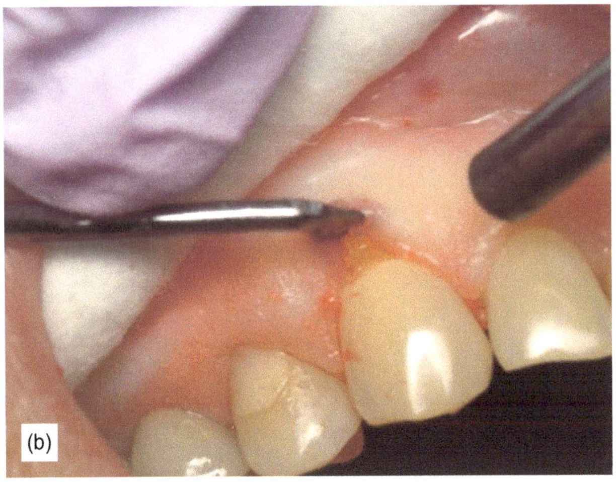

Figure 12.21 (a) This tooth has a subgingival abfraction, not caused by tooth paste abrasion. (b) Using a gingival retractor, the abfraction becomes evident; this patient had group function and was a heavy bruxer.

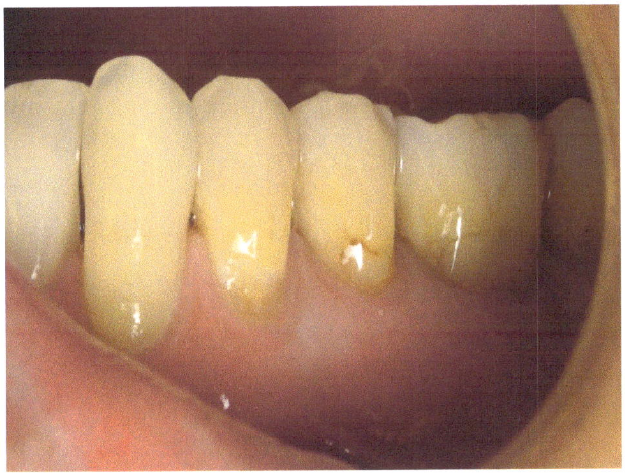

Figure 12.22 Failed class V.

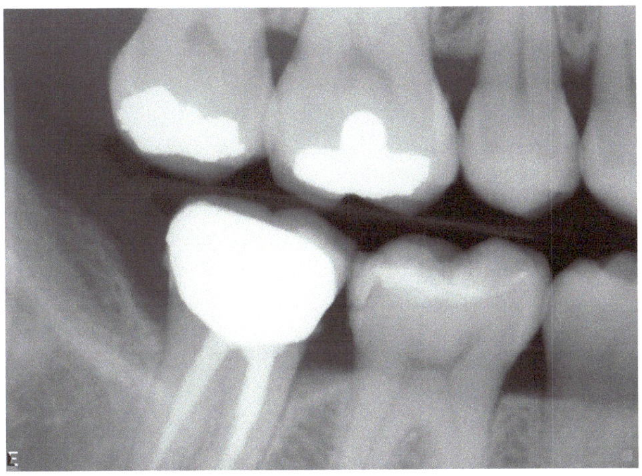

Figure 12.23 X-ray showing accelerated bone loss around a single tooth.

accelerated periodontal destruction, mobility, and premature tooth loss. Educating the patient about the link between occlusal disease and bone loss is important.

Sign: Muscle Pain and Temporomandibular Joint Pain

Pain associated to occlusal problems is a powerful motivator for treatment. Apart from wear, it is the most recognizable and obvious symptom of occlusal disease. Conversely, patients may exhibit severe headaches and pain and never link it to their dentition (Figure 12.24). This is why it is important to have a methodical system where the right questions are asked to prompt the disclosure of a symptom that the patient otherwise would

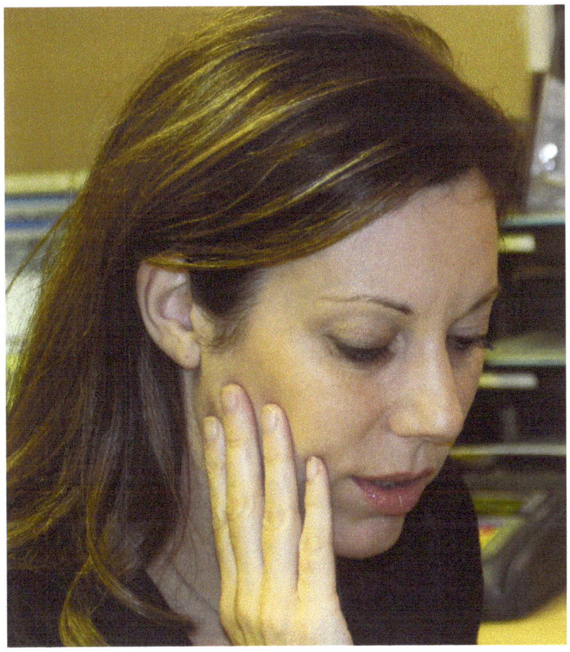

Figure 12.24 Severe muscle pain.

not feel the need to disclose to their dentist, like headaches or migraines. While muscle pain and temporomandibular disorder has a controversial etiology, and many suggest that it has no link to occlusion, clinical experience shows otherwise [33,34]. A well-adjusted splint has been shown to be an extremely effective way of managing some of these symptoms, as well as a correctly performed equilibration.

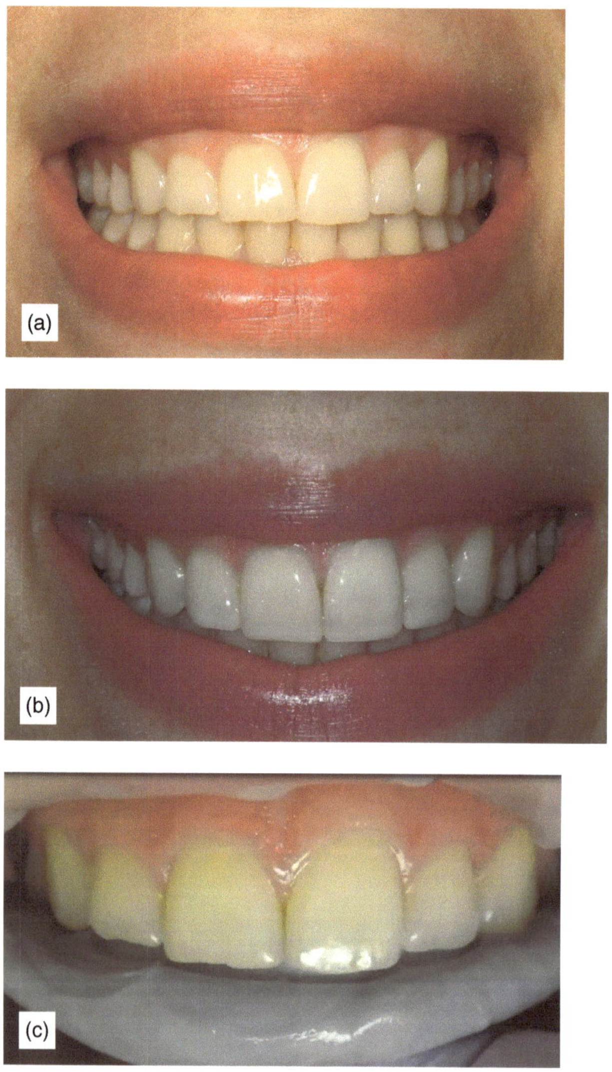

Figure 12.25 (a) A 23-year-old patient with severe signs and symptoms of occlusal disease, including cracked tooth syndrome on a virgin first molar, severe sensitivity, daily headaches, especially in the morning. She was facing a very bad dental future owing to her severe occlusal disease. (b) Four-year postoperative image of the patient, who was treated with minimally invasive equilibration, plus six direct composite restorations, to rebuild anterior and canine guidance, with no tooth preparation. Four years later, there have been no fractures of the restorations, no sensitivity and headaches have been drastically reduced. (c) Silicon matrix used to do fast direct composite restorations for anterior and canine guidance.

Course of Action

After an initial diagnosis is accomplished, a course of treatment should be assigned based on the presence and severity of the signs and symptoms: No treatment, a simple preventative night guard, or further examination for more severe cases, which includes occlusal analysis. Early diagnosis and good knowledge of proper minimally invasive occlusal management can improve the quality of the patient's dental life, as well as giving clinicians confidence in treatment success (Figure 12.25a–c). Of course, the clinician's goal is to treat every disease we are presented with, but the patient must first allow us to do so. Education is key, but if after proper education the patient is reluctant to accept that a problem exists or to accept treatment, it is acceptable to continue to treat such patients with some modifications. The patient should be informed that just as their natural teeth are suffering and wearing excessively, any restoration we place will have a tougher life and may have a shorter durability. Single-tooth supragingival minimally invasive bonded restorations are extremely successful when the restoration is well adjusted for occlusion [35,36,37]. There are some cases in the anterior or posterior areas in which patients may only want to treat a single damaged or fractured tooth with a direct composite and does not acknowledge any occlusal parafunctional activity, exposing the clinician to unpredictable results. Routine occlusal diagnosis and expertise in occlusion will allow the clinician to identify a risky case and then refuse to treat it, unless the patient accepts occlusal therapy along with the appropriate restorative procedure.

The final chapter (Chapter 13) presents the principles needed to provide the patient with a mechanically and physiologically healthy occlusion.

References

1 van Dijken JW, Hasselrot L. A prospective 15-year evaluation of extensive dentin-enamel-bonded pressed ceramic coverages. *Dent Mater*, 2010; 26(9): 929–923.

2 Ekfeldt A, Karlsson S. Changes of masticatory movement characteristics after prosthodontic rehabilitation of individuals with extensive tooth wear. *Int J Prosthodont*, 1996; 9(6): 539–546.

3 Bakeman EM, Kois JC. Posterior, all ceramic adhesively retained restorations. *Inside Dent*, 2009; 5(5): 20–23.

4 Kois DE, Chaiyabutr Y, Kois JC. Comparison of load fatigue performance of posterior ceramic onlay restorations under different preparation designs. *Compend Contin Educ Dent*, 2012 ; 33(Spec No 2): 2–9.

5 Barghi N, Berry TG. Clinical evaluation of etched porcelain onlays, a 4 year report. *Compend Contin Educ Dent*, 2002; 23(7): 657–674.
6 Meyer A Jr, Cardoso LC, Araujo E, Baratieri LN. Ceramic inlays and onlays: clinical procedures for predictable results. *J Esthet Restor Dent*, 2003; 15(6): 338–352.
7 Ruiz JL. Occlusal disease: restorative consequences and patient education. *Dent Today*, 2007; 26(9): 90–95.
8 Dawson PE. Occlusal disease. In *Functional Occlusion: From TMJ to Smile Design*. St Louis, MO: Mosby Elsevier; 2007, pp. 17–26.
9 Christensen GJ. Abnormal occlusion conditions: A forgotten part of dentistry. *J Am Dent Assoc*, 1995; 126(12): 1667–1668.
10 Merriam-Webster Online. Merriam-Webster, Inc. 2016. https://www.merriam-webster.com (accessed December 12, 2016).
11 Barker DK. Occlusal interferences and temporomandibular dysfunction. *Gen Dent*, 2004; 52: 56–62.
12 Telles D, Pegoraro LF, Pereira JC. Incidence of noncarious cervical lesions and their relation to the presence of wear facets. *J Esthetic Restorative Dent*, 2006; 18: 178–183.
13 Ruiz JL. Achieving longevity in esthetics by proper diagnosis and management of "occlusal disease." *Contemp Esthet*, 2007; 11(6): 24–30.
14 Ruiz JL, Coleman TA. Occlusal disease management system: the diagnosis process. *Compend Contin Educ Dent*, 2008; 29(3): 148–152.
15 Ratcliff S, Becker IM, Quinn L. Type and incidence of cracks in posterior teeth. *J Prosthet Dent*, 2001; 86(2): 168–172.
16 Veitz-Keenan A, Barna JA, Strober B, Matthews AG, Collie D, Vena D, Curro FA, Thompson VP. Treatments for hypersensitive noncarious cervical lesions: a Practitioners Engaged in Applied Research and Learning (PEARL) Network randomized clinical effectiveness study. *J Am Dent Assoc*, 2013; 144(5): 495–506.
17 Freitas Sda S, Sousa LL, Moita Neto JM, Mendes RF, Prado RR. Dentin hypersensitivity treatment of non-carious cervical lesions: A single-blind, split-mouth study. *Braz Oral Res*, 2015; 29(1): 45. doi: 10.1590/1807-3107BOR-2015.vol29.0045.
18 Cunha-Cruz J, Wataha JC, Heaton LJ, Rothen M, Sobieraj M, Scott J, Berg J; Northwest Practice-based Research Collaborative in Evidence-based DENTistry. The prevalence of dentin hypersensitivity in general dental practices in the northwest United States. *J Am Dent Assoc*, 2013; 144(3): 288–296.
19 Senna P, Del Bel Cury A, Rösing C. Non-carious cervical lesions and occlusion: a systematic review of clinical studies. *J Oral Rehabil*, 2012; 39(6): 450–462.
20 Coleman TA, Grippo JO, Kinderknecht KE. Cervical dentin hypersensitivity: Part III: Resolution following occlusal equilibration. *Quintessence Int*, 2003; 34: 427–434.
21 Ishigaki S, Kurozumi T, Morishige E, Yatani H. Occlusal interference during mastication can cause pathological tooth mobility. *J Periodontal Res*, 2006; 41(3): 189–192.
22 Greenstein G, Grenstein B, Cavallaro J. Prerequisite for treatment planning implant dentistry: Periodontal prognostication of compromised teeth. *Compend Contin Educ Dent*, 2007; 28(6): 436–447.
23 Abrahamsen TC. The worn dentition – pathognomonic patterns of abrasion and erosion. *Int Dent J*, 2005; 55: 268–276.
24 Grippo JO, Simring M, Coleman TA. Abfraction, abrasion, biocorrosion, and the enigma of noncarious cervical lesions: A 20-year perspective. *J Esthet Restor Dent*, 2012; 24(1): 10–23.
25 Grippo JO. Abfractions: A new classification of hard tissue lesions of the teeth. *J Esthetic Dent*, 1991; 3(1): 14–19.
26 Jakupovic S, Cerjakovic E, Topcic A, Ajanovic M, Prcic AK, Vukovic A. Analysis of the abfraction lesions formation mechanism by the finite element method. *Acta Inform Med*, 2014; 22(4): 241–245.
27 Ichim I, Schmidlin PR, Kieser JA, Swain MV. Mechanical evaluation of cervical glass-ionomer restorations: 3D finite element study. *J Dent*, 2007; 35(1): 28–35.
28 Borcic J, Anic I, Smojver I, Catic A, Miletic I, Ribaric SP. 3D finite element model and cervical lesion formation in normal occlusion and in malocclusion. *J Oral Rehabil*, 2005; 32: 504–510.
29 Tyras MJ. The class V lesion – aetiology and restoration. *Aust Dent J*, 1995; 40(3): 167–170.
30 Harrel SK, Nunn ME, Hallmon WW. Is there an association between occlusion? Yes, occlusal forces can contribute to periodontal destruction. *J Am Dent Assoc*, 2006; 137(10): 1380–1392.
31 Deas DE, Mealey BL. Is there an association between occlusion and periodontal destruction?: Only in limited circumstances does occlusal force contribute to periodontal disease progression. *J Am Dent Assoc*, 2006; 137(10): 1381–1385.
32 Gher ME. Changing concepts. The effects of occlusion on periodontitis. *Dent Clin North Am*, 1998; 42(2): 285–299.
33 Sipila K, Ensio K, Hanhela H, Zitting P, Pirttiniemi P, Raustia A. Occlusal characteristics in subjects with facial pain compared to a pain-free control group. *Cranio*, 2006; 24: 245–251.
34 Komazaki Y, Fujiwara T, Ogawa T, Sato M, Suzuki K, Yamagata Z, Moriyama K. Association between malocclusion and headache among 12- to 15-year-old adolescents: A population-based study. *Community Dent Oral Epidemiol*, 2014; 42(6): 572–580.
35 Christensen GJ. A look at state-of-the-art tooth-colored inlays and onlays. *J Am Dent Assoc*, 1992; I23(9): 66–67, 70.
36 Ruiz JL. Achieving optimal esthetics in a patient with severe trauma: Using a multidisciplinary approach and an all-ceramic fixed partial denture. *J Esthetic Restor Dentistry*, 2005; 17(5): 285–291.
37 Ruiz JL, Christensen GJ. Rationale for the utilization of bonded nonmetal onlays as an alternative to PFM crowns. *Dent Today*, 2006; 25(9): 80–83.

13

A Healthy Occlusion and the Occlusal Analysis

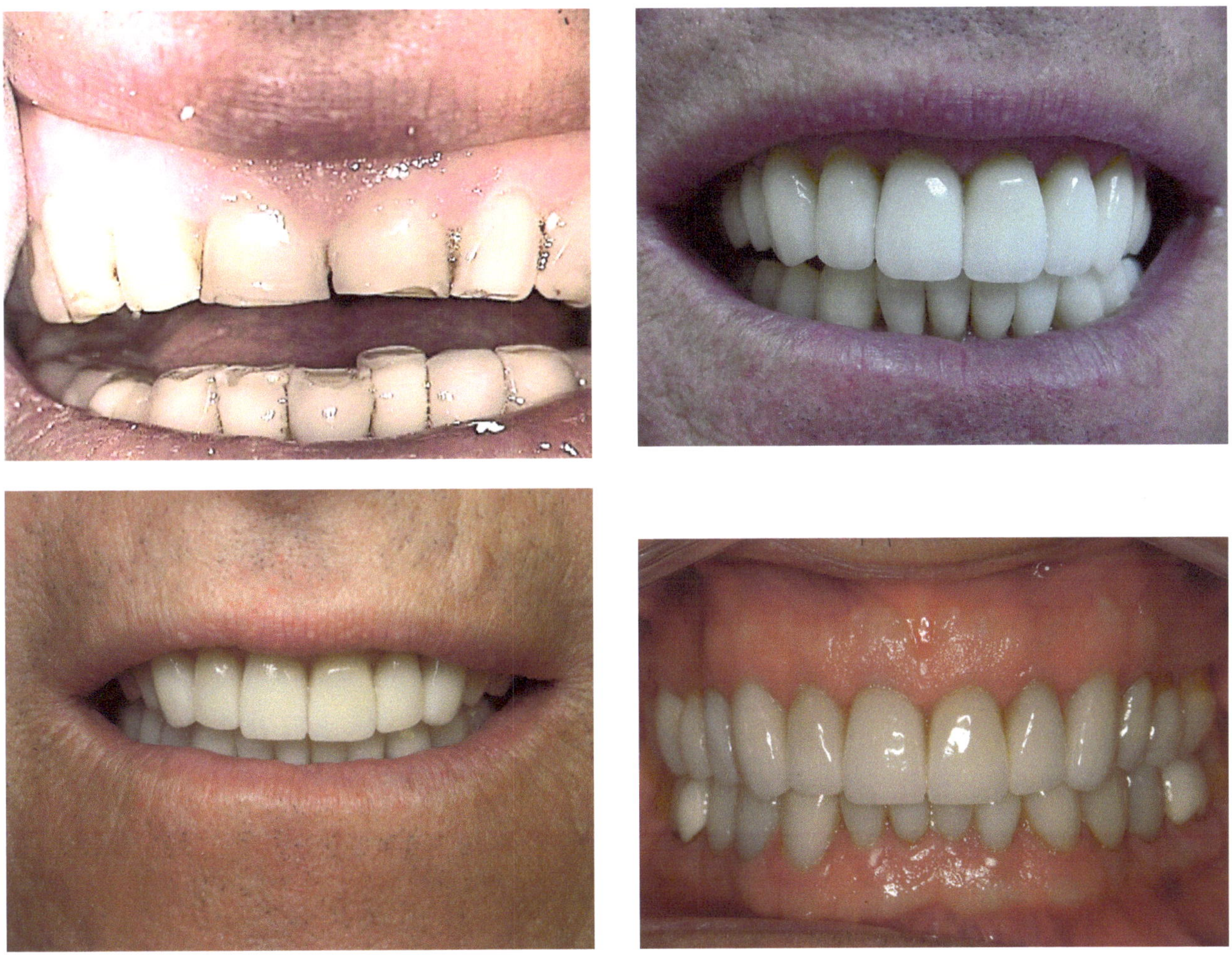

A badly damaged occlusion dating from 1997, 20 years postoperatively, showing good results.

Introduction

Understanding how to provide a physiologically and mechanically sound occlusion greatly serves the patient's overall oral health needs, and is a necessary asset for the clinician. As difficult as it has been historically for the profession to understand occlusion, it is a disservice to the patient to ignore it altogether, as occlusal disease continues to destroy dentition and restorations young and old (Figure 13.1). Unfortunately, not only has occlusion been complicated to learn but it has also become one of the most controversial subjects in dentistry. There are many occlusal methods, ranging in complexity from an intricate gnathological approach, a myofunctional approach, or even an overly-simplified natural bite approach. Each approach has its own following of

Supra-Gingival Minimally Invasive Dentistry: A Healthier Approach to Esthetic Restorations, First Edition. By Jose-Luis Ruiz.

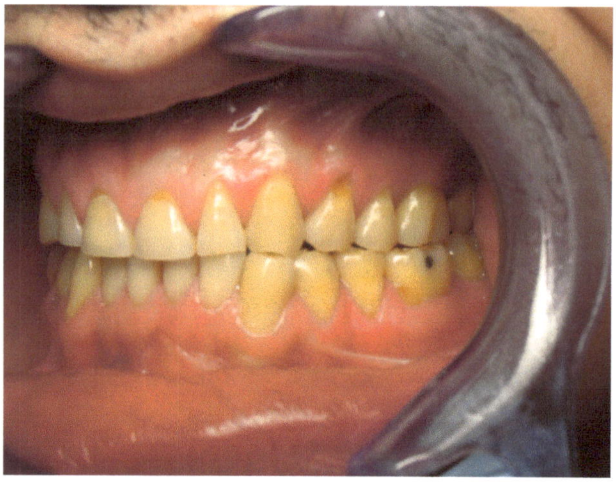

Figure 13.1 Severe occlusal disease in a young patient.

clinicians, who interpret the literature to back their opinion. Owing to the intense controversy, a large sector of overwhelmed dentists is confused as to which is the correct path and often choose to limit their involvement to single-tooth bite adjustment after a procedure and may choose to avoid occlusal therapy altogether. The literature points to three important rules for a harmonious occlusion, which encompass many other considerations. I call them the three golden rules of occlusion (Box 13.1). These rules are simple to remember and are the scientifically based goals of occlusal therapy. When used, the rules will give the patient a sound bite and will make the process less intimidating for the dentist.

Box 13.1 The three golden rules of occlusion

1) Bilateral, even occlusal contact, ideally in a centric relationship.
2) Posterior disocclusion (anterior and canine guidance).
3) An unobstructed envelope of function.

When Should the Three Golden Rules be Implemented?

These rules become very important for diagnosis and therapy only when the patient has clear signs and symptoms of occlusal disease, demonstrating that they have not adapted well to their current bite, and corrections would be desirable (Figure 13.2a). Additionally, when extensive dentistry is being planned, or the bite will be altered due to the partial or full rehabilitation (Figure 13.2b). These three rules make for a mechanically and physiologically sound bite.

It is important to remember that many patients may not fulfill one or more of the golden rules and may not show signs and symptoms of occlusal disease. This would suggest that they are well adapted to their current bite and no treatment is necessary or advisable. The mandible and its musculature have dozens of different movements and intricate relationships which govern the way in which the masticatory system functions, and just as when using a computer it is not necessary to know its internal workings, also it is not necessary to memorize all jaw movements and relationships. Fulfilling the three golden rules of occlusion encompasses all elements, and greatly simplifies the approach.

First Golden Rule: Equal Contacts

Ideally, all teeth must touch at the same time when a patient is in occlusion, forming bilateral equal contacts (Figure 13.3). Humans, when biting, exert hundreds of pounds of force per square inch, and it only makes sense that equal contacts during occlusion will allow for the forces to be

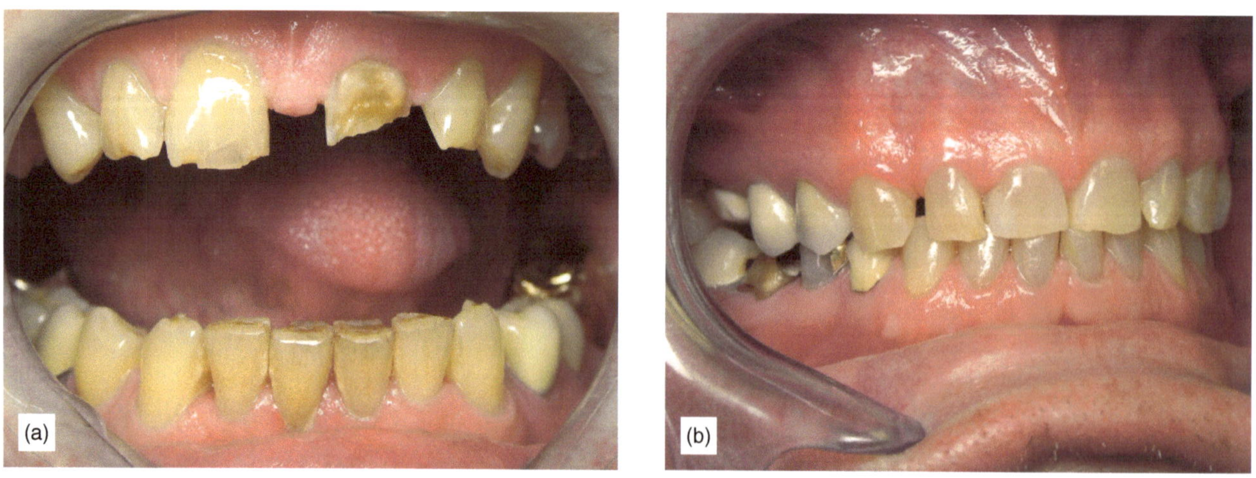

Figure 13.2 (a) Occlusal disease in an older patient (c. 50 years). (b) Case needing extensive rehabilitation.

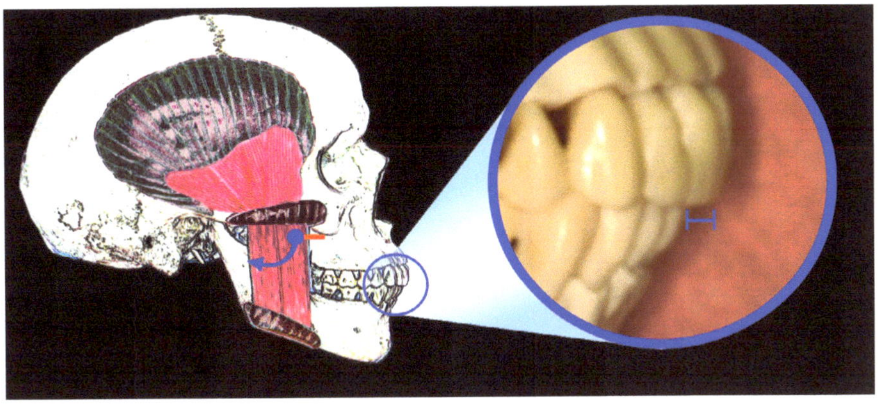

Figure 13.3 Jaw showing equal contact throughout.

shared among all teeth [1]. When one of the teeth interferes with equal contact, it can lead to severe damage to these teeth, as they will absorb excessive forces [2]. Additionally, the literature shows that if a patient develops or receives an interference in their bite, they will develop transient muscle discoordination and other problems (Figure 13.4) [3,4]. When an interference to the centric bite exists, the patient may develop a deflective interference, which will cause a permanent deviation to the centric bite and lead to uneven destructive wear, similar to the uneven wear that occurs with an unbalanced tire in a car.

All clinicians have had a patient tell them, "That filling we did a while back felt really high at first, but now it feels fine." It would be important to consider how did the bite adapt to the high contact? Most often what happened is that the deflective interference caused a permanent change in their bite in order for them to adapt and function (Figure 13.5a–c) [5]. This occurs when a patient's musculature develops engrams to avoid the dangerous interference and permanently changes the position of their mandible, mostly forward, as a defense mechanism [6]. The interference forces the mandible to find a new, safe way to bite, chew and clench without damaging that high spot. Unfortunately, something else in the masticatory system will pay the price for this change [7]. Whatever is the weakest link in the patient's mouth is what ends up paying the price for this deflective interference. If there is a weak tooth, it will fracture (Figure 13.6). If the patient has weak muscles or joints, they may develop headaches. They can also easily develop any of the other signs and symptoms of occlusal disease, such as hypermobility, abfractions, or wear.

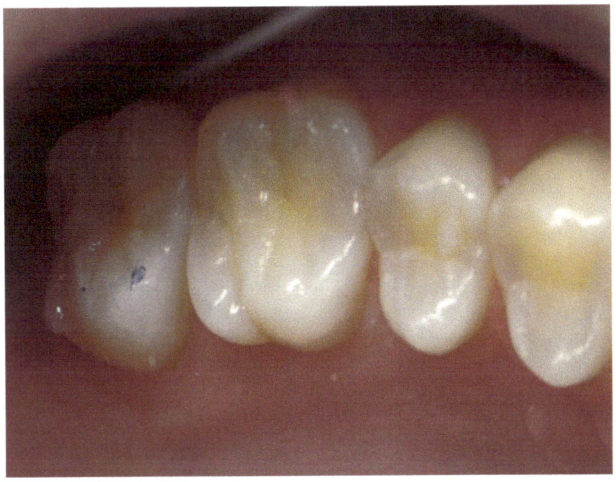

Figure 13.4 Centric interference; only one tooth touches in centric relationship.

While research is clear that when the patient occludes, all teeth should touch at the same time, there are many opinions as to where the mandible should be while this occurs. The mandible has almost infinite possibilities for movement, so there must be some means of reliably reproducing the location of the mandible in relationship to the maxilla. The centric relationship is a reproducible jaw relationship unrelated to the teeth, as it is the place where both condyles seat high up, tightly against the fossa. The centric relationship is considered to be a physiological position because, when the masticatory muscles are contracting, they will guide the condyle to sit in the fossa as long as there is no dental interference. In extensive rehabilitations and equilibration, it is ideal to adjust the teeth to ensure that the patient's centric occlusion, or natural bite, coincides with their centric relationship [8,9]. I adopt a non-strict centric relationship philosophy, meaning that as long as the patient has no signs or symptoms of occlusal disease, it is not necessary to adjust or equilibrate the patient into a centric relationship, as they have clearly adapted their natural bite. Additionally, the centric relationship is not a perfect, unmovable place in space [10].

Second Golden Rule: Posterior Disocclusion

Posterior disocclusion occurs when the canines and anterior teeth will immediately disclude the posterior teeth in any eccentric movements (Figure 13.7a,b). As previously discussed, humans exert hundreds of pounds of force per square inch when biting. While biting on the centric position where the forces are mostly axial and all the teeth

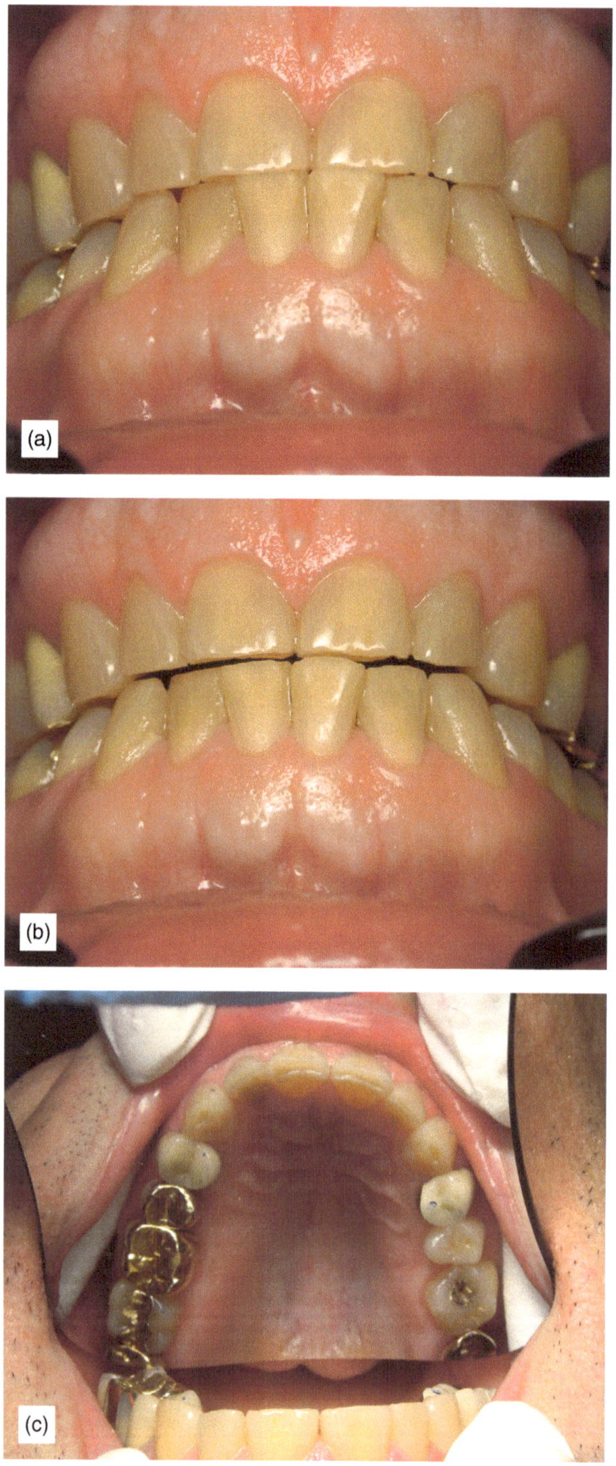

Figure 13.5 (a) Natural bite showing severe anterior wear. (b) Centric relationship bite showing more overjet. (c) Mandible in forward position because of centric sliding interference.

touch at the same time, the forces are shared and any damage to the teeth is minimized. A different scenario occurs when the mandible goes into eccentric movement (forward or to the sides). This is, of course, a natural occurrence when eating, as the mandible goes in the direction of the food, and of course this also happens during parafunctional

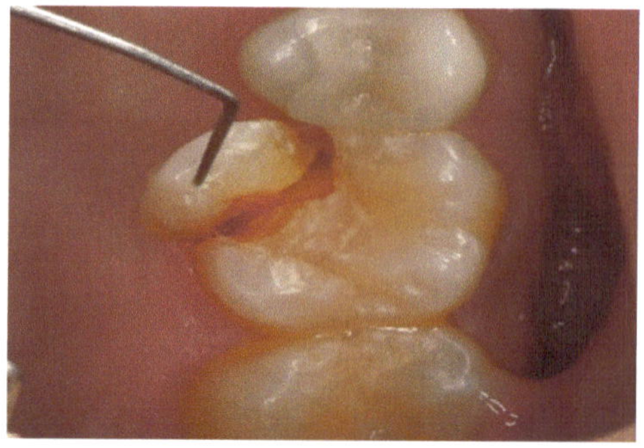

Figure 13.6 Virgin tooth fractured due to tooth being in severe interference.

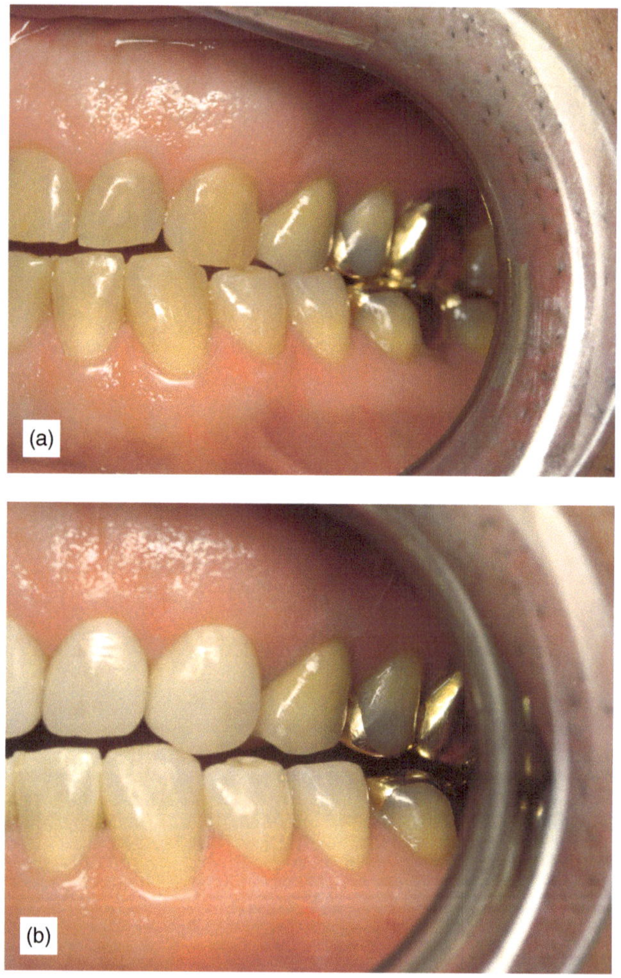

Figure 13.7 Lateral movement showing: (a) Group function. (b) Canine guidance.

movements. It is in these lateral eccentric movements where only a few teeth touch, mostly in off-center directions (shear), that damage occurs when the full forces of the masticatory muscles are exerted.

Is there a way in which the forces could be minimized or controlled while the mandible is in eccentric movements? Researchers have found that once anterior teeth separate from posterior teeth, the forces are diminished dramatically, and thus the possible damage is decreased [11,12,13].

Ideally, when the mandible swings outside the centric position, the canines and anterior teeth should immediately disclude the back teeth; when this happens, the forces decrease dramatically. This becomes a significant benefit to the patient in protecting their dentition. Therefore, to adhere to the second golden rule, the molars cannot touch anywhere outside the centric relationship (no red outside of blue; Figure 13.8).

For canine guidance to be successful, no posterior interference should be present, and disocclusion must be immediate. This means that a strong palatal ridge must be present on the canines (Figure 13.9a–c). If this is not accomplished,

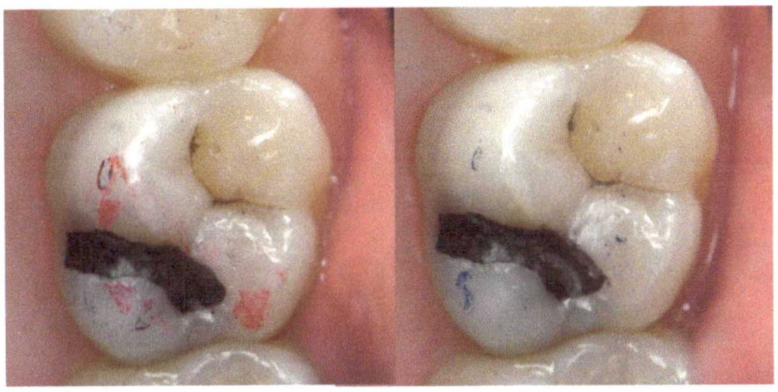

Figure 13.8 Red outside blue during occlusal adjustment, showing lateral interference during eccentric movements.

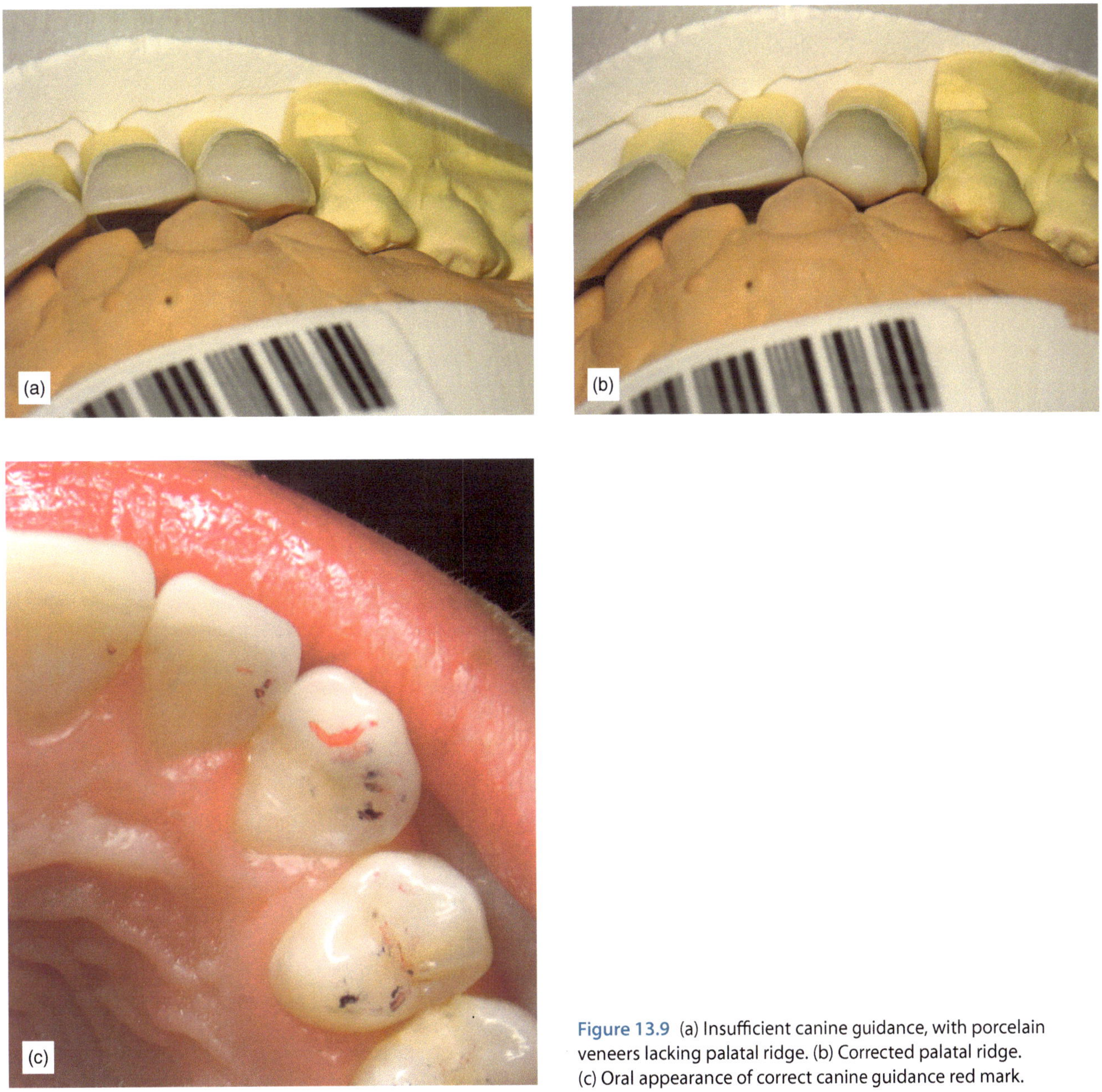

Figure 13.9 (a) Insufficient canine guidance, with porcelain veneers lacking palatal ridge. (b) Corrected palatal ridge. (c) Oral appearance of correct canine guidance red mark.

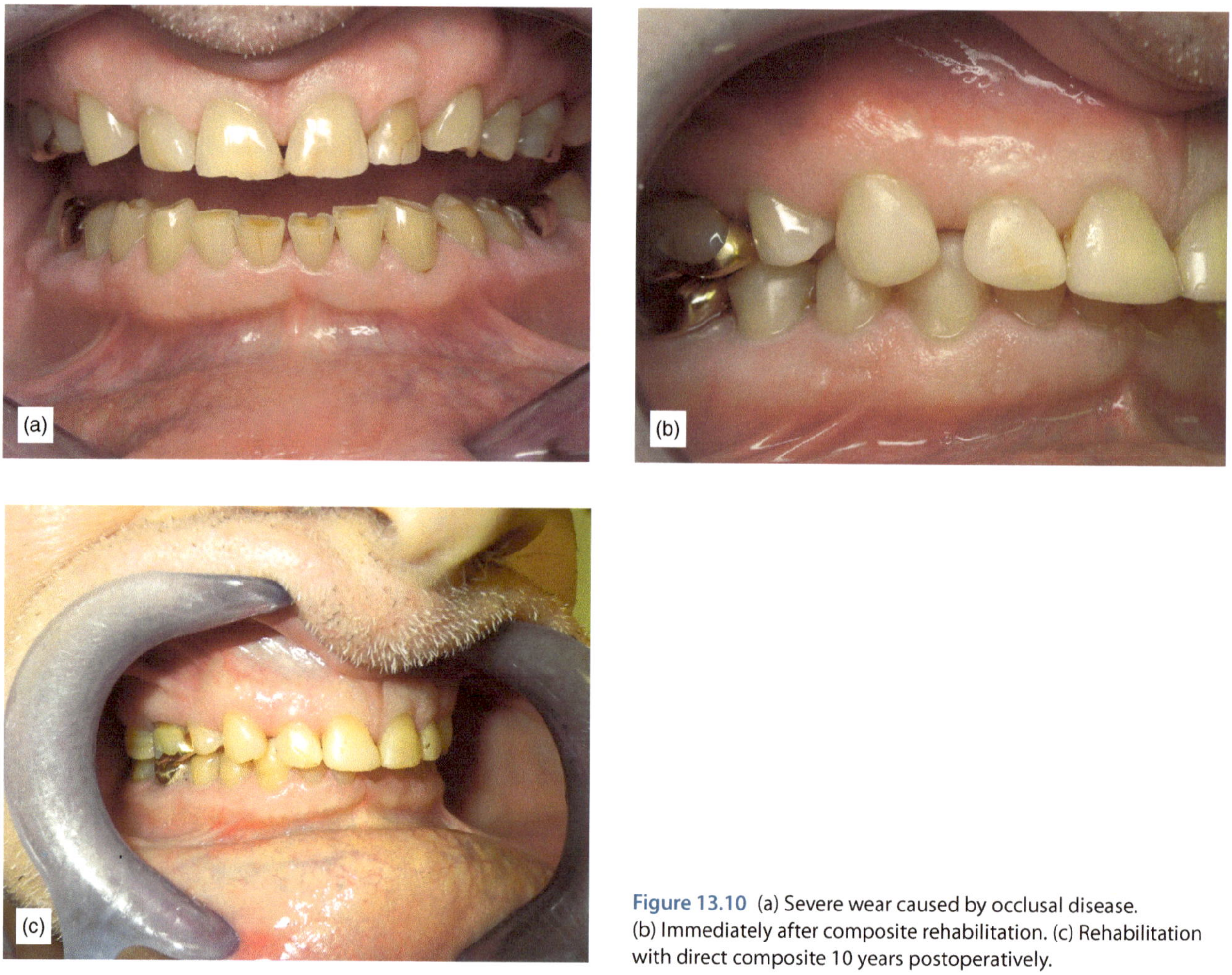

Figure 13.10 (a) Severe wear caused by occlusal disease. (b) Immediately after composite rehabilitation. (c) Rehabilitation with direct composite 10 years postoperatively.

as soon as there is an interference, or a posterior tooth can touch outside of centric, the muscles will be able to exude those hundreds of pounds of force [14,15], with the ability to cause damage to the involved structures. When there is simultaneous contact between multiple posterior teeth on the working or non-working side of the mouth during the swinging of the mandible, this is called group function. Group function occurs when the second golden rule is absent, and is the instigator of wear, fractures, loose teeth, abfractions, and even muscle pain.

When a patient presents with group function and severe occlusal disease, regaining posterior disocclusion is very successful [16] and can be achieved by equilibrating the posterior teeth or lengthening the anterior teeth to improve guidance with porcelain or composite. Evidence from the literature points to the successful use of direct composite as a viable alternative in treating even severe wear cases, although wear and durability will not match porcelain, but because of lower cost and easier patient acceptance, it can be used as a long-term transitional procedure (Figure 13.10a–c) [17,18,19]. Regardless of the choice of material, fulfilling the three golden rules will maximize durability.

It is possible to become confused between anterior guidance and envelope of function. These are separate principles that need to be understood and implemented in each case. Therefore, to clarify, anterior guidance is the protrusive motion of the mandible, such as in chewing, which provides immediate posterior disocclusion that can be altered with restorations (Figure 13.11). The envelope of function is the small amount of play or freedom that the mandible has in the centric opening and closing, not related to eccentric movements, as will be seen next.

Third Rule: The Envelope of Function

The envelope of function is the natural play or freedom in movement of the mandible during opening and closing. When a human opens and closes their mouth, the jaw does not act like a straight-path hinge. When the mouth is opened, the jaw moves down and slightly back. When closing, the jaw moves up and forward, returning to centric. If that motion were to be drawn on a diagram, it would almost be similar to a teardrop-shaped motion. This requires that there be space in the front of the occlusion,

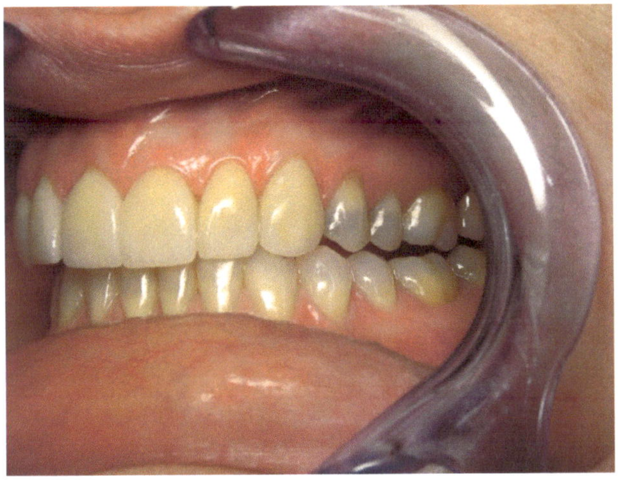

Figure 13.11 The mandible is moved forward to check anterior guidance and the lack of posterior interference.

or overjet, for the mandible to swing in this fashion (Figure 13.12).

When the patient lacks sufficient overjet, severe damage and wear to the anterior teeth will be a lifelong problem, until it is corrected (Figures 13.13, 13.14). If patients with this problem come into a practice seeking esthetic treatment, it is imperative that the dentist does not jump right into lengthening their teeth without planning to provide sufficient overjet. Those longer restorations will be worn down or broken the same way that the natural teeth were if the envelope of function violation is not corrected [20].

Although incisal overjet is necessary to provide clearance for the envelope of function movement, overjet in the incisal area alone is not sufficient. Having or creating the space necessary for the freedom or slight variation on the centric contact during opening and closing in front of the centric contact is equally necessary. Lundeen and Gibbs state that this variation is approximately 0.3 mm (Figure 13.15) [15]. Other people have

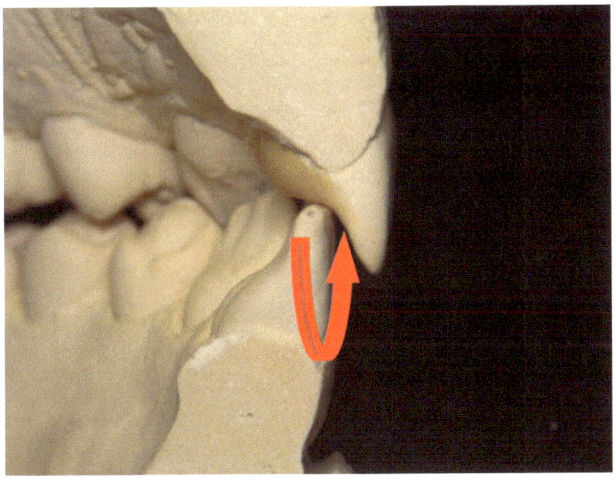

Figure 13.12 Envelope of function path.

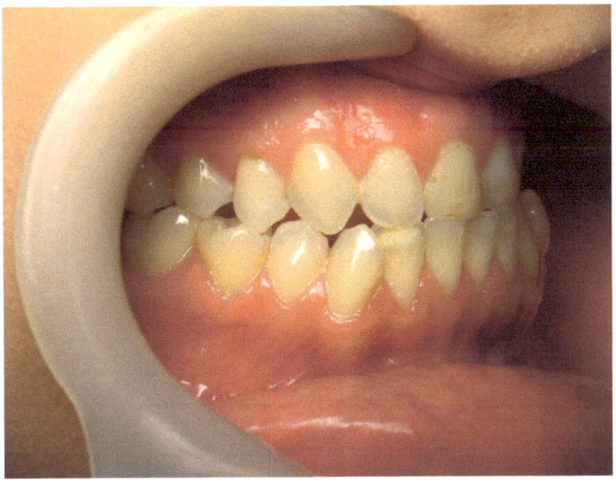

Figure 13.13 Lack of overjet leading to damage caused by an envelope of function violation.

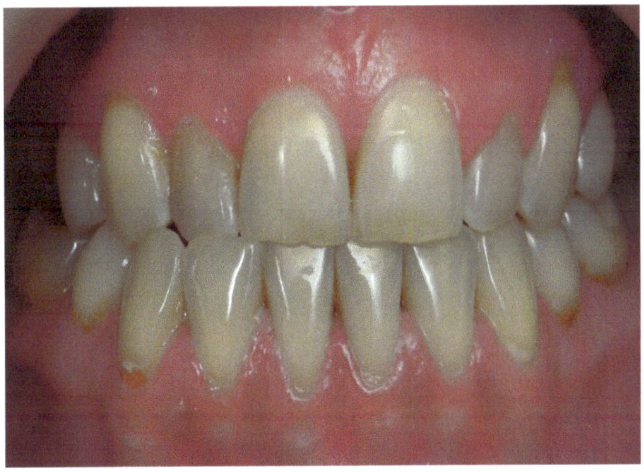

Figure 13.14 Lack of overjet leading to damage caused by an envelope of function violation.

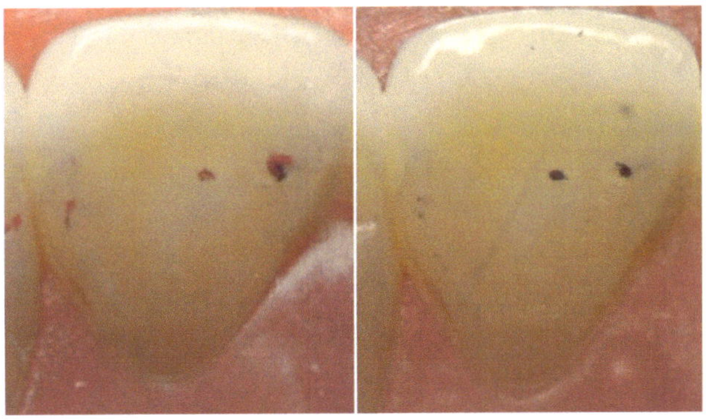

Figure 13.15 Envelope of function violation on the cingulum area.

called this long centric. Sometimes a violation to the envelope of function can be discovered, either when patients state that their front teeth are getting in the way of their bite, or when a significant amount of wear is visible in the lingual surface of the maxillary teeth. Fremitus is an excellent way of assessing envelope of

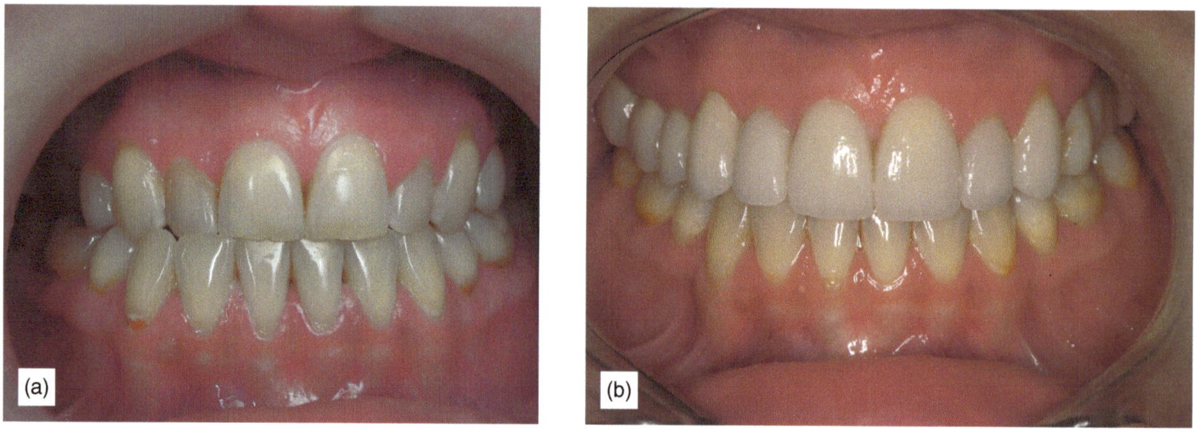

Figure 13.16 (a) Lack of overbite and overjet. (b) After veneers and onlays.

function violation. If there is movement on any tooth, there is an envelope of function violation. This can lead to fractures, and other signs and symptoms. Envelope of function violations alter muscle activity and can easily trigger parafunctional activity [21,22].

Envelope of function violations are managed by creating the necessary space to allow for the unrestricted opening and closing movement of the mandible during centric closure. Sufficient overjet and centric contact space is the answer (Figure 13.16a,b). Gaining overjet will, in many cases, require some changes to the anterior teeth. This requires decisions on esthetic preferences (Chapter 8), financial investment, and length of treatment preferences, so options should be given to the patient to enable them to make a decision. The main three ways to alter overjet are:

1) Orthodontic correction.
2) Opening the vertical dimension.
3) Restorative alteration of the shape of teeth.

All three methods have positive and negative aspects, and each case is unique as to which option or options will best suit the needs of that specific patient (Figure 13.17a–d).

Vertical Dimension of Occlusion and Minimally Invasive Rehabilitation

Contrary to many assumptions, the vertical dimension of occlusion is not a golden rule, and can be altered if necessary [23,24,25]. Patients can accommodate changes in the vertical dimension of occlusion within reason [26]. In some cases with severe wear, expanding the vertical dimension of occlusion can be a good option, as it will dramatically decrease the need for excessive occlusal and incisal tooth reduction. This, combined with supragingival minimally invasive techniques, can allow for a truly "minimally invasive rehabilitation" of the worn dentition (Figures 13.18a–g,

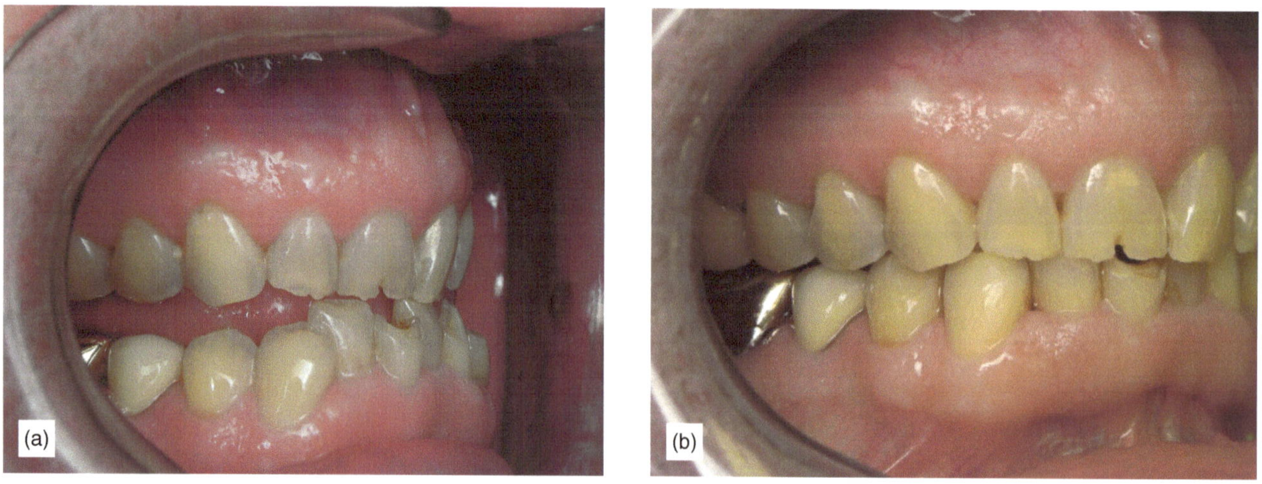

Figure 13.17 (a) Patient with severe lack of overjet and envelope of function violation. (b) After orthodontics to align and provide more overjet. (*Continued*)

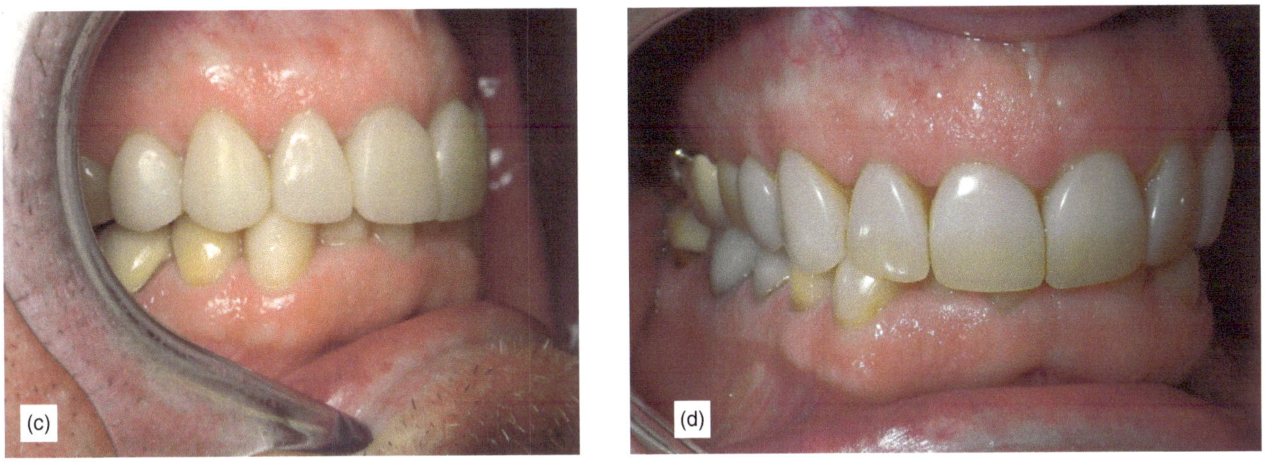

Figure 13.17 (*Continued*)
(c) After porcelain veneers to rehabilitate his smile with proper overjet and free envelope of function. (d) After 11 years.

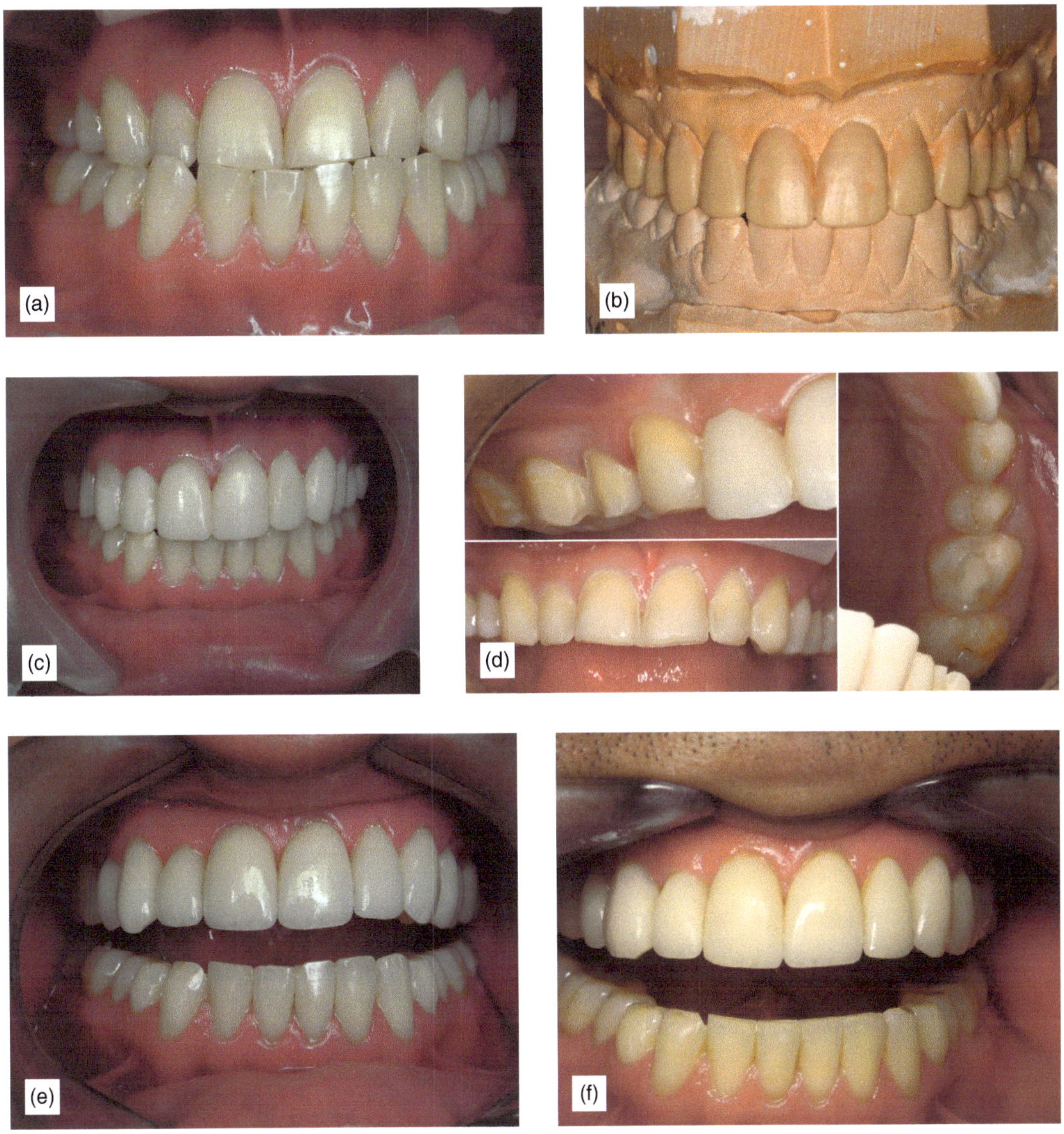

Figure 13.18 (a) Minimally invasive rehabilitation requiring opening of the vertical dimension of occlusion. (b) Maxillary wax-up showing the longer teeth and opening of the vertical dimension of occlusion (c) Provisionals in the mouth. (d) Supragingival minimally invasive tooth preparation. (e) Immediately after bonded cementation. (f) Ten years postoperatively. (*Continued*)

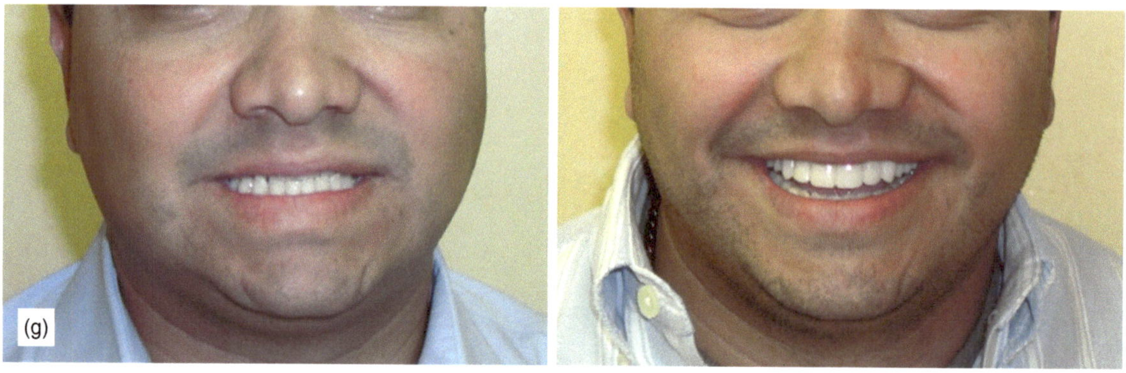

Figure 13.18 (*Continued*)
(g) Before and after smile.

13.19a–f). Knowing that the three golden rules allow for a physiologically and mechanically sound bite and using the above described minimally invasive worn dentition rehabilitation will allow for healthier dentistry for the patient.

Data Gathering and Developing a Treatment Plan

Discovering that a patient has occlusal disease by taking a few minutes in each examination to notice any of the

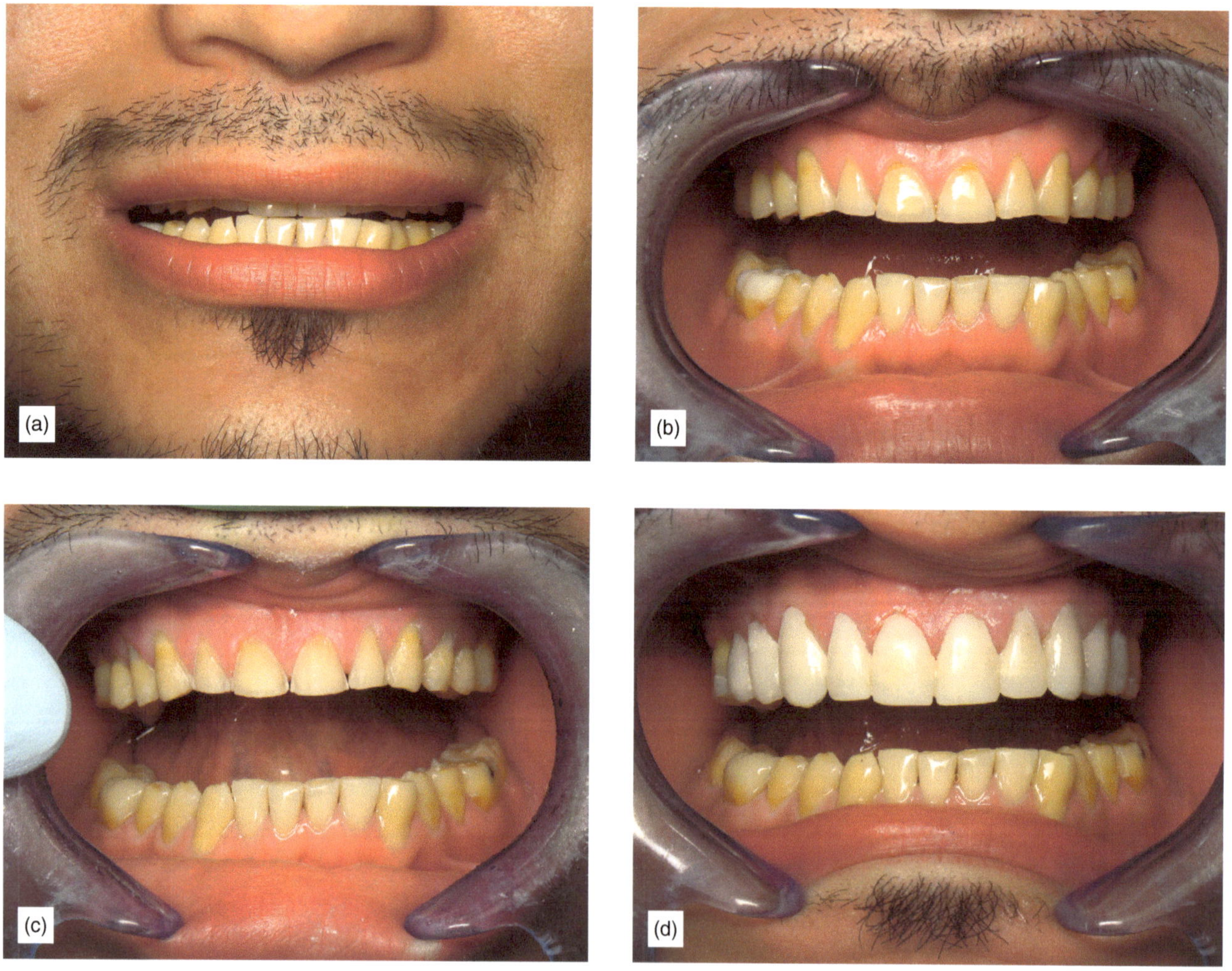

Figure 13.19 (a) Severely worn dentition, with short anterior teeth, needing opening of the vertical dimension of occlusion. (b) Severe wear evident before preparation. (c) Teeth after preparation showing the supragingival minimum preparation. (d) After provisionals. (*Continued*)

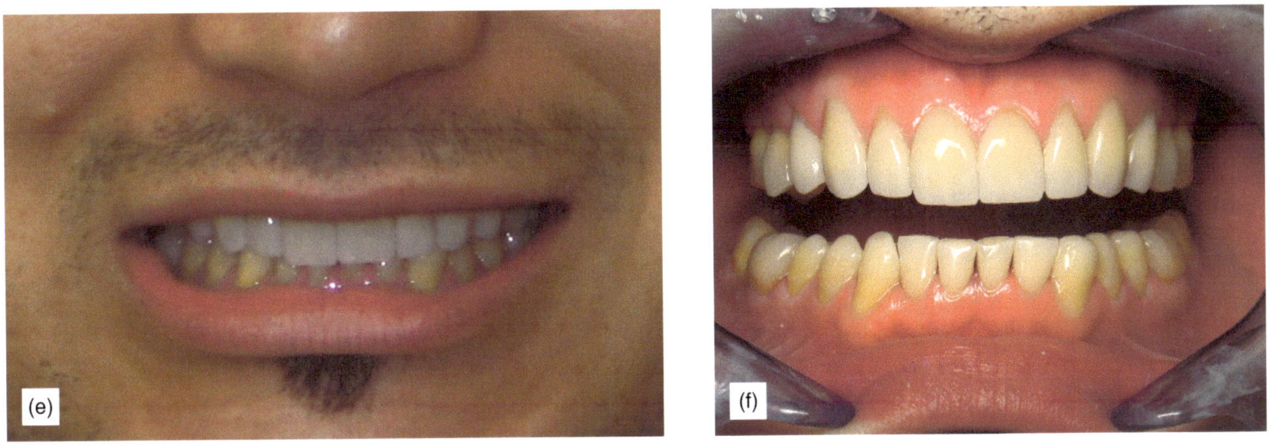

Figure 13.19 (*Continued*)
(e) Smile after finished rehabilitation, with feldspathic porcelain. (f) Five years postoperatively, with no chips or fractures.

seven signs and symptoms is only the first step in diagnosis. Once the need for occlusal therapy is discovered, it is necessary to have a methodical process in place to take a patient who is only interested in basic care to accepting and completing occlusal and maybe esthetic treatment (Figure 13.20a–d) [27]. The record-taking visit, which includes an occlusal analysis and, if necessary, an esthetic diagnosis, allows for a few elements to come together to

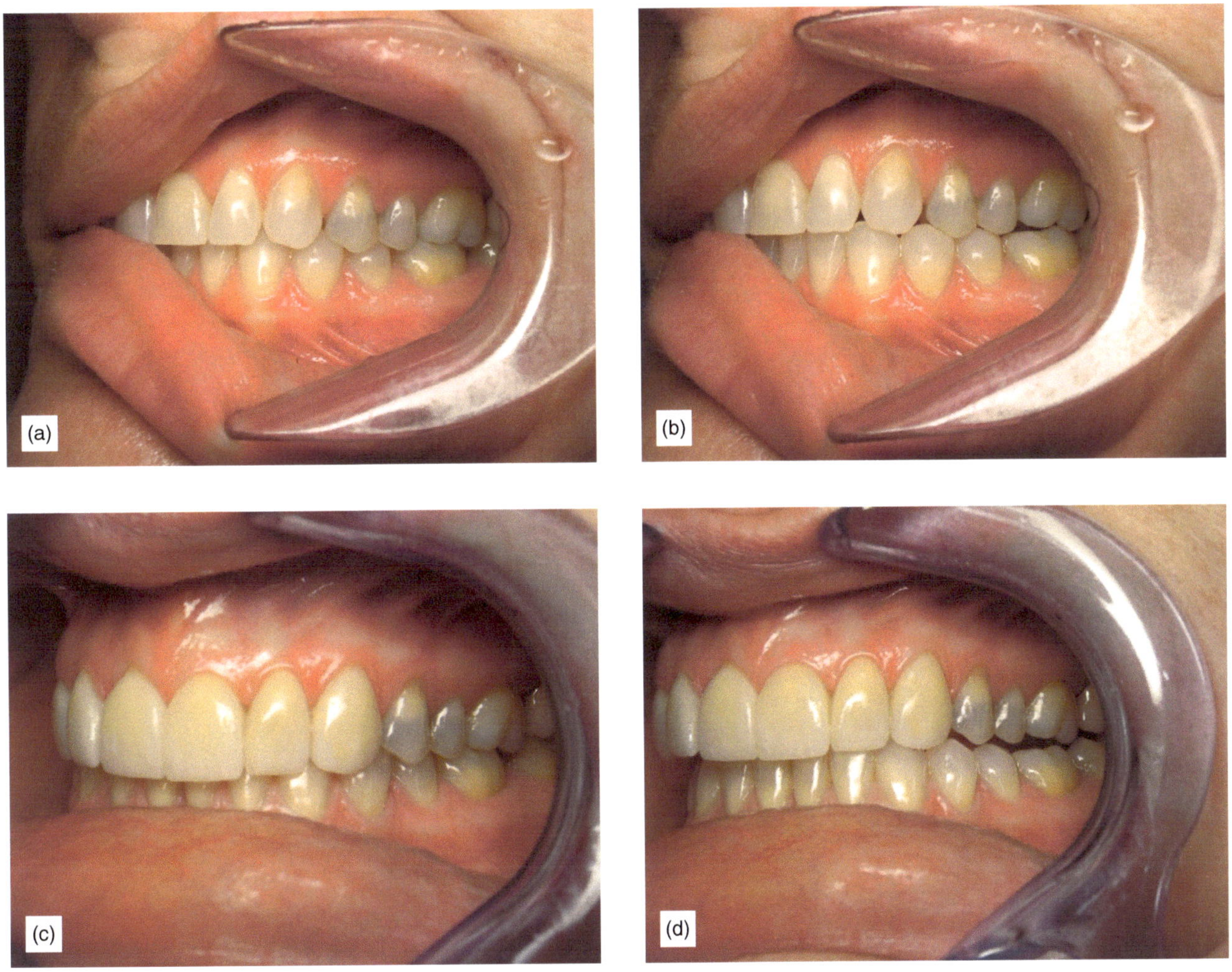

Figure 13.20 (a) Patient with severe migraines, biting in her natural bite. (b) Patient performing a lateral movement, showing group function. (c) Patient on centric after equilibration and porcelain veneers for esthetic and occlusal purposes. (d) Lateral showing good posterior disocclusion; the patient's migraines disappeared after occlusal therapy.

make treatment more predictable: the gathering of information for final diagnosis; the opportunity for both parties to communicate goals and limitations for occlusal and esthetic therapy.

Records should be taken and comprehensive diagnosis should be performed when a patient has been diagnosed with occlusal disease, and any time that a patient requires extensive restorative dentistry or esthetic treatment, including several anterior restorations, to ensure more predictable results for the patient and a reassurance to the clinician of longevity of restorations being placed [28]. The records should include a dentofacial diagnostic photographic series, a panoramic x-ray, a Silginate impression to make study cast models, a facebow recording using a good articulator with well-designed facebow (Figure 13.21a–h), a muscle deprogrammer (Figure 13.22), a good comprehensive questionnaire (Figure 13.23). This should be followed by a clinical examination which may include load testing, assessment of the first point of contact and occlusal slide, range of motion assessment, listening for temporomandibular joint noise using a stethoscope.

The data recorded above, and with a set of casts mounted on a semi-precision articulator, a good cast evaluation and trial equilibration, or even a diagnostic wax-up, can yield much information towards a final diagnosis and treatment planning with good occlusal principles (Figure 13.24a–j) [29]. The diagnosis can range in complexity, and options should be given. From least to most invasive, patients who have damaged their dentition owing to occlusal disease can be managed with the following interventions:

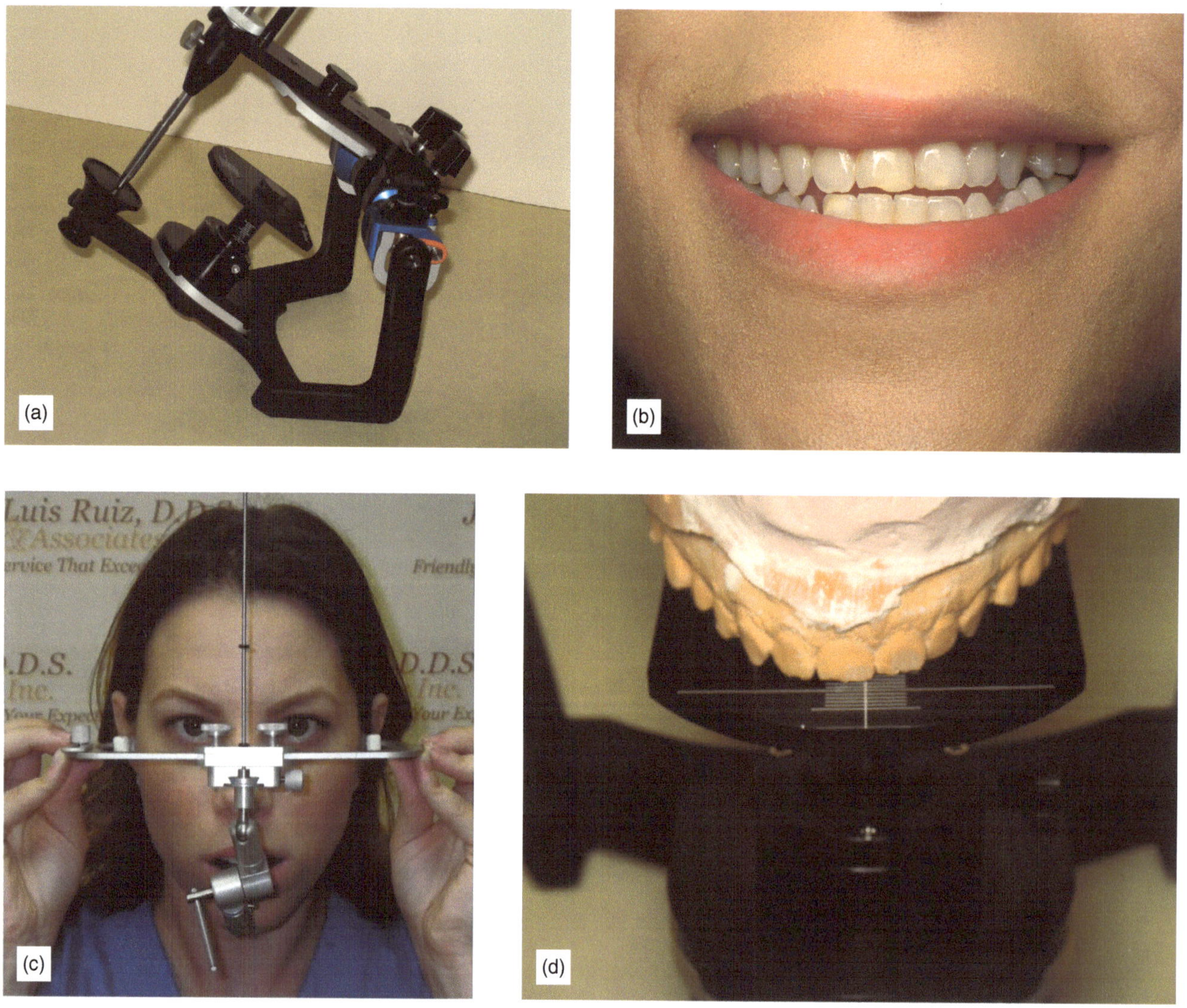

Figure 13.21 (a) The Director Articulator and Diagnostic System. (b) Patient with severe asymmetries needing proper diagnostic tools. (c) Facebow correctly used to evaluate midline, occlusal plane, as well as axis of rotation to dentition. (d) Correct facebow-mounted cast evaluated with a coordinated diagnostic plate from the Director system. (*Continued*)

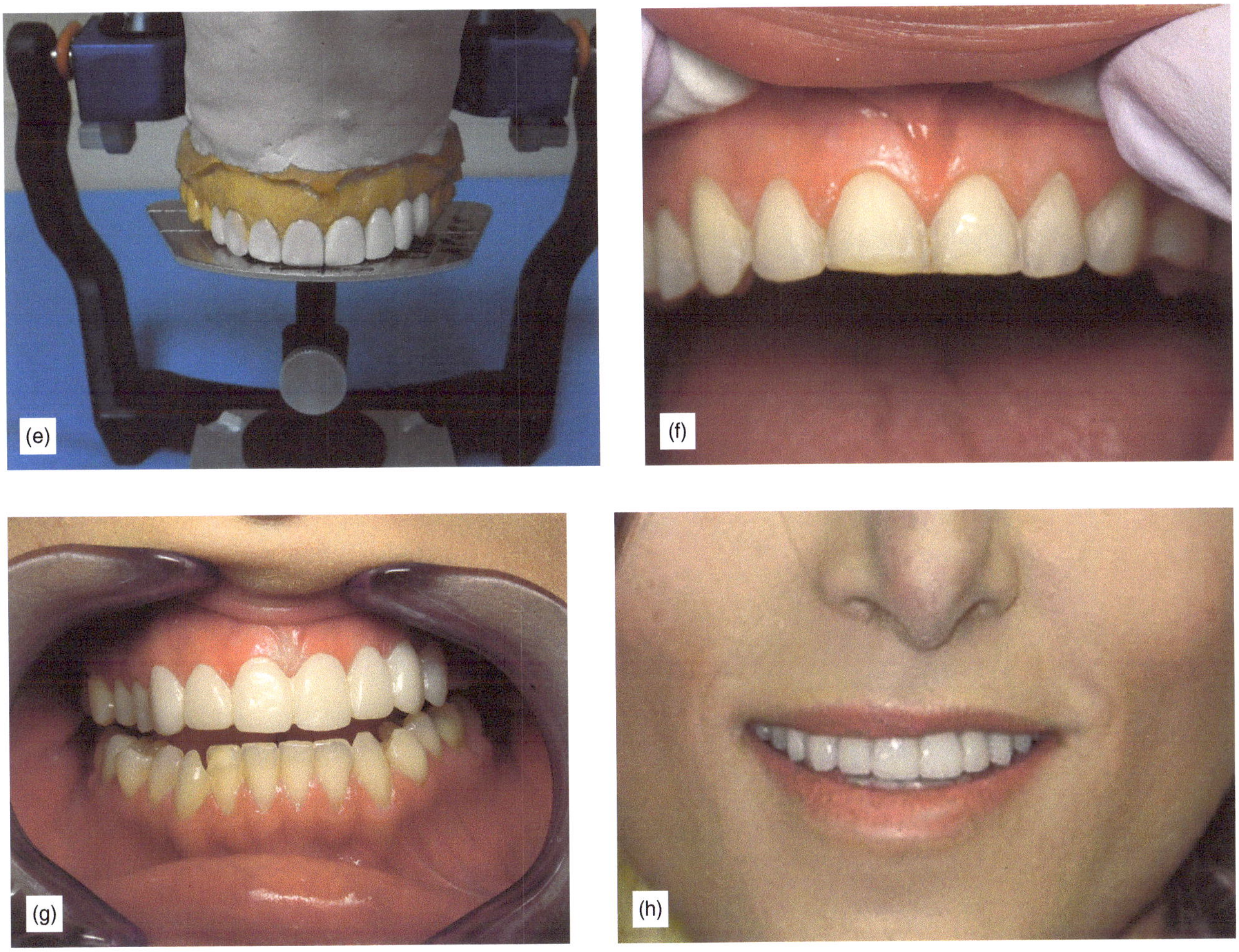

Figure 13.21 (*Continued*)
(e) Wax-up was easily fabricated by laboratory using the diagnostic plate (prototype depicted) to evaluated amount of cant and midline correction needed. (f) Supragingival minimally invasive preparations. (g) Provisionals at the time of esthetic check; correction can easily be made before final restorations. (h) Final restoration showing the dramatic improvement.

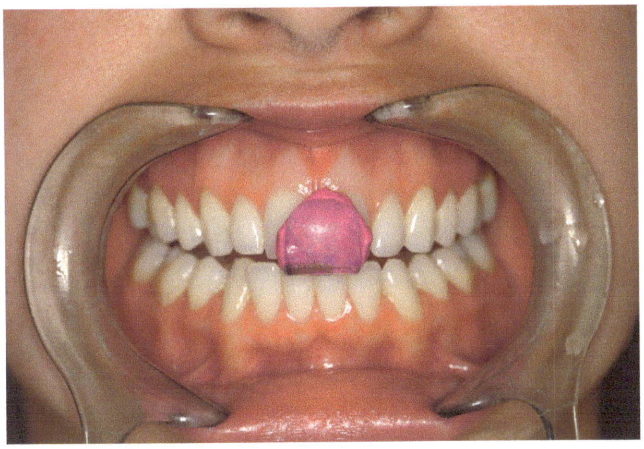

Figure 13.22 Pankey jig used as a deprogrammer.

- night guard or occlusal splint
- simple subtractive equilibration plus night guard
- subtractive and additive equilibration night guard
- occlusal rehabilitation night guard.

Combining the findings from the occlusal analysis, the esthetic smile design, and any caries and periodontal diagnosis, a clinician can achieve an ideal global treatment plan that will benefit a patient's overall health. It is important to remember that minimally invasive treatment is the goal, which includes minimally invasive occlusal therapy as well as minimally invasive esthetic treatment.

Implementing a minimally invasive occlusal diagnosis and therapy should take the following into consideration:

- The consequences of untreated occlusal disease are far more than temporomandibular joint disease or pain.
- Occlusal diagnosis must be practical if it is going to be implemented routinely.

OCCLUSION & TMJ ANALYSIS

PATIENT NAME: **DATE:**

Please answer by checking, circling and/or describing all that apply: CIRCLE

INITIAL EXAM

YES NO

____ ____ 1) Do you have frequent headaches? Migraines?______ 1-10?______

____ ____ 2) Do you have pain in or around the jaw joint? 1-10?______ L R

When did you first notice the jaw pain? ______________________

____ ____ 3) Has the pain recently become more severe?

____ ____ 4) When is the pain worse? Mornings Evenings At Meals

____ ____ 5) Do you have tired jaw muscles? Mornings Evenings

____ ____ 6) Do you have tooth sensitivity to: Cold?__ Air?__ Chewing?__ Tooth/Teeth?______

____ ____ 7) Do you have clicking, popping, or grating noises in your jaw joint? L R

When did you first notice the noise? ______________________

1ST FOLLOW UP

____ ____ 8) Does your jaw problem interfere with your normal activities?

____ ____ 9) Have you had treatment(s) for this problem? When? ______ Where? ______

____ ____ 10) Are you taking, or have you taken, medication for this problem?

____ ____ 11) Are you taking antidepressants or any medication that may affect muscle activity or cause dry mouth?

____ ____ 12) Have you ever had a severe blow or trauma to the head, neck or jaw?

Explain: ______________________

____ ____ 13) Do you have difficulty chewing? This is a result of: Pain in joint Pain in teeth Limited opening Other (specify): ______________________

____ ____ 14) Has your mouth ever locked open or closed? When?______________

2ND FOLLOW UP

____ ____ 15) Are you aware of: clenching and/or: grinding your teeth? (Please circle)

____ ____ 16) Do you think nervous tension seems to affect this problem?

____ ____ 17) Have there been recent changes in your lifestyle or other stressful events?

____ ____ 18) Have you had problems with other joints? Pain? ______________

____ ____ 19) Have you ever felt or do you feel like your bite is changing? Y N When?______

20) What are your main Goals for "Occlusal" & TMJ treatment? ______________

____

CLINICAL EVALUATION **DATE:**

1. Load Test Pain ______ **2. Initial Contact (Mouth)** ______ **3. Occlusal Slide** ***Take Bite*** ______

4. Ant. Guidance ______ **Canine Guide. R:** ______ **L:** ______

5. Max Opening ______ **Lat. R:** ______ **L:** ______ **Pain On: Opening:** ______ **R:** ______ **L:** ______

6. Fremitus:/Mobility 2+ ______ **7. CD Hypersensitivity (CDH)** ______

8. TMJ Noise R: ______ **L:** ______

9. Envelope Violation ______ **10. Cross Bite** ______ **Open Bite** ______

11.Parafuction: Brux Clench 12. Angle Bite Class: I IID1 IID2 III

MOUNTED CAST EVALUATION / Specify Tooth, Surface, Location

CHECK BITE first **CR Interf:** ______ **Lat. Interf:** ______ **Occlusal Plane:** ______

Severe Wear: **Abfraction:** ***Is It Close Enough*?** **Wax-Up Needed?**

TRIAL OCCLUSAL EQUILIBRATION (Specify tooth, surface, location)

Initial Incisal Pin Setting: ______ **Final Pin Setting:** ______ **Bite Close?** ______

Teeth Needing Plasty: ______________________

Teeth Needing Restoration: ______________________

DIAGNOSIS: Dawson Class I II III IV	TREATMENT

Figure 13.23 Occlusal examination form (LA Institute).

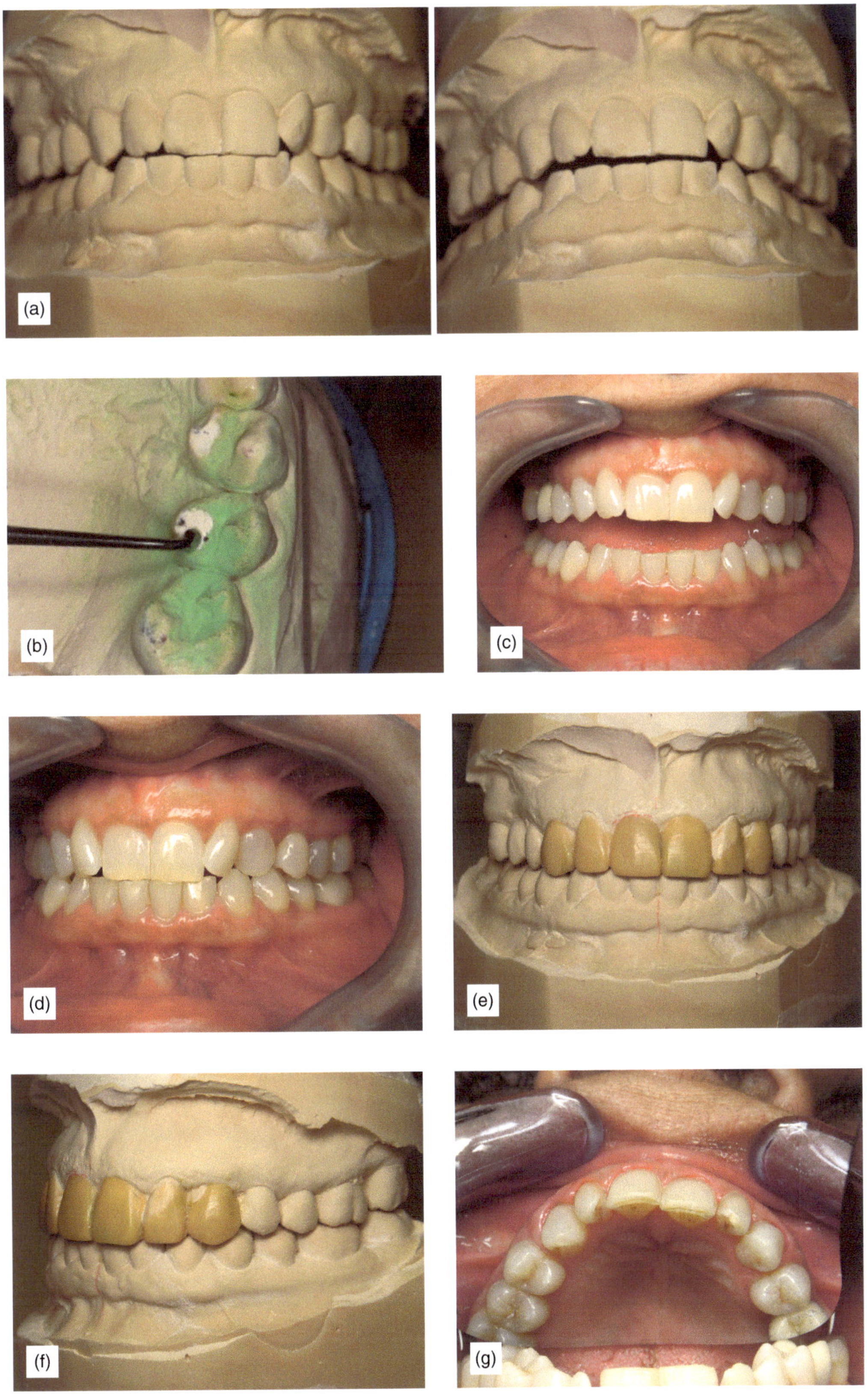

Figure 13.24 (a) Patient showing lack of overjet on her natural bite; after trial equilibration, the bite shows more overjet. (b) Trial equilibration showing deflective interferences. (c) Incisal edge wear caused by lack of overjet and parafunctional activity. (d) Observe the lack of noticeable overjet in side view. (e) Wax-up of equilibrated cast. (f) Side view of wax-up. (g) Observe the minimum facial reduction of preparations. (*Continued*)

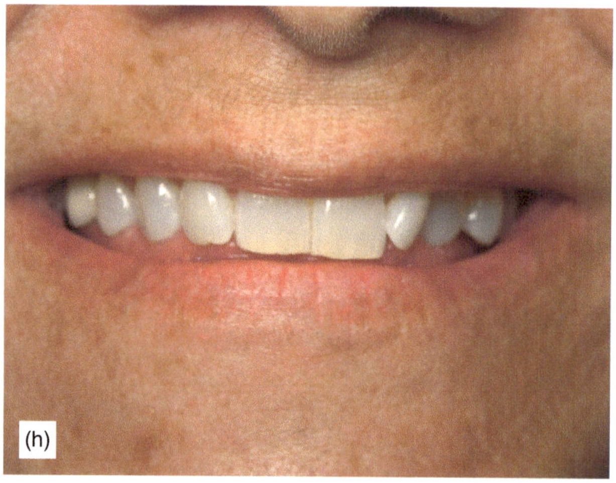

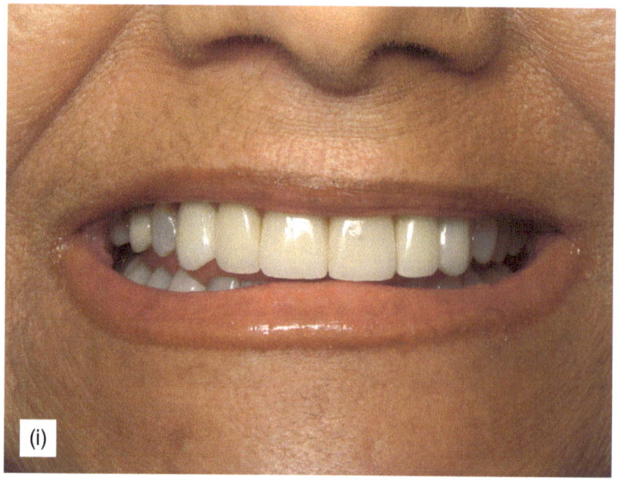

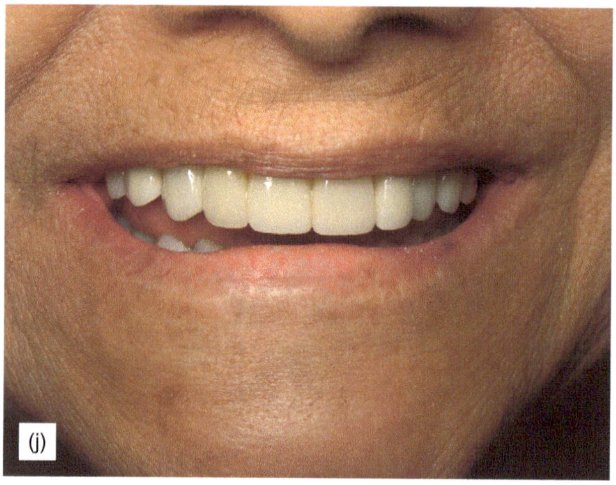

Figure 13.24 *(Continued)*
(h) Before veneers and occlusal equilibration. (i) After treatment. (j) Seven years postoperatively.

- "Ideal dentistry" is an illusion and leads to overtreatment.
- Occlusal disease is not curable, but it can be managed.
- There must be a realistic and definable end point for occlusal treatment, which cannot be perfection. The three golden rules of occlusion make a sound end point.
- Managing occlusal disease should not be more destructive than the disease itself; the most minimally invasive approach is always best.
- Occlusal treatment does not require expensive instrumentation.

An entire book can be written on occlusal disease and how to manage it, but that is not the focus of this book. This section is very relevant and indispensable to restorative dentistry, though. By ensuring that the patient's occlusion adheres to the three golden rules of occlusion, the clinician is able to manage occlusal forces and help the patient to preserve their dentition and restorations for a much longer period.

References

1 Gibbs CH, Mahan PE, Mauderli A, Lundeen HC, Walsh EK. Limits of human bite strength. *J Prosthet Dent*, 1986; 56(2): 226–229.
2 Ishigaki S, Kurozumi T, Morishige E, Yatani H. Occlusal interference during mastication can cause pathological tooth mobility. *J Periodontal Res*, 2006; 41(3): 189–192.
3 Sheilholeslam A, Riise C. Influence of experimental interfering occlusal contacts on the activity of the anterior temporal and masseter muscles during submaximal and maximal bite in the intercuspal position. *J Oral Rehab*, 1983; 10: 207–214.
4 Clark GT, Tsukiyama Y, Baba K, Watanabe T. Sixty-eight years of experimental occlusal interference studies: What have we learned? *J Prosthet Dent*, 1999; 82(6): 704–713.
5 Piehslinger E, Celar RM, Horejs T, Slavicek R. Recording orthopedic jaw movements. Part IV: The rotational component during mastication. *Cranio*, 1994; 12(3): 156–160.

6 Gibbs CH, Lundeen HC, Mahan PE, Fujimoto J. Chewing movements in relationship to border movements at first molar. *J Prosthet Dent*, 1981; 46(308–322.

7 Barker DK. Occlusal interferences and the temporomandibular dysfunction. *Gen Dent*, 2004: 52(1): 56–62.

8 Becker CM, Kaiser DA, Schwalm C. Mandibular centricity: centric relation. *J Prosthet Dent*, 2000; 83(2): 158–160.

9 Fleigel JD III, Sutton AJ. Reliable and repeatable centric relation adjustment of the maxillary occlusal device. *J Prosthodont*, 2013; 22(3): 233–236.

10 Kandasamy S, Boeddinghaus R, Kruger E. Condylar position assessed by magnetic resonance imaging after various bite position registrations. *Am J Orthod Dentofacial Orthop*, 2013; 144(4): 512–517.

11 Mann A, Miralles R. Influence of variation in anteroposterior occlusal contacts on electromyographic activity. *J Prosth Dent*, 1989; 61(5): 617–623.

12 Mansour RM, Reynik RJ. In vivo occlusal forces and moments: I. Forces measured in hinge position and associated moments. *J Dent Res*, 1975; 54(1): 114–120.

13 Williamson EH, Lundquist DO. Anterior guidance: its effect on electromyographic activity of the temporal and masseter muscles. *J Prosthet Dent*, 1983; 49(6): 816–823.

14 Mann A, Chan C, Miralles R. Influence of group function and canine guidance on electromyographic activity of elevator muscles. *J Prosthet Dent*, 1987; 57(4): 494–501.

15 Lundeen HC, Gibbs CH. *The Function of Teeth: The Physiology of Mandibular Function Related to Occlusal Form and Esthetics*. Gainsville, FL: L and G Publishers, 2005.

16 Belser UC, Hannam AG. The influence of altered working-side occlusal guidance on masticatory muscles and related jaw movement. *J Prosthet Dent*, 1985; 53(3): 406–413.

17 Hamburger JT, Opdam NJ, Bronkhorst EM, Kreulen CM, Roeters JJ, Huysmans MC. Clinical performance of direct composite restorations for treatment of severe tooth wear. *J Adhes Dent*, 2011; 13(6): 585–593.

18 Deliperi S, Bardwell DN. Clinical evaluation of direct cuspal coverage with posterior composite resin restorations. *J Esthet Restor Dent*, 2006; 18(5): 256–257.

19 Peumans M, Van Meerbeek B, Lambrechts P, Vanherle G. The 5-year clinical performance of direct composite additions to correct tooth form and position. I. Esthetic qualities. *Clin Oral Investig*, 1997; 1(1): 12–18.

20 Dawson PE. *Evaluation, Diagnosis and Treatment of Occlusal Problems*, 2nd ed. St Louis, MO: Mosby; 1989.

21 Kloprogge MJ, van Griethuysen AM. Disturbances in the contraction and co-ordination pattern of the masticatory muscles due to dental restorations. An electromyographic study. *J Oral Rehabil*, 1976; 3(3): 207–216.

22 Trovato F, Orlando B, Bosco M. Occlusal features and masticatory muscles activity. A review of electromyographic studies. *Stomatologija*, 2009; 11(1): 26–31.

23 Rugh JD, Drago CJ. Vertical dimension: A study of clinical restoration position and jaw muscle activity. *J Prosthet Dent*, 1991; 45(6): 670–675.

24 Wyke BD. Neuromuscular mechanisms influencing mandibular posture: a neurologist's review of current concepts. *J Dent*, 1974; 2(3): 111–120.

25 Helsing G. Functional adaptation to changes in vertical dimension. *J Prosthet Dent*, 1984; 52(6): 867–870.

26 McNeill C. *Vertical Dimension: A Study of Clinical Restoration Position*. Chicago, IL: Quintessence Pub. Co; 1997, p. 409.

27 Ruiz JL, Coleman TA. Occlusal disease management system: The diagnosis process. *Compend Clin Educ Dent*, 2008; 29(3): 154–158.

28 Ruiz JL. Achieving longevity in esthetics by proper diagnosis and management of "occlusal disease". *Contemp Esthet*, 2007; 11(6): 24–30.

29 Komiyama O, Obara R, Lida T, Asano T, Masuda M, Uchida T, De Laat A, Kawara M. Comparison of direct and indirect occlusal contact examinations with different clenching intensities. *J Oral Rehabil*, 2015; 42(3): 185–191.

Index

Note: Page numbers in *italics* refer to Figures, those in **bold** to Tables.

d

www.ingramcontent.com/pod-product-compliance
Lightning Source LLC
LaVergne TN
LVHW071242210926
848486LV00007B/327

* 9 7 8 1 1 1 8 9 7 6 4 1 8 *